MW00846307

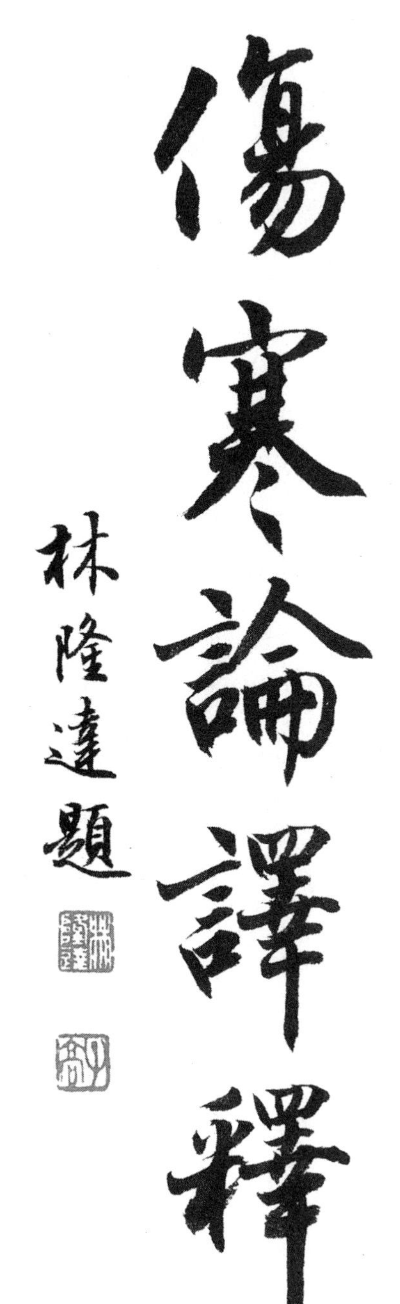

SHĀNG HÁN LÙN
ON COLD DAMAGE

TRANSLATION AND COMMENTARIES

CRAIG MITCHELL, FÉNG YÈ, NIGEL WISEMAN

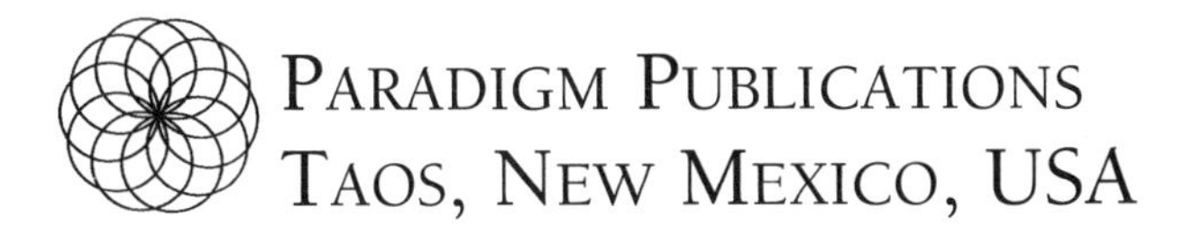
PARADIGM PUBLICATIONS
TAOS, NEW MEXICO, USA

SHĀNG HÁN LÙN
ON COLD DAMAGE
Translation and Commentaries

CRAIG MITCHELL, FÉNG YÈ, NIGEL WISEMAN

Council of Oriental Medical Publishers (C.O.M.P.) Designation
Compiled from primary Chinese sources. English terminology from Wiseman N.
and Feng Y., *A Practical Dictionary of Chinese Medicine*, published by Paradigm Publications, Brookline, Massachusetts and Taos, New Mexico

Library of Congress Cataloging-in-Publication Data:
Chang, chung-ching, fl. 168-196.
[Shang han Lun. English]
Shang han lun = On cold damage / transation and commentaries
Craig Mitchell, Féng Yè, and Nigel Wiseman
p. cm.
Includes index.
ISBN 0-912111-57-7 (alk. paper)
Medicine, Chinese. I. Mitchell, Craig, 1966- . II. Féng Yè, 1967-
III Wiseman, Nigel. IV. Title. V. Title: On cold damage.
R601.C42513 1999
610'.951- -dc21 99-21069
CIP

Library of Congress Number: 99-201069
International Standard Book Number (ISBN-13):
9780912111-575
Printed in the United States of America

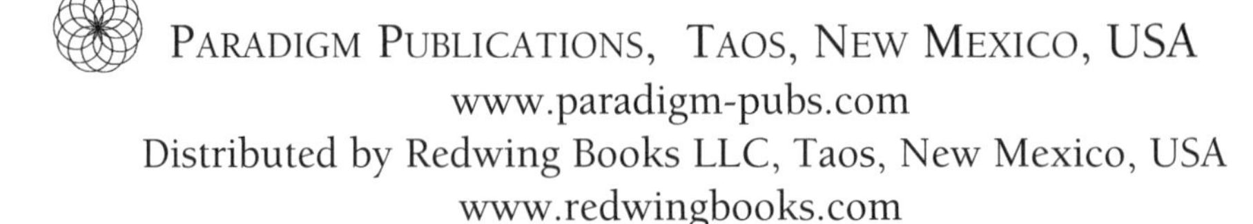

PARADIGM PUBLICATIONS, TAOS, NEW MEXICO, USA
www.paradigm-pubs.com
Distributed by Redwing Books LLC, Taos, New Mexico, USA
www.redwingbooks.com

Contents

Acknowledgements

致 谢

First and foremost, we would like to thank the many students at Pacific College of Oriental Medicine, New York, for their enthusiastic cooperation in improving the didactic aspect of the book. We wish to acknowledge the feedback and input given by our colleagues, and especially those within the New York community of practitioners of Chinese medicine. We thank Thomas Dey for his careful editing of the text, Guō Nián-Fēng (郭年峰) for helping to compute character frequency, and Lín Yí-Qiàn (林怡倩) for helping with the appendixes. Finally, we express our appreciation to China Medical College for granting financial assistance to this project, and to China Medical College Lifu Museum of Chinese Medicine for permission to reproduce the water-color painting by Jiǎng Zhào-Hé (蒋兆和) of Zhāng Jī appearing in the cover.

Preface
自 序

Over the last five decades, attempts have been made in the People's Republic of China to distill all that is valuable amid the vast mass of traditional medical literature into a systematized body of knowledge. This is the inevitable outcome of the challenge by Western medicine and the Western sciences. Throughout the Chinese-speaking world, Western medicine has established itself as the mainstream medicine; scientific values dominate all fields of learning, and education is based very closely on Western models. Despite this, there are hopes in China that by discovering its scientific bases, traditional medicine will evolve into a scientific discipline that can be integrated with modern medicine. So far, however, such efforts, valid and necessary though they may be, have been unable to escape the fact that Chinese medicine, rooted in the past, has for centuries looked back to its formative period as a golden age, and that even today a sound knowledge of the classics is still needed to gain a firm understanding of Chinese medicine.

The impressive array of Chinese medical literature now available in English largely derives from the recent Chinese effort to distill what is valuable from the knowledge of the past. In content and presentation, English textbooks of Chinese medicine are English versions, for the most part simplified, of the primers used in China. Nevertheless, the lamentable fact that remains is that while traditional approaches to Chinese medicine are still accessible to modern Chinese people, they are unavailable to Westerners without linguistic access to the wealth of Chinese texts. Anyone who, penetrating the language barrier, engages in the study of Chinese texts, and goes to China to witness the teaching and practice of Chinese medicine in the Chinese-language environment soon realizes that the classical literature continues to provide an invaluable source of information for advanced students. The sheer volume of Chinese medical thought makes its complete transmission to the West almost impossible. Nonetheless, until the seminal classical texts and traditional commentaries are translated and widely read, Chinese medicine as transmitted to the West will continue to lack an essential element that it has on its home soil.

The earliest classics generally deemed to be the greatest seminal works of Chinese medicine are the *Nèi Jīng*, the *Nàn Jīng*, and the *Shāng Hán Lùn*. Of these, the *Shāng Hán Lùn* "On Cold Damage," attributed to Zhāng Jī (张机, style 仲景 Zhòng-Jǐng), who lived about 150–219 C.E., is undoubtedly the text of greatest clinical relevance to the majority of those Chinese practitioners who use medicinal therapy rather than acupuncture as their principal method of treatment. While the *Nèi Jīng* and the *Nàn Jīng* are studied for the theoretical elements that were considered important by successive generations of physicians, the *Shāng Hán Lùn* is studied very much for its clinical value. Not only was the *Shāng Hán Lùn* the first comprehensive and detailed treatise on externally contracted disease, it was also the first attempt to incorporate medicinal therapy, previously practiced with a minimum of theory, into the medicine of systematic correspondences and the channels and network vessels. It is a seminal work in the development of a holistic understanding of disease conditions that considers not only the offending disease evil but also the patient's resistance to it; that is, an understanding of disease in which the focus is on patterns (证 *zhèng*)—groups of related symptoms—rather than specific "diseases." The *Shāng Hán Lùn* was far ahead of its time in both theory and practice, and, not surprisingly therefore, the medicinal formulae it contains constitute an important part of the modern formulary. Given the Western interest in the clinical application of Chinese medicine rather than the historical evolution of medical thought in China, the *Shāng Hán Lùn*, of all the classical texts, is without doubt the one that stands the greatest chance of evoking interest among Westerners, at least those interested in Chinese medicinal therapy.

Despite the clinical interest that it attracts, the *Shāng Hán Lùn*, as indeed other ancient texts, is not easy reading—even for Chinese students. It is an ancient text whose original form in the *Shāng Hán Zá Bìng Lùn* (伤寒杂病论 "On Cold Damage and Miscellaneous Diseases") has been lost. The exact order of the original lines is no longer known, and their content may have been changed through mistranscription and possible deliberate reworking. Material is not presented as systematically as in modern literature; there are many ambiguities that have given rise to endless annotation and commentary over the centuries. Nonetheless, a rich body of commentary that has appeared over the last millennium, now as much a part of *Shāng Hán Lùn* thought as what survives of the original text itself, constitutes valuable reading matter for the present-day student.

Presenting classical literature to a clinically oriented Western readership is no easy task. The difficulties in translating an ancient text containing numerous ambiguities is the least of the problems. The greatest is providing notes and commentaries that make the text interesting and relevant to the modern Western student and practitioner. In the past, translators have erred on the side of insufficient commentary. With the sole exception of Paul Unschuld's translation and commentary of the *Nàn Jīng*, no complete translation of any Chinese medical classic provides any commentary sufficiently comprehensive to enable the Western reader to understand the issues that have traditionally surrounded texts. Other translations of classic texts provide an idea of the contents of the original texts, but fail to enable the Westerner acquainted with Chinese medicine to make full sense of the work. Many of these translations eliminate all the original ambiguities, while the commentaries on the one hand are scant and fail to explain the underlying theories in terms of current Western understanding of Chinese medicine, and on the other hand offer overly simplified explanations that obscure the variety of traditional interpretation.

The aim of our present volume is to enable the modern Western student and practitioner to gain access to a classical text written eighteen hundred years ago and to the corpus of medical thought to which it gave rise. To that end we have translated the original text with commentary, both modern and classical. Our translation of the text is intended to be an accurate reflection of the original. It is highly literal and avoids any idiomatic English paraphrasing that might obscure any facet of meaning of the original text or enshrine in the translation any one interpretation at the expense of all others. Although this may make reading more difficult in certain places, we felt that it was the most appropriate approach to take with this type of text. Difficulties that the reader may have in an initial literal understanding of any line of the text, such as those posed by technical terms, are dealt with in text notes that follow it. The commentaries consist of two different types of information: a compilation of textual interpretations from the modern literature, and direct translations of classical commentary. The modern material is not a direct translation of any one source, but an attempt to present the major schools of thought that one finds in current textbooks. The classical commentary is translated directly to allow the reader to gain some understanding of the complexity of material present in the related literature. In the commentaries we explain the technical significance of each line, discussing textual problems in greater depth and major differences of interpretation among scholars. Yet since our aim has been to reach the modern Western student and practitioner of Chinese medicine, we have not dwelt excessively on the minutiae of traditional debate that might only interest the medical historian, and have concentrated our main effort on detailed explanation of widely recognized interpretations.

Neither the original text of the *Shāng Hán Zá Bìng Lùn* nor Wáng Shū-Hé's original text of the *Shāng Hán Lùn* survives. Consequently, the sequence of the lines is subject to considerable doubt. The Sòng version became the standard version up until the modern era. Modern scholars, as indeed scholars of the past, doubt the reliability of the Sòng order, and have attempted a new order based on the logic of the treatments. This order makes much greater clinical sense of the text than the Sòng order. Although it separates some lines containing references to foregoing lines that are not separated in the Sòng version, and therefore cannot be regarded as a reliable historical reconstruction of the original text, it presents a clinical understanding of the *Shāng Hán Lùn* that encourages modern readers to appreciate the value of this work. Since our intended readership is one for whom the clinical relevance is of greater interest than historical detail, we have—albeit somewhat hesitantly—chosen the modern order for this volume. We nevertheless include the text in the Sòng order in Appendix I.

The choice as to whether to set the Chinese text in the traditional complex characters or the simplified form recently adopted by the PRC was difficult. Even in the PRC there is a continuing tendency to typeset ancient classics in complex characters, in order to preserve for the modern reader the original form of the text. Nevertheless, since most Western students studying Chinese learn the simplified characters first, we have set the Chinese text of each line in the main chapters of the book in simplified characters, but have set the Sòng version in Appendix I in complex characters.

We have taken every opportunity to help the growing number of people who recognize the need to learn Chinese in order to gain access to primary literature. In addition to including the original Chinese text of each line and its Pīnyīn transcription, we have also included in Appendix 2 an analysis of the grammatical structures and the vocabulary used in the text. Students possessing a rudimentary knowledge of basic Chinese characters and their components should find this material helpful in approaching the original Chinese text.

The English terminology used in the present volume is, with few exceptions, that appearing in *A Practical Dictionary of Chinese Medicine* (Wiseman and Feng, Paradigm Publications, 1998), in which Chinese terms are given largely literal equivalents that can be used in the various senses in which the Chinese terms are used, or have been used, over the centuries. Readers should note, however, that certain terms appearing in the *Shāng Hán Lùn* are used in senses that may not have been recorded in *A Practical Dictionary*.

Although this present volume neither represents the full body of knowledge relating to the *Shāng Hán Lùn*, nor offers any fresh insights into it, we are nevertheless confident that it will facilitate access to the original text and foster understanding of its clinical value.

Introduction
总 论

The *Shāng Hán Lùn* (伤寒论 "On Cold Damage") is the oldest surviving, the most copiously commented, and the most revered Chinese medical text devoted to externally contracted disease (外感病 *wài gǎn bìng*). It also presents the oldest extant systematized body of knowledge concerning the origin and development of such diseases and their treatment, not by acupuncture, but principally by a highly sophisticated use of medicinals combined in formulae that are skillfully modulated to deal with a vast variety of disease manifestations.

The *Shāng Hán Lùn* originally formed part of the now inextant *Shāng Hán Zá Bìng Lùn* (伤寒杂病论 "On Cold Damage and Miscellaneous Diseases"), a comprehensive clinical manual written by the Eastern Hàn physician Zhāng Jī (circa 150–219 C.E.). The sections relating to externally contracted disease, which Zhāng Jī ascribed chiefly to contraction of wind and cold ("cold damage"), were reorganized by Wáng Shū-Hé (王叔和) (210–285) in the Western Jìn period (265–316) to form the *Shāng Hán Lùn*, and the sections relating to other diseases of internal medicine ("miscellaneous diseases") were later arranged to form the *Jīn Guì Yào Lüè* (金匮要略 "Essential Prescriptions of the Golden Coffer"). Wáng Shū-Hé's original version of the *Shāng Hán Lùn* has been lost, but several versions were handed down to the Sòng period (960–1279), when the text was edited and printed. Medical scholars of the Sòng onwards showed great interest in the text and produced a large body of commentary. The corpus of knowledge concerning "cold damage" that has been passed down to us is a large and complex elaboration of Zhāng Jī's original ideas, to which many medical writers have contributed over the last millennium. In the Míng and Qīng Dynasties, the *Shāng Hán Lùn* further provided the basis for a new systematic analysis of externally contracted disease, the doctrine of warm disease (温病学说, *wēn bìng xué shuō*), in which heat rather than cold was identified as the major cause of disease. Despite the emergence of this new doctrine, the *Shāng Hán Lùn* has never been eclipsed, and in the curricula of Chinese medical schools in China today, it occupies an equally if not more important place.

The *Shāng Hán Lùn*'s descriptions of externally contracted diseases and their treatment reflect a theoretical understanding which ostensibly descends from the *Huáng Dì Nèi Jīng* (黄帝内经 "The Yellow Emperor's Inner Canon"), *Nàn Jīng* (难经 "The Classic of Difficult Issues") and *Běn Cǎo Jīng* (本草经 "The Materia

Medica Canon"), but which evinces major advances in the integration of theoretical knowledge with clinical observation and practice. In the *Shāng Hán Lùn*, externally contracted disease in all its varied manifestations and possible courses is understood in terms of evils, most notably wind and cold, which invade the body from outside and pass through the channels and network vessels (经络 *jīng luò*), causing disturbances of aspects of bodily function that can be recognized by distinct constellations of signs known as 证 *zhèng*, "patterns." Each pattern can be treated by a variety of methods (sweating, vomiting, precipitation, harmonization, warming, clearing, dispersion, and supplementation), using medicinal drugs that are combined on the basis of their therapeutic effects into a limited number of formulae whose constituents can be varied to address different presentations. It is for this reason that the *Shāng Hán Lùn* is regarded as the basis of the approach to diagnosis and treatment that in the Qīng dynasty came to be called "determining treatment on the basis of patterns identified" (辨证论治 *biàn zhèng lùn zhì*), which is now considered to be the quintessence of Chinese medical genius, yet is somewhat erroneously regarded as having been the mainstream of healing practices in China since time immemorial.

The Author

Zhāng Jī, whose style was Zhòng-Jǐng (仲景), lived in the Eastern Hàn (东汉 *dōng hàn*) Dynasty, from circa 150 to 219 C.E. No record of him from his own time survives, and the earliest records date from the Jìn Dynasty. He is believed to have been born in Niè-Yáng (涅阳) in what is today Nán-Yáng (南阳) county of Hé-Nán (河南) Province. According to Sòng records, he was the Grand Protector (太守 *tài shǒu*) of Cháng-Shā (长沙).

As to Zhāng Jī's medical training, we have little definitive knowledge. He is believed to have studied medicine under Zhāng Bó-Zǔ (张伯祖). Nevertheless, what texts he studied, indeed what texts were available to him, are not fully known.

In the *Zhēn Jiǔ Jiǎ Yǐ Jīng* ("The Systematized Canon of Acupuncture and Moxibustion"), Huáng-Fǔ Mì (皇甫谧) states that Zhāng Jī (张机, style 仲景 Zhòng-Jǐng) had expanded the (no longer extant) *Yī Yǐn Tāng Yè* ("Yī Yǐn's Decoctions") into several tens of fascicles, providing very effective remedies, and that Imperial Physician Wáng Shū-Hé, in reediting and selecting from Zhāng Jī's work, enhanced its essence.

Huáng-Fǔ Mì elsewhere expresses his high opinion of Zhāng Jī's medical skills with the following anecdote:

> [Zhòng-Jǐng] had an audience with the Privy Secretary (侍中 *shì zhōng*) Wáng Zhòng-Xuān (王仲宣), who that year was over twenty. He said to him, "Sir, you are sick. [At the age of] forty, [your] eyebrows will fall out and within half a year [you] will die. If [you] take Five Stones Decoction now, [you] can avoid [this]. Wáng Zhòng-Xuān took his words as an offense, [and although] he accepted the formula, did not ingest it. Three days later, upon seeing Wáng Zhòng-Xuān, Zhòng-Jǐng asked, "Have you taken the formula?" Wáng Zhòng-Xuān replied [that he had] already taken it. Zhòng-Jǐng said, "[Your] complexion is not that of [one who] has taken [a medicinal] decoction. Why [do you thus] make light of [your] life?" Wáng Zhòng-Xuān remained in-

> credulous. Twenty years later, sure enough, [Wáng Zhòng-Xuān's] eyebrows did fall out, [and] on the 187th day he died. [Thus], in the end, it was as [Zhòng-Jǐng had] said.

As to Zhāng Jī's personal motive for writing *Shāng Hán Zá Bìng Lùn*, we know that during the final years of the Eastern Hàn Dynasty, continual war and strife led to the outbreak of many epidemics. According to Zhāng Jī's original preface, which is not fully authenticated (see p. 29), we learn that he apparently lost approximately two thirds of his family members during this period and he reported that seven tenths of these deaths were due to externally contracted disease. He sought the counsel of ancient books, reviewed the remedies applied in his time, and combined these findings with his own clinical experience. Out of that process grew the sixteen fascicles of *Shāng Hán Zá Bìng Lùn*.

THE HISTORY OF THE TEXT

The original *Shāng Hán Zá Bìng Lùn* covered a broad area including the interpretation of pulses, cold damage and six channel pattern identification of treatment, miscellaneous disease (including women's and children's disease), and dietary contraindications. The text of the *Shāng Hán Zá Bìng Lùn* did not survive the turbulence of the Three Kingdoms period (220–265) fully intact, but in the Western Jìn period which followed, Wáng Shū-Hé collected and arranged surviving fragments, and is believed to have organized all the parts relating to externally contracted disease into the book we know as the *Shāng Hán Lùn*. From the various extant versions of the text and parts of it included in other works, it is no longer possible to determine the exact contents and sequence of either the *Shāng Hán Lùn* or *Shāng Hán Zá Bìng Lùn*. Wáng Shū-Hé included elements of the *Shāng Hán Lùn* in his *Mài Jīng* ("The Pulse Canon"), but in the order of methods of treatment. Modern scholars believe that this is most likely to have been the order of *Shāng Hán Zá Bìng Lùn* and that, in the creation of the independent *Shāng Hán Lùn*, the contents dealing with externally contracted disease were reordered to follow the sequence of the channels.

During the upheavals of the Eastern Jìn and Northern and Southern dynasties, the *Shāng Hán Lùn* text was not widely available. In the Táng Dynasty, Sūn Sī-Miǎo (孙思邈) drew from the *Shāng Hán Lùn* in *Bèi Jí Qiān Jīn Yào Fāng* ("A Thousand Gold Pieces Prescriptions for Emergencies"), but the full text was apparently not available to him until later. When compiling the *Qiān Jīn Yì Fāng* ("Wings to the Thousand Gold Pieces Prescriptions") toward the end of his life, he included most of the text, and this therefore constitutes the earliest known version of the *Shāng Hán Lùn*.

Since the *Wài Tái Mì Yào* ("Essential Secrets from Outside the Metropolis") quotes over 200 lines of the *Shāng Hán Lùn*, we infer that its author, Wáng Tāo (王涛) (707–772 C.E., Táng), placed great emphasis on the contribution of the *Shāng Hán Lùn* to the understanding of externally contracted disease. The first fascicle gives the views of eight medical scholars on the *Shāng Hán Lùn*, while the second brings together the views of different scholars on twenty cold damage patterns. Wáng Tāo's importance with regard to the *Shāng Hán Lùn* thus lies in his presentation of a diverse group of pre-Táng writings discussing the *Shāng Hán*

Lùn. Nevertheless, he did influence later scholars greatly since he did not include the full text, but only quoted it.

In the Sòng Dynasty, the government established a Medical Literature Editing Bureau (校正医书局 *jiào zhèng yī shū jú*) responsible for collecting, editing, and publishing medical works, which now, with the invention of wood-block printing, could enjoy a wider circulation than had previously been possible. The Bureau's official version of the *Shāng Hán Lùn* was prepared under the supervision of Lín Yì (林亿) and subsequently published. Unfortunately, no copy of this first printing survives, and the earliest extant text is a Míng reprint (1056 C.E.) by Zhào Kāi-Měi (赵开美), which nevertheless is believed to be identical. The term "Sòng version" now refers to this.

The Sòng version contains more than most modern versions of the *Shāng Hán Lùn*. Míng scholars argued that the first four and the last seven fascicles should be discarded on the grounds that they contained matter that either did not relate to externally contracted disease or that was more representative of Wáng Shū-Hé's thought than Zhāng Jī's.

The Relationship of the Shāng Hán Lùn to the Sù Wèn

In his original preface, Zhāng Jī mentions a number of books he had studied. All of these but the *Nèi Jīng* and the *Nàn Jīng* are no longer extant. Consequently, our picture of the theoretical origins of the *Shāng Hán Lùn* is not entirely clear. The *Nèi Jīng* devotes considerably more text to discussion of externally contracted disease than the *Nàn Jīng*, and given the importance accorded to it over history, considerable effort has been made to tie the theories of the *Shāng Hán Lùn* in with it.

Below we present three passages from the *Sù Wèn* ("Elementary Questions"), the first part of the *Nèi Jīng*, discussing externally contracted disease:

Sù Wèn (Rè Lùn):

> The Yellow Thearch says: Now [as we know], all heat [effusion] disease is of the cold damage category....
>
> Qí-Bó says:
>
> On the first day of cold damage, greater yáng (*jù yáng*) is affected, and signs include stiffness and pain in the head and nape, and stiffness in the lumbar spine.
>
> On the second day, yáng brightness (*yáng míng*) is affected. Since the yáng brightness governs the flesh, and its channel passes up the side of the nose to connect with the eyes, there is generalized heat effusion (i.e., fever), eye pain, and dry nose.
>
> On the third day, the lesser yáng (*shào yáng*) is affected. Since the lesser yáng governs the gallbladder, and its channel passes through the rib-side and connects with the ears, signs include pain in the chest and rib-side, and tinnitus.
>
> On the fourth day, the greater yīn (*tài yīn*) is affected. Since the greater yīn channel passes through the stomach and connects with the throat, signs include fullness in the stomach and dry throat.

On the fifth day, the lesser yīn (*shào yīn*) is affected. Since the lesser yīn channel passes through the kidney, connects with the lung, and penetrates through to the root of the tongue, signs include dry mouth and tongue, and thirst.

On the sixth day, the reverting yīn (*jué yīn*) is affected. Since the reverting yīn channel passes through the genitals and connects with the liver, signs include agitation and retracted scrotum.

Sù Wèn (Yīn Yáng Yìng Xiàng Dà Lùn):

[When there are] irregularities of joy and anger, and excesses of heat and cold, life is insecure. Hence weighted yīn must [become] yáng, and weighted yáng must [become] yīn. Therefore it is said that in winter [there is] damage by cold and in spring there must disease [caused by] warmth.

Sù Wèn (Tiáo Jīng Lùn):

The Thearch says: The classics say that when yáng is vacuous, there is external cold, when yīn is vacuous, there is internal heat; when yáng is exuberant there is external heat, when yīn is exuberant there is internal cold. I have already asked about this, [but] I do not know why it is so.

Qí-Bó says: Yáng receives qì from the upper burner to warm the area of the skin and the divided flesh. Now, [when] cold qì is in the outer body, the upper burner is blocked. When the upper burner is blocked, cold qì alone remains in the outer body, hence there is cold shivering.

The Thearch says: What of yīn [being] vacuous [and] engendering internal heat?

Qí-Bó says: [When] there is taxation fatigue, the body's qì becomes debilitated, and grain qì is not exuberant; the upper burner fails to move, and the lower [stomach] duct is blocked; stomach qì is hot, and heat qì fumes into the chest, hence there is internal heat.

The Thearch says: What of yáng [being] exuberant and engendering external heat?

Qí-Bó says: When the upper burner is blocked and inhibited, the skin becomes tight, the interstices become blocked, and the mysterious houses [sweat pores] are blocked, [so that] defense qì cannot discharge outward; hence there is external heat.

The Thearch says: What of yīn [being] exuberant [and] engendering internal cold?

Qí-Bó says: Reverse qì ascends counterflow, cold qì accumulates in the chest and does not drain [away]; [because] its does not drain [away], warm qì departs; cold alone remains, so blood congeals; [when blood] congeals, the vessels become blocked, and the pulse becomes exuberant and large, and rough; hence [there is] cold strike.

From the first of these quotations, we see that the *Nèi Jīng* agrees with the *Shāng Hán Lùn* in categorizing heat disease as cold damage, and in understanding cold damage as a progression through the six channels. The names of the channels are the same except that greater yáng is referred to as 巨阳 *jù yáng* in the *Nèi Jīng*.

Furthermore, the two texts both ascribe unique sets of signs to disease in each of the channels. Nevertheless, they agree only partially on which signs are associated with each channel. In the comparison set out below, we provide full enumerations of the channel disease signs listed in the *Nèi Jīng*, but, for the sake of simplicity, we have chosen only the main signs given in the *Shāng Hán Lùn*.

Greater yáng

NJ: Stiffness and pain of the head and nape; stiff lumbar spine

SH: Floating pulse; stiffness and pain in the head and nape; aversion to cold; heat effusion

Yáng brightness

NJ: Generalized heat effusion; eye pain; dry nose; sleeplessness

SH: Generalized heat effusion; spontaneous sweating; thirst with desire to drink; dry bound stool; tidal heat effusion; delirious speech

Lesser yáng

NJ: Chest and rib-side pain; deafness

SH: Bitter taste in the mouth; dry throat; dizzy vision; chest and rib-side fullness; alternating [aversion to] cold and heat [effusion]

Greater yīn

NJ: Abdominal fullness and dry throat

SH: Abdominal fullness; vomiting; inability to get food down; diarrhea; periodic abdominal pain

Lesser yīn

NJ: Dry mouth and tongue with thirst

SH: Pulse that is faint and fine; desire only for sleep; aversion to cold; lying curled up; counterflow cold of the extremities

Reverting yīn

NJ: Vexation and fullness; retracted scrotum

SH: Dispersion-thirst; qì surging up into the heart; pain and heat in the chest; hunger with no desire to eat; vomiting of roundworms after eating; incessant diarrhea

The signs differ in that in the *Nèi Jīng* they are all classifiable as heat or repletion; in the *Shāng Hán Lùn*, repletion and heat signs are associated with three yáng, while cold and vacuity signs are associated with the three yīn. The *Shāng Hán Lùn* therefore envisages a much larger scope for externally contracted disease. Furthermore, by associating heat and repletion patterns with the three yáng, and cold and vacuity signs with the three yīn, it represents a more systematic application of the yīn-yáng doctrine.

The signs given in the *Sù Wèn* are clearly associated with the channel pathways (or associated with the bowels and viscera to which the channels home). Those given in the *Shāng Hán Lùn* are less consistently associated with particular locations on channel pathways. For example, the signs given for greater yáng in the *Sù Wèn* are located on the pathway of the greater yáng channel (stiffness and pain of the head and nape, stiff lumbar spine); those given in the *Shāng Hán Lùn* (floating pulse, stiffness and pain in the head and nape, aversion to cold, heat effusion) are predominantly general exterior signs. Such differences prompted Měi Chūn-Huá (美春华) to comment, "One cannot use the six channels... of the *Sù Wèn* to explain the six channels of *Shāng Hán Lùn*."

A further major difference between the *Shāng Hán Lùn* and *Sù Wèn* is seen in the timing of passage from channel to channel. The *Sù Wèn* places the timing of developments in the foreground, describing signs in a one-channel-per-day scheme. The timing of channel passage in the *Shāng Hán Lùn* is much more complex. Although many lines state what signs occur at a specified number of days after onset, the timing is much less rigid, and is certainly not one of daily change. Attempts have been made to reconcile the differences in timing by suggesting that *Sù Wèn* presents a standard pattern that is not always seen in practice. A more cogent view, however, is that while the *Sù Wèn* statements represent a neat theoretical scheme, Zhāng Jī worked from clinical observation. Although the degree to which numbers of days given by Zhāng Jī are to be taken literally has given rise to much unresolved debate, it is obvious that the *Shāng Hán Lùn* does not follow a one-channel-per-day scheme.

We can therefore conclude that although similarities do exist between the *Shāng Hán Lùn* and *Sù Wèn*, they are only partial, and that however much Zhāng Jī drew on the *Sù Wèn*, the *Shāng Hán Lùn* represents a thorough reworking of ideas contained in it. Kē Qín sums up the differences in the following words:

> In the *Sù Wèn* ("Elementary Questions"), the six channels [the three yīn and three yáng] only have exterior and interior repletion and heat patterns, no vacuity and cold patterns. As to treatment, we see only treatment by sweating and precipitation, no use of supplementation and warming. In Zhòng-Jǐng, the six channels are broader in scope, including different aspects: cold, wind, warmth, and heat evils; diseases caused either by external or internal evils; the passage of diseases from exterior to interior; and diseases that are due to cold or heat and to vacuity or repletion. The *Shāng Hán Lùn* is totally inclusive.

A further major difference between the *Nèi Jīng* and the *Shāng Hán Lùn* lies in the relative importance of drug and acupuncture therapy. The *Nèi Jīng* provides considerably more detail on needle therapy than on medicinal therapy, while the reverse is the case in the *Shāng Hán Lùn*.

The Development of Shāng Hán Lùn Thought

Before the appearance of the Sòng version, the value of the *Shāng Hán Lùn* was asserted by influential figures in the development of Chinese medicine over the centuries, such as Huáng-Fǔ Mì (皇甫谧), Sūn Sī-Miǎo (孙思邈), and Wáng Tāo (王涛). According to Sūn Sī-Miǎo, in southern China in the 7th century (Táng Dynasty), the *Shāng Hán Lùn* was jealously guarded by those who possessed copies. In the 8th century (Táng Dynasty), it was designated as an examination text for medical officials. Yet it was in the Sòng-Jīn-Yuán (宋金元, 960–1368) that the *Shāng Hán Lùn* began to make its fullest impact. This is partly due to the invention of printing, which allowed the text to become widely available. More importantly, however, developments in medical thought provided an environment more conducive to the recognition of Zhāng Jī's ideas. Before that period, medicinal therapy in general remained conservatively based on a pragmatic, symptomatic approach.

> Although they held their classic, the Han *Shen-nung pents'ao ching* [*Shén Nóng Běn Cǎo Jīng*], in great respect, its insights represented only a starting point for their own concerns and not, as was the case for followers of the *Huang-ti nei-ching/Nan-ching* [*Huáng Dì Nèi Jīng/Nàn Jīng*], the ultimate and complete stage in a particular field of knowledge.
> Unschuld 1985: 167

In the Sòng-Jīn-Yuán, efforts were made to apply the yīn-yáng and five-phase doctrines in the analysis of drug actions.

> While the interest generated by Wang Shu-ho [Wáng Shū-Hé] (210–285), for example, in pulse diagnosis had been continued in more than seventy titles by the beginning of the Sung [Sòng] period, and while during the same interval more than ninety works had been devoted to acupuncture and more than fifty to physiology, not even ten authors followed the direction taken by Chang Chi [Zhāng Jī]. It was only during the Sung [Sòng] and Chin [Jīn] epochs that a larger circle of scholars became interested in the surviving fragments of Chang Chi; during the course of these two dynasties alone, so many revisions or commentaries appeared on the problems of cold-related illness that more than eighty titles have survived to the present day. The contrast becomes even more striking when we compare the ten titles devoted specifically to the treatment of such illness written before the Sung period with the more than three hundred encyclopedic works containing prescriptions for all kinds of illnesses that appeared during the same time. The Chang Chi renaissance during the Sung-Chin-Yüan [Sòng-Jīn-Yuán] era was due primarily to two characteristics of his writings. To scholars of the twelfth, thirteenth, and fourteenth centuries, it was significant that Chang Chi had been the first to combine the use of drug therapy with the theory of systematic correspondence. In addition, Chang Chi, with his interest in the effects of cold on illness, was the first and virtually only author whose work was devoted exclusively to a specific etiology. All authors of the Sung-Chin-Yüan medical texts adopted these elements, which had virtually lain dormant for some 1,000 years, as the point of departure for their own, further-reaching deliberations. Consequently, in almost all of their works, drug prescriptions and theoretical considerations are linked on the basis of systematic correspondence.
> Unschuld 1985: 168

Sòng scholars approached the *Shāng Hán Lùn* in a number of different ways. In the early period after the publication of the Sòng version, scholars such as Páng Ān-Shí (庞安时, style 安常 Ān-Cháng) and Zhū Gōng (朱肱, style 翼中 Yì-Zhòng) believed that since Zhāng Jī's original text had not survived intact and had been reworked by Wáng Shū-Hé and others, the Sòng version could be improved by reordering the lines and filling in apparent gaps in the content. These scholars took as their basis not only the text of the *Shāng Hán Lùn* but all of what had allegedly survived from the *Shāng Hán Zá Bìng Lùn*. In some cases, they even introduced parts of the *Jīn Guì Yào Lüè*, and incorporated ideas concerning externally contracted disease that had developed over the eight centuries since Zhāng Jī's time. This approach, however, was eventually superseded by that of Chéng Wú-Jǐ (成无己), who believed that the Sòng version in its order and contents was, if not the original text, the most faithful representation of Zhāng Jī's understanding of externally contracted disease, and that the text could be made clearer by carefully researched commentary. Chéng Wú-Jǐ was highly influential because his *Zhù Jiě Shāng Hán Lùn* (注解伤寒论 "Annotated *Shāng Hán Lùn*"), which contained the text of the Sòng version altered in minor details and furnished with a detailed commentary, came to replace the Sòng version.

Over recent decades, commentated editions of the *Shāng Hán Lùn* have established a new order that makes the clinical study of the text much easier. This is the sequence adopted in the present volume, although the Chinese text in Sòng order is presented in Appendix I. In this new order, the basic six-channel order of the Sòng version is retained, but the individual lines are ordered according to the various formulae used. In the process of rearrangement, some lines appear in a chapter relating to a different channel than in the original Sòng version. Lines that cannot be ordered according to this schema are related to appendixes, mostly placed at the end of each chapter. Notably relegated to these appendices are lines containing inconsistencies and ambiguous phrases, lines suspected of having been added by transcribers, and lines that do not contain formulae or any clear indications as to where they might belong in the sequence. The meanings of such lines have been subject to ceaseless debate among medical scholars over the centuries. For students whose aim is a clinical grasp of the doctrine of cold damage, these appended lines can be ignored. It should be noted that in the present volume the lines are numbered according to their order in the Sòng version. Since these do not coincide with the order of their appearance, a Sòng Version Line Number Index has been included at the end of the book.

THE CONTENTS OF THE SHĀNG HÁN LÙN

The Concept of Cold Damage

The term "cold damage" (伤寒 *shāng hán*) has both broad and narrow meanings. *Sù Wèn* states, "Now all heat diseases are of the cold damage kind." The 58th difficulty of the *Nàn Jīng* states, "There are five [types of] cold damage: wind stroke, cold damage, damp warmth, heat disease, and warm disease." According to Zhāng Zǐ-Hé (张子和), "In spring, it is warm disease. In summer, it is summer-heat disease. In fall, it is malaria and diarrhea. In winter, it is cold qì and cough. In the four seasons, all qì that is not right qì is called cold damage." The broad meaning of cold damage is all externally contracted disease; the narrow meaning is external contraction of wind-cold and the resultant diseases. The text of the *Shāng Hán Lùn* provides a great deal of information regarding the pathological changes, patterns, and treatment of diseases resulting from external contraction of wind-cold, but more importantly, it deals with cold damage in the broad sense. It discusses the six excesses as the cause of disease and combines internal and external factors in an analysis of pathomechanisms, signs, and treatment.

Six-Channel Pattern Identification

The *Shāng Hán Lùn* attributes cold damage to the invasion of the body by evils such as wind and cold, and explains the vast variety of manifestations of cold damage in terms of the way in which these evils affect various parts of the channel and network vessel system. As a rule, evils first affect the greater yáng (*tài yáng*), and then, if the disease does not terminate there, they progress through the various channels according to certain partially predictable patterns. In some cases, however, disease evils directly affect channels other than the greater yáng.

Disease in any of the six channels takes the form of different disease patterns that are reflected in various constellations of signs and pulse conditions. It is for this reason that each chapter title contains the words "Pulses and Signs." These disease patterns reflect certain specific etiologies.

The brief outline below presents the various patterns arising in disease of each of the six channels. Readers should note that many of the technical terms appearing in this outline are explained in the chapters ahead and may be accessed through the index.

Greater Yáng Disease (太阳病 *tài yáng bìng*): The greater yáng controls the construction and defense, and governs the exterior of the body, which serves as the body's external barrier. Externally contracted evils usually first affect the exterior. Accordingly, many of the signs associated with greater yáng appear in the early stages of disease. The essential features of greater yáng disease are a pulse that is floating, headache, stiffness and pain of the head and nape, heat effusion, and aversion to cold.

The most important forms of greater yáng disease exterior disease are wind strike and cold damage, which are differentiated on the basis of the patient's constitution and the strength of the evil. Wind strike (中风 *zhòng fēng*) is attributed to "construction-defense disharmony" (营卫不和 *yíng wèi bù hé*) characterized by "strength in defense and weakness in construction" (卫强营弱 *wèi qiáng yíng ruò*). The major signs are aversion to wind and cold, heat effusion (发热 *fā rè*, i.e., fever), stiffness and pain of the head and nape, spontaneous sweating, noisy nose, dry retching, and a pulse that is floating and moderate. The special signs associated with this pattern are spontaneous sweating and a pulse that is floating and moderate; hence it is also called exterior vacuity. Cold damage (伤寒 *shāng hán*) is characterized by aversion to cold, heat effusion, stiffness and pain of the head and nape, generalized pain in the body and/or bones and joints, absence of sweating, panting (any form of difficult breathing or breathlessness), retching counterflow, and a pulse that is floating and tight. The defensive yáng is obstructed and the construction yīn is stagnant; consequently sweat cannot issue, and the pulse is floating and tight. This form of greater yáng disease is often referred to as exterior repletion.

Greater yáng disease can undergo a variety of irregular developments, which are known as transmuted patterns (变证 *biàn zhèng*). These include heat patterns (热证 *rè zhèng*), vacuity cold patterns (虚寒证 *xū hán zhèng*), chest bind patterns (结胸证 *jié xiōng zhèng*), and glomus patterns (痞证 *pǐ zhèng*). Also figuring among the transmuted patterns are the interior patterns of greater yáng disease affecting the greater yáng bowel—the bladder—these being water amassment and blood amassment. In greater yáng water amassment (太阳蓄水 *tài yáng xù shuǐ*), an unresolved external evil enters the bladder and the yáng qì is unable to transform water. The major signs are heat effusion, sweating, vexation thirst or thirst with desire to drink, vomiting immediately upon the ingestion of water, inhibited urination, lesser abdominal fullness, and a pulse that is floating and rapid. In greater yáng blood amassment, (太阳蓄血 *tài yáng xù xuè*), heat evil penetrates deep into the lower burner and binds the blood. The signs are a tense, bound lesser abdomen or lesser abdominal hardness and fullness, mania or similar conditions, and uninhibited urination.

In greater yáng disease, there are also concurrent patterns, such as exterior vacuity with concurrent stiffness of the nape and back, or with cough and panting, or with water-rheum. There are also transmuted patterns due to incorrect treatment, such as inappropriate promotion of sweating, use of precipitation, and/or use of fire therapies.

Yáng Brightness Disease (阳明病 *yáng míng bìng*): The main feature of yáng brightness disease is yáng hyperactivity and heat exuberance. An evil can directly enter the yáng brightness channel from the exterior, but it usually passes into the channel from the greater yáng. Yáng brightness disease is generally characterized by generalized heat effusion, spontaneous sweating, aversion not to cold but to heat, and a pulse that is large. Distinction is made between a heat pattern and a repletion pattern. In the yáng brightness heat pattern (阳明热证 *yáng míng rè zhèng*), also called a yáng brightness channel pattern (阳明经证 *yáng míng jīng zhèng*), an evil enters the channel, transforms to heat, and scorches liquid and humor. In addition to the general yáng brightness disease signs just listed, this pattern is characterized by dry mouth and tongue, and a great thirst that is unquenchable. If the evil transforms into heat and causes waste matter in the intestines to form a repletion bind, this is called a yáng brightness repletion pattern (阳明实证 *yáng míng shí zhèng*), also known as a yáng brightness bowel pattern (阳明腑证 *yáng míng fǔ zhèng*). Here, the generalized heat effusion takes the form of tidal heat effusion (fever at a certain time each day). Other specific signs include delirious speech, sweat streaming from the extremities, abdominal distention with fullness and pain, hard stool, and a pulse that is sunken and replete.

Lesser Yáng Disease (少阳病 *shào yáng bìng*): Lesser yáng disease manifests as a half exterior half interior pattern (半表半里证 *bàn biǎo bàn lǐ zhèng*), perhaps more accurately described as a "halfway pattern" since it is correctly conceived as disease located neither in the exterior nor in the interior, but between the two. It can be the result of an evil passing into the lesser yáng from another channel or may originate in this channel itself. The essential features are bitter taste in the mouth, dry throat, and dizzy vision. Other major signs are alternating aversion to cold and heat effusion, fullness in the chest and rib-side, taciturnity with no desire for food or drink, heart vexation, frequent retching, and white tongue fur. The pulse of lesser yáng disease is one that is fine and stringlike. There is neither the aversion to cold that typically marks greater yáng exterior patterns nor the exuberant heat that characterizes yáng brightness disease. Accordingly, promotion of sweating and precipitation cannot be used; the appropriate treatment is harmonization.

The lesser yáng is often referred to as the "pivot" (枢 *shū*), the central element of the three yáng. When disease evil enters the lesser yáng, it causes inhibition of the pivot (枢机不利 *shū jī bù lì*). Alternating aversion to cold and heat effusion, for example, is a manifestation of "right and evil struggling by turns" (正邪分争 *zhèng xié fēn zhēng*). Aversion to cold occurs when evil qì prevails; heat effusion occurs when right qì prevails, but right qì is unable to repel the evil through the exterior, and the evil qì is unable to advance into the interior. Thus in lesser yáng, the disease, as it were, oscillates on the pivot. Basically, the pivot is one aspect of the "qì dynamic" (气机 *qì jī*). Inhibition of the qì dynamic in lesser yáng disease can have varied consequences, notably disturbance of spleen and stomach function. It is for this reason that retching is one of the main signs of lesser yáng disease.

Though lesser yáng disease is typically a halfway pattern, there may be concurrent exterior or interior patterns. Lesser yáng with a concurrent exterior pattern may manifest in heat effusion, mild aversion to cold, vexation pain of the joints and extremities, mild retching, and propping bind below the heart; lesser yáng with a concurrent interior pattern can manifest in alternating aversion to cold and heat effusion, interior heat bind, persistent retching, distress below the heart, depression and vexation, and absence of stool.

Greater Yīn Disease (太阴病 *tài yīn bìng*): Greater yīn disease is an interior vacuity cold pattern of spleen yáng vacuity, and is characterized by abdominal fullness, vomiting, inability to get food down, severe diarrhea, and occasional abdominal pain. Greater yīn disease can result from an unresolved yáng channel disease damaging spleen yáng, from direct invasion of wind-cold, or from internal damage engendering cold-rheum. When the spleen yáng is vacuous, cold and dampness become exuberant, and movement and transformation are impaired. If greater yīn disease progresses further, it may become spleen-kidney vacuity cold and form a lesser yīn vacuity cold pattern.

Lesser Yīn Disease (少阴病 *shào yīn bìng*): Lesser yīn disease, a pattern of interior vacuity, usually develops from disease that starts in one of the other channels, although it can be the result of an evil penetrating directly into the interior in someone with a vacuous constitution. It includes serious conditions that may be fatal. The major manifestations of lesser yīn disease are a pulse that is fine and faint, and a desire to sleep. Distinction is made between cold transformation and heat transformation patterns. Cold transformation (寒化 *hán huà*) is the result of heart-kidney yáng qì debility and in addition to the above signs also includes aversion to cold, curled-up lying posture, heart vexation, vomiting and diarrhea, thirst with desire for hot fluids, small intake of fluids, clear uninhibited urination, and reversal cold of the extremities. In severe cases, when the yáng qì is repelled by the yīn cold, one may see no aversion to cold, heat effusion, red face, and vexation and agitation, which indicates true cold and false heat (真寒假热 *zhēn hán jiǎ rè*). Heat transformation (热化 *rè huà*), a result of yīn vacuity, is characterized by heart vexation and inability to sleep, dry sore throat, diarrhea, thirst, crimson tongue, and a pulse that is fine and rapid.

Reverting Yīn Disease (厥阴病 *jué yīn bìng*): Reverting yīn disease generally develops some time after the onset of cold damage disease. It is more complicated and severe than disease of any other channel. The main forms are as follows: upper-body heat and lower-body cold patterns; reverse-flow patterns; and patterns characterized by either diarrhea, reverse-flow, retching, or hiccup. The **upper-body heat and lower-body cold** (上热下寒 *shàng rè xià hán*) complex is characterized by dispersion-thirst (severe thirst unallayed by fluid intake), qì surging upward to the heart, vexing heat in the heart, hunger with inability to eat and vomiting of roundworms, and unceasing diarrhea. **Reversal-heat exuberance and retaliation** (厥热胜复 *jué rè shèng fù*) patterns are characterized by reverse-flow and heat effusion. The reverse-flow (厥逆 *jué nì*), which is severe palpable coldness of the extremities stretching up to the elbows and knees (also called "reversal cold of the extremities" 手足厥冷 *shǒu zú jué lěng*), is accompanied by diarrhea, and alternates with heat effusion. The reverse-flow marks the prevalence of yīn, whereas the heat effusion marks the retaliation of yáng. **Diarrhea**, as it occurs in reverting yīn disease, can occur in cold or heat patterns, or in cold-heat complexes. **Reverse-flow** is the single most important sign of reverting yīn disease. It occurs not only in the reversal-heat exuberance and retaliation pattern described above, but is also seen in a number of other conditions: visceral reversal, cold reversal, heat reversal, roundworm reversal, collected water reversal, and phlegm repletion reversal. **Retching** can be differentiated into lower burner cold vacuity type, counterflow ascent of turbid yīn type, and a third type observed in heat patterns when a shift to the lesser yáng takes place. **Hiccup** can be differentiated into vacuity cold and repletion heat types.

Eight-Principle Pattern Identification

The notion of the eight principles, though it was not formalized until much later in history, is implicit in *Shāng Hán Lùn* pattern identification. Externally contracted disease ("cold damage" in the broad sense) is the result of disease evils entering the body and the body's response to them. The different manifestations of disease are explained in terms of the outcome of the struggle between right and evil. Six-channel pattern identification provides the framework for understanding the specific ways in which externally contracted disease develops. Underlying it, however, are the notions of exterior-interior, cold-heat, vacuity-repletion, and yīn-yáng, which constitute a more general framework. This is reflected in line 7, p. 50, which says: "When an illness [is characterized by] heat effusion and aversion to cold, it is springing from yáng; when [an illness is characterized by] the absence of heat effusion and [the presence of] aversion to cold, it is springing from yīn."

In the theory of the *Shāng Hán Lùn*, greater yáng, yáng brightness, and lesser yáng are called the three yáng; greater yīn, lesser yīn, and reverting yīn are called the three yīn. Broadly speaking, disease of the three yáng is characterized by exuberant right qì (strong resistance) and repletion of evil qì (powerful threat to resistance), and takes the form of heat or repletion, which in the eight principles are both yáng patterns. By contrast, disease of the three yīn is generally characterized by debilitation of right qì with the continuing presence of evil qì, and largely takes the form of cold or vacuity patterns, which in the eight principles are both yīn patterns.

The first of the eight principles are exterior and interior. These two terms are somewhat confusing because they are used in different senses. In the *Shāng Hán Lùn*, the greater yáng is exterior, the lesser yáng lies between exterior and interior, and the other channels are all interior. In another sense, however, the three yáng are all exterior, while the three yīn are all interior. In this sense, the greater yáng is exterior while the greater yīn is interior. Within the yáng channels, the difference between exterior and interior is reflected in a sharp difference in treatment: effusing the exterior (promoting sweating) in the one case and attacking the interior (precipitation) in the second. For this reason, the concepts of interior and exterior are of great importance in deciding treatment.

Cold and heat are the principles by which the nature of a disease is identified. Acute conditions attributable to exuberant yáng evil usually manifest in heat patterns; chronic conditions and ones due to exuberant yīn evil are mostly cold patterns. Diarrhea, for example, can be due either to cold or to heat, which have to be differentiated by the presence or absence of thirst. In some cases, either the cold or heat may be false (see line 350, p. 545, and line 317, p. 478).

The importance of vacuity and repletion is reflected not only in the overall difference between the three yáng and three yīn, as explained above. Judging the precise state of right qì in relation to evil qì can be of crucial importance even within one channel. For example, line 70, p. 133, states, "After sweating is promoted, if [there is] aversion to cold, [this] is because of vacuity. If aversion to cold is absent, and only heat [effusion] [is present], this indicates repletion."

Bowel and Visceral Pattern Identification

Like eight-principle pattern identification, the notion of bowel and visceral pattern identification was not formulated until later in the development of Chinese medicine. Yet, like the eight principles, it also helps our understanding of the *Shāng Hán Lùn* since diseases of the channels can affect their associated bowels and viscera.

In greater yáng disease, an exterior evil that fails to resolve can pass into the bladder, the bowel of the greater yáng. This evil can impair qì transformation and cause water-qì to collect internally, manifesting in inhibited urination or thirst with desire to drink, but with immediate vomiting of fluids ingested.

The stomach and the large intestine are both yáng brightness bowels. When evils enter the yáng brightness and damage the fluids, manifestations can include generalized heat, sweating, and dry mouth and tongue. When dryness-heat in the stomach and intestines causes stoppage of bowel qì, there is constipation with abdominal distention and fullness with pain that refuses pressure.

The gallbladder and the triple burner are the bowels of the lesser yáng. When gallbladder fire flames upward, there is bitter taste in the mouth, dry throat, and visual dizziness. When regulated flow through the waterways of the triple burner is impaired, one of several things may happen: water may collect below the heart giving rise to heart palpitations and inhibited urination; water-cold may invade the lung, giving rise to cough; or inhibition of the lesser yáng pivot could prevent cold rheum from transforming, giving rise to alternating aversion to cold and heat effusion, heart vexation, chest and rib-side fullness with slight bind, inhibited urination, thirst and retching, and sweating only from the head.

The spleen is the viscus of the greater yīn. When it is affected by externally contracted disease, spleen yáng is devitalized, and movement and transformation is impaired. When the spleen viscus is vacuous, and cold, cold-damp collects and causes abdominal fullness and vomiting, inability to get food down, spontaneous diarrhea, and periodic spontaneous abdominal pain.

The heart and kidney are the viscera of the lesser yīn. When in externally contracted disease they become vacuous, and qì and blood become insufficient, there is a faint pulse, desire only for sleep, aversion to cold, curled-up lying posture (in severe cases, reversal cold of the extremities), diarrhea, and retching counterflow. If the heart fire becomes hyperactive and kidney yīn is insufficient, signs of yīn vacuity heat such as vexation in the heart, sleeplessness, dry throat, red tongue body, and a pulse that is fine and rapid may be observed.

The liver is the viscus of the reverting yīn. When it is affected by disease, a cold-heat complex arises and liver qì ascends counterflow, giving rise to dispersion-thirst (a thirst unallayed by drinking), heat and pain in the heart, hunger with no desire to eat, and vomiting of roundworms on ingestion of food, or diarrhea.

Diagnostic Difficulties

The major difficulty in learning the *Shāng Hán Lùn* approach to externally contracted diseases lies in the correct identification of patterns. Single signs rarely provide conclusive evidence for diagnosis and a basis for treatment. While a pulse that is stringlike and chest and rib-side fullness are each more or less a sure sign of lesser yáng disease in the context of externally contracted disease (not beyond this, however), aversion to cold, sweating, or vexation, for example, can be observed in diseases of all channels. The majority of major signs can occur in the disease of more than one channel. Since in each case the pathomechanism is different, the precise nature of a specific sign and combinations in which it occurs can vary. The art of diagnosis therefore lies in viewing each sign in its wider context and grasping the pathomechanism from a synthesis of all signs present.

Below are a number of examples of such signs, the different conditions in which they may be observed, and their different pathomechanisms.

Aversion to wind/aversion to cold (恶风、恶寒 *wù fēng, wù hán*): Aversion to wind is a feeling of cold when exposed to wind; aversion to cold is a feeling of cold. The distinction between aversion to wind and aversion to cold is ambiguous because in greater yáng disease the two terms seem to be used indiscriminately. It is, however, worth noting that "aversion to wind" does not occur in the lines presenting disease of the three yīn.

GREATER YÁNG: Aversion to wind or to cold is a basic sign of greater yáng. It is due to impairment of the normal function of defense qì when evil qì is in the exterior of the body.

YÁNG BRIGHTNESS: Yáng brightness disease is typically characterized by heat effusion with aversion to heat rather than cold. Nevertheless, heat effusion is sometimes accompanied by aversion to cold, as in line 168, p. 323, where heat in both the interior and exterior manifests in great thirst, dry tongue fur, vexation, and aversion to cold. Aversion to cold here results from damage to liquid and qì on the one hand causing the interstices of the flesh to loosen, and on the other causing yáng qì to become depressed in the interior.

LESSER YÁNG: In line 99, p. 418, aversion to wind occurs with heat effusion, stiffness and pain of the head and nape, and fullness below the rib-side. This pattern is not a pure lesser yáng pattern, and the aversion to wind is considered to be a greater yáng sign.

Heat effusion (热、发热 *rè, fā rè*): In this text, we render 发热 *fā rè* as "heat effusion" rather than "fever," since the Chinese term is somewhat wider in meaning than the familiar English term. Heat effusion is associated with many conditions and occurs both in externally contracted disease and miscellaneous disease (杂病 *zá bìng*, disease due to causes other than external evils). In externally contracted diseases of the three yáng channels, heat effusion is a manifestation of the struggle between right qì and evil qì; it does not necessarily indicate the presence of evil heat. In diseases of the three yīn, right qì is not strong enough to counter evil qì; hence heat effusion is absent, and instead only aversion to cold is present.

GREATER YÁNG: In exterior patterns, evil qì is in the exterior of the body, impairing the normal function of defense qì; hence heat effusion is accompanied by aversion to wind or cold.

YÁNG BRIGHTNESS: In yáng brightness disease, the disease evil transforms into heat and enters the interior. In heat patterns, heat effusion is accompanied by aversion to heat rather than aversion to cold. In repletion patterns, the heat is not so exuberant, and so the heat effusion is tidal, i.e., occurs in the afternoon.

LESSER YÁNG: In lesser yáng disease, the struggle is taking place between the interior and exterior, so heat effusion alternates with aversion to cold.

Sweating (汗出 *hàn chū*): Sweating occurs in a variety of patterns. A distinction is made between spontaneous and night sweating. Spontaneous sweating (自汗 *zì hàn*) is so called because it occurs spontaneously without exertion. It has numerous causes. Night sweating (盗汗 *dào hàn*) is sweating during sleep that ceases on awakening. The Chinese term literally means "thief sweating," reflecting that it occurs when the patient is unaware of it. The English term "night sweating" is somewhat unsatisfactory because it suggests that sweating during daytime sleep is excluded, which is not the case. Night sweating is usually a sign of yīn vacuity, but examples of this are not found in the *Shāng Hán Lùn*. In the externally contracted disease patterns described in the *Shāng Hán Lùn*, spontaneous sweating is much more common, although it is often simply referred to as sweating. Night sweating in the *Shāng Hán Lùn* is mentioned only in yáng brightness disease and lesser yáng disease.

GREATER YÁNG: Here, sweating is observed in exterior vacuity wind strike, while absence of sweating is a sign of exterior repletion cold damage. In exterior vacuity, the defense qì is vacuous and is easily damaged when an external evil is contracted. When this happens, it fails to contain construction-yīn, which discharges outward in the form of sweat. This is known as "insecurity of the defensive exterior" (卫表不固 *wèi biǎo bù gù*). Conversely, in exterior repletion, the interstices and fleshy exterior are secure.

YÁNG BRIGHTNESS: Sweating is copious and streams outward, in contrast to that which occurs in greater yáng wind strike, which is scant and issues slowly. In heat patterns, the sweat is said to be copious over the whole body, whereas in repletion patterns, it is said to stream from the limbs. In both these cases, sweating is spontaneous sweating. Line 201, p. 390, and line 268, p. 448, describe conditions in which night sweating is a sign of exuberant internal heat forcing the fluids out to the exterior. In yáng brightness disease, there is also sweating only from the head after heat has been reduced by precipitation.

LESSER YÁNG: Line 269, p. 442, the last line of lesser yáng in the present text, speaks of "sweating after the eyes close," which is the same as night sweating. It is explained there as being a sign of yáng exuberance. During sleep, yáng enters the interior so defense yáng decreases. Consequently, interior heat becomes exuberant and distresses humor, which discharges outward in the form of sweat.

Pulse that is floating (脉浮 *mài fú*): A pulse that is pronounced at the superficial level.

GREATER YÁNG: A floating pulse in greater yáng disease reflects exterior evil in the exterior being resisted by right qì.

YÁNG BRIGHTNESS: In yáng brightness disease, the pulse is typically large. Nevertheless, line 221, p. 312, describes a condition of rampant dryness-heat in both the interior and exterior that gives rise to a pulse that is floating and tight; line 176, p. 316, describes a similar condition where a pulse that is floating and slippery is an outward manifestation of exuberant internal heat.

GREATER YĪN: In greater yīn disease, a pulse that is floating may indicate a concurrent greater yáng exterior pattern (as in line 276, p. 456).

LESSER YĪN: A pulse that is floating is not normally observed in lesser yīn disease. When the cubit pulse is floating as described in line 290, p. 521, it means that the yáng qì is returning.

REVERTING YĪN: A pulse that is slightly floating in reverting yīn can be a sign that the disease is moving outwards prior to recovery (line 280, p. 460).

Passage and Transmutation

Passage (传 *chuán*) means the development of the disease along a particular course; transmutation (变 *biàn*) means change in the nature of disease contrary to the normal laws. These are dependent upon a number of factors:

- relative strength of right and evil qi
- administration of appropriate or inappropriate treatment
- constitution of the patient
- presence or absence of other illnesses

As a general rule, externally contracted disease begins in the exterior, and if it fails to resolve there, passes to the interior. Greater yáng exterior patterns give way to either yáng brightness or lesser yáng disease. Lesser yáng often progresses to yáng brightness. Disease of the three yīn is usually a later development occurring when the body is severely weakened by the struggle against the disease evil. This is the general pattern, but in some cases, if right qì is restored and the evil qì weakens, the disease may pass from the interior to the exterior.

Combination disease and dragover disease both involve more than one channel. Any pattern of two or three channels is called combination disease (合病 *hé bìng*). There is greater yáng and yáng brightness combination disease, greater yáng and lesser yáng combination disease, and three-yáng combination disease. When the signs of one channel abate as those of another develop, this is called dragover disease (并病 *bìng bìng*). In the *Shāng Hán Lùn*, there is greater yáng and yáng brightness dragover disease and greater yáng and lesser yáng dragover disease. In addition, in debilitated patients, disease evils under some circumstances do not go through the three yang, but instead enter the three yīn channels directly. This is called direct strike [on the yīn channels] (直中 *zhí zhòng*).

Treatment

The *Shāng Hán Lùn* text makes reference to several different forms of treatment including acupuncture, moxibustion, fuming, and drug therapy. Zhāng Jī mostly recommends medicinal treatments; only occasionally does he suggest acupuncture. Other treatments mentioned in the *Shāng Hán Lùn* are those that patients have previously received, and often they are specifically stated to have been inappropriate.

The medicinal therapy applied by Zhāng Jī is based on the notion that each drug has certain properties that affect the body in a specific way. Different medicinals are combined in innumerable ways to cope with the complex manifestations of externally contracted disease. The treatments are not symptomatic, but address specific pathomechanisms.

One treatment alone stands out as being based on different notions. The formula Burnt Pants Decoction (*shāo kūn sǎn*), a decoction made from the ash of the crotch of underpants, seems to based on an older, magical conception of yīn and yáng. According to *Shāng Hán Lùn*, when the body is severely weakened by externally contracted disease, the disease is easily transmitted through sexual intercourse. A condition transmitted to a person in this way is treated by the burnt crotch of the underpants of a person of the opposite sex. This formula is not applied in modern practice.

Zhāng Jī uses medicinal formulae to promote sweating (汗 *hàn*), promote vomiting (吐 *tù*), precipitate (下 *xià*), harmonize (和 *hé*), warm (温 *wēn*), clear (清 *qīng*), supplement (补 *bǔ*), and disperse (消 *xiāo*), although the last three of these terms do not appear in the therapeutic sense in the *Shāng Hán Lùn*. Through the lines of the *Shāng Hán Lùn*, we can see that the notions of "supporting yáng qì" (扶阳气 *fú yáng qì*) and "preserving yīn humor" (存阴液 *cún yīn yè*) constitute the basic approach to dispelling evil. In other words, the spearhead of Zhāng Jī's treatments consists in enhancing the body's power to dispel evil. In diseases of the three yáng, the object is to dispel evil, but the treatments are mostly designed to adjust bodily functions in such a way as to release or expel the evil. For greater yáng disease, the main approach is to resolve the exterior. In exterior repletion this involves opening the interstices, causing cold to dissipate by the promotion of sweating. In exterior vacuity, it entails harmonizing construction and defense in order to resolve the flesh and dispel wind. In yáng brightness disease, heat patterns are treated by clearing, whereas repletion patterns are treated by precipitation. In lesser yáng disease, where inhibition of the pivot gives rise to half exterior half interior patterns, the treatment is harmonization and resolution. Disease of the three yīn mostly manifests in vacuity patterns, for which the treatment is primarily to support right qì. For example, greater yīn disease manifests in vacuity cold-damp patterns, so that the treatment is primarily to warm the center, dissipate cold, and dry dampness. Lesser yīn disease manifests in heart-kidney debilitation with insufficiency of qì and blood, there being, however, a distinction between cold transformation and heat transformation. Cold transformation is treated by supporting yáng and repressing yīn, while heat transformation is treated by fostering yīn and clearing heat. Reverting yīn disease manifests in a variety of complex patterns, where heat is treated by clearing, cold is treated by warming, and cold-heat complexes are treated by dual application of warming and clearing.

THE LANGUAGE OF THE SHĀNG HÁN LÙN

The main body of the *Shāng Hán Lùn* is divided into short lines describing patterns and their treatment, and sometimes their etiology. The content is not only clinically oriented and matter-of-fact, but is also reasonably uniform. Accordingly, its expression is also quite consistent as regards both terminology and sentence patterns. Since our translation is highly literal, these and other features of the language of the *Shāng Hán Lùn* will also be apparent to the English-speaking reader. Nevertheless, certain variations in terminology and certain specific sentence patterns may be troublesome to the English-speaking reader, and these are discussed here. Learners of Chinese wishing to read the original text are referred to Appendix II for a comprehensive analysis of the grammar and vocabulary of the *Shāng Hán Lùn*.

Terms

The *Shāng Hán Lùn* is a book offering treatments for various different manifestations of cold damage. Accordingly, terms can be divided into three broad categories: sign names, pattern names, and formula (and drug) names. Pattern names and formula and drug names are the most consistent; each term denotes only one concept and, discounting abbreviated forms, is the only term to denote that concept.

Sign names are more numerous and more variable. The notion of heat effusion appears as 发热 *fā rè* and 身热 *shēn rè*, and simply as 热 *rè*. Other clusters of terms to a greater or lesser degree synonymous include:

（口）不能食 *(kǒu) bù néng shí*, inability to eat
食不下 *shí bù xià*, inability to get food down
不欲饮食 *bù yù yǐn shí*, no desire for food or drink

不得眠 *bù dé mián*, inability to sleep
不得卧 *bù dé wò*, inability to sleep
不得卧寐 *bù dè wò mèi*, inability to sleep

手足冷 *shǒu zú lěng*, cold extremities
手足厥冷 *shǒu zú jué lěng*, reversal cold of the extremities
手足逆冷 *shǒu zú nì lěng*, counterflow cold of the extremities

喘 *chuǎn*, panting
短气 *duǎn qì*, shortness of breath
少气 *shǎo qì*, shortage of qì

Many terms contained in the *Shāng Hán Lùn* are to this day used in the same sense. 发热 *fā rè* and 恶寒 *wù hán* denote the same sign now as they did in the time of Zhāng Jī. A few terms, however, have changed in their meaning. Readers should be warned against reading into terms contained in the *Shāng Hán Lùn* definitions and connotations that they accrued later in history.

The term dispersion-thirst (消渴 *xiāo kě*) appears in reverting yīn disease, and describes a thirst that is unallayed by fluid intake. The same term also is more commonly encountered outside the *Shāng Hán Lùn* as denoting a disease entity that corresponds in large measure to diabetes. Interestingly, the thirst in greater yáng disease is sometimes unquenchable, but "dispersion-thirst" is not used to describe it.

Terms whose meaning have undergone change notably include certain pulse terms that were given specific definitions that are not known to have applied in Zhāng Jī's writings. Most of the pulse terms used in Chinese medicine are commonly used adjectives, and the absence in early literature of definitions for these terms suggests that writers believed they were not using these terms in a technical sense that required special explanation. The first attempt to systematically define pulse terms was made by Wáng Shū-Hé, who, it will be remembered, gathered together the parts of the *Shāng Hán Zá Bìng Lùn* relating to cold damage to form the *Shāng Hán Lùn*. Wáng Shū-Hé based his *Mài Jīng* largely on Zhāng Jī's work, but gave definitions for the pulse that were clearly more specific than the sense in which Zhāng Jī had used them.[1] For example, Wáng Shū-Hé defined 动 *dòng*, "stirred," as being a rapid quality of the pulse felt only at the bar (关 *guān*) point, despite the fact that in one instance in the *Shāng Hán Lùn* a "stirred" quality is explained to be palpable over an area not limited to the bar. Wáng Shū-Hé's narrower definition, which was accepted by many physicians of subsequent generations, does not apply in the *Shāng Hán Lùn*.

The Chinese 微 *wēi* is sometimes used adverbially in the sense of "slightly" (before line 23, p. 122), and sometimes adjectivally to describe a pulse quality (after line 23, p. 122). 促 *cù*, "skipping," is sometimes taken to mean "rapid and urgent" (line 34, p. 158), and sometimes to mean "rapid and interrupted" (line 21, p. 85). 缓 *huǎn*, "moderate," is sometimes taken to be the opposite of "tight" (line 2, p. 43) and sometimes to be slower than normal in speed (line 187, p. 462). 阴阳 *yīn yáng*, "yīn and yáng," are sometimes taken to mean inch and cubit respectively (line 4, p. 52, and line 6, p. 47), and sometimes taken to mean superficial level and deep level (line 12, p. 60).

[1]Wáng Shū-Hé also introduced the innovation of referring to single pulse qualities in the format "adjective (or qualifying noun) + pulse," e.g., "floating pulse" as compared with descriptive "the pulse is floating" used by Zhāng Jī and earlier writers.

The usage of the terms yīn and yáng also deserves our attention. In the *Shāng Hán Lùn*, these terms are rarely used to denote the two aspects of physiological function (yīn blood and yáng qì) as they are in other literature. Rather, they most commonly appear in the names of the channels and, as individual terms, are most frequently used to name pulse conditions or positions. In the context of the pulse, the terms are polysemous. As classes of pulse types, yīn refers to sunken, rough, weak, stringlike, and faint pulses, while yáng refers to large, floating, rapid, stirred, and slippery pulses. In other pulse contexts, however, yīn and yáng refer to the cubit and inch pulse (cf. line 290, p. 521).

Finally, the various terms denoting jaundice deserve some attention. In the *Shāng Hán Lùn*, jaundice is usually referred to as 发黄 *fā huáng*, "yellowing," or 身发黄 *shēn fā huáng*, "generalized yellowing." The word 黄疸 *huáng dǎn*, most commonly used in modern texts, does not appear, but the 瘅, *dǎn*, a synonym of 疸 *dǎn*, appears in the term 谷瘅 *gǔ dǎn*, "grain jaundice." These terms have always meant the same thing since Zhāng Jī's time. Nevertheless, understanding of the causes has changed. Throughout most of the history of Chinese medicine, jaundice was considered to be a disease of the spleen arising when damp-heat or damp-cold obstructing the normal movement of fluids in the center burner affected spleen function. The yellowness was considered to be a direct reflection of spleen disease, since yellow is the color associated with spleen-earth. Zhāng Jìng-Yuè (张景岳) of the Míng Dynasty may have been the first physician in China to propose the term 胆黄 *dǎn huáng*, "gallbladder jaundice," claiming that this disease arose when damage to gallbladder qì caused bile to discharge, i.e., leak from the gallbladder and flow to the skin. In the Qīng Dynasty, Yè Guì (叶桂, style 天士 Tiān-Shì), in his *Lín Zhèng Zhǐ Nán Yī Àn* (临证指南医案 "Case Studies for Clinical Guidance") of 1766, combined the theories of damp-heat and gallbladder involvement. Nevertheless, no writer before the modern era ever stated that yellowing of the skin and the sclerae, whatever the root cause, was always the manifestation of stray bile. It is only in this century that the notion of jaundice has become central to the concept of jaundice, so much so that even modern commentators introduce it into their explanations of pathomechanisms in the *Shāng Hán Lùn*.

Stylistic Features

With the sole exception of Zhāng Jī's preface, the *Shāng Hán Lùn* is written in straightforward style with no literary adornment. Given the similarity of Chinese syntax to English, the word order can be almost perfectly replicated in English. Nevertheless, two rather peculiar stylistic features deserve our attention. Intercalation and inversion are two features of Hàn Dynasty Chinese that caused interpretation difficulties in later ages. In the translation, we have reproduced these features in English with the aid of parentheses. We give a few examples to warn the unsuspecting reader.

Intercalation: Sometimes additional qualifying or explanatory phrases are included in the text. In the English translation, in accordance with modern custom, we have placed such phrases in brackets.

阳明病，谵语，有潮热，反不能食者，胃中必有燥屎五六枚也。若能食者，但硬耳，宜大承气汤下之。

[Line 215, p. 347:] When in yáng brightness disease, [there is] delirious speech and tidal heat effusion, but inability to eat, [this means that] there must be five or six pieces of dry stool in the stomach. (If [the person] is able to eat, [there is] only hard [stool].) Major Qì-Coordinating Decoction (*dà chéng qì tāng*) is appropriate for precipitation.

Inversion: The appearance of a note or comment that can only be understood after reading the predicate of the sentence that follows is called inversion. We have marked inversions by placing them in parentheses.

太阳病，脉浮紧，无汗发热，身疼痛，八九日不解，表证仍在，此当发其汗。服药已，微除，其人发烦目瞑，剧者必衄，衄乃解。所以然者，阳气重故也。麻黄汤主之。

[Line 46, p. 96:] In greater yáng disease, when a pulse that is floating and tight, absence of sweating, heat effusion, and generalized pain are unresolved after eight or nine days, the exterior pattern is still present and one should promote sweating. (After taking medicine, [the condition] is slightly relieved, and the person is vexed and the eyes are heavy. If it is acute, there will be spontaneous external bleeding, which will bring about resolution. Why [this] is so is because the yáng qì is weighted.) Ephedra Decoction (*má huáng tāng*) governs.

The parenthesized section in the above example is an inversion since "medicine" refers to Ephedra Decoction (*má huáng tāng*), which is not mentioned until the end of the sentence.

伤寒心下有水气，咳而微喘，发热不渴；服汤已，渴者，此寒去欲解也；小青龙汤主之。

[Line 41, p. 120:] When in cold damage, [there is] water qì below the heart, cough, mild panting, and heat effusion without thirst, (thirst, after taking the decoction, means the cold is going and [the disease] is about to resolve) Minor Green-Blue Dragon Decoction (*xiǎo qīng lóng tāng*) governs.

Here, the word "decoction" in the parenthesis refers to Minor Green-Blue Dragon Decoction, which has not yet been mentioned. The author jumps ahead of his own thoughts, and the prompt to do so apparently comes from the word "thirst": the decoction treats a pattern without thirst, but may in fact cause thirst.

太阳病，发热恶寒，热多寒少，脉微弱者，此无阳也，不可发汗，宜桂枝二越婢一汤。

[Line 27, p. 127:] When in greater yáng disease [there is] heat effusion and aversion to cold [with] more heat and less cold (a pulse that is faint and weak means that yáng is absent and one cannot promote sweating), Two Parts Cinnamon Twig and One Part Spleen-Effusing Decoction (*guì zhī èr yuè bì yī tāng*) is appropriate.

发汗后，不可更行桂枝汤，汗出而喘，无大热者，可与麻黄杏仁甘草石膏汤。

[Line 63, p. 154:] After the promotion of sweating, ([one] cannot again use Cinnamon Twig Decoction (*guì zhī tāng*)) if sweat issues, and [there is] panting and great heat is absent, one can use Ephedra, Apricot Kernel, Licorice, and Gypsum Decoction (*má huáng xìng rén gān cǎo shí gāo tāng*).

Solving Ambiguities

The *Shāng Hán Lùn* contains a considerable number of textual ambiguities that are clarified by considering contextual information. For example, the pattern can be determined from the formula or from the pulse, or the formula can be determined from the pattern.

Determining the pattern from the formula: Many if not most of the lines of the *Shāng Hán Lùn* discuss a particular constellation of signs prefaced by a generic pattern (e.g., "wind strike," "greater yáng disease"). Generally speaking, the generic pattern is intended to evoke the basic signs, even when these are not explicitly stated. Thus whenever the text of a line starts as "[When] in greater yáng disease...," we can usually be sure that whatever signs follow, we are to understand that the basic signs of greater yáng disease (floating pulse, stiffness and pain of head and nape, etc.) are also implied. Sometimes, however, there is no generic reference. Given the speculation as to the original order of the lines, the absence of a generic reference introduces potential ambiguity. In such cases, the formula mentioned in the line very often provides the desired reference. Much interpretation of ambiguous lines is based on the principle of working backwards from the formula. Let us look at the following example:

脉浮者，病在表，可发汗，宜麻黄汤。

[Line 51, p. 93:] When the pulse is floating, the disease is in the exterior, [and if] one can promote sweating, Ephedra Decoction (*má huáng tāng*) is appropriate.

Although it is not clear from the signs given here whether this is a cold damage or wind strike pattern, the use of Ephedra Decoction (*má huáng tāng*) clarifies the issue since this formula is only appropriate when there is no sweating, i.e., for cold damage patterns.

大病差后，从腰以下有水气者，牡蛎泽泻散主之。

[Line 395, p. 601:] When after a major illness has been cured, [there is] water qì from the lumbus down, Oyster Shell and Alisma Powder (*mǔ lì zé xiè sǎn*) governs.

This line is ambiguous because the appearance of water-qì after an illness can be a sign of vacuity or repletion. An analysis of the formula, however, shows that this line discusses a repletion pattern of water swelling from the lumbus down due to damp-heat congestion and a loss of normal qì transformation in the lower burner.

Determining the pattern from the pulse: In some instances, the pulse provides information about the nature of the pattern.

问曰：病有结胸，有藏结，其状何如？答曰：按之痛，寸脉浮，关脉沉，名曰结胸也。

[Line 128, p. 211:] Question: There is a disease [called] chest bind, and there is [one called] storehouse bind. What form do they take? Answer: [If there is] pain when pressure is applied, and the inch pulse is floating, and the bar pulse is sunken, this is called chest bind.

何谓藏结？答曰：如结胸状，饮食如故，时时下利，寸脉浮，关脉小细沉紧，名曰藏结。舌上白胎滑者，难治。

[Line 129, p. 225:] What is storehouse bind? Answer: [When there are] signs like chest bind, eating and drinking are normal, [and there is] frequent diarrhea, an inch pulse that is floating, and a bar pulse that is small, fine, sunken, and tight, it is called storehouse bind. When the tongue fur is white and slippery, this [pattern] is difficult to treat.

Both chest bind and storehouse bind manifest in hard fullness below the heart that is painful when pressed and in a pulse that is floating at the inch. Chest bind is characterized by a pulse that is sunken at the bar, while storehouse bind is characterized by a pulse that is small and fine, sunken, and tight. The pulses clearly reflect the pathomechanisms: Chest bind is usually a yáng or heat pattern that arises when heat and water bind in the chest and rib-side and below the heart. Because the bar pulse governs the center, it reflects the location of the disease qì in the chest and diaphragm. Because this is a repletion pattern, the pulse that is sunken at the bar is also forceful. In contrast, storehouse bind is a yīn or cold pattern that arises when, owing to center burner vacuity cold and debilitation of yáng qì, yīn cold evil binds in the treasuries. Because the right is vacuous and evil is exuberant, this is difficult to treat. The pulse that is small and fine at the bar reflects debilitation of right qì, and the sunkenness and tightness reflect the yīn evil binding internally.

Determining the formula from the pattern: Sometimes the context provides information about a formula name.

太阳病，项背强几几，反汗出恶风者，桂枝加葛根汤主之。

[Line 14, p. 79:] When in greater yáng disease [there is] stretched stiff nape and back, but also sweating and aversion to wind, it is treated with Cinnamon Twig Decoction Plus Pueraria (*guì zhī jiā gé gēn tāng*).

The formula prescribed contains ephedra (*má huáng*), which is not appropriate if there is sweating. From the context, therefore, it has been suggested that Cinnamon Twig Decoction Plus Pueraria (*guì zhī jiā gé gēn tāng*) means Cinnamon Twig Decoction (*guì zhī tāng*) with the addition of gé gēn.

There are many places where the Chinese text is ambiguous at the level of conceptual understanding. Although the wording of the text in such places may be clear, different interpretations as to the clinical significance are given. Line 353, p. 546, provides an example:

大汗出，热不去，内拘急，四肢疼，又下利，厥逆而恶寒者，四逆汤主之。

> [Line 353, p. 546:] When great sweat issues, the heat has not gone, and [there is] internal hypertonicity, pain in the limbs, diarrhea, reverse-flow and aversion to cold, Counterflow Cold Decoction (*sì nì tāng*) governs.

It is generally clear that this line presents a condition of interior yīn exuberance, but whether this is accompanied by exterior yáng collapse, or an unresolved exterior pattern, has been a matter of debate.

Yet there are also places where the literal meaning of the text is unclear. Here the problem may lie in the grammatical ambiguity of phrases or the referential ambiguity of words.

For example in line 17, p. 76, which reads 若酒客病，不可与桂枝汤 *ruò jiǔ kè bìng, bù kě yǔ guì zhī tāng*, it is not clear if this is to be understood as "If a liquor drinker is sick [with greater yáng disease], [one] cannot give Cinnamon Twig Decoction" or "If [the patient has] liquor drinker sickness (i.e., alcoholism, without greater yáng disease), [one] cannot give Cinnamon Twig Decoction." In such cases, we have tried to make the English translation as ambiguous as the Chinese text, so that it supports either interpretation.

Ambiguity in the referential meaning is most commonly found in the words yīn and yáng.

> 凡厥者，阴阳气不相顺接，便为厥。厥者，手足逆冷者是也。
>
> [Line 337, p. 542:] In all reversal [patterns], yīn and yáng qì are not connecting smoothly, which means reversal. Reversal means counterflow cold of the extremities.

Here, yīn and yáng are variously interpreted as meaning qì in the channels, the relationship between organs, or the relationship between organ qì and channel qì.

Finally, we should also mention the word 必 *bì*, which is generally understood to mean "must," "ought to," "bound to." Zhāng Jī uses this word, for example, in line 32, p. 111, to indicate the likelihood of spontaneous diarrhea in greater yáng and yáng brightness combination disease. Nonetheless, if one looks ahead to line 33, p. 112, it is clear that in the same combination disease, diarrhea does not occur. This and other apparent incongruities have led some commentators to suggest that 必 *bì* should be understood to mean "might" or "may." Since we have found no lexicographical source that notes 必 possesses this sense, the suggestion can only be based on belief in Zhāng Jī's infallibility. Of course, logical inconsistency in the original text and transcription error are just as likely possibilities. In the translation, we leave the question open by rendering the 必 *bì* as "will."

Zhāng Jī's Preface

张机原序

㈠余每览越人入虢之诊，望齐侯之色，未尝不慨然叹其才秀也。㈡怪当今居世之士，曾不留神医药，精究方术，上以疗君亲之疾，下以救贫贱之厄，中以保身长全，以养其生，但竞逐荣势，企踵权豪，孜孜汲汲，惟名利是务，崇饰其末，忽弃其本，华其外而悴其内，皮之不存，毛将安附焉？㈢卒然遭邪风之气，婴非常之疾，患及祸至，而方震栗，降志屈节，钦望巫祝，告穷归天，束手受败，赍百年之寿命，持至贵之重器，委付凡医，恣其所措，咄嗟呜呼！㈣厥身已毙，神明消灭，变为异物，幽潜重泉，徒为啼泣。痛夫！㈤举世昏迷，莫能觉悟，不惜其命，若是轻生，彼何荣势之云哉！㈥而进不能爱人知人，退不能爱身知己，遇灾值祸，身居厄地，蒙蒙昧昧，惷若游魂。哀乎！㈦趋世之士，驰竞浮华，不固根本，忘驱徇物，危若冰谷，至于是也。

(1) *Yú měi lǎn yuè rén rù guó zhī zhěn, wàng qí hòu zhī sè, wèi cháng bù kǎi rán tàn qí cái xiù yě.* (2) *Guài dāng jīn jū shì zhī shì, céng bù liú shén yī yào, jīng jiù fāng shù, shàng yǐ liáo jūn qīn zhī jí, xià yǐ jiù pín jiàn zhī è, zhōng yǐ bǎo shēn cháng quán, yǐ yǎng qí shēng, dàn jìng zhú róng shì, qì zhǒng quán háo, zī zī jí jí, wéi míng lì shì wù, chóng shì qí mò, hū qì qí běn, huá qí wài ér cuì qí nèi, pí zhī bù cún, máo jiāng ān fù yān?* (3) *Zú rán zāo xié fēng zhī qì, yīng fēi cháng zhī jí, huàn jí huò zhì, ér fāng zhèn lì, jiàng zhì qū jié, qīn wàng wū zhù, gào qióng guī tiān, shù shǒu shòu bài, jī bǎi nián zhī shòu mìng, chí zhì guì zhī zhòng qì, wěi fù fán yī, zì*

qí suǒ cuò, duō jiē wū hū! (4) *Jué shēn yǐ bì, shēn míng xiāo miè, biàn wéi yì wù, yōu qián zhòng quán, tú wéi tí qì. Tòng fū!* (5) *Jǔ shì hūn mí, mò néng jué wù, bù xí qí mìng, ruò shì qīng shēng, bǐ hé róng shì zhī yún zāi.* (6) *Ér jìn bù néng ài rén zhī rén, tuì bù néng ài shēn zhī jǐ, yù zāi zhí huò, shēn jū è dì, méng méng mèi mèi, chún ruò yóu hún. Aī hū!* (7) *Qù shì zhī shì, chí jìng fú huá, bù gù gēn běn, wàng qū xún wù, wéi ruò bīng gǔ, zhì yú shì yě.*

(1) Each time I read about Yuè-Rén[1] entering [the Kingdom of] Guó to examine [patients] and inspect the complexion of the Marquis of Qí, I always sigh with great emotion about his superb talents. (2) [It is] bewildering that the learned men of our age never pay attention to medicine [and are not] proficiently versed in the remedial arts, [which would enable them] to treat the illnesses of the sovereign and of [their] elders above, to relieve the suffering of the poor and destitute below, and to safeguard [their own] body and sustain health at center,[2] [all] in order to cultivate life. Instead, [they] only compete and pursue glory and power. [They] stand on the tiptoe of expectancy for influential officials and families of power, diligently and untiringly devoting their efforts only to fame and profit. Revering and refining nonessentials, [they] neglect and abandon the root. While embellishing the external, they impoverish the internal.[3] [If] the skin is absent, [how] can the hair be securely attached? (3) [When they then] suddenly suffer [an attack of] evil wind qì and [consequently] develop an extraordinary illness, meeting misfortune and disaster, [they] tremble and shake. Abandoning their integrity, they lower themselves to grovel before magical healers. Declaring [their] helplessness, [they] attribute [their misfortune to fate ordained by] heaven;[4] with hands tied, they accept defeat. Holding a life[-span] of [potentially a] hundred years, their most valuable posession, they entrust themselves to common physicians, who treat recklessly, without regard [for life's value]. Oh woe! (4) The body already dead and the spirit destroyed, they transmute into weird beings, and descend to roam in the underworld, weeping and sobbing to no avail. Oh, what pain! (5) The whole world is stuporous, nobody is aware, [nobody] cherishes life. Making light of life in this way, why [all] that talk of glory and power? (6) Moving forward [into society, they are] unable to love and know others; retreating [into themselves, they are] unable to love and know themselves. Meeting disaster and encountering misfortune, placed in precarious position, [they are still] clouded by

ignorance, blind as wandering souls. What sorrow! (7) Men who pursue the ways of the world race in competition for vain ostentation, failing to secure the root. Neglecting the body in pursuit of material possessions, [their situation is as] dangerous as if [they were walking on thin] ice [in the bottom of a deep] valley, so serious is it.

㈠余宗族素多，向余二百，建安纪年以来，犹未十稔，其死亡者，三分有二，伤寒十居其七。㈡感往昔之沦丧，伤横夭之莫救，乃勤求古训，博采众方，撰用《素问》、《九卷》、《八十一难》、《阴阳大论》、《胎胪药录》并《平脉辨证》，为《伤寒杂病论》合十六卷。㈢虽未能尽愈诸病，庶可以见病知源。㈣若能寻余所集，思过半矣。

(1) *Yú zōng zú sù duō, xiàng yú èr bǎi, Jiàn Ān jì nián yǐ lái, yóu wèi shí rěn, qí sǐ wáng zhě, sān fēn yǒu èr, shāng hán shí jū qí qī.* (2) *Gǎn wǎng xí zhī lún sāng, shāng hèng yāo zhī mò jiù, nǎi qín qiú gǔ xùn, bó cǎi zhòng fāng, zhuàn yòng 《sù wèn》, 《jiǔ juàn》, 《bā shí yī nàn》, 《yīn yáng dà lùn》, 《tāi lú yào lù》, bìng 《píng mài biàn zhèng》, wéi 《shāng hán zá bìng lùn》 hé shí liǔ juàn.* (3) *Suī wèi néng jìn yù zhū bìng, shù kě yǐ jiàn bìng zhī yuán.* (4) *Ruò néng xún yú suǒ jí, sī guò bàn yǐ.*

(1) My family was formerly large, once [counting] over two hundred members, [but] from [the beginning of] the Jiàn-Ān reign,[5] in less than ten years, two thirds have died, seven tenths of them from cold damage. (2) Lamenting the fall of [our glorious] past and the untimely loss of so many lives that could not be saved, I have diligently sought the guidance of the ancients, widely collected the various remedies, and consulted the *Sù Wèn* ("Plain Questions"), *Jiǔ Juàn* ("The Nine Fascicles"), *Bā Shí Yī Nán* ("The Eighty-One Difficult Issues"), *Yīn Yáng Dà Lùn* ("The Great Treatise on Yīn-Yáng"), *Tài Lú Yào Lù* ("The Tài Lú Record of Medicinals"), and the *Píng Mài Biàn Zhèng* ("The Assessment of Pulses and Identification of Patterns") to create the *Shāng Hán Zá Bìng Lùn*, totaling sixteen fascicles. (3) Although this book cannot completely cure all diseases, it provides the means to understand the origin of illnesses encountered. (4) If [the reader] follows the materials herein collected, [he should be able to] think out over half [of all medical problems].

㈠ 夫天布五行，以运万类；人禀五常，以有五藏；经络府俞，阴阳会通，玄冥幽微，变化难极。㈡ 自非才高识妙，岂能探其理致哉！㈢ 上古有神农、黄帝、岐伯、伯高、雷公、少俞、少师、仲文、中世有长桑、扁鹊、汉有公乘阳庆及仓公，下此以往，未之闻也。㈣ 观今之医，不念思求经旨，以演其所知，各承家技，终始顺旧，省疾问病，务在口给，相对斯须，便处汤药。按寸不及尺，握手不及足；人迎趺阳，三部不参；动数发息，不满五十。㈤ 短期未知决诊，九候曾无髣髴，明堂阙庭，尽不见察，所谓窥管而已。㈥ 夫欲视死别生，实为难矣。

(1) *Fū tiān bù wǔ xíng, yǐ yùn wàn lèi; rén bǐng wǔ cháng, yǐ yǒu wǔ zàng; jīng luò fǔ shū, yīn yáng huì tōng, xuán míng yōu wēi, biàn huà nán jí.* (2) *Zì fēi cái gāo shì miào, qǐ néng tàn qí lǐ zhì zāi!* (3) *Shàng gǔ yǒu Shén Nóng, Huáng Dì, Qí Bó, Bó Gāo, Léi Gōng, Shào Yú, Shào Shī, Zhòng Wén, zhōng shì yǒu Cháng Sāng, Biǎn Què, Hàn yǒu Gōng Shéng Yáng Qìng jí Cāng Gōng, xià cǐ yǐ wáng, wèi zhī wén yě.* (4) *Guān jīn zhī yī, bù niàn sī qiú jīng zhǐ, yǐ yǎn qí suǒ zhī, gè chéng jiā jì, zhōng shǐ shùn jiù, xǐng jí wèn bìng, wù zài kǒu jǐ, xiāng duì sī xū, biàn chǔ tāng yào. Àn cùn bù jí chǐ, wò shǒu bù jí zú; rén yíng dié yáng, sān bù bù cān; dòng shù fā xī, bù mǎn wǔ shí.* (5) *Duǎn qí wèi zhī jué zhěn, jiǔ hòu zēng wú fǎng fú, míng táng què tíng, jìn bù jiàn chá, suǒ wèi kuī guǎn ér yǐ.* (6) *Fū yù shì sǐ bié shēng, shí wéi nán yǐ.*

(1) Heaven is woven with the five phases which move [to produce] the myriad types. Man is constituted by the five constants,[6] and therefore has five viscera,[7] as well as channels and network vessels and the points. Yīn and yáng interact with each other in dark and subtle [ways and in] transmutations hard to fathom. (2) Naturally, without high talent to understand [these] mysteries, how can [anyone] probe the logic to its limits! (3) In high antiquity, there were Shén-Nóng, Huáng-Dì, Qí-Bó, Bó-Gāo, Léi-Gōng, Shào-Shū, Shào-Shī, and Zhòng-Wén; in middle antiquity, there were Cháng-Sāng and Biǎn-Què; in the Hàn, there have been Gōng-Shèn Yáng-Qìng and Cāng-Gōng. After these, we know of no [famous physicians]. (4) Looking at the physicians of today, [we see that they] do not ponder on the meaning of the [medical] classics to develop their knowledge, [but instead] each inherits the skills passed down in their family, constantly following traditional ways. In reflecting

on illnesses and inquiring of patients' suffering, their effort is placed on the gift of the gab, and after a brief consultation, give a simple prescription for a decoction. (5) They feel the inch pulse and do not bother with the cubit, feel the hand [pulse] and neglect the foot [pulse]. They do not correlate the three positions, [the wrist pulse with] Man's Prognosis and Instep Yáng. When counting the beats and controlling their breath, they do not complete the fifty [beats].[8] (6) They are unable to diagnose when the patient will die, and even have no understanding of the nine indicators. They do not look at the bright hall[9] and the tower gate[10] at all. This is what is [proverbially] called "looking [at the world] through a tube." (7) If they expect to be able to differentiate life from death in this way, they indeed have a hard task.

㈠ 孔子云，生而知之者上，学则亚之，多闻博识，知之次也。㈡ 余宿尚方术，请事斯语。

(1) *Kǒng Zǐ yún, shēng ér zhī zhī zhě shàng, xué zé yǎ zhī, duō wén bó shì, zhī zhī cì yě.* (2) *Yú sù shàng fāng shù, qǐng shì sī yǔ.*

(1) Confucius says: Those who know naturally from birth are greatest; those who [understand through] study are second to them; those who understand through listening broadly to learned opinion are inferior. (2) I have always prized remedial arts, in the hope of putting these words into practice.

TEXT NOTES

1. The story of Biǎn Què (Qín Yuè-Rén) entering the Kingdom of Guó relates how he revived the Prince of Guó from "deathlike reversal" (尸厥 *shī jué*), i.e., from an incurable state close to death.
2. Above, below, at center 上、下、中 *shàng, xià, zhōng*: In Confucian philosophy, above, below, and center describe social levels relative to the individual: above the individual are the sovereign and the individual's parents; below the individual are those less fortunate; the center is the individual himself.
3. While embellishing the external, they impoverish the internal 华其外而悴其内 *huà qí wài ér cuì qí nèi*: Foster overt ostentation at the expense of their inner life.
4. Declaring [their] helplessness, [they] attribute [their misfortune to fate ordained by] heaven 告穷归天 *gào qióng guī tiān*: 告 *gào* means "to declare" 穷 *qióng* means "to run out," "come to an end," "to be impoverished." 归天 *guī tiān* can be interpreted to mean "go (back), return to heaven" (to die), or "to trace back (here, their misfortune) to the will of heaven." Both specific interpretations imply an acceptance of ill fate.

5. Jiàn Ān [reign] 建安 *Jiàn-Ān*: Literally, "The Establishment of Peace," the title of the reign of Emperor Hàn-Xiàn (汉献帝), which began in 196 C.E.
6. Five constants 五常 *wǔ cháng*: The five phases.
7. Five viscera 五藏 *wǔ zàng*: The heart, liver, spleen, lung, and kidney.
8. Fifty beats 五十 *wǔ shí*: Literally, "fifty," the Chinese is understood to mean 五十动 *wǔ shí dòng*, the fifty beats of the pulse considered to mark the minimum time devoted to feeling the pulse. This theory comes from the *Nàn Jīng*.
9. Bright hall 明堂 *míng táng*: The nose.
10. Tower-gate court 阙庭 *què tíng*: The area between the two eyebrows. (The "court" 庭 *tíng*, is the forehead.) Inspection of this area was formerly a point of attention when examining patients.

COMMENTARY

Zhāng Jī's original preface to the *Shāng Hán Zá Bìng Lùn*, which is here divided into four paragraphs, has not been completely authenticated.

In the first paragraph, Zhāng Jī comments on the practice of medicine in his time. In it we can see a Confucianist axiom that the learned have a social and moral obligation to be conversant with medicine. For Zhāng Jī, medicine is ideally not a service provided by a specialist, but a branch of knowledge in which learned people should be knowledgeable for the benefit of society as a whole. Society apparently does not come up to his standards, because men of learning do not concern themselves with medicine and, when they fall ill, resort to magical healers.

In the second paragraph, the author tells us that he was motivated to write this book by the rampant disease that had brought a severe toll on his own family and presumably on the population in general. His solution consisted not in resorting to magical healers but to studying the medical literature available at the time. When we recall that this is the preface of a larger, more comprehensive work than the *Shāng Hán Lùn*, we realize that Zhāng Jī's intention was to write a comprehensive medical text for very real clinical needs.

Paragraph three, which in the Kāng Píng edition appears in small print to indicate that it is annotation, stresses the importance of yīn and yáng and the five phases in medicine elucidating the mysteries of health and sickness that allegedly had received waning attention over the centuries. There is specific criticism here of diagnostic practices, in particular the failure of contemporary physicians to apply diagnostic techniques of which there is little or no mention in the *Shāng Hán Lùn*.

The final paragraph is a statement of Confucian faith in learning.

Chapter One

Greater Yáng Disease

Pulses and Signs; Treatment

辨太阳病脉证并治

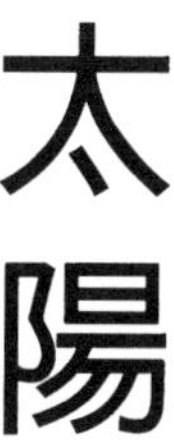

1 OVERVIEW

Externally contracted disease (cold damage in the broad sense) is caused by evils entering the body from outside. Since the greater yáng channel governs the exterior of the body, it is usually the first to be affected. For this reason, the discussion of greater yáng disease forms the first chapter of the *Shāng Hán Lùn*. External evils may enter other channels directly, but very often, externally contracted disease begins with the greater yáng contracting the evil. Greater yáng disease is much more varied in its manifestations than disease of any other channel. This is reflected in the fact that the lines devoted to greater yáng disease make up nearly half of the entire book.

In greater yáng disease, an evil invades the fleshy exterior. There are three basic forms of greater yáng disease—wind strike, cold damage (in the narrow sense), and warm disease—reflecting Zhāng Jī's understanding that externally contracted disease is attributable to wind, cold, or warmth. Diseases attributed to external contraction of cold form the main body of information presented in this chapter. Warmth is accorded relatively insignificant status, since only one line of greater yáng disease deals with it.

Greater yáng disease arises when external evil invades the fleshy exterior and impairs the normal functioning of the defense qì. Wind strike is characterized by fever—or as we refer to it in this text, "heat effusion"—together with aversion to cold or wind, and spontaneous sweating; cold damage is characterized by heat effusion, aversion to cold, and absence of sweating; and warm disease is characterized by heat effusion, thirst, and mild aversion to wind and cold or, in some cases, absence of aversion to cold. Which of these three basic patterns occurs depends on the constitution of the patient and the nature of the evil.

In modern literature, exterior patterns are usually presented in a primary division of wind-heat and wind-cold. This represents a later development in the understanding of externally contracted disease. Neither of these terms occurs in the *Shāng Hán Lùn*.

Inappropriate treatment or lack of treatment can give rise to a transmuted pattern (变证 *biàn zhèng*) or cause the evil to shift into another channel. These changes depend on the type of inappropriate treatment, the patient's constitution and the nature of the evil. Although greater yáng disease is associated with exterior patterns, many transmuted patterns are interior in nature. These patterns are varied in nature, as will be seen below, due to the combination of factors producing them.

If an exterior evil falls inward and binds with phlegm-rheum, stagnant food, or static blood, bind patterns may be observed, including water amassment, blood amassment, chest bind, and glomus patterns.

1.1 SIGNS AND PULSES

The main signs of greater yáng disease are a pulse that is floating, stiffness and pain of the head and nape, and aversion to cold. Whatever the disease evil or the duration of the disease, the simultaneous presence of this pulse and these signs is a certain indication of greater yáng disease. Also important are heat effusion (fever) and the presence or absence of sweating.

A pulse that is floating 脉浮 *mài fú*: A pulse that is felt when light pressure is applied is called "floating." In greater yáng disease, a pulse that is floating usually reflects a condition in which an external evil has invaded the fleshy exterior and right qì is resisting the evil and pushing it out of the body.

Stiffness and pain of the head and nape 头项强痛 *tóu xiàng jiàng tòng*: The greater yáng channel stretches from head to foot, passing over the back of the body. When the greater yáng channel contracts an evil, it invades the fleshy exterior, and regardless of whether it is wind strike, in which the evil causes disharmony between defense and construction, or cold damage, in which the defense and construction become depressed and blocked, the greater yáng channel qì becomes congested and cannot move properly. When the movement of channel qì is impaired, the channel loses its suppleness which, in this case, gives rise to stiffness and pain of the head and nape.

Aversion to cold 恶寒 *wù hán*: The Chinese term 恶寒 *wù hán* is wider in meaning than the usual translation "chill." Unlike "chill," it is not limited to shivering, but includes sensitivity to cold. Hence we consistently render it as "aversion to cold." Aversion to cold is often specifically defined as a pronounced sensation of cold that is felt even in the absence of external wind or cold and is undiminished by adding extra clothing or bedclothes, and is often contrasted with **aversion to wind**, which denotes a feeling of cold experienced on exposure to wind or drafts. In practice, this is usually a distinction of degree. The pathomechanism producing aversion to cold is an inability of yáng qì to warm the body, either because it is blocked and depressed or vacuous. In both exterior repletion and exterior vacuity patterns, defensive yáng, that is, the warming function of defensive qì, is blocked and depressed by the exterior evil, while in exterior vacuity, defensive yáng may also be slightly vacuous. In interior patterns, the appearance of aversion to cold is usually attributable to yáng qì vacuity.

Heat effusion 发热 *fā rè*: The Chinese term 发热 *fā rè* is usually rendered as "fever." However, unlike "fever," it includes subjective sensations of heat as well as a palpable increase in body temperature. For this reason, we consistently render it literally as "heat effusion." Heat effusion is associated with many conditions and occurs both in externally contracted disease and miscellaneous disease (杂病 *zá bìng*, disease due to causes other than external evils). In externally contracted diseases of the three yáng channels, heat effusion is a manifestation of the struggle between right qì and evil qì; it does not necessarily indicate the presence of evil heat. In the exterior patterns of greater yáng disease, it occurs even in patterns caused by the contraction of cold, which constitute the majority of patterns discussed in this chapter. In exterior patterns, evil qì is in the exterior of the body, impairing the normal function of defense qì; hence heat effusion is accompanied by aversion to wind or cold. Heat effusion also occurs in yáng brightness and lesser yáng disease. Here, however, different pathomechanisms and locations of the struggle between right qì and evil qì are reflected in different accompanying signs. In yáng brightness disease, the disease evil transforms into heat and enters the interior, so heat effusion is accompanied by aversion to heat rather than aversion to cold. In lesser yáng disease, the struggle is taking place between the interior and exterior, so heat effusion alternates with aversion to cold. In diseases of the three yīn, right qì is not strong enough to counter evil qì; hence heat effusion is absent, and instead only aversion to cold is present.

Sweating/absence of sweating 汗出／汗不出 *hàn chū/hàn bù chū*: Depending on the relative strength of the evil and the patient's constitution, greater yáng disease takes one of two major forms: exterior vacuity wind strike and exterior repletion cold damage. These are primarily differentiated by the presence or absence of sweating. In exterior vacuity, the defense qì is vacuous, and is easily damaged when an external evil is contracted. When this happens, it fails to contain construction-yīn, which discharges outward in the form of sweat. This is known as "insecurity of the defensive exterior." Conversely, in exterior repletion, the interstices and fleshy exterior are secure. When an exterior evil is contracted, the defense qì struggles against evil qì, resulting in obstruction of the defense qì. The construction-yīn becomes stagnant and sweat cannot issue. In greater yáng disease that has persisted for a long time, an exterior depression pattern may arise.

1.2 TREATMENT

The two basic patterns of greater yáng exterior disease, wind strike and cold damage, are each treated with a basic formula. For wind strike exterior vacuity patterns, Cinnamon Twig Decoction (*guì zhī tāng*) is used to resolve the fleshy exterior and dispel wind, and harmonize construction and defense. Ephedra Decoction (*má huáng tāng*) is used in cold damage exterior repletion patterns to open the interstices and promote sweating, diffuse the lung, and calm panting. These two formulae are modified to treat variations on the basic patterns. In mild patterns of exterior depression, a combination of the two formulae above is used to promote mild sweating. If heat is depressed in the interior, these formulae are modified to include medicinals that clear interior heat.

The greater yáng disease patterns other than the two basic exterior patterns are transmuted patterns (变证 *biàn zhèng*). These are highly varied and are treated in very different ways.

If yīn humor have been damaged, the evil will generally shift to the lesser yáng or yáng brightness channel, or become a pattern of repletion heat. The main formulae used in these patterns include Gardenia and Fermented Soybean Decoction (*zhī zǐ chǐ tāng*), Ephedra, Apricot Kernel, Licorice, and Gypsum Decoction (*má huáng xìng rén gān cǎo shí gāo tāng*), White Tiger Decoction Plus Ginseng (*bái hǔ jiā rén shēn tāng*), Pueraria, Scutellaria, and Coptis Decoction (*gé gēn huáng qín huáng lián tāng*), Scutellaria Decoction (*huáng qín tāng*), and Scutellaria Decoction Plus Pinellia and Fresh Ginger (*huáng qín jiā bàn xià shēng jiāng tāng*).

If the yáng qì is damaged, the evil may shift to the yīn channels or become a pattern of vacuity cold. When this damage affects the heart yáng, formulae such as Cinnamon Twig and Licorice Decoction (*guì zhī gān cǎo tāng*), Cinnamon Twig Decoction Plus Extra Cinnamon (*guì zhī jiā guì tāng*), Cinnamon Twig Minus Peony Plus Dichroa Leaf, Dragon Bone, and Oyster Shell Counterflow-Stemming Decoction (*guì zhī qù sháo yào jiā shǔ qī mǔ lì lóng gǔ jiù nì tāng*) and Cinnamon Twig, Licorice, Dragon Bone, and Oyster Shell Decoction (*guì zhī gān cǎo lóng gǔ mǔ lì tāng*) are suggested.

When yáng vacuity and water qì appear simultaneously, one of the following formulae are suggested: Poria (Hoelen), Cinnamon Twig, Licorice, and Jujube Decoction (*fú líng guì zhī gān cǎo dà zǎo tāng*), Poria (Hoelen), Cinnamon Twig, Ovate Atractylodes, and Licorice Decoction (*fú líng guì zhī bái zhú gān cǎo tāng*), and Cinnamon Twig Decoction Minus Cinnamon Twig Plus Poria (Hoelen) and Ovate Atractylodes (*guì zhī qù guì jiā fú líng bái zhú tāng*).

For greater yáng disease that involves spleen vacuity, Magnolia Bark, Fresh Ginger, Pinellia, Licorice, and Ginseng Decoction (*hòu pò shēng jiāng bàn xià gān cǎo rén shēn tāng*), Minor Center-Fortifying Decoction (*xiǎo jiàn zhōng tāng*), and Cinnamon Twig and Ginseng Decoction (*guì zhī rén shēn tāng*) are suggested.

For greater yáng disease with kidney vacuity, Dried Ginger and Aconite Decoction (*gān jiāng fù zǐ tāng*), Poria (Hoelen) Counterflow Cold Decoction (*fú líng sì nì tāng*), and True Warrior Decoction (*zhēn wǔ tāng*) are suggested.

In greater yáng disease with yīn-yáng dual vacuity, one can use Licorice and Dried Ginger Decoction (*gān cǎo gān jiāng tāng*), Peony and Licorice Decoction (*sháo yào gān cǎo tāng*), Peony, Licorice, and Aconite Decoction (*sháo yào gān cǎo fù zǐ tāng*), and Honey-Fried Licorice Decoction (*zhì gān cǎo tāng*).

Water amassment, blood amassment, chest bind, and glomus patterns are complex and are treated with a range of formulas to wide to be summarized here.

1.3 SCHEMATIC OVERVIEW

Basic Greater Yáng Disease Patterns

- **Essential features**
  - Pulse that is floating, stiffness and pain of the head and nape, aversion to cold, and heat effusion
- **Pattern types**
  - Wind strike: Heat effusion, aversion to wind or cold, spontaneous sweating, and a pulse that is floating and moderate
  - Cold damage: Heat effusion, aversion to wind or cold, absence of sweating, and a pulse that is floating and tight
  - Warm disease: Heat effusion, thirst, and absence of aversion to cold
- **Treatment principles and primary formulae**
  - Wind strike: Harmonize construction and defense; resolve the exterior and dispel wind: Cinnamon Twig Decoction (*guì zhī tāng*)
  - Cold damage: Open the interstices and promote sweating; diffuse the lung and calm panting: Ephedra Decoction (*má huáng tāng*)
  - Warm disease: Resolve the exterior with coolness and acridity
- **Mild patterns of exterior depression**
  - A condition like malaria with red face and generalized itching: Cinnamon Twig and Ephedra Half-and-Half Decoction (*guì zhī má huáng gè bàn tāng*)
  - Heart vexation and thirst: Two Parts Cinnamon Twig and One Part Spleen-Effusing Decoction (*guì zhī èr yuè bì yī tāng*)

Identification and Treatment of Transmuted Patterns

- **Heat patterns**
  - Heat depressed in the chest and diaphragm with vexation heat in the chest and anguish
    * Basic pattern with inability to sleep: Gardenia and Fermented Soybean Decoction (*zhī zǐ chǐ tāng*)
    * With shortage of qì: Gardenia, Licorice, and Fermented Soybean Decoction (*zhī zǐ gān cǎo chǐ tāng*)
    * With retching and vomiting: Gardenia, Fresh Ginger, and Fermented Soybean Decoction (*zhī zǐ shēng jiāng chǐ tāng*)

  * With abdominal fullness: Gardenia and Magnolia Bark Decoction (*zhī zǐ hòu pò tāng*)
  * With decreased food intake, sloppy stool, abdominal fullness, and abdominal pain: Gardenia and Dried Ginger Decoction (*zhī zǐ gān jiāng tāng*)
- Other heat patterns
  * Evil heat congesting the lung and counterflow ascent of lung qì with sweating, panting, and heat effusion: Ephedra, Apricot Kernel, Licorice, and Gypsum Decoction (*má huáng xìng rén gān cǎo shí gāo tāng*)
  * Exterior disease failing to resolve and evil entering the yáng brightness with heat effusion, diarrhea, sweating, and panting: Pueraria, Scutellaria, and Coptis Decoction (*gé gēn huáng qín huáng lián tāng*)
  * Exuberant yáng brightness heat with damage to qì and yīn with great heat, great sweating, great vexation, and thirst, and a pulse that is large and surging: White Tiger Decoction Plus Ginseng (*bái hǔ jiā rén shēn tāng*)
  * Lesser yáng evil heat distressing yáng brightness with diarrhea, abdominal pain, and scorching heat in the anus: Scutellaria Decoction (*huáng qín tāng*)
  * Lesser yáng evil heat distressing yáng brightness with vomiting: Scutellaria Decoction Plus Pinellia and Fresh Ginger (*huáng qín jiā bàn xià shēng jiāng tāng*)

- **Vacuity cold patterns**
  - Heart yáng vacuity
    * Damage to heart yáng with palpitations and in serious cases deafness: Cinnamon Twig and Licorice Decoction (*guì zhī gān cǎo tāng*)
    * Disquieted heart spirit with vexation and agitation: Cinnamon Twig, Licorice, Dragon Bone, and Oyster Shell Decoction (*guì zhī gān cǎo lóng gǔ mǔ lì tāng*)
    * Straying of the heart spirit with fright mania, and fidgetiness whether lying or sitting: Cinnamon Twig Minus Peony Plus Dichroa Leaf, Dragon Bone, and Oyster Shell Counterflow-Stemming Decoction (*guì zhī qù sháo yào jiā shǔ qī mǔ lì lóng gǔ jiù nì tāng*)
    * Counterflow ascent of water and cold evil with running piglet (qì from the lesser abdomen surging upward to the heart): Cinnamon Twig Decoction Plus Extra Cinnamon (*guì zhī jiā guì tāng*)
  - Yáng vacuity with water qì
    * Insufficiency of heart yáng with water collecting in the lower burner with palpitations below the umbilicus and running piglet about to occur: Poria (Hoelen), Cinnamon Twig, Licorice, and Jujube Decoction (*fú líng guì zhī gān cǎo dà zǎo tāng*)

  * Spleen failing to move and transform with water qì collecting internally with counterflow fullness below the heart, qì surging up into the chest, dizzy head upon standing, and a pulse that is sunken and tight: Poria (Hoelen), Cinnamon Twig, Ovate Atractylodes, and Licorice Decoction (*fú líng guì zhī bái zhú gān cǎo tāng*)
  * Spleen vacuity with collected water and an unresolved exterior pattern with fullness and slight pain below the heart, and inhibited urination: Cinnamon Twig Decoction Minus Cinnamon Twig Plus Poria (Hoelen) and Ovate Atractylodes (*guì zhī qù guì jiā fú líng bái zhú tāng*)
- Spleen vacuity
  * Spleen vacuity with turbid qì stagnation with abdominal distention and fullness: Magnolia Bark, Fresh Ginger, Pinellia, Licorice, and Ginseng Decoction (*hòu pò shēng jiāng bàn xià gān cǎo rén shēn tāng*)
  * Center burner vacuity cold with qì and blood vacuity with palpitations in the heart, vexation, and pain in the abdomen: Minor Center-Fortifying Decoction (*xiǎo jiàn zhōng tāng*)
  * An unresolved exterior evil and spleen stomach vacuity cold with aversion to cold, heat effusion, diarrhea, and hard glomus below the heart: Cinnamon Twig and Ginseng Decoction (*guì zhī rén shēn tāng*)
- Kidney yáng vacuity
  * Exuberant internal yīn cold and yáng qì floating astray with vexation in the daytime and peacefulness at night, a pulse that is sunken and faint, and absence of great heat: Dried Ginger and Aconite Decoction (*gān jiāng fù zǐ tāng*)
  * Extreme vacuity of yīn and yáng with true yīn about to desert, vexation and agitation, aversion to cold, counterflow cold of the limbs, diarrhea, and a pulse that is faint and fine: Poria (Hoelen) Counterflow Cold Decoction (*fú líng sì nì tāng*)
  * Debilitation of heart and kidney yáng with palpitations, dizzy head, generalized twitching, quivering, and the person about to fall: True Warrior Decoction (*zhēn wǔ tāng*)

• **Dual vacuity of yīn and yáng**
- Yáng qì vacuity and stomach qì disharmony with retching counterflow and reverse flow in the limbs: Licorice and Dried Ginger Decoction (*gān cǎo gān jiāng tāng*)
- Insufficiency of yīn-blood with hypertonicity of the legs and dryness in the throat: Peony and Licorice Decoction (*sháo yào gān cǎo tāng*)
- Vacuity of the exterior and interior, and of yīn and yáng with aversion to cold, sweating, hypertonicity of the legs, and a pulse that is faint and fine: Peony, Licorice, and Aconite Decoction (*sháo yào gān cǎo fù zǐ tāng*)

- Insufficiency of heart yīn and devitalized heart yáng with a pulse that is bound and intermittent, and stirring heart palpitations: Honey-Fried Licorice Decoction (*zhì gān cǎo tāng*)

- **Water amassment and blood amassment patterns**
  - Water amassment
    * Inhibited urination with lesser abdominal fullness, a pulse that is floating and rapid, and in severe cases immediate vomiting of ingested fluids: Poria (Hoelen) Five Powder (*wǔ líng sǎn*)
  - Blood amassment
    * Mild pattern of blood heat bound in the lower burner with uninhibited urination, mania, and tense, bound lesser abdomen: Peach Kernel Qì-Coordinating Decoction (*táo hé chéng qì tāng*)
    * Severe pattern of blood heat bound in the lower burner with uninhibited urination, mania, hardness and fullness of the lesser abdomen, and generalized yellowing: Dead-On Decoction (*dǐ dàng tāng*)

- **Chest bind patterns**
  - Major chest bind with pain below the heart that is as hard as stone when pressed, and sweating only from the head: Major Chest Bind Decoction (*dà xiàn xiōng tāng*)
  - Minor chest bind with fullness and oppresion below the heart that is painful when pressed: Minor Chest Bind Decoction (*xiǎo xiàn xiōng tāng*)
  - Cold repletion chest bind with hardness, fullness, and pain below the heart, inability to defecate, and absence of heat signs: Three Agents White Powder (*sān wù bái sǎn*)

- **Glomus patterns**
  - Heat glomus
    * Evil heat congested in the stomach duct with glomus below the heart that is soft when pressed and a pulse that is floating above the bar: Rhubarb and Coptis Heart-Draining Decoction (*dà huáng huáng lián xiè xīn tāng*)
    * Evil heat congested in the stomach duct and yáng vacuity with glomus below the heart, aversion to cold, and sweating: Aconite Heart-Draining Decoction (*fù zǐ xiè xīn tāng*)
  - Heat and cold complex glomus (Disharmony of the spleen and stomach)
    * Counterflow ascent of stomach qì with glomus and fullness below the heart, retching, and rumbling intestines: Pinellia Heart-Draining Decoction (*bàn xià xiè xīn tāng*)

    * Stomach vacuity with hard glomus below the heart, dry belching and food malodor, rumbling intestines, and diarrhea: Fresh Ginger Heart-Draining Decoction (*shēng jiāng xiè xīn tāng*)

    * Spleen vacuity with glomus, hardness and fullness below the heart, diarrhea, dry retching, and heart vexation: Licorice Heart-Draining Decoction (*gān cǎo xiè xīn tāng*)

  - Water glomus with glomus below the heart, inhibited urination, dry mouth and thirst, and heart vexation: Poria (Hoelen) Five Powder (*wǔ líng sǎn*)

  - Phlegm glomus with hard glomus below the heart, and incessant belching: Inula and Hematite Decoction (*xuán fù dài zhě tāng*)

- **Upper body heat and lower body cold**

  - Desire to vomit and pain in the abdomen: Coptis Decoction (*huáng lián tāng*)

- **Patterns similar to greater yáng disease**

  - Water-rheum collected and bound in the chest and rib-side with glomus, hardness and fullness below the heart, and dry retching: Ten Jujubes Decoction (*shí zǎo tāng*)

  - Phlegm-drool obstructing the chest and diaphragm with hard glomus in the chest, and qì surging up into the throat and inability to breath: Melon Stalk Powder (*guā dì sǎn*)

2 ESSENTIAL FEATURES OF GREATER YÁNG DISEASE

The essential features of greater yáng disease are presented in line 1. The greater yáng governs the fleshy exterior. When an exterior evil invades, it generally affects the exterior first. Right qì rises up against the evil and generally the first signs are of greater yáng disease, also referred to as an exterior pattern. Signs of greater yáng disease include stiffness and pain of the head and nape, aversion to cold, possibly heat effusion, possibly sweating, and a pulse that is commonly floating and that may also be tight or moderate. These signs represent those commonly seen in greater yáng disease, but should not be seen as absolute indicators of any one pattern because specific presentations vary widely. Greater yáng disease represents the early stages of an externally contracted disease, although this period cannot be strictly defined.

Line 1

太阳之为病，脉浮，头项强痛而恶寒。

Tài yáng zhī wéi bìng, mài fú, tóu xiàng jiàng tòng ér wù hán.

In disease of the greater yáng, the pulse is floating, the head and nape are stiff and painful,[1] and [there is] aversion to cold.[2]

Text Notes

1. Head and nape are stiff and painful, 头项强痛 *tóu xiàng jiàng tòng*: Headache, and pain and stiffness in the back of the neck.
2. Aversion to cold, 恶寒 *wù hán*: Sensitivity to cold or a subjective sensation of cold. Aversion to cold is now often specifically defined as a pronounced sensation of cold that is felt even in the absence of external wind or cold and is undiminished by adding extra clothing or bedclothes, and is often contrasted with aversion to wind, which denotes a feeling of cold experienced on exposure to wind or drafts (see line 2, p. 43). However, this distinction is not always clearly made in *Shāng Hán Lùn* and other literature.

   In the *Shāng Hán Lùn*, "aversion to cold" often occurs with heat effusion (see note accompanying line 2, p. 43), as a sign of wind-cold. In the absence of heat effusion or other exterior signs, it is a sign of cold arising from within due to yáng qì vacuity.

   The Chinese term 恶寒 *wù hán* is often translated as "chill." Strictly speaking, however, it is wider in meaning, including not only an acute feeling of cold with shivering, but general sensitivity to the cold. For this reason we consistently render it as "aversion to cold." Aversion to cold is often specifically defined as a pronounced sensation of cold that is felt even in the absence of external wind or cold and is undiminished by adding extra clothing or bedclothes, and is often contrasted with aversion to wind (恶寒 *wù hán*), which denotes a feeling of cold experienced on exposure to wind or drafts.

   The term 恶寒 *wù hán*, aversion to cold, would appear to be a misnomer, if we accept the definition conventionally given in Chinese medical literature as a "sensation of cold that is felt even in the absence of wind and cold and that is undiminished by adding extra clothing or bedclothes" since 恶 *wù*, aversion, implies a response to the external stimulus 寒 *hán*, cold, which the traditional definition specifically states to be irrelevant.

Synopsis

A general outline of the pulse and signs of greater yáng disease.

Commentary

The basic pattern associated with greater yáng disease includes a pulse that is floating, headache, pain and stiffness in the back of the neck, and aversion to cold. The greater yáng governs the exterior and rules the construction and defense, providing protection for the body. When an exterior evil attacks the body, right qì is excited and rises up to contend with the evil. The signs of exterior disease are evidence of the contention between right qì and evil qì. When right qì contends with evil qì, the qì and blood quickly gather in the exterior of the body. The vessels become full and the qì of the pulse is stirred. Thus the pulse is felt easily with light pressure and is described as "floating." The greater yáng channel passes through the head and neck. Wind-cold attacks and fetters the exterior, the channel receives the evil, and the movement of qì and blood is blocked. This manifests as headache and pain and stiffness in the back of the neck. The defense qì is damaged by the evil and unable to warm the fleshy exterior and interstices normally; consequently, aversion to cold arises.

This line presents the basic features of greater yáng disease. In clinical practice, however, variations are often observed, as we shall see in the lines ahead. Moreover, the same signs may occur in other patterns. While a pulse that is floating and aversion to cold occurring together indicate an exterior disease, either of the two can, in the presence of other signs, also indicate other patterns. For example, a pulse that is floating and moderate, and accompanied by warm extremities (line 278, p. 461), occurs in greater yīn disease. Aversion to cold occurs with a pulse that is faint (line 385, p. 585) in a pattern of severe yáng vacuity in sudden turmoil disease.

The basic pulse and signs given in this line apply to all greater yáng disease, even when they are not specifically stated. The *Shāng Hán Lùn* is terse in its expression. Basic pulses and signs are often not repeated in pattern descriptions.

LINE 2

太阳病，发热汗出，恶风，脉缓者， 名为中风。

Tài yáng bìng, fā rè hàn chū, wù fēng, mài huǎn zhě, míng wéi zhòng fēng.

When in greater yáng disease [there is] heat effusion,[1] sweating,[2] aversion to wind,[3] and a pulse that is moderate,[4] it is called wind strike.[5]

TEXT NOTES

1. Heat effusion, 发热 *fà rè*: Abnormal heat in the body that can be detected by palpation or that is experienced subjectively. The English term "fever," which is often used to render this term, implies an objective elevation of body temperature only. To cover the broader meaning of 发热 *fā rè*, we consistently translate the term literally as "heat effusion," even though in the context of the present line, fever detectable by palpation is intended.

   The Chinese 热 *rè*, heat, is used in the sense of 发热 *fā rè*, heat effusion, that is the manifestation of illness, in a number of terms including 烦热 *fán rè*, "heat vexation" (line 77, p. 148) and 潮热 *cháo rè*, "tidal heat effusion" (line 104, p. 434). In other contexts, it denotes a cause of illness, e.g., heat entering the blood chamber, 热入血室 *rè rù xuè shì* (line 216, p. 378) and heat binding the bladder, 热结膀胱 *rè jié páng guāng* (line 106, p. 202).

2. Sweating, 汗出 *hàn chū*: The expulsion of sweat from the skin. Literally "sweat issuing," this is a sign that should be differentiated from "promotion of sweating" (发汗 *fā hàn*) as a method of treatment.

3. Aversion to wind, 恶风 *wù fēng*: A sensation of cold experienced upon exposure to wind or drafts that abates when the patient is no longer exposed. Compare "aversion to cold" (line 1, p. 41).

4. A pulse that is moderate, 脉缓 *mài huǎn*: A pulse that is loose, soft, and harmonious; hence opposite to a pulse that is tight. "Moderate" does not refer to the speed of the pulse, as it usually does in modern usage.

It is important to note that in greater yáng disease patterns, a pulse that is floating is usually assumed present, even if it is not explicitly stated.

5. Wind strike, 中风 *zhòng fēng*: An exterior pattern caused by externally contracted wind-cold. Note that in other literature, the same term is used denote stroke (apoplexy).

SYNOPSIS

An outline of the pulse and signs of greater yáng wind strike pattern.

COMMENTARY

Greater yáng disease takes different forms. Heat effusion, sweating, aversion to wind, and a pulse that is floating and moderate is known as greater yáng wind strike and also referred to as a greater yáng exterior vacuity pattern. Exterior vacuity refers to the constitution of the patient and means a slack quality in the fleshy exterior and interstices. When a patient with this type of constitution contracts an exterior evil, the exterior of the body easily becomes insecure. Heat effusion is an indication that the defensive yáng rises to the exterior of the body to contend with the evil and it is in this struggle that the defensive yáng is damaged. The defensive yáng, already weak in this type of patient, is further weakened by this struggle. Construction fails to be contained in the interior and construction-yīn discharges outward, giving rise to sweating. The exterior is insecure and cannot overcome wind; consequently, aversion to wind arises.

Spontaneous sweating is a key diagnostic feature of greater yáng wind strike. This kind of sweating is a pathological reaction, and not the same as that resulting from the promotion of sweating using medicinals. It cannot reduce the body temperature, and cannot expel the exterior evil. A pulse that is floating indicates evil in the exterior, and a pulse that is moderate means that construction-yīn is weak. Hence the pathomechanism of the pulse is directly related to that of spontaneous sweating.

LINE 3

太阳病，或已发热，或未发热，必恶寒，体痛，呕逆，脉阴阳俱紧者，名为伤寒。

Tài yáng bìng, huò yǐ fā rè, huò wèi fā rè, bì wù hán, tǐ tòng, ǒu nì, mài yīn yáng jù jǐn zhě, míng wéi shāng hán.

Greater yáng disease, whether heat has effused or not, as long as there is aversion to cold,[1] with generalized pain,[2] retching counterflow,[3] and yīn and yáng [pulses] both tight,[4] is called cold damage.[5]

TEXT NOTES

1. As long as [there is] aversion to cold, 必恶寒 *bì wù hán*: Aversion to cold is a primary sign when identifying cold damage patterns. This phrase literally means "there must be aversion to cold," but here is interpreted as introducing a condition for qualification of cold damage, irrespective of whether heat effusion has developed or not. Aversion to cold is generally taken to be the only

essential condition, but it is not clear from the text, when taken literally, whether the signs subsequently enumerated are also necessary.

2. Generalized pain, 体痛 *tǐ tòng*: Pain that is felt throughout the body, not in any specific place. This term is synonymous with 身痛 *shēn tòng*.
3. Retching counterflow, 呕逆 *ǒu nì*: The act of vomiting, 呕 *ǒu*, without necessarily producing any vomitus, and attributed to counterflow ascent of qì (气逆 *qì nì*).
4. The yīn and yáng pulses, 脉阴阳 *mài yīn yáng*: Either: a) the cubit (尺 *chǐ*) and inch (寸 *cùn*) positions or b) the deep-level and superficial-level pulses. Because the basic pulse associated with greater yáng disease is floating, any change in the form of the pulse is indistinct at the deep level, so that the first of the two possible interpretations is more reasonable. This interpretation holds that "yīn and yáng," though literally referring to the inch and cubit positions, means the inch-cubit axis as a whole and, consequently, that the pulse at the bar as well as the inch and cubit is tight. Compare line 283, p. 473, for another occurrence of this pulse description.
5. Cold damage, 伤寒 *shāng hán*: In the broad sense, all externally contracted diseases, and in the narrow sense, the group of signs resulting from externally contracted wind-cold and treated with Ephedra Decoction (*má huáng tāng*). Within the *Shāng Hán Lùn*, externally contracted wind-cold disease is frequently discussed, but many patterns also involve other types of externally contracted disease, as well as miscellaneous internal diseases. It should be noted that the Chinese term 伤寒 *shāng hán*, has been adopted in modern medicine as the equivalent of the English "typhoid" (an acute infectious disease caused by the bacillus *Salmonella typhi* and acquired by ingesting food or water contaminated by excreta). It is is sometimes erroneously translated as "typhoid" in the Chinese medical literature. See the introduction for further discussion of the issues surrounding the definition of this term.

SYNOPSIS

An outline of the pulse and signs of greater yáng cold damage pattern.

COMMENTARY

As line 1, page 41, states, aversion to cold is a major distinguishing characteristic of greater yáng disease. The evil invades the exterior, depressing and fettering the defense qì. The defense qì is unable to warm the fleshy exterior and this causes aversion to cold. When aversion to cold, generalized pain, retching counterflow, and a pulse that is tight are present, it is not necessary to observe heat effusion to diagnose a cold damage pattern. Furthermore, at the beginning of a cold damage pattern, heat effusion may be absent if the evil has severely blocked the exterior. A short period of time may pass after contraction of the evil before heat effusion develops. Typically, in patients whose constitutions tend toward yáng exuberance, heat effusion develops earlier. Whether or not heat effusion has developed, there must nevertheless be aversion to cold if cold damage is to be diagnosed.

When the exterior is blocked by an evil and the defense qì is fettered, generalized pain often occurs, as a result of blockage of the normal movement of qì in the channels. When the movement of qì is blocked, the pulse may become tight at the inch, bar, and cubit. Abnormal qì movement often results in qì counterflow and retching, in addition to the other signs.

In this line, the defense qì is blocked and the construction-yīn is depressed and stagnant. This pattern is different from wind strike, in which the defensive exterior is insecure and the construction-yīn discharges to the exterior. An important concept, first introduced in the *Nèi Jīng* and elucidated further in *Shāng Hán Lùn*, is that both the patient's constitution and the strength of the evil influence the course of a disease. From clinical experience, one of the characteristics distinguishing wind strike from cold damage is the constitution of the patient. Wind strike is more commonly seen in patients with weak constitutions, whereas cold damage is more common in patients with strong constitutions. A patient with a weak constitution becomes sick more easily and the pulse is moderate because the yáng qì is not sufficient to counter evil qì strongly. A patient with a strong constitution will have a tight pulse because the yáng qì offers strong resistance to the evil. Although this line contains no mention of sweating, the formula prescribed, Ephedra Decoction (*má huáng tāng*), is specifically noted to be for patients in whom sweating is absent (see line 35, p. 91). Thus, the key criterion for distinguishing between wind strike and cold damage is that the former is associated with spontaneous sweating and the latter is associated with the absence of sweating.

So far, we have explained the difference between wind strike and cold damage in terms of constitutional differences. However, the naming of the two patterns suggests that the author considered them to have different causes (wind or cold). However, since wind and cold as evils in the body cannot be detected directly, the cause is a matter of speculation. Modern writers tend to attribute both patterns to "wind-cold" and explain the difference between the two patterns in terms of both constitutional differences and the strength of the wind-cold evil, attributing cold damage to a stronger constitution and a stronger evil.

The difference between wind strike and cold damage is also to some extent mirrored in the difference between "aversion to wind" and "aversion to cold." Wind strike and cold damage are both greater yáng patterns. According to line 2, aversion to wind is associated with wind strike, and according to line 3, aversion to cold is associated with cold damage. However, in the basic outline given in line 1, greater yáng disease is said to be characterized by "aversion to cold" rather than "aversion to wind or to cold." The distinction between aversion to wind and aversion to cold seems to be based as much on the supposed cause of illness, wind or cold, as it is on any subjective difference between these two signs.

LINE 6

(一) 太阳病，发热而渴，不恶寒者，为温病。 (二) 若发汗已，身灼热者，名风温。 (三) 风温为病，脉阴阳俱浮，自汗出，身重，多眠睡，鼻息必鼾，语言难出。 (四) 若被下者，小便不利，直视失溲；若被火者，微发黄色，剧则如惊痫，时瘛疭， 若火熏之；一逆尚引日，再逆促命期。

(1) *Tài yáng bìng, fā rè ér kě, bù wù hán zhě, wéi wēn bìng.* (2) *Ruò fā hàn yǐ, shēn zhuó rè zhě, míng fēng wēn.* (3) *Fēng wēn wéi bìng, mài yīn yáng jù fú, zì hàn chū, shēn zhòng, duō mián shuì, bí xī bì hān, yǔ yán nán chū.* (4) *Ruò bèi xià zhě, xiǎo biàn bù lì, zhí shì shī sōu, ruò bèi huǒ zhě, wēi fā huáng sè, jù zé rú jīng xián, shí jì zòng, ruò huǒ xūn zhī; yí nì shàng yǐn rì, zài nì cù mìng qī.*

(1) When in greater yáng disease [there is] heat effusion and thirst, without aversion to cold, [this] is warm disease.[1] (2) If, after sweating has been promoted,[2] there is generalized scorching heat,[3] this is called wind-warmth.[4] (3) [When] wind-warmth causes disease, the yīn and yáng pulses are both floating,[5] [there is] spontaneous sweating,[6] generalized heaviness,[7] a tendency to sleep,[8] the breath [from the] nose will [make a] snoring [sound],[9] and speech is difficult.[10] (4) If precipitation has been used,[11] [there is] inhibited urination,[12] forward staring eyes, and fecal incontinence;[13]if fire has been used,[14] [there is] slight yellowing, and in acute cases [there is] fright epilepsy,[15] periodic tugging and slackening,[16] and [the skin] appears as if fumed by fire;[17]one [instance of] of adverse [treatment][18] will lengthen the time [of disease], and further adverse [treatment] will lead to the term of life.[19]

TEXT NOTES

1. Warm disease, 温病 *wēn bìng*: An externally contracted disease characterized at onset by heat effusion, thirst, and absence of aversion to cold.
2. Promote sweating, 发汗 *fā hàn*: In the *Shāng Hán Lùn*, 发汗 *fā hàn* means the therapeutic action of promoting sweating. Sweating as a manifestation of disease is usually referred to has 汗出 *hàn chū*. In modern Chinese medical texts, 发汗 *fā hàn* can also denote this sign.
3. Generalized scorching heat, 身灼热 *shēn zhuó rè*: The body feels hot to the touch.
4. Wind warmth, 风温 *fēng wēn*: A transmuted pattern caused by the inappropriate use of warm, acrid medicinals to promote sweating in warm disease. It is not the concept of wind warmth developed later in the warm disease school.

5. Yīn and yáng [pulses] both floating, 阴阳俱浮 *yīn yáng jù fú*: The cubit and inch pulses are both floating. The floating pulse here does not reflect an exterior pattern; it is attributed to a heat evil in the interior, with heat being expressed in the exterior of the body.
6. Spontaneous sweating, 自汗出 *zì hàn chū*: Sweating that occurs in the absence of any treatment.
7. Generalized heaviness, 身重 *shēn zhòng*: A subjective feeling of increased weight and loss of agility. This sign occurs in three conditions:
   a) Following the use of precipitation, debilitation of interior qì may result in generalized heaviness, which is often accompanied by palpitations and a pulse that is faint.
   b) Heat congestion and qì stagnation may result in obstruction of the qì and blood and inhibition of the channels, which causes generalized heaviness. This pattern is frequently seen with tidal fever, abdominal fullness, and panting.
   c) In warm disease, as defined above, the inappropriate promotion of sweating can cause fluid damage and exacerbate the heat. The qì is damaged by the heat, resulting in generalized heaviness.
8. Tendency to sleep, 多眠睡 *duō mián shuì*: A desire to sleep and tendency to sleep for long periods of time. This term means the presence of heat evil congested in the interior, harassing the heart spirit.
9. The breath from the nose will [sound of] snoring, 鼻息必鼾 *bí xí bì hān*: Inhibited breathing with an audible sound accompanying the breath. Although not necessarily occurring during sleep, inhibited breathing is related to tendency to sleep, because when an interior heat evil, which can cause an increased tendency to sleep, becomes congested in the lungs, it can cause an inhibition of the lung qì, resulting in congestion of heat and phlegm, and snoring.
10. Speech is difficult, 语言难出 *yǔ yán nán chū*: Inability to speak with normal ease and fluency. Here, it is associated with lack of mental clarity, due to severe heat harassing the heart.
11. Precipitation, 下 *xià*: To cause expulsion of stool; to eliminate evil through the bowels.
12. Inhibited urination, 小便不利 *xiǎo biàn bù lì*: Difficult voiding of scant urine.
13. Fecal incontinence, 失溲 *shī sōu*: According to *Rì Běn Yī Jiā Shāng Hán Lùn Zhù Jiě Jì Yào* (日本医家伤寒论注解辑要 "Collected Commentaries of Japanese Medical Scholars on the *Shāng Hán Lùn*") this term may mean either fecal or urinary incontinence. In the explanation of this line, the authors of *Gāo Děng Zhōng Yī Yán Jiū Cān Kǎo Cóng Shū* (高等中医研究参考丛书 "Advanced-Level Chinese Medical Reference Series") concur with this opinion. Nonetheless, because inhibited urination is mentioned previously, the authors of *Shāng Hán Lùn Jiǎng Yì* (伤寒论讲义 "*Shāng Hán Lùn* Lectures") suggest that here it only refers to fecal incontinence.
14. Fire, 火 *huǒ*: Any method of treatment involving the application of heat, i.e., warm needling, moxibustion, fuming, hotpack, etc.

15. Fright epilepsy, 惊痫 *jīng xián*: A disease pattern characterized by clouding and loss of consciousness, convulsions, and forward-staring eyes.
16. Tugging and slackening, 时瘈疭 *shí jì zòng*: Convulsive spasm characterized by alternating tensing and relaxing of the muscles; clonic spasm. The character 瘈 *jì* is now usually written as 瘛 *jì*.
17. [The skin] appears as if fumed by fire, 若火熏之 *ruò huǒ xūn zhī*: The skin appears darkened as though fumed by fire. According to another interpretation, 若 is taken to mean not "appears as if" but simply "if," introducing a condition for the final part of the line: "If [the patient has been] fumed by fire, one [instance] of adverse [treatment] will...." Fuming is a method of treatment that uses the smoke generated by burning medicinal ingredients or steam to force sweating (generally considered by Zhāng Jī to be a mistreatment). In this latter interpretation, fuming by fire appears as another mistreatment in addition to the others previously described (precipitation and fire treatment). This interpretation is considered less likely since a) fuming is in itself one form of fire treatment, b) no signs are given as for the other two mistreatments, and c) the grammatical construction is not parallel with the previous two descriptions of mistreatment (the phrase reads 火熏之 *huǒ xūn zhī*, not 被火熏 *bèi huǒ xūn*).
18. Adverse [treatment], 逆 *nì*: A treatment that is contrary to proper treatment strategy. The character 逆 *nì* means to oppose, contrary to, go against, to rebel. It is most commonly used in medicine to describe movement in the wrong direction (counterflow). In the *Shāng Hán Lùn*, it is also used to mean going against normal therapeutic procedures.
19. Term of life, 命期 *mìng qí*: The termination of life; death.

SYNOPSIS

The primary distinguishing features of warm disease and transmuted patterns occurring after mistreatment.

COMMENTARY

Warm disease is characterized by heat effusion and thirst, without aversion to cold, whereas in greater yáng disease, aversion to wind or cold is present but thirst is generally absent. Wind-warmth evil, the cause of warm disease, easily damages the fluids; consequently, early in these patterns, at the same time as heat effusion occurs, thirst is also observed. Because warm evil tends to damage not yáng qì but yīn humor, aversion to cold is generally absent in these patterns. If, in the course of greater yáng or cold damage disease, one sees heat effusion, thirst, and no aversion to cold, these signs may signify a transmuted pattern. These transmuted patterns, although similar in appearance to the group of diseases known as warm disease, have a completely different pathomechanism, treatment method, and disease course.

Warm disease should be treated through cool acrid exterior-resolution. Because the warm-heat evil invades the lung, it may cause the loss of normal defensive qì function and the temporary appearance of slight aversion to wind-cold. If this aversion is mistaken for an indication of wind-cold fettering the exterior and sweating is promoted, it will result in more severe damage to the fluids because the warmth of the formula will assist the interior heat and the body will become scorching hot.

Exuberant internal heat damages the fluids and causes palpable heat in wind-warmth disease. In this disease, the pulse is floating and forceful, since the heat effuses towards the exterior. The exuberant heat forces the construction-yīn to be discharged outward, resulting in the spontaneous issuing of sweat. The heat damages both the qì and the fluids and this damage results in a feeling of generalized heaviness. Heat has a tendency to rise and become congested in the upper burner, where it can harass the heart and the lung. This harassment results in a tendency to sleep, and inhibited breathing and snoring. This type of sleeping is stuporous and not restful. Because the heart governs speech and the tongue is the sprout of the heart, harassment of the heart spirit also results in difficulty speaking.

Wind warmth disease is characterized by exuberant heat and fluid damage. It should be treated by clearing heat and nourishing yīn. If precipitation is used, the fluids will become desiccated and the urination will be inhibited. Fluid depletion in the lower burner results in insufficient yīn essence to nourish the eyes. There is also exuberant heat harassing the spirit. The combination of these two factors results in forward-staring eyes and an inability to move the eyes with normal ease.

If wind warmth is treated with fire, the result will be yellowing, fright tetany, and tugging and slackening. Yellowing is a result of exuberant heat scorching the blood. The construction aspect of the blood is forced out to the exterior and the skin yellows. If the condition is severe, the heat may stir liver wind and cause an epileptic-like state and spasmodic movement of the limbs. In addition, the skin is darkened as if it had been fumed by fire.

Zhāng Jī records the results of mistreatment. He cautions that one mistreatment may lengthen the course of the disease and further mistreatment may be fatal.

(This line is line 6, and in this version it follows line 3. Note that the line numbers given are those of their appearance in the Sòng text, not of their appearance in this text.)

LINE 7

(一) 病有发热恶寒者，发于阳也；无热恶寒者，发于阴也。(二) 发于阳，七日愈。(三) 发于阴，六日愈。(四) 以阳数七、阴数六故也。

(1) *Bìng yǒu fā rè wù hán zhě, fā yú yáng yě; Wú rè wù hán zhě, fā yú yīn yě.* (2) *Fā yú yáng, qī rì yù.* (3) *Fā yú yīn, liù rì yù.* (4) *Yǐ yáng shù qī、 yīn shù liù gù yě.*

(1) When an illness [is characterized by] heat effusion and aversion to cold, it is springing from yáng; when [an illness is characterized by] the absence of heat effusion and [the presence of] aversion to cold, it is springing from yīn. (2) [In illness] springing from yáng, [the patient] recovers in seven days. (3) [In illness] springing from yīn, [the patient]

recovers in six days. (4) This is because yáng numbers seven and yīn numbers six.*

TEXT NOTE

* Yáng numbers seven and yīn numbers six: 以阳数七，阴数六故也 *yáng shù qī, yīn shù liù gù yě*: Seven, as all odd numbers, is yáng, and six, as all even numbers, is yīn.

SYNOPSIS

A differentiation of the two main types of externally contracted disease (yīn and yáng), and determination of the recovery period.

COMMENTARY

In externally contracted heat disease, heat effusion with aversion to cold constitutes a yáng sign; absence of heat effusion with aversion to cold is a yīn sign. Right qì, when it is exuberant, contends with the evil, giving rise to a yáng pattern with heat effusion. When right qì is vacuous, it is incapable of struggling against the evil; hence we observe a yīn pattern of aversion to cold and absence of heat effusion.

The terms "yīn" and "yáng" in this line have been interpreted in different ways:

1. Yóu Yí (尤怡, style 在泾 Zài-Jīng) and Zhāng Lù (张璐, style 路玉 Lù-Yù) write that the terms "yīn" (阴 *yīn*) and "yáng" (阳 *yáng*) represent the three yīn channels and the three yáng channels. Thus, "springing from yīn" or "springing from yáng" refers to disease which starts in either a yīn or a yáng channel, respectively. In the *Shāng Hán Lùn*, pattern identification is based on the six channels: greater yáng (太阳 *tài yáng*), yáng brightness (阳明 *yáng míng*), lesser yáng (少阳 *shào yáng*), greater yīn (太阴 *tài yīn*), lesser yīn (少阴 *shào yīn*), and reverting yīn (厥阴 *jué yīn*). Heat effusion is associated with diseases of all three yáng channels, signifying that right qì is still effulgent and able to oppose the evil strongly. In these basic patterns, right qì is exuberant and the evil is replete. Absence of heat effusion and presence of aversion to cold is associated with disease of all three yīn channels. It signifies yáng vacuity, yīn exuberance, and debilitation of right qì.
2. In the *Yī Zōng Jīn Jiàn* (医宗金鉴 "The Golden Mirror of Medicine") these terms are interpreted more specifically, so that "yīn" represents construction-yīn, and "yáng" represents defensive yáng. Greater yáng wind strike with wind evil damaging the defensive yáng is "springing from yáng" and greater yáng cold damage with cold evil damaging the construction-yīn is "springing from yīn."
3. Kē Qín (柯琴, style 韵伯 Yùn-Bó) comments that yīn and yáng refer not to construction and defense or the different channels, but simply to cold and heat seen in externally contracted disease patterns.

Yīn and yáng are relative concepts which may be applied in many different ways from various perspectives. The three interpretations presented differ one from the other, but they are not mutually conflicting or irreconcilable.

2.1 Identification of Disease Passage and Periods of Resolution

This section presents information that can be used to determine if an evil has passed from the greater yáng channel into another channel. The final group of lines discuss the period of the day when a certain pattern should resolve. This final group takes as its foundation the relationship between the channels and the earthly branches, such that by knowing in which of the channels an evil is located, one can predict the hour of the day during which it will resolve.

Line 4

伤寒一日，太阳受之，脉若静者，为不传；颇欲吐，若躁烦，脉数急者，为传也。

Shāng hán yí rì, tài yáng shòu zhī, mài ruò jìng zhě, wéi bù chuán; pǒ yù tù, ruò zào fán, mài shuò jí zhě, wéi chuán yě.

On the first day[1] of cold damage, greater yáng contracts [the disease]. If the pulse is tranquil,[2] this means no passage;[3] a strong desire to vomit, if [there is] agitation and vexation,[4] and the pulse is rapid and urgent, means passage.

Text Notes

1. On the first day, 一日 *yí rì*: At the onset.
2. The pulse is tranquil, 脉若静 *mài ruò jìng*: "Tranquil" is the opposite of "stirred" and means that the pulse has not undergone any changes and is congruent with the current signs.
3. No passage, 不传 *bù chuán*: The disease does not pass to another channel. Implicit in this is that the disease does not enter the interior.
4. Agitation and vexation, 燥烦 *zào fán*: The terms "vexation," "agitation," and their combinations "agitation and vexation" and "vexation and agitation," all of which appear in the *Shāng Hán Lùn*, have distinct meanings. "Agitation" means a subjective feeling of restlessness outwardly expressed by pronounced abnormal movement. "Vexation" means a feeling of restlessness in the area of the heart. When these two terms are combined, as in "vexation and agitation," it refers to a subjective feeling of heat and disquietude in the chest (vexation) and objective fidgetiness of the limbs (agitation). There is not complete agreement on whether or not "agitation and vexation" is different from "vexation and agitation," although some commentators suggest that the first term in the pair is the more predominant sign of the two.

Synopsis

How to determine, on the basis of the pulse and signs, whether a greater yáng disease will pass [to another channel].

Commentary

When wind-cold first attacks the body, the greater yáng contracts the evil.

Differences not only in the strength or weakness of the evil, but also in the patient's constitution will determine the progression of the disease. When determining whether or not passage has taken place, the pulse and signs are the main criteria. In cold damage, the pulse is floating and tight. If it does not change, it is described as being "tranquil" and one knows that passage has not occurred. The presence of this pulse suggests that right qì is prevailing, evil qì is retreating, and no treatment is necessary to resolve the disease. It may also mean that right qì is contending with evil qì in the exterior and that the disease is contained in the greater yáng. If the pulse becomes rapid and urgent, and if a desire to vomit and agitation and vexation arise, one knows that passage has already occurred. Desire to vomit and vexation and agitation are explained in several different ways. According to Huáng Yuán-Yù (黄元御, style 坤载 Kūn-Zài) desire to vomit is a lesser yáng sign and vexation is a yáng brightness sign. Thus the disease is passing through the lesser yáng into the yáng brightness. Shěn Jīn-Aó (沈金鳌, style 芊绿 Qiān-Lǜ) ascribes all of the signs to the yáng brightness, and contends that the disease is passing directly into the yáng brightness. Zhāng Zhì-Cōng (张志聪, style 隐庵 Yǐn-Ān) considers these to be lesser yīn signs, indicating exuberance of yīn cold. Thus the disease is passing from the exterior, greater yáng, directly into the interior, lesser yīn. The original text is quite short and the information is limited; therefore the opinions of the authors above should be thought of as references to be considered in the light of clinical presentation, not definitive answers to the questions which the line raises.

LINE 5

伤寒二三日，阳明、少阳证不见者，为不传也。

Shāng hán èr sān rì, yáng míng、shào yáng zhèng bù jiàn zhě, wéi bù chuán yě.

When on the second or third day of cold damage, yáng brightness and lesser yáng signs* are absent, it means no passage [has occurred].

TEXT NOTE

* Signs, 证 *zhèng*: Individual pathological "signs," such as pain or localized discomfort, heat effusion, poor appetite, abnormalities of stool, urine, menses, etc. This character 证 *zhèng* is also used in the sense of a group of signs, comprising a manifestation of human sickness understood to reflect the nature, location, and the constitution of the patient. Hence the character 证 *zhèng* is translated as "sign" or "pattern," depending on context.

The concept of pattern is distinct from that of "disease" 病 *bìng*, in the sense of a disease entity (e.g., measles or cholera) as a specific kind of morbid condition that is recognizable as such in all patients it affects. A disease entity may manifest in different patterns during its course and may vary to some extent from one patient to another.

SYNOPSIS

Further discussion of a greater yáng disease in which passage does not occur, continuing from the preceding line.

COMMENTARY

The preceding line describes the situation in which the patient has just contracted an exterior evil, which manifests as greater yáng cold damage. In this line, the patient has already had the disease for a short period of time. The phrase "two or three days" is generally considered to be an approximation and is not taken literally. When determining whether or not the disease has shifted to another channel, one must be familiar with the major signs associated with the other patterns. The text states, "yáng brightness and lesser yáng signs are absent." The major yáng brightness signs are generalized heat effusion, spontaneous sweating, no aversion to cold, aversion to heat, thirst, vexation, and a large pulse. The major signs of lesser yáng disease are bitter taste in the mouth, alternating aversion to cold and heat effusion, dry throat, dizzy vision, fullness in the chest and rib-side, and a pulse that is stringlike. Although the *Sù Wèn* states, "Cold damage for one day, greater yáng contracts [the disease]... the second day, yáng brightness contracts [it]... the third day, lesser yáng contracts [it]...," it is clear that in clinical practice, diseases do not progress with such regularity. Line 4, p. 52, and line 5, p. 53, emphasize that one must examine the patient carefully in order to determine the progress of the disease, not simply count the number of days. For a discussion of the relationship of the *Shāng Hán Lùn* to *Sù Wèn*, see the Introduction, p. 9.

LINE 8

(一) 太阳病，头痛至七日以上自愈者，以行其经尽故也。(二) 若欲作再经者，针足阳明，使经不传则愈。

(1) *Tài yáng bìng, tóu tòng zhì qī rì yǐ shàng zì yù zhě, yǐ xíng qí jīng jìn gù yě.* (2) *Ruò yù zuò zài jīng zhě, zhēn zú yáng míng, shǐ jīng bù chuán zé yù.*

(1) When in greater yáng disease, a headache lasts for more than seven days, [and then the patient] spontaneously recovers, this is because [the evil] has gone right through the channel. (2) If it is about to pass to another channel, and [one] needles the foot yáng brightness* to prevent passage, then [the patient will] recover.

TEXT NOTE

* The foot yáng brightness, 足阳明 *zú yáng míng*: The foot yáng brightness channel.

SYNOPSIS

The mechanism of spontaneous recovery in greater yáng disease and a method for blocking passage of a greater yáng disease.

COMMENTARY

Headache is the only sign explicitly mentioned in this line, although others are implied. Yú Wú-Yán (余无言) explains this in the following way: "Greater yáng disease includes a floating pulse, headache, pain and stiffness in the back of the neck, and aversion to cold." When an evil attacks the greater yáng, but the bowels and viscera are not damaged, it is possible for the body's regulatory and defense mechanisms to contend with and expel the evil. The disease may resolve spontaneously, that is without the patient taking medicinals or receiving other treatment. It is not uncommon for diseases of this nature to resolve spontaneously in approximately one week; hence the number "seven" should be taken as an approximation. The number seven is possibly an allusion to the line of the *Nèi Jīng* that reads: "In seven days the greater yáng disease is weakened and the headache [has undergone a] slight recovery." If the disease does not resolve spontaneously, the physician should take the necessary steps to prevent the shift of the disease. Following the typical progression of greater yáng disease inward to the yáng brightness, one can first needle the foot yáng brightness channel. In this way, one can course the channel qì, rouse the stomach yáng, support the right, dispel the evil, and prevent the shift.

2.2 SECTION APPENDIX: PERIODS OF RESOLUTION FOR THE SIX CHANNELS

Generally, lines are placed in chapter or section appendices such as this one either because commentators have been unable to explain them, or, as in the present case, because their authorship is doubtful. Although the meaning of lines below is clear, they reflect the influence of the *Sù Wèn* and many commentators believe that they were added by a later author. Furthermore, they appear to be inconsistent with clinical reality and therefore are considered to be less important for modern clinicians.

LINE 9

太阳病，欲解时，从巳至未上。

Tài yáng bìng, yù jiě shí, cóng sì zhì wèi shàng.

The time when greater yáng disease is about to resolve is from *sì* (B6) to *wèi* (B8).*

TEXT NOTE

* B6 to B8, 从巳至未上 *cóng sì zhì wèi shàng*: 9 A.M.–3 P.M. See the table below.

THE TWELVE HOURS

子时 *zǐ shí* B1, 11 P.M.–1 A.M.	午时 *wǔ shí* B7, 11 A.M.–1 P.M.
丑时 *chǒu shí* B2, 1 A.M.–3 A.M.	未时 *wèi shí* B8, 1 P.M.–3 P.M.
寅时 *yín shí* B3, 3 A.M.–5 A.M.	申时 *shēn shí* B9, 3 P.M.–5 P.M.
卯时 *mǎo shí* B4, 5 A.M.–7 A.M.	酉时 *yǒu shí* B10, 5 P.M.–7 P.M.
辰时 *chén shí* B5, 7 A.M.–9 A.M.	戌时 *xū shí* B11, 7 P.M.–9 P.M.
巳时 *sì shí* B6, 9 A.M.–11 A.M.	亥时 *hài shí* B12, 9 P.M.– 11 P.M.

SYNOPSIS

On the basis of the intimate relationship between humans and the natural world, inferring the favorable periods (three of the 12 two-hour periods into which the day was traditionally divided) during which a greater yáng disease will resolve.

LINE 193

阳明病，欲解时，从申至戌上。

Yáng míng bìng, yù jiě shí, cóng shēn zhì xū shàng.

The time when yáng brightness disease is about to resolve is from *shēn* (B9) to *xū* (B11).*

TEXT NOTE

* B9 to B11, 从申至戌上 *cóng shēn zhì xū shàng*: 3 P.M.–9 P.M.

SYNOPSIS

How to predict the favorable period during which yáng brightness disease will resolve.

LINE 272

少阳病，欲解时，从寅至辰上。

Shào yáng bìng, yù jiě shí, cóng yín zhì chén shàng.

The time when lesser yáng disease is about to resolve is from *yín* (B3) to *chén* (B5).*

TEXT NOTE

* B3 to B5, 从寅至辰上 *cóng yín zhì chéng shàng*: 3 A.M.–9 A.M.

SYNOPSIS

How to predict the favorable period during which lesser yáng disease will resolve.

LINE 275

太阴病，欲解时，从亥至丑上。

Tài yīn bìng, yù jiě shí, cóng hài zhì chǒu shàng.

The time when greater yīn disease is about to resolve is from *hài* (B12) to *chǒu* (B2).*

Text Note

* B12 to B2, 从亥至丑上 *cóng hài zhì chǒu shàng*: 9 p.m.–3 a.m.

Synopsis

How to predict the favorable period during which greater yīn disease will resolve.

Line 291

少阳病，欲解时，从寅至辰上。

Shào yīn bìng, yù jiě shí, cóng zǐ zhì yín shàng.

The time when lesser yīn disease is about to resolve is from *zǐ* (B1) to *yín* (B3).*

Text Note

* B1 to B3 从子至寅上 *cóng zǐ zhì yín shàng*: from 11 p.m.–5 a.m.

Synopsis

How to predict the favorable period during which lesser yīn disease will resolve.

Line 328

厥阴病，欲解时，从丑至卯上。

Jué yīn bìng, yù jiě shí, cóng chǒu zhì mǎo shàng.

The time when reverting yīn disease is about to resolve is from *chǒu* (B2) to *mǎo* (B4).*

Text Note

* B2 to B4, 从丑至卯上 *cóng chǒu zhì mǎo shàng*: from 1 a.m.–7 a.m.

Synopsis

How to predict the favorable period during which reverting yīn disease will resolve.

Line 10

风家，表解而不了了者，十二日愈。

Fēng jiā, biǎo jiě ér bù liǎo liǎo zhě, shí èr rì yù.

Wind patients[1] in whom the exterior has resolved, but not clearly,[2] will recover in twelve days.

TEXT NOTES

1. Wind patients, 风家 *fēng jiā*: Three interpretations of this term have been offered, but modern commentators generally agree that the third is most likely the author's intended meaning.
   a) According to Fāng Yǒu-Zhí (方有执, style 中行 Zhōng-Xíng), "wind patients [means those patients with] wind strike disease."
   b) Gāo Xué-Shān (高学山) explains that the use of 家 *jiā* means abiding disease. Thus, this term means a person prone to wind disease.
   c) Chéng Yìng-Máo (程应旄, style 程郊倩 Chéng Jiāo-Qiàn) writes that the origin of this patient's disease is wind and that the disease could be any greater yáng disease, such as wind strike or cold damage.
2. Not clearly, 不了了 *bù liǎo liǎo*: Not decisively, not definitively. Although the exterior signs have resolved, the patient has not recovered completely.

SYNOPSIS

After the exterior resolves, when the person still does not feel well, one can wait for spontaneous recovery.

COMMENTARY

A patient who no longer has any exterior signs but still does not feel completely well may simply need some time to rest, eat well, and allow the body to recuperate naturally. This patient does not need to take more medicinals. Again, the use of the number twelve should be understood as an approximate measurement of the time needed for full recovery.

3 BASIC GREATER YÁNG DISEASE PATTERNS

Greater yáng disease is differentiated into wind strike exterior vacuity and cold damage exterior repletion. These patterns are identified on the basis of observed pulses and signs, as described below.

3.1 WIND STRIKE EXTERIOR VACUITY PATTERNS

The primary signs of wind strike are headache, heat effusion, aversion to wind and cold, spontaneous sweating, and a pulse that is floating and moderate. The pathomechanism of these signs can be summed up by the phrase, "weakness in the construction and strength in the defense." The defense is yáng and defends the exterior of the body. The construction is yīn and nourishes the fleshy exterior. When an evil invades the exterior, the defense yáng floats exuberantly to the exterior to resist the evil, giving rise to heat effusion. Thus, here "strength in the defense" means that the defense has contracted the evil. It is not a statement of the physiological strength of the defense yáng. (If this were the case, the exterior would be secure and the evil would be unable to invade.) In fact, here, the defense yáng is less effective in performing its basic functions and when the evil invades, it is unable to secure the exterior; consequently, construction-yīn is not contained and spontaneous sweating occurs. Sweating is called "weakness in the construction," referring to the vacuity of the defense qì and its inability to contain the construction. As a result of sweating, the interstices of the flesh become loose and construction-yīn becomes insufficient, causing the pulse to be not only floating, but also moderate, a quality that indicates weakness. As a result of vacuity of defense qì (yáng qì) and an evil blocking the exterior of the body, the patient experiences aversion to cold and wind. In summary, wind strike patterns are characterized by spontaneous sweating, which indicates that the interstices of the flesh are open and right qì is relatively weak; therefore this pattern is also called an "exterior vacuity pattern."

3.1.1 Cinnamon Twig Decoction Patterns

In greater yáng exterior vacuity patterns, treatment focuses on harmonizing the construction and defense, and Cinnamon Twig Decoction (*guì zhī tāng*) is the representative formula. The signs associated with Cinnamon Twig Decoction (*guì zhī tāng*) patterns are aversion to wind and cold, heat effusion, sweating, headache, pain and stiffness in the back of the neck, nasal congestion, possibly dry retching, and a pulse that is floating and moderate. The cause of the disease is external contraction of wind-cold evil. The pathomechanism is one of wind-cold evil fettering the exterior and defense qì resisting the evil. In this process the defense qì strives to confront the evil and the construction qì is weakened by this struggle. Construction and defense lose normal regulation and the channel qì becomes inhibited. When evil qì and right qì contend, the evil may interfere with the lungs. Treatment consists in using warm acrid medicinals to resolve the fleshy exterior, dispel wind, and harmonize the construction and defense. In cases where the evil is more severe, acupuncture may be used to strengthen the treatment. Cinnamon Twig Decoction (*guì zhī tāng*) is the formula of choice.

Cinnamon Twig Decoction (*guì zhī tāng*) is appropriate for the following conditions:

a) greater yáng disease with unresolved exterior signs in which the pulse is floating and weak

b) greater yáng cold damage in which sweating has been promoted, but the evil has not been completely eliminated and the promotion of further mild sweating is required

c) greater yáng disease in which erroneous precipitation has not caused a shift to another disease pattern and the exterior signs are still present

d) greater yáng disease in which the patient has not defecated for six or seven days, but the urine is still clear

e) miscellaneous diseases in which, in the absence of internal organ disease, the construction and defense are disharmonious and frequent spontaneous sweating or intermittent heat effusion and sweating occur.

Line 12

(一) 太阳中风，阳浮而阴弱，阳浮者，热自发，阴弱者，汗自出。(二) 啬啬恶寒，淅淅恶风，翕翕发热，鼻鸣干呕者，桂枝汤主之。

(1) *Tài yáng zhòng fēng, yáng fú ér yīn ruò, yáng fú zhě, rè zì fā, yīn ruò zhě, hàn zì chū.* (2) *Sè sè wù hán, xī xī wù fēng, xì xì fā rè, bí míng gān ǒu zhě, guì zhī tāng zhǔ zhī.*

(1) In greater yáng wind strike with floating yáng and weak yīn,[1] floating yáng is spontaneous heat effusion,[2] and weak yīn is spontaneous issue of sweat.[3] (2) If [there is] huddled aversion to cold,[4] wetted aversion to wind,[5] feather-warm heat effusion,[6] noisy nose,[7] and dry retching, Cinnamon Twig Decoction (*guì zhī tāng*) governs.

Text Notes

1. Floating yáng and weak yīn, 阳浮阴弱 *yáng fú yīn ruò*: There are two interpretations of this phrase, one from the perspective of the pulse and the other considering the pathomechanism. The interpretation relative to the pathomechanism provides greater insight into these patterns, and consequently may be given precedence.
   a) The superficial pulse felt by applying light pressure is yáng, the deep pulse felt by applying heavy pressure is yīn. "Floating yáng and weak yīn" means a floating moderate pulse. This pulse is forceful when light pressure is applied and forceless when heavy pressure is applied. Chéng Yìng-Máo writes, "'Yīn [and] yáng' describe floating and deep [qualities of the pulse]; [they] do not describe the cubit and inch [positions]."
   b) A pathomechanism in which wind-cold fetters the exterior and exuberant defensive yáng floats up to contend with an evil. The defensive exterior becomes insecure and the construction cannot be contained. This phrase is the same as strength in the defense and weakness in the construction. Chéng Wú-Jǐ writes, "Yáng is an indicator of defense; yīn is an indicator of construction. When the yáng pulse is floating, [there is] wind in the defensive [exterior]. When the yīn pulse is weak, the construction qì is weak. Wind merges with the defense so [there is] strength in the defense and weakness in the construction. Thus, [there is] heat effusion and spontaneous sweating."
2. Floating yáng is spontaneous heat effusion, 阳浮者，热自发 *yáng fú zhě, rè zì fā*: Describes the pathomechanism of greater yáng wind strike and the production of heat effusion. When wind evil fetters the exterior, exuberant defensive yáng floats to the exterior and contends with the evil. This struggle produces heat which effuses from the surface of the body.
3. Weak yīn is spontaneous issue of sweat, 阴弱者，汗自出 *yīn ruò zhě, hàn zì chū*: Describes the pathomechanism of greater yáng wind strike involving the production of sweat. When the defensive yáng is striving to contend with the

evil, its normal function of securing the exterior and regulating the opening and closing of the interstices is compromised. Consequently, the construction-yīn is not contained in the interior and sweat issues. Here weak yīn refers to weak construction, 营弱 *yíng ruò*.

4. Huddled aversion to cold, 啬啬恶寒 *sè sè wù hán*: Severe aversion to cold. The Chinese 啬 *sè*, usually meaning stingy, is here used to describe how the patient huddles up to preserve his own bodily warmth. Fāng Yǒu-Zhí writes, "'Huddled' means aversion to cold that stems from dispirited qì, which is insufficient to delay [inward] percolation [of the exterior evil], and so the aversion is severe."
5. Wetted aversion to wind, 淅淅恶风 *xī xī wù fēng*: Acute aversion to wind. 淅 *xī*, which usually means to wash or soak rice, is taken in this context to mean to spray or to splash. When the surface of the body is splashed with water, it is more sensitive to wind. Fāng Yǒu-Zhí writes, "'Wetted' refers to aversion to wind owing to looseness of the external body, as if there is fear and hatred of rain-water suddenly splashing the body, and means the feeling of aversion."
6. Feather-warm heat effusion, 翕翕发热 *xì xì fā rè*: Gentle heat effusion, felt in the skin and fleshy exterior, as if the body were wrapped in feathers. It does not mean a great sweltering heat effusion. Fāng Yǒu-Zhí writes, "... [this means] warm heat and not a great steaming heat."
7. Noisy nose, 鼻鸣 *bí míng*: Nasal congestion which results in audible breathing.

Formula

Cinnamon Twig Decoction (*guì zhī tāng*)

○ Resolve the flesh and dispel wind; harmonize construction and defense.

桂枝三两（去皮） 芍药三两 甘草二两（炙） 生姜三两（切） 大枣十二枚（擘）

(一) 右五味，㕮咀三味，以水七升，微火煮取三升，去滓，适寒温，服一升。(二) 服已须臾，歠热稀粥一升余，以助药力。(三) 温覆令一时许，遍身漐漐微似有汗者益佳，不可令如水流漓，病必不除。(四) 若一服汗病差，停后服，不必尽剂。(五) 若不汗，更服依前法。(六) 又不汗，后服小促其间，半日许令三服尽。(七) 若病重者，一日一夜服，周时观之。(八) 服一剂尽，病证犹在者，更作服。(九) 若汗不出，乃服至二、三剂。(十) 禁生冷、粘滑、肉面、五辛、酒酪，臭恶等物。

Guì zhī sān liǎng (qù pí) sháo yào sān liǎng gān cǎo èr liǎng (zhì) shēng jiāng sān liǎng (qiè) dà zǎo shí èr méi (bò)

(1) *Yòu wǔ wèi, fǔ jǔ sān wèi, yǐ shuǐ qī shēng, wēi huǒ zhǔ qǔ sān shēng, qū zǐ, shì hán wēn, fú yī shēng.* (2) *Fú yǐ xū yú, chuò rè xī zhōu yī shēng yú, yǐ zhù yào lì.* (3) *Wēn fù lìng yī shí xǔ, piān shēn zhé zhé wēi sì yǒu hàn zhě yì jiā, bù kě lìng rú shuǐ liú lí, bìng bì bù chú.* (4) *Ruò yī fú hàn bìng chài, tíng hòu fú, bù bì jìn jì.* (5) *Ruò bù hàn, gèng fú yī qián fǎ.* (6) *Yòu bù hàn, hòu fú xiǎo cù qí jiān, bàn rì xǔ lìng sān fú jìn.* (7) *Ruò bìng zhòng zhě, yī rì yī yè fú, zhōu shí guān zhī.* (8) *Fú yī jì jìn, bìng zhèng yóu zài zhě, gèng zuò fú.* (9) *Ruò hàn bù chū, nǎi fú zhì*

èr、 sān jì. (10) *Jìn shēng lěng、 nián huá、 ròu miàn、 wǔ xīn、 jiǔ luò、 chòu è děng wù.*

cinnamon twig (桂枝 *guì zhī*, Cinnamomi Ramulus) 3 liǎng (remove bark)[1]
peony (芍药 *sháo yào*, Paeoniae Radix)[2] 3 liǎng
mix-fried[3] licorice (甘草 *gān cǎo*, Glycyrrhizae Radix) 2 liǎng
fresh ginger (生姜 *shēng jiāng*, Zingiberis Rhizoma Recens) 3 liǎng (cut)
jujube (大枣 *dà zǎo*, Ziziphi Fructus) 12 pieces (broken)

(1) [For] the preceding five ingredients, break the [first] three ingredients into small pieces and use seven shēng of water. Boil over a mild flame to get three shēng and remove the dregs. Take one shēng at moderate temperature. (2) Shortly after taking [the first dose] drink approximately one shēng of hot, thin gruel to reinforce the strength of the medicinals. (3) Warm [the body] by covering [with a blanket] for a short period, ideally until the whole body is moist, as if sweating very lightly. One cannot allow [the sweat] to flow like water, since the disease will not be eliminated [in this way]. (4) If one dose [causes] sweating and the disease is diminished, cease taking further [doses]. One need not finish the whole packet. (5) If sweating is absent, take another dose according to the previous method. (6) If sweating is again absent, reduce the time between doses, finishing three doses in half a day. (7) If the disease is severe, take [doses] throughout the whole day, and observe [the patient] the whole time. (8) After finishing one packet, [if] the disease signs are still evident, take again. (9) If sweating is absent, one can take up to two or three packets. (10) Foods contraindicated [while taking the formula] include raw and cold foods, sticky and slimy foods, meat and noodles, the five acrids,[4] liquor, milk products, and foods with a peculiar or spoiled flavor or odor.

FORMULA NOTES

1. Remove bark, 去皮 *qù pí*: Because the flavor (and hence the medicinal strength) cinnamon twig (*guì zhī*) is contained in the bark, the instruction to remove the bark has led to different interpretations. According to Kē Qín, "removing the bark" refers to the removal of the rough outer bark of Cinnamon twig (*guì zhī*). According to Zhāng Zhì-Cōng, it means using tender twigs without skin. Both interpretations are considered acceptable.
2. Peony, 芍药 *sháo yào*: Peony (*sháo yào*) is taken to mean white peony (*bái sháo yào*).
3. Mix-fried, 炙 *zhì*: In modern terms, this refers to stir-frying with liquid adjuvants, but it is unclear what it means in this text. It may simply mean that the medicinal agent is roasted, not necessarily stir-fried with honey, vinegar, or wine, as is common today.
4. Five acrids, 五辛 *wǔ xīn*: This term refers generally to foods with a penetrating and stimulating odor or flavor, but it has been the subject of much disagreement among authors. Below are some of the main lists as recorded in the *Shāng Hán Lùn Yán Jiū Dà Cí Diǎn* (伤寒论研究大辞典 "*Shāng Hán Lùn* Studies Dictionary").
   a) According to the authors of the dictionary: scallion (*cōng*), Chinese chive (*xiè*), Chinese leek (*jiǔ*), garlic (*suàn*), and asafetida (*qú*).

b) Lǐ Shí-Zhēn (李时珍, sobriquet 滨湖 Bīn Hú), in the *Běn Cǎo Gāng Mù* (本草纲目 "The Comprehensive Herbal Foundation") writes, "The five strong-smelling vegetables are the five acrid; those that are acrid, malodorous, and cloud the spirit with an attacking nature. [According to] those who cultivate their bodies, the five strong-smelling vegetables are sand garlic (*xiǎo suàn*), garlic (*dà suàn*), oil rape (*yún tái*), and coriander (*hú suī*). [According to] Taoist [teaching], the five strong-smelling vegetables are Chinese leek (*jiǔ*), Chinese chive (*xiè*), garlic (*suàn*), oil rape (*yún tái*), and coriander (*hú suī*). [According to] Buddhist [teaching], the five strong-smelling vegetables are garlic (*dà suàn*), sand garlic (*xiǎo suàn*), asafetida (*xīng qú*), scallion (*cí cōng*), Chinese leek (*jiǔ*), and victorialis (*gè cōng*).

According to *Gāo Děng Cóng Shū*, the significance of the contraindication is that one must avoid foods that have a penetrating fragrance and a stimulating or irritating taste.

SYNOPSIS

The pathology, clinical manifestation, and treatment of the greater yáng wind strike pattern.

COMMENTARY

The signs of greater yáng wind strike include heat effusion, aversion to wind and cold, sweating, stiffness and pain of the head and nape, noisy nose, dry retching, and a pulse that is floating and moderate. The pulse is not only moderate, but also floating since this quality is common to greater yáng disease. In this pattern, wind-cold fetters the exterior and defensive yáng floats to the exterior to resist the evil. Because of existing yáng qì (defense qì) vacuity, the exterior becomes insecure and construction-yīn is not contained. This pathomechanism is described in the text as "floating yáng and weak yīn." The struggle between defense qì and the exterior evil produces heat effusion. The presence of an evil in the exterior and vacuity of defense qì gives rise to wetted aversion to wind and huddled aversion to cold. The construction-yīn issues outward in the form of sweat and the nourishment normally provided by the construction-yīn is lost or diminished. This loss of nourishment results in stiffness and pain. The evil may also interfere with the lung and/or stomach. If it attacks the lung, inhibiting lung qì, the patient will have a noisy nose. If it attacks the stomach, causing counterflow ascent of qì, retching will be observed.

Cinnamon Twig Decoction (*guì zhī tāng*) is the formula of choice for greater yáng wind strike. Cinnamon twig (*guì zhī*) is acrid and warm. Because acrid-flavored medicinals dissipate and warm-natured medicinals dispel cold and free yáng, cinnamon twig (*guì zhī*) resolves exterior wind and cold from the fleshy exterior and interstices. Peony (*sháo yào*) is sour and cold. Because sour-flavored medicinals contract and cold-natured medicinals penetrate the construction-yīn, peony (*sháo yào*) contracts yīn and harmonizes construction. These two medicinals used together harmonize construction and defense, which is the basic action of Cinnamon Twig Decoction (*guì zhī tāng*). Acrid and warm, fresh ginger (*shēng jiāng*) not only assists cinnamon twig (*guì zhī*) in resolving the exterior, but also downbears counterflow and checks retching. This last action is particularly useful when the exterior evil impairs the function of the stomach. Sweet jujube (*dà zǎo*) boosts the center and assists peony (*sháo yào*) in boosting yīn and harmonizing construction. Sweet, balanced, mix-fried licorice (*gān cǎo*) harmonizes all the ingredients in the formula and promotes interaction between the construction and defense. This formula can be used for any disharmony of the construction and defense, not just greater yáng wind strike.

After taking the decoction, the patient should drink a bowl of thin, warm gruel. Eating rice gruel provides fluid nourishment and stomach qì, which supports right qì; hence sweating occurs easily. If after the first dose sweat issues, no more doses should be taken. If sweating is absent, another dose may be taken, up to three times in a roughly twelve hour period. Zhāng Jī cautions against the excessive promotion of sweating. Generally, the sweat should issue very lightly, and as soon as it does, the patient is not allowed to take the decoction again. If the illness is severe, doses may be given continuously and two to three whole packets may be used in one day. When Cinnamon Twig Decoction (*guì zhī tāng*) is prepared, it is divided into three doses. A dose is one-third of the whole decoction prepared from one packet. The terms used in the Hàn Dynasty to denote weights and measures are largely the same as those used in modern texts, but the amounts are different. For example, in the Hàn Dynasty, a liǎng was equivalent to 15.625 grams, whereas today a liǎng is equivalent to 31.25 grams. Many authors have written commentaries on this issue and after researching historical commentaries and modern clinical ingredient dosages, Kē Xuě-Fán (柯雪帆) suggests the following equivalents:

one jīn = 250 grams
one liǎng = 15.625 grams
one zhū = 1/24 of a liǎng
one gě = 20 milliliters
one shēng = 200 milliliters = 6.76 fluid ounces
one dǒu = 10 shēng

Note: Shēng is a unit of volume used for any liquid as well as for solid materials, such as pinellia (*bàn xià*) or schisandra (*wǔ wèi zǐ*), which can be conveniently measured with a scoop.

LINE 13

太阳病，头痛，发热，汗出，恶风，桂枝汤主之。

Tài yáng bìng, tóu tòng, fā rè, hàn chū, wù fēng, guì zhī tāng zhǔ zhī.

[For] greater yáng disease with headache, heat effusion, sweating, and aversion to wind, Cinnamon Twig Decoction (*guì zhī tāng*) governs.

SYNOPSIS

The primary manifestations and treatment of greater yáng wind strike patterns.

COMMENTARY

In this line, no pulse is described. Nevertheless, if the patient has the four basic signs of headache, heat effusion, sweating, and aversion to wind, the pulse need not be floating and moderate for one to use Cinnamon Twig Decoction (*guì zhī tāng*) or to classify this pattern as greater yáng wind strike. A comparison of this set of signs with those of cold damage shows that the only difference is the presence or absence of sweating, an important point in the differentiation of these two patterns.

LINE 95

太阳病，发热汗出者，此为荣弱卫强，故使汗出，欲救邪风者，宜桂枝汤。

Tài yáng bìng, fā rè hàn chū zhě, cǐ wéi róng ruò wèi qiáng, gù shǐ hàn chū, yù jiù xié fēng zhě, yí guì zhī tāng.

When in greater yáng disease [there is] heat effusion and sweating, this means weakness in the construction and strength in the defense,[1] [which] consequently causes sweat to issue; to eliminate the evil wind,[2] Cinnamon Twig Decoction (*guì zhī tāng*) is appropriate.

TEXT NOTES

1. Weakness in the construction and strength in the defense, 荣弱卫强 *róng ruò wèi qiáng*: 荣 *róng* is interchangeable with 营 *yíng*, construction. There are different interpretations of this phrase, but common to all is the notion that "weakness in the construction" means weakness in the construction-yīn and inability to contain the interior. "Strength in the defense" means that the defensive yáng rises up to meet a repletion evil that is in the defensive exterior. The commentaries below provide additional insight into this phrase.

   Fāng Yǒu-Zhí: "In line 3, it says floating yáng and weak yīn. Here it says weakness in the construction and strength in the defense. Strength in the defense is floating yáng and weakness in the construction is weak yīn. Each explains the other."

   Yī Zōng Jīn Jiàn: "This explains the meaning of floating yáng and weak yīn from the line above. In the *Huáng Dì Nèi Jīng*, [it states that] 'Exuberant evil qì is repletion. Despoliation of essence qì is vacuity.' The defense is entered by the wind and then [there is] heat effusion. The cause is repletion evil qì. Thus, strength in the defense is strong evil qì in the defensive [exterior]. The construction receives the evil and is steamed, then sweat issues. The cause is weak essence qì. Thus weakness in the construction is weak yīn qì in the construction [aspect]."

2. Evil wind, 邪风 *xié fēng*: Wind evil.

SYNOPSIS

Further discussion of the cause, pathology, and treatment of greater yáng wind strike patterns.

COMMENTARY

In greater yáng disease, the presence of heat effusion and sweating means that this is a wind strike pattern as compared with a cold damage pattern, in which heat effusion may or may not have developed and in which sweating is absent. The pathomechanism of greater yáng wind strike is described in the phrase, "weakness in the construction and strength in the defense." When a wind-cold evil fetters the exterior, the defensive yáng floats to the outer body. This phenomenon is described as "strength in the defense." "Weakness in the construction" means that when the defensive exterior becomes insecure, the construction-yīn is not contained and issues outwards as sweat. "Weakness in the construction and strength in the defense" is a concrete explanation of the phrase, "floating yáng and weak yīn" from line 12, p. 60. In these patterns, wind evil is often involved. Cinnamon Twig Decoction (*guì zhī tāng*) resolves the fleshy exterior and expels wind.

LINE 24

太阳病，初服桂枝汤，反烦不解者，先刺风池、风府，却与桂枝汤则愈。

Tài yáng bìng, chū fú guì zhī tāng, fǎn fán bù jiě zhě, xiān cì fēng chí、fēng fǔ, què yǔ guì zhī tāng zé yù.

When in greater yáng disease, [the patient] has initially taken Cinnamon Twig Decoction (*guì zhī tāng*),* but is vexed and [the exterior] is unresolved, first needle Wind Pool (*fēng chí,* GB-20) and Wind Mansion (*fēng fǔ,* GV-16), then give Cinnamon Twig Decoction (*guì zhī tāng*), and [the patient] will recover.

TEXT NOTE

* In which [the patient] has initially taken Cinnamon Twig Decoction (*guì zhī tāng*), 初服桂枝汤 *chū fú guì zhī tāng*: According to Kē Qín and Chén Niàn-Zǔ, this phrase may be taken to mean that only the initial dose of the formula has been given. In the directions for Cinnamon Twig Decoction (*guì zhī tāng*), one is cautioned against giving more than one dose of the formula, unless all of the signs remain unchanged. The precise meaning in Chinese is unclear and, according to the *Gāo Děng Cóng Shū* , it would be reasonable to explain this phrase as meaning that a few doses or even a whole packet has already been taken. It simply means that it is early in the disease process and the patient has started taking Cinnamon Twig Decoction (*guì zhī tāng*).

SYNOPSIS

In greater yáng wind strike patterns, when evil qì is severe, one should treat using needles and medicinals.

COMMENTARY

After the initial ingestion of Cinnamon Twig Decoction (*guì zhī tāng*), not only has the exterior not resolved, but the patient is now also experiencing vexation. Two explanations are possible. The first is that the formula was not strong enough for the strength of the evil and the second is that the evil has already passed into another channel. If the evil has transformed to heat and entered the interior, harassing the spirit and causing vexation, one would expect changes in the pulse and other signs to be described. However, this line speaks only of vexation and mentions no pulse or other signs. Furthermore, it speaks only of "vexation" (also called "heart vexation"); it does not speak of the more severe "agitation and vexation," which would be more likely in the case of internal heat. One may conclude therefore that the evil is still in the greater yáng, right qì and evil qì are contending with each other, and that the vexation is a consequence of an unresolved evil qì depressed in the exterior. When the evil is stronger than the formula used, right qì acts to assist the medicinals in expelling the evil. If the formula is not strong enough to expel a strong evil, when right qì and evil qì contend, vexation occurs. Furthermore, the injunction to apply acupuncture before giving Cinnamon Twig Decoction (*guì zhī tāng*) gives a further indication that this pattern is a more severe form of greater yáng wind strike, since needling the points suggested has the effect of dispelling wind and resolving the exterior, thus strengthening the treatment.

Line 42

太阳病，外证未解，脉浮弱者，当以汗解，宜桂枝汤。

Tài yáng bìng, wài zhèng wèi jiě, mài fú ruò zhě, dāng yǐ hàn jiě, yí guì zhī tāng.

When in greater yáng disease the exterior pattern has not resolved and the pulse is floating and weak,* this should be resolved through [the promotion of] sweating; [therefore,] Cinnamon Twig Decoction (*guì zhī tāng*) is appropriate.

Text Note

* The pulse is floating and weak, 脉浮弱 *mài fú ruò*: A pulse that is felt with the application of only light pressure and that is forceless. The term "weak pulse" is taken at face value to mean forceless, lacking in strength. The more specific definition of "sunken and forceless" that usually applies in modern texts was a later development. See the Introduction, for a further discussion of this issue.

Synopsis

In greater yáng wind disease, when the pulse is floating and weak, it is appropriate to use Cinnamon Twig Decoction (*guì zhī tāng*).

Commentary

Chéng Wú-Jǐ and Fāng Yǒu-Zhí both write that "the pulse is floating and weak" means the same as "floating yáng and weak yīn," referring to weakness in the construction and strength in the defense. This pulse is the basic one expected in greater yáng wind strike and it means that although the disease has not resolved, no transmutation has occurred. A slight variation on this idea is presented by Kē Qín and the authors of *Yī Zōng Jīn Jiàn*, who take "the pulse is floating and weak" to mean not "floating yáng and weak yīn," but a pulse that is floating and moderate, as distinct from a pulse that is floating and tight seen in greater yáng cold damage. One of the important differences between greater yáng wind strike and greater yáng cold damage is a pulse that is floating and moderate, as opposed to a pulse that is floating and tight. Thus, since Cinnamon Twig Decoction (*guì zhī tāng*) is suggested, this pattern is probably wind strike with its associated pulse. The two interpretations presented above are not contradictory, since the clinical significance of both is the same. Since the exterior pattern has not resolved, the basic signs of greater yáng wind strike are still present, so that Cinnamon Twig Decoction (*guì zhī tāng*) is appropriate for the mild promotion of sweating.

Line 57

伤寒发汗已解，半日许复烦，脉浮数者，可更发汗，宜桂枝汤。

Shāng hán fā hàn yǐ jiě, bàn rì xǔ fù fán, mài fú shuò zhě, kě gèng fā hàn, yí guì zhī tāng.

When in cold damage, sweating has already brought resolution, and then after half a day or so [there is] again vexation and a pulse that is rapid and floating, [one] can again promote sweating; [therefore,] Cinnamon Twig Decoction (*guì zhī tāng*) is appropriate.

Synopsis

After the promotion of sweating in a greater yáng cold damage pattern, when a residual evil has not been exhausted, it is still appropriate to resolve the exterior through the promotion of sweating.

Commentary

In greater yáng cold damage, the promotion of sweating is the appropriate treatment method. Nevertheless, in this case, after resolution of the disease, vexation appears. One might conclude that the evil has shifted to the yáng brightness channel and that the vexation is a sign of an exterior evil entering the interior and transforming into heat. This transformation is further suggested by the presence of a rapid pulse. The pulse, however, is also floating and no other signs of internal heat are present. Furthermore, vexation, also known as heart vexation, is considered a mild sign of the contention between right qì and residual evil qì that has not been completely eliminated and is depressed in the exterior because of a particularly strong evil qì, weakened right qì, or some combination of these factors. The pathomechanism associated with this transmutation has been described by various commentators.

Zhāng Zhì-Cōng writes, "An unfinished residual evil passes [into] and abides in the fleshy exterior and interstices."

According to Chéng Yìng-Máo, "The cold evil abates and then gathers again."

Fāng Yǒu-Zhí (方有执, style 中行 Zhōng-Xíng) explains that, "[When] sweating is promoted improperly, after sweating, [if] one is not careful, it is easy for wind evil to reenter [the exterior]."

Finally, Zhōu Yáng-Jùn (周扬俊) comments, "[There has] been sweating, [so] the old evil is already gone. [Because there is] new vacuity, [there is] again an attack from evil wind."

According to all these interpretations it would be an error to use a treatment for an interior heat condition. The text tells us that sweating can be promoted again. Cinnamon Twig Decoction (*guì zhī tāng*) is used rather than Ephedra Decoction (*má huáng tāng*) because we assume that the latter formula has already been used once. Although the text does not tell us if the newly appearing signs constitute a greater yáng cold damage pattern, the fact that Cinnamon Twig Decoction (*guì zhī tāng*) is suggested means that mild sweating is appropriate, rather than the strong sweating induced by Ephedra Decoction (*má huáng tāng*).

LINE 44

太阳病，外证未解，不可下也，下之为逆，欲解外者，宜桂枝汤。

Tài yáng bìng, wài zhèng wèi jiě, bù kě xià yě, xià zhī wéi nì, yù jiě wài zhě, yí guì zhī tāng.

Greater yáng disease in which the exterior pattern has not resolved cannot be precipitated [since] precipitation would be an adverse [treatment]. When [one] desires to resolve the exterior, Cinnamon Twig Decoction (*guì zhī tāng*) is appropriate.

SYNOPSIS

It is a treatment principle that in greater yáng disease the promotion of sweating is appropriate and the use of precipitation is not.

COMMENTARY

In any pattern with exterior signs, promotion of sweating is the appropriate treatment. When interior signs are present as well as exterior signs, precipitation may be used, but it should only be used before promotion of sweating if the interior signs require more urgent treatment than the exterior signs. Prior to resolution of exterior signs, the use of precipitation usually constitutes an error in treatment, since it causes the exterior evil to fall inward and gives rise to such signs as panting, fullness in the chest, glomus, and diarrhea. According to *Gāo Děng Cóng Shū*, Cinnamon Twig Decoction (*guì zhī tāng*) is just one example of an appropriate exterior-resolving formula. It is still necessary to examine the signs before choosing the formula and one should not be restricted to Cinnamon Twig Decoction (*guì zhī tāng*).

Line 45

(一) 太阳病，先发汗不解，而复下之，脉浮者不愈。(二) 浮为在外，而反下之，故令不愈，今脉浮，故在外，当须解外则愈，宜桂枝汤。

(1) *Tài yáng bìng, xiān fā hàn bù jiě, ér fù xià zhī, mài fú zhě bù yù.* (2) *Fú wéi zài wài, ér fǎn xià zhī, gù lìng bù yù, jīn mài fú, gù zài wài, dāng xū jiě wài zé yù, yí guì zhī tāng.*

(1) When in greater yáng disease initial promotion of sweating fails to resolve [the disease] and precipitation then is used, [so that] the pulse is floating; [there will be] no recovery. (2) [A pulse that is] floating means location in the outer body, and [if] instead precipitation [is used], it will prevent recovery. The pulse is now* floating so [we know that the disease is] located in the outer body and this requires resolution of the outer body to achieve recovery; [therefore,] Cinnamon Twig Decoction (*guì zhī tāng*) is appropriate.

Text Note

* Now, 今 *jīn*: In the present case.

Synopsis

In a greater yáng disease, after sweating has been promoted and precipitation has been used, if the disease is still in the exterior and has not become a transmuted pattern, one should still treat by resolving the exterior.

Commentary

In this line, the patient has already been treated through sweating and precipitation. The evil is still in the exterior, as indicated by the presence of a pulse that is still floating, even after erroneous precipitation, which can cause an evil to fall into the interior. This line illustrates an important principle of the *Shāng Hán Lùn*, namely that one should choose the treatment on the basis of the observed signs. This patient still has the signs of greater yáng disease and no transmuted pattern has arisen from mistreatment. Since the evil is still in the exterior, it is appropriate to promote sweating. It would be wrong to assume that because promotion of sweating and precipitation have already been used the promotion of sweating cannot be used again. Nevertheless, it is important to bear in mind that in view of the damage to right qì caused by both sweating and precipitation, although the promotion of sweating is the correct treatment method, a mild formula must be used rather than a strong one. The formula of choice is Cinnamon Twig Decoction (*guì zhī tāng*), which will not further damage right qì.

LINE 56

㈠ 伤寒不大便六七日，头痛有热者，与承气汤。 ㈡ 其小便清者，知不在里，仍在表也，当须发汗；若头痛者，必衄，宜桂枝汤。

(1) *Shāng hán bù dà biàn liù qī rì, tóu tòng yǒu rè zhě, yǔ chéng qì tāng.* (2) *Qí xiǎo biàn qīng zhě, zhī bù zài lǐ, réng zài biǎo yě, dāng xū fā hàn; ruò tóu tòng zhě, bì nǜ, yí guì zhī tāng.*

(1) When cold damage[1] [is characterized by] inability to defecate for six or seven days, headache, and heat [effusion], give a Qì-Coordinating Decoction (*chéng qì tāng*).[2] (2) If the urine is clear, [we] know [the disease] is not located in the interior, [but] is still in the exterior, and should [be treated by] the promotion of sweating, [and] (if [there is still] a headache, [after taking the decoction], there will be spontaneous external bleeding), Cinnamon Twig Decoction (*guì zhī tāng*) is appropriate.[3]

TEXT NOTES

1. Cold damage, 伤寒 *shāng hán*: In this context, "cold damage" is used in its broader sense of any externally contracted disease because the treatment used for the resolution of the exterior disease is Cinnamon Twig Decoction (*guì zhī tāng*). If it were used in the narrow sense of exterior repletion, Ephedra Decoction (*má huáng tāng*) would be the formula.
2. Qì-coordinating decoction, 承气汤 *chéng qì tāng*: Any of the formulae whose name contains "qì-coordinating." These formulae clear heat and free the stool.
3. Cinnamon Twig Decoction (*guì zhī tāng*) is appropriate, 宜桂枝汤 *yí guì zhī tāng*: This, according to Yóu Yí (尤怡, style 在泾 Zài-Jīng), is an example of grammatical inversion. The clause containing the formula belongs directly after the clause, "should be treated by the promotion of sweating," 当须发汗 *dāng xū fā hàn*, since it indicates what should be used to promote sweating. In that case, this line would be, "In cold damage with inability to defecate for six or seven days, headache, and heat effusion, give Qì-Coordinating Decoctions (*chéng qì tāng*). If the urine is clear, [one] knows [the disease] is not located in the interior, [but] is still in the exterior, and should [be treated by] the promotion of sweating. Cinnamon Twig Decoction (*guì zhī tāng*) is appropriate. If [there is still] a headache [after taking the decoction], there will be spontaneous external bleeding."

SYNOPSIS

a) On the basis of whether or not the urine is clear, one can differentiate exterior and interior patterns.

b) If the urine is clear, the pattern belongs to the exterior and it is appropriate to use Cinnamon Twig Decoction (*guì zhī tāng*).

COMMENTARY

When defecation is absent for about a week, one might conclude that the evil has entered the interior and transformed to heat. In that case, in addition to a headache, the patient's urine would be turbid, dark yellow or reddish and/or feel hot, suggesting the presence of interior heat bind repletion for which offensive precipitation can be used. When, as is actually the case here, the urine is clear or light colored, one knows that the evil is not in the interior, but is still in the exterior; hence precipitation is inappropriate and the promotion of sweating is appropriate. Urination is one important indicator used to determine whether an evil is located in the interior or exterior. In the line above, Cinnamon Twig Decoction (*guì zhī tāng*) is used to promote sweating.

If, after giving the decoction, the headache is still present or actually becomes more severe, one knows that the evil is depressed in the exterior. The evil may then damage the channels and cause spontaneous external bleeding. "Spontaneous external bleeding" is blood issuing from the nose, gums, or skin, without the presence of exterior damage or injury. In the *Shāng Hán Lùn*, it commonly refers to nosebleed, but not exclusively. Spontaneous external bleeding occurs in three basic patterns. The first is in a greater yáng disease without sweating when the evil becomes depressed in the exterior and damages the yáng channels, causing impaired movement of the blood and fluids. The second is when yáng brightness heat distresses the blood aspect and scorches the yáng channels, causing the hot blood to move recklessly and leave the channels. The third possibility is that the erroneous use of a heating method to force sweating scorches the yáng channels, causing bleeding.

LINE 15

㈠ 太阳病，下之后，其气上冲者，可与桂枝汤，方用前法。㈡ 若不上冲者，不得与之。

(1) *Tài yáng bìng, xià zhī hòu, qí qì shàng chōng zhě, kě yǔ guì zhī tāng, fāng yòng qián fǎ.* (2) *Ruò bù shàng chōng zhě, bù dé yǔ zhī.*

(1) When in greater yáng disease, after precipitation, qì surges upward,[1] [one] may give Cinnamon Twig Decoction (*guì zhī tāng*), according to the previously mentioned method.[2] (2) If [there is] no upsurge, [one] cannot give this formula.

TEXT NOTES

1. Qì surges upward, 气上冲 *qì shāng chōng*: A subjective feeling of qì ascending counterflow into the heart and chest. This pattern is different from running piglet qì, 奔豚气 *bēn tún qì*, in which the qì counterflow starts lower, in the lesser abdomen. Running piglet qì will be discussed further in line 117, p. 167.
2. According to the previously mentioned method, 方用前法 *fāng yòng qián fǎ*: The method of decocting and taking Cinnamon Twig Decoction (*guì zhī tāng*), described in line 12, p. 60.

Synopsis

After the inappropriate use of precipitation in a greater yáng disease, if the exterior pattern is still present, one should treat by resolving the exterior, but if the exterior evil has fallen into the interior, the promotion of sweating is contraindicated.

Commentary

In greater yáng disease, precipitation is usually inappropriate and its use may result in a transmutation, the patterns above being two possibilities. The key diagnostic point is the presence or absence of qì surging upward. When this is present, it means that right qì is still strong and is contending with evil qì and the exterior evil has not yet fallen inward. The exuberant right qì attempts to push evil qì out, and because evil qì is still blocking the exterior, right qì rises up. One should resolve the exterior to allow the outward passage of evil qì. Following the inappropriate use of precipitation, one must be careful not to further damage right qì. Therefore, it is suggested that the exterior be resolved using Cinnamon Twig Decoction (*guì zhī tāng*), which is mild and harmonizing, not Ephedra Decoction (*má huáng tāng*), which might damage right qì. The absence of any feeling of upsurge means that the evil has already sunk into the interior; consequently, resolving the exterior is inappropriate. Once the evil falls into the interior, the possible transmutations are varied. No particular treatment method is suggested, since one must choose an appropriate treatment on the basis of presenting signs.

Line 53

㈠病常自汗出者，此为荣气和，荣气和者，外不谐，以卫气不共荣气谐和故尔。㈡以荣行脉中，卫行脉外，复发其汗，荣卫和则愈，宜桂枝汤。

(1) *Bìng cháng zì hàn chū zhě, cǐ wéi róng qì hé, róng qì hé zhě, wài bù xié, yǐ wèi qì bù gòng róng qì xié hé gù ěr.* (2) *Yǐ róng xíng mài zhōng, wèi xíng mài wài, fù fā qí hàn, róng wèi hé zé yù, yí guì zhī tāng.*

(1) When illness [is characterized by] frequent spontaneous sweating, it means construction qì is in harmony* and when [in such cases] construction qì is in harmony, [it is] the outer body [that] is not harmonious; that is [to say] it is because defense qì is not in harmony with construction qì. (2) Because construction [qì] moves in the vessels, and defense [qì] moves outside the vessels, by the further promotion of sweating, construction and defense will harmonize, bringing about recovery; [therefore,] Cinnamon Twig Decoction (*guì zhī tāng*) is appropriate.

TEXT NOTE

* Construction qì is in harmony, 荣气和 *róng qì hé*: The construction qì is not affected by the disease. According to Xú Dà Chūn (徐大椿, style 灵胎 Líng-Tāi), although the construction qì is not affected by the disease, it is not harmonious in the sense of harmony between the construction and defense.

SYNOPSIS

a) The pathology and treatment of disease characterized by frequent spontaneous sweating.

b) This is a suitable pattern for treatment with Cinnamon Twig Decoction (*guì zhī tāng*).

COMMENTARY

This line does not specifically refer to greater yáng disease, but instead refers to diseases with frequent spontaneous sweating. The pathomechanism of this is explained as defense qì not being in harmony with construction qì. Xú Dà Chūn makes a distinction between spontaneous sweating and the promotion of sweating: "Spontaneous sweating is the separation of construction and defense. The promotion of sweating causes construction and defense to unite." Coordination between the construction qì within the vessels and the defense qì outside the vessels is impaired. Cinnamon Twig Decoction (*guì zhī tāng*) is the primary formula for harmonizing construction and defense. It can be used whenever there is construction-defense disharmony, and its use is not restricted to treatment of wind strike.

LINE 54

病人藏无他病，时发热自汗出 而不愈者，此卫气不和也，先其时发汗则愈，宜桂枝汤。

Bìng rén zàng wú tā bìng, shí fā rè zì hàn chū ér bù yù zhě, cǐ wèi qì bù hé yě, xiān qí shí fā hàn zé yù, yí guì zhī tāng.

When patients whose viscera have no other disease[1] have periodic heat effusion and spontaneous sweating, and are failing to recover, this means defense qì is disharmonious and the promotion of sweating ahead of time[2] will bring about recovery; [therefore,] Cinnamon Twig Decoction (*guì zhī tāng*) is appropriate.

TEXT NOTES

1. Patients whose viscera have no other disease 病人藏无他病 *bìng rén zàng wú tā bìng*: There is no disease in the bowels or viscera; no interior pattern.
2. Promotion of sweating ahead of time, 先其时发汗 *xiān qí shí fā hàn*: Promotion of sweating while the patient is not experiencing the signs of heat effusion and sweating.

SYNOPSIS

a) The pathology and treatment of patterns with periodic heat effusion and spontaneous sweating.

b) This is a suitable pattern for treatment with Cinnamon Twig Decoction (*guì zhī tāng*).

COMMENTARY

This pattern is characterized by the presence of periodic heat effusion and spontaneous sweating, and the absence of interior signs. The pathomechanism of this exterior pattern is disharmony of the defense qì, as in the previous line.

Although this is an exterior pattern in which construction and defense are in disharmony, the periodicity of the heat effusion indicates a difference from greater yáng wind strike patterns. The use of Cinnamon Twig Decoction (*guì zhī tāng*) should not be construed as indicating the presence of wind strike exterior vacuity. The promotion of sweating with Cinnamon Twig Decoction (*guì zhī tāng*), which harmonizes construction and defense, is suggested in this line and the previous one to treat spontaneous sweating. In this line, the formula is given prior to an episode of heat effusion. Once sweat issues, construction and defense will become harmonious and heat effusion will cease.

3.1.2 Contraindications for Cinnamon Twig Decoction

The contraindications for Cinnamon Twig Decoction (*guì zhī tāng*) are as follows:

a) Patients with greater yáng cold damage signs

b) Patients with interior damp-heat

c) Patients with hyperactivity of exuberant interior heat

d) Greater yáng disease in which precipitation has been used erroneously and no exterior signs are present.

LINE 16B

㈠ ...桂枝本为解肌，若其人脉浮紧，发热汗不出者，不可与之也。㈡ 常须识此，勿令误也。

(1) ... *guì zhī běn wéi jiě jī, ruò qí rén mài fú jǐn, fā rè hàn bù chū zhě, bù kě yǔ zhī yě.* (2) *Cháng xū shì cǐ, wù lìng wù yě.*

(1) ... Cinnamon Twig [Decoction][1] is basically for resolving the flesh;[2] if the person's[3] pulse is tight and floating, [and there is] heat effusion, and sweating is absent, it cannot be given. (2) [One] needs always to be aware of this, so as not to cause this error.

TEXT NOTES

1. Cinnamon Twig, 桂枝 *guì zhī*: An ellipsis of Cinnamon Twig Decoction (*guì zhī tāng*).

2. Resolving the flesh, 解肌 *jiě jī*: To resolve the fleshy exterior of wind evil, through the mild promotion of sweating. This is different from the action of Ephedra Decoction (*má huáng tāng*), which strongly promotes sweating.
3. The person, 其人 *qí rén*: Literally, "this person," but here meaning "the patient."

SYNOPSIS

Cinnamon Twig Decoction (*guì zhī tāng*) should not be used in greater yáng cold damage patterns.

COMMENTARY

The resolution of the fleshy exterior and the regulation of the construction and defense are the chief actions of Cinnamon Twig Decoction (*guì zhī tāng*), which promotes mild sweating. In the line above, the patient has a pulse that is floating and tight, heat effusion, and absence of sweating, indicating greater yáng cold damage, which should be treated with Ephedra Decoction (*má huáng tāng*). The promotion of strong sweating is appropriate and a mild formula such as Cinnamon Twig Decoction (*guì zhī tāng*) must not be given. This line suggests that when using promotion of sweating to resolve the exterior, the formula should be sufficiently strong, since if it is not strong enough, the opportunity for the most effective dispelling of evil will be lost. Previous lines have also emphasized that if a formula is too strong, right qì will be damaged. If a formula is not strong enough or is too strong, transmuted patterns can arise.

This line and line 16A, p. 132, are, in some texts, written as a single line.

LINE 17

若酒客病，不可与桂枝汤，得之则呕，以酒客不喜甘故也。

Ruò jiǔ kè bìng, bù kě yǔ guì zhī tāng, dé zhī zé ǒu, yǐ jiǔ kè bù xǐ gān gù yě.

If a drinker is sick,[1] Cinnamon Twig Decoction (*guì zhī tāng*) cannot be given, since it will cause retching. This is because drinkers do not like sweet things.[2]

TEXT NOTES

1. If a drinker is sick, 若酒客病 *ruò jiǔ kè bìng*: The Chinese phrase can actually be read in two different ways.
   a) If [a] drinker [is] sick, i.e., if a person given to drinking liquor [contracts greater yáng] disease...
   b) If [this is] drinkers" sickness, i.e., if the condition is due to drinking...

   The term 酒客 *jiǔ kè* seems to imply disapproval (客 *kè*, literally "visitor," is often used to describe a person engaged in a specific activity, often one that is frowned upon); but it is not clear if it refers to someone given to drinking or one who is habitually drunk.
2. Do not like sweet things, 不喜甘 *bù xǐ gān*: Cannot tolerate sweet things.

SYNOPSIS

Using the example of a drinker, this line points out that Cinnamon Twig Decoction (*guì zhī tāng*) is contraindicated when there is damp-heat in the interior.

COMMENTARY

The grammatical meaning of the opening clause is not clear since we do not know if 酒客病 *jiǔ kè bìng* is intended to be read as a disease name ("drinker's sickness," i.e., alcoholism) or whether it is a drinker (酒客 *jiǔ kè*) who is sick (病 *bìng*). If the latter interpretation is correct, the referential meaning is still not clear, since we do not know whether the drinker is sick from drinking or from contracting greater yáng disease. According to the *Yī Zōng Jīn Jiàn*, the patient described in this line is sick not from greater yáng disease, but from excessive consumption of liquor; in other words, no exterior evil is present. According to the other view, which is attributed to Wèi Lì-Tóng (魏荔彤, style 念庭 Niàn-Tíng), the patient is a person given to drinking who has contracted greater yáng disease. Nevertheless, this distinction is not critical from a clinical perspective because the underlying principle of this line is not fundamentally changed by the different interpretations. The key point is that a person given to drinking has a tendency towards interior damp-heat. Cinnamon Twig Decoction (*guì zhī tāng*) is an acrid, sweet formula. Acrid flavors reinforce heat and sweet flavors reinforce dampness. Any patient with interior damp-heat, due to drinking liquor or to other causes, should not be given Cinnamon Twig Decoction (*guì zhī tāng*).

The contraindication stated here, like many others appearing in the *Shāng Hán Lùn*, should not be taken as absolute, but should be considered as a strong caution against using this formula. When a patient with interior damp-heat contracts greater yáng disease and one desires to resolve the exterior through the promotion of sweating, a cool acrid exterior-resolving formula should be given.

LINE 19

凡服桂枝汤吐者，其后必吐脓血也。

Fán fú guì zhī tāng tù zhě, qí hòu bì tù nóng xuè yě.

Whenever taking Cinnamon Twig Decoction (*guì zhī tāng*) [makes the person] vomit, there will be vomiting of pus and blood afterwards.

SYNOPSIS

a) Cinnamon Twig Decoction (*guì zhī tāng*) is not appropriate for use in patterns with interior heat.

b) An example of contraindications for the use of this formula.

COMMENTARY

Vomiting following the ingestion of Cinnamon Twig Decoction (*guì zhī tāng*) means exuberance of interior heat. Cinnamon Twig Decoction (*guì zhī tāng*) is a warm acrid formula, and warm acrid medicinals cannot be given to patients with interior heat since they reinforce yáng, causing exuberant heat and stomach counterflow, which manifest in vomiting. The vomiting of pus and blood following the inappropriate use of Cinnamon Twig Decoction (*guì zhī tāng*) is the result of exuberant heat damaging the blood network vessels. The main point of the line is that Cinnamon Twig Decoction (*guì zhī tāng*) should not be given when there is internal heat.

3.1.3 Concurrent Patterns

Concurrent patterns are those in which the main signs of a pattern are still present, but significant new signs also are observed. The six concurrent patterns related to greater yáng wind strike can be differentiated by formula, as below.

1. Cinnamon Twig Decoction Plus Pueraria (*guì zhī jiā gé gēn tāng*) pattern: Greater yáng wind strike signs plus distinct hypertonicity in the nape and back. This is the simultaneous appearance of greater yáng wind strike (disharmony of the construction and defense) and constrained greater yáng channel qì. The fluids are damaged and cannot moisten and nourish the channels normally. The treatment method is to resolve the fleshy exterior and dispel wind, and engender liquid and soothe channels.
2. Cinnamon Twig Decoction Plus Magnolia Bark and Apricot Kernel (*guì zhī jiā hòu pò xìng zǐ tāng*) pattern: Greater yáng wind strike signs plus panting. It is the simultaneous appearance of greater yáng wind strike and lung cold causing qì counterflow. This pattern can occur through the inappropriate use of precipitation, which allows evil qì to fall inward, distress the lungs, and inhibit downbearing of lung qì. It can also arise when a patient who originally had breathing difficulty contracts an exterior evil, which causes the panting to recur. The treatment method consists in resolving the fleshy exterior and dispelling wind and in downbearing lung qì and stabilizing panting.
3. Cinnamon Twig Decoction Plus Aconite (*guì zhī jiā fù zǐ tāng*) pattern: Greater yáng wind strike signs plus aversion to wind-cold, incessant leaking sweat, hypertonicity of the extremities, and difficult scant urination. Greater yáng wind strike and yáng vacuity simultaneously appear. If sweating is promoted excessively, it damages the defensive yáng and the fluids. The fluids are further depleted through leaking sweat and are unable to nourish the extremities. The treatment method is to support yáng and resolve the exterior.
4. Cinnamon Twig Decoction Minus Peony (*guì zhī qù sháo yào tāng*) pattern: Greater yáng wind strike signs plus fullness in the chest and a pulse that is short and skipping. This pattern is the result of erroneous precipitation. The exterior is not resolved and instead the evil falls into the chest, the chest yáng is devitalized, and the evil qì and right qì contend. The treatment method consists in resolving the fleshy exterior and dispelling wind and in eliminating yīn and freeing yáng.
5. Cinnamon Twig Decoction Minus Peony Plus Aconite (*guì zhī qù sháo yào jiā fù zǐ tāng*) pattern: Greater yáng wind strike signs plus chest fullness, severe aversion to cold, and a pulse that is faint and weak. This pattern is also the result of erroneous precipitation. The exterior is not resolved and the evil falls into the chest; the chest yáng is damaged and the yáng qì is insufficient. The treatment method consists in resolving the fleshy exterior and dispelling wind and in warming the channels and restoring yáng.

6. Cinnamon Twig Decoction Newly Supplemented with One Liǎng Each of Peony and Fresh Ginger and Three Liǎng of Ginseng (*guì zhī jiā sháo yào shēng jiāng gè yī liǎng rén shēn sān liǎng xīn jiā tāng*) pattern: Greater yáng wind strike signs plus generalized pain and a pulse that is sunken and slow. This pattern is caused either by the excessive promotion of sweating, which damages the qì and blood, or by contraction of an exterior evil when qì and blood are insufficient. The treatment method consists in harmonizing construction and defense and boosting the qì.

LINE 14

太阳病，项背强几几，反汗出恶风者，桂枝加葛根汤主之。

Tài yáng bìng, xiàng bèi jiàng shū shū, fǎn hàn chū wù fēng zhě, guì zhī jiā gé gēn tāng zhǔ zhī.

When in greater yáng disease [there is] stretched stiff nape and back,* but also sweating and aversion to wind, it is treated with Cinnamon Twig Decoction Plus Pueraria (*guì zhī jiā gé gēn tāng*).

TEXT NOTE

* Stretched stiff nape and back, 项背强几几 *xiàng bèi jiàng shū shū*: Hypertonicity of the neck and back and discomfort when looking up and down, as if the neck were forcefully stretched, a condition that is considered more severe than simple stiffness and pain in the neck. The reduplication 几几 *shū shū* is said to describe a short-feathered bird stretching its neck to fly but unable to.

FORMULA

Cinnamon Twig Decoction Plus Pueraria (*guì zhī jiā gé gēn tāng*)

○ Resolve the fleshy exterior and expel wind; engender fluids and soothe channels.

葛根四两　麻黄三两（去节）　桂枝二两（去皮）　芍药二两　生姜三两（切）　甘草二两（炙）　大枣十二枚（擘）

右七味，以水一斗，先煮麻黄、葛根，减二升，去上沫，内诸药，煮取三升，去滓，温服一升，覆取微似汗，不须歠粥，余如桂枝法将息及禁忌。

Gé gēn sì liǎng má huáng sān liǎng (qù jié) guì zhī èr liǎng (qù pí) sháo yào èr liǎng shēng jiāng sān liǎng (qiē) gān cǎo èr liǎng (zhì) dà zǎo shí èr méi (bò)

Yòu qī wèi, yǐ shuǐ yī dǒu, xiān zhǔ má huáng、gé gēn jiǎn èr shēng, qù shàng mò, nà zhū yào, zhǔ qǔ sān shēng, qù zǐ, wēn fú yī shēng, fù qǔ wēi sì hàn, bù xū chuò zhōu, yú rú guì zhī fǎ jiāng xī jí jìn jì.

pueraria (葛根 *gé gēn*, Puerariae Radix) 4 liǎng
ephedra (麻黄 *má huáng*, Ephedrae Herba) 3 liǎng (remove nodes)

cinnamon twig (桂枝 *guì zhī*, Cinnamomi Ramulus) 2 liǎng (remove bark)
peony (芍药 *sháo yào*, Paeoniae Radix) 2 liǎng
fresh ginger (生姜 *shēng jiāng*, Zingiberis Rhizoma Recens) 3 liǎng (cut)
mix-fried licorice (甘草 *gān cǎo*, Glycyrrhizae Radix) 2 liǎng
jujube (大枣 *dà zǎo*, Ziziphi Fructus) 12 pieces (broken)

For the preceding seven ingredients use one dǒu of water. First boil ephedra (*má huáng*) and pueraria (*gé gēn*) to reduce [the water] by two shēng. Remove the foam [collecting] on top and add all [the other] ingredients. Boil to get three shēng and remove the dregs. Take one shēng warm. Cover [with bedclothes] to obtain slight sweating. [The patient] does not need to sip gruel. The remainder is as for Cinnamon Twig Decoction (*guì zhī tāng*) [with regard to] rest and contraindications.

SYNOPSIS

The signs and treatment of greater yáng wind strike with inhibited greater yáng channel qì.

COMMENTARY

The use of 反 *fǎn*, "but" in this line suggests an important clinical distinction made between this line and line 31, p. 109. A stretched stiff nape and neck is considered a severe form of the stiff nape mentioned in the outline of greater yáng disease given in line 1, p. 41. It generally occurs in greater yáng cold damage as the result of an evil fettering the exterior to the point that the channel qì is unable to flow smoothly. When the qì does not flow, the fluids cannot moisten and nourish the channels. The presence of sweating, however, means that this is not cold damage, in which sweating is generally absent, but greater yáng wind strike with constrained channel qì. A formula based on Cinnamon Twig Decoction (*guì zhī tāng*) would seem the most likely choice, whereas in line 31, p. 109, in a pattern without sweating, Pueraria Decoction (*gé gēn tāng*), which contains ephedra (*má huáng*), is used. The formula Cinnamon Twig Decoction Plus Pueraria (*guì zhī jiā gé gēn tāng*) is used for the treatment of greater yáng wind strike with constrained greater yáng channel qì. The addition of pueraria (*gé gēn*), which resolves the fleshy exterior, abates heat effusion, upbears yáng, and engenders fluids, seems completely reasonable. Ephedra (*má huáng*), however, also appears in the formula. This inclusion seems unreasonable, since the patient is already sweating. In the Sòng Dynasty version of the *Shāng Hán Lùn*, Lín Yì and his team added the following commentary to this formula:

> We have carefully followed the original text of Zhāng Jī. In greater yáng wind strike with spontaneous sweating, [one should] use Cinnamon Twig [Decoction]. In cold damage without sweating, [one should] use Ephedra [Decoction]. [In this line] the signs are sweating and aversion to wind and the formula contains ephedra (*má huáng*). [We] fear this is not the original idea. The fascicle contains the Pueraria Decoction (*gé gēn tāng*) pattern [with the signs of] absence of sweating and aversion to wind. It is correct to give this formula, since the use of ephedra (*má huáng*) is proper. This says [the name of the formula above is] Cinnamon Twig Decoction Plus Pueraria (*guì zhī jiā gé gēn tāng*), [but] we fear that [the formula of this name should be] Cinnamon Twig Decoction (*guì zhī tāng*) plus only pueraria (*gé gēn*).

Thus, according to this interpretation, the formula should simply be Cinnamon Twig Decoction (*guì zhī tāng*) plus pueraria (*gé gēn*).

LINE 18

喘家作桂枝汤，加厚朴、杏子佳。

Chuǎn jiā zuò guì zhī tāng, jiā hòu pò、xìng zǐ jiā.

For panting patients[1] suffering from[2] Cinnamon Twig Decoction (*guì zhī tāng*) [pattern], it is best to add magnolia bark (*hòu pò*) and apricot kernel (*xìng zǐ*).[3]

TEXT NOTES

1. Panting patients, 喘家 *chuǎn jiā*: Patients ordinarily suffering from panting. Panting is hasty, rapid, labored breathing with discontinuity between inhalation and exhalation and in severe cases with gaping mouth, raised shoulders, flaring nostrils, and inability to lie down.
2. Suffering from a Cinnamon Twig Decoction [pattern], 作桂支汤 *zuò guì zhī tāng*: 作 is here taken to mean 发作 to have an attack of, to be afflicted by. The word "pattern" does not appear in the Chinese.
3. Apricot kernel, 杏子 *xìng zǐ*: An alternate name for apricot kernel (*xìng rén*).

FORMULA

Cinnamon Twig Decoction Plus Magnolia Bark and Apricot Kernel (*guì zhī jiā hòu pò xìng zǐ tāng*)

○ Resolve the fleshy exterior and dispel wind; downbear qì and stabilize panting.

桂枝三两（去皮） 甘草二两（炙） 生姜三两（切） 芍药三两 大枣十二枚（擘） 厚朴二两（炙，去皮） 杏仁五十枚（去皮尖）

右七味，以水七升，微火煮取三升，去滓，温服一升，覆取微似汗。

Guī zhī sān liǎng (qù pí) gān cǎo èr liǎng (zhì) shēng jiāng sān liǎng (qiē) sháo yào sān liǎng dà zǎo shí èr méi (bò) hòu pò èr liǎng (zhì, qù pí) xìng rén wǔ shí méi (qù pí jiān)

Yòu qī wèi, yǐ shuǐ qī shēng, wēi huǒ zhǔ qǔ sān shēng, qù zǐ, wēn fú yī shēng, fù qǔ wēi sì hàn.

cinnamon twig (桂枝 *guì zhī*, Cinnamomi Ramulus) 3 liǎng (remove bark)
mix-fried licorice (甘草 *gān cǎo*, Glycyrrhizae Radix) 2 liǎng
fresh ginger (生姜 *shēng jiāng*, Zingiberis Rhizoma Recens) 3 liǎng (cut)
peony (芍药 *sháo yào*, Paeoniae Radix) 3 liǎng
jujube (大枣 *dà zǎo*, Ziziphi Fructus) 12 pieces (broken)
magnolia bark (厚朴 *hòu pò*, Magnoliae Cortex) 2 liǎng (remove bark and mix-fry[1])

apricot kernel (杏子 *xìng zǐ*, Armeniacae Semen) 50 pieces (remove skin and tips[2])

(1) [For] the above seven ingredients use seven shēng of water. Boil over a mild flame to get three shēng. Remove the dregs and take one shēng, warm. Cover [with bedclothes] to obtain slight sweating.

Formula Notes

1. Magnolia bark (*hòu pò*): "Removing the bark" refers to removing the coarse outer bark. The inner bark is used here. Traditionally, it is mix-fried with fresh ginger (*shēng jiāng*), although it is unclear as to whether that particular process is specified in this case. In the context of the *Shāng Hán Lùn*, what is referred to as mix-frying may simply be dry frying. The frying process moderates the more stimulating nature of the agent; using fresh ginger (*shēng jiāng*) increases its ability to harmonize and warm the center burner.
2. Apricot kernel (*xìng rén*): The tips and the skin are considered to have a powerful effusing and dissipating action; therefore they are generally removed for clinical use. This agent is fried in order to increase its ability to warm the lung and dissipate cold. This process reduces the oil and increases the efficacy for diffusing the lung, eliminating phlegm, and stabilizing panting. Frying is done by placing the agent in a metal pan and lightly stir frying until the color changes to a deep yellow or slightly burnt appearance.

Synopsis

The treatment of panting, when it is an abiding ailment that is caused to recur by contraction of an exterior wind-cold pattern.

Commentary

This line describes a situation in which a patient who ordinarily has some breathing difficulty contracts wind-cold, giving rise to Cinnamon Twig Decoction (*guì zhī tāng*) greater yáng wind strike pattern, manifesting in panting respiration, heat effusion, sweating, aversion to wind, headache, and a pulse that is floating and moderate. The pathomechanism is one of wind-cold distressing the lungs, causing lung cold and qì counterflow and impaired diffusion and downbearing of the lung, manifesting in panting. Magnolia bark (*hòu pò*) and apricot kernel (*xìng zǐ*) are bitter, acrid, and warm medicinals that diffuse the lung and disinhibit qì. Cinnamon Twig Decoction (*guì zhī tāng*) with the addition of these two medicinals resolves the flesh and dispels wind, and downbears qì and stabilizes panting.

Rather than using the customary "govern" (主 *zhǔ*), here it is written that "it is best" (佳 *jiā*), to add magnolia bark (*hòu pò*) and apricot kernel (*xìng zǐ*) since the addition of these two medicinals treats only the present pattern; it does not eradicate the patient's panting problem.

Line 43

太阳病，下之微喘者，表未解故也，桂枝加厚朴杏子汤主之。

Tài yáng bìng, xià zhī wēi chuǎn zhě, biǎo wèi jiě gù yě, guì zhī jiā hòu pò xìng zǐ tāng zhǔ zhī.

When in greater yáng disease, [there is] mild panting following precipitation, it means that the exterior has not resolved; [therefore,] Cinnamon Twig Decoction Plus Magnolia Bark and Apricot Kernel (*guì zhī jiā hòu pò xìng zǐ tāng*) governs.

Synopsis

The treatment of panting that is the result of lung qì counterflow ascent, which occurs after the inappropriate use of precipitation, when the exterior evil has not resolved.

Commentary

A comparison between this line and the preceding line is instructive. In this line, greater yáng wind strike is not treated by promotion of sweating in the proper way. Instead, it is inappropriately treated by precipitation, which causes the patient to pant, because the exterior evil is forced into the lung, giving rise to dual disease of the exterior and interior. In the previous line, panting in a patient who ordinarily tends to suffer from panting, is induced by the contraction of an exterior evil. Both lines describe cases of greater yáng disease with panting. Although their pathomechanisms, signs, and treatment are the same, the cause and history are different.

Inappropriate precipitation often causes the disease to enter the interior, and, in such cases, all exterior signs disappear; therefore, promotion of sweating is no longer appropriate. This line, however, describes a case in which inappropriate precipitation has given rise to dual disease of the interior and exterior, with the continuing presence of exterior signs. For this reason, promotion of sweating is still appropriate, albeit with the addition of Magnolia bark (*hòu pò*) and apricot kernel (*xìng zǐ*) to diffuse the lung and disinhibit qì.

Line 20

太阳病，发汗，遂漏不止，其人恶风，小便难，四肢微急，难以屈伸者，桂枝加附子汤主之。

Tài yáng bìng, fā hàn, suì lòu bù zhǐ, qí rén wù fēng, xiǎo biàn nán, sì zhī wēi jí, nán yǐ qū shēn zhě, guì zhī jiā fù zǐ tāng zhǔ zhī.

When in greater yáng disease, sweating is promoted and then gives way to incessant leaking,* the person is averse to wind, has difficult urination, and the limbs are slightly tensed so that they bend and stretch with difficulty, Cinnamon Twig Decoction Plus Aconite (*guì zhī jiā fù zǐ tāng*) governs.

TEXT NOTE

* Sweating is promoted and then gives way to incessant leaking, 发汗，遂漏不止 *fā hàn, suì lòu bù zhǐ*: Sweating that fails to run a normal course and develops into an incessant flow of a small amount of sweat. This kind of sweating is now called "leaking sweat" (漏汗 *lòu hàn*).

FORMULA

Cinnamon Twig Decoction Plus Aconite (*guì zhī jiā fù zǐ tāng*)

○ Support yáng and resolve the exterior. (Harmonize construction and defense; supplement yáng and constrain sweat.)

桂枝三两（去皮） 芍药三两 甘草三两（炙） 生姜三两（切） 大枣十二枚（擘） 附子一枚（炮，去皮，破八片）

(一) 右六味，以水七升，煮取三升，去滓，温服一升。(二) 本云，桂枝汤，今加附子。(三) 将息如前法。

Guì zhī sān liǎng (qù pí) sháo yào sān liǎng gān cǎo sān liǎng (zhì) shēng jiāng sān liǎng (qiē) dà zǎo shí èr méi (bò) fù zǐ yī méi (pào, qù pí, pò bā piàn)

(1) *Yòu liù wèi, yǐ shuǐ qī shēng, zhǔ qǔ sān shēng, qù zǐ, wēn fú yī shēng.* (2) *Běn yún: guì zhī tāng, jīn jiā fù zǐ.* (3) *Jiāng xī rú qián fǎ.*

cinnamon twig (桂枝 *guì zhī*, Cinnamomi Ramulus) 3 liǎng (remove bark)
peony (芍药 *sháo yào*, Paeoniae Radix) 3 liǎng
mix-fried licorice (甘草 *gān cǎo*, Glycyrrhizae Radix) 3 liǎng
fresh ginger (生姜 *shēng jiāng*, Zingiberis Rhizoma Recens) 3 liǎng (cut)
jujube (大枣 *dà zǎo*, Ziziphi Fructus) 12 pieces (broken)
aconite (附子 *fù zǐ*, Aconiti Tuber Laterale) 1 piece (blast-fry, remove skin, break into eight pieces*)

(1) [For] the above six ingredients, use seven shēng of water. Boil to get three shēng, remove the dregs and take one shēng, warm. (2) [This is] Cinnamon Twig Decoction (*guì zhī tāng*) with the addition of aconite (*fù zǐ*). (3) One should rest [as described] in the method [for Cinnamon Twig Decoction (*guì zhī tāng*)].

FORMULA NOTE

* Aconite (*fù zǐ*): Blast-frying involves stir-frying vigorously in an iron wok over a fierce fire until the medicinal smokes and the surface becomes scorched, swollen, and cracked. Medicinals are blast-fried to reduce harshness and toxicity.

SYNOPSIS

The clinical manifestation and treatment of a greater yáng disease pattern in which excessive sweating is promoted, leading to yáng vacuity leaking sweat and an unresolved exterior pattern.

COMMENTARY

In greater yáng disease, the promotion of sweating is the treatment of choice. Nevertheless, excessive promotion of sweating is clearly inappropriate. One may refer back to the directions for Cinnamon Twig Decoction (*guì zhī tāng*) in which the decoction is to be taken: "... until the body is moist, as if sweating very lightly... One cannot allow [the patient to sweat] like water flowing. The disease will not be eliminated [this way]." When sweating is promoted excessively, it damages both yáng qì and yīn liquid. Leaking sweat means that the yáng qì has been damaged, and vacuous exterior yáng on the one hand fails to check the flow of sweat, and on the other fails to warm and secure the exterior, so that there is aversion to wind. These signs, when analyzed in the light of the formula, indicate yáng vacuity, but difficult urination and slight tension of the sinews indicate that yīn liquid has also been damaged. However, although yīn liquid is depleted, the treatment does not address this directly. The treatment method is primarily that of supporting yáng, and secondarily resolving the exterior. This is because with the restoration of yáng qì and resolution of the exterior evil, the exterior will be secure, sweating will stop, and yīn liquid will be engendered. Once yīn liquid is sufficient, the other signs will resolve spontaneously. The formula, Cinnamon Twig Decoction Plus Aconite (*guì zhī jiā fù zǐ tāng*), is simply Cinnamon Twig Decoction (*guì zhī tāng*) plus aconite (*fù zǐ*), which can be used either raw or blast-fried. Raw, it returns yáng and stems counterflow. Blast-fried, it warms the channels and restores yáng. In this formula, blast-fried aconite (*fù zǐ*) is used in order to secure the exterior and check sweating. This addition to Cinnamon Twig Decoction (*guì zhī tāng*) eliminates the evil and returns yáng so that liquid and humor are spontaneously restored.

LINE 21

太阳病，下之后，脉促，胸满者，桂枝去芍药汤主之。

Tài yáng bìng, xià zhī hòu, mài cù, xiōng mǎn zhě, guì zhī qù sháo yào tāng zhǔ zhī.

In greater yáng disease, when after precipitation the pulse is skipping* and [there is] fullness in the chest, Cinnamon Twig Decoction Minus Peony (*guì zhī qù sháo yào tāng*) governs.

TEXT NOTE

* Skipping, 脉促 *mài cù*: Urgent and forceful. It does not here mean rapid and periodically interrupted, as it does in modern texts. See the Introduction for a further discussion of this issue.

FORMULA

Cinnamon Twig Decoction Minus Peony (*guì zhī qù sháo yào tāng*)

○ Resolve the fleshy exterior and expel wind; eliminate yīn and free yáng.

桂枝三两（去皮） 甘草二两（炙） 生姜三两（切） 大枣十二枚（擘）

(一) 右四味，以水七升，煮取三升，去滓，温服一升。(二) 本云，桂枝汤，今去芍药。(三) 将息如前法。

Guì zhī sān liǎng (qù pí) gān cǎo èr liǎng (zhì) shēng jiāng sān liǎng (qiē) dà zǎo shí èr méi (bò)

(1) *Yòu sì wèi, yǐ shuǐ qī shēng, zhǔ qǔ sān shēng, qù zǐ, wēn fú yī shēng.* (2) *Běn yún: guì zhī tāng, jīn qù sháo yào.* (3) *Jiāng xī rú qián fǎ.*

cinnamon twig (桂枝 *guì zhī*, Cinnamomi Ramulus) 3 liǎng (remove bark)
mix-fried licorice (甘草 *gān cǎo*, Glycyrrhizae Radix) 2 liǎng
fresh ginger (生姜 *shēng jiāng*, Zingiberis Rhizoma Recens) 3 liǎng (cut)
jujube (大枣 *dà zǎo*, Ziziphi Fructus) 12 pieces (broken)

(1) [For] the above four ingredients, use seven shēng of water. Boil to get three shēng, remove the dregs and take one shēng, warm. (2) This is Cinnamon Twig Decoction (*guì zhī tāng*) [after] removing peony (*sháo yào*). (3) One should rest [as described] in the previous method [for Cinnamon Twig Decoction (*guì zhī tāng*)].

SYNOPSIS

The distinguishing features and treatment of a greater yáng disease pattern, in which, after the inappropriate use of precipitation, the exterior pattern is unresolved and the chest yáng is devitalized.

COMMENTARY

In greater yáng disease the appropriate treatment is exterior resolution, not precipitation. Here, after precipitation, the pulse becomes skipping and fullness in the chest is observed. We also know that Cinnamon Twig Decoction (*guì zhī tāng*) is still used, but without peony (*sháo yào*). In general, when precipitation is used in cases of an exterior evil, one expects that the evil will fall into the interior. The following interpretations of this pathomechanism are given:

Chéng Wú-Jǐ states, "In greater yáng disease, [after] precipitation, [when] the pulse is skipping and [there is] no chest bind, this means [the disease] is about to resolve. Here, [after] precipitation, the pulse is skipping and also [there is] fullness in the chest. This means that [the disease] is not about to resolve. [In this case] after precipitation yáng vacuity [exists], the exterior evil gradually enters [the interior] and [this] visiting [evil] is in the chest. Give Cinnamon Twig Decoction (*guì zhī tāng*) in order to dissipate the visiting evil and free the yáng qì. Peony (*sháo yào*) boosts yīn, and [when there is] yáng vacuity it is not appropriate, so it is removed."

Kē Qín presents the view that "[When] yáng is exuberant, [the pulse may be] skipping.... After precipitation, a pulse that is skipping, [accompanied by] absence of sweating, fullness in the chest and absence of panting, does not [indicate] exuberant yáng, [but indicates] a cold evil bound in the interior."

In contrast, Chén Niàn-Zǔ (陈念祖, style 修园 Xiū-Yuán) explains that fullness in the chest represents qì stagnation in the chest.

Thus these three authors present three different interpretations: yáng vacuity with an evil falling into the chest, cold evil bound in the interior, and qì stagnation in the chest. These commentators agree that in exterior diseases, since the right and evil are in contention, the use of precipitation will cause right qì to be damaged and evil qì to fall inward. After this, the transmutations and pathomechanisms can be explained differently. The formula reveals several key points. The first is that this is still considered an exterior condition, so Cinnamon Twig Decoction (*guì zhī tāng*) is used. The second is that the movement in the chest is impaired, so cinnamon twig (*guì zhī*), which warms the channels and frees yáng, is used to open the chest and resolve the chest fullness. Peony (*sháo yào*) is not used because not only does it boost yīn, but it also promotes contraction, and if used in this situation, would prevent the evil from moving out of the chest.

LINE 22

若微寒者，桂枝去芍药加附子汤主之。

Ruò wēi hán zhě, guì zhī qù sháo yào jiā fù zǐ tāng zhǔ zhī.

When [the pulse is] faint and [there is aversion to] cold,* Cinnamon Twig Decoction Minus Peony Plus Aconite (*guì zhī qù sháo yào jiā fù zǐ tāng*) governs.

TEXT NOTE

* [The pulse is] faint and [there is aversion to] cold, 微寒 *wēi hán*: For a discussion of the interpretation of this phrase, see the commentary below.

FORMULA

Cinnamon Twig Decoction Minus Peony Plus Aconite (*guì zhī qù sháo yào jiā fù zǐ tāng*)

○ Resolve the fleshy exterior and expel wind; warm the channels and restore yáng.

桂枝三两（去皮） 甘草二两（炙） 生姜三两（切） 大枣十二枚（擘） 附子一枚（炮，去皮，破八片）

(一) 右五味，以水七升，煮取三升，去滓，温服一升。(二) 本云，桂枝汤，今去芍药加附子。(三) 将息如前法。

Guì zhī sān liǎng (qù pí) gān cǎo èr liǎng (zhì) shēng jiāng sān liǎng (qiē) dà zǎo shí èr méi (bò) fù zǐ yī méi (pào, qù pí, pò bā piàn)

(1) *Yòu wǔ wèi, yǐ shuǐ qī shēng, zhǔ qǔ sān shēng, qù zǐ, wēn fú yī shēng.* (2) *Běn yún: guì zhī tāng, jīn qù sháo yào jiā fù zǐ.* (3) *Jiāng xī rú qián fǎ.*

cinnamon twig (桂枝 *guì zhī*, Cinnamomi Ramulus) 3 liǎng (remove bark)
mix-fried licorice (甘草 *gān cǎo*, Glycyrrhizae Radix) 2 liǎng
fresh ginger (生姜 *shēng jiāng*, Zingiberis Rhizoma Recens) 3 liǎng (cut)
jujube (大枣 *dà zǎo*, Ziziphi Fructus) 12 pieces (broken)
aconite (附子 *fù zǐ*, Aconiti Tuber Laterale) 1 piece (blast-fry, remove skin, break into eight pieces)

(1) [For] the above five ingredients, use seven shēng of water. Boil to get three shēng, remove the dregs and take one shēng, warm. (2) This is Cinnamon Twig Decoction (*guì zhī tāng*) with the addition of aconite (*fù zǐ*) and without peony (*sháo yào*). (3) One should rest [as described] in the previous method [for Cinnamon Twig Decoction (*guì zhī tāng*)].

Synopsis

Continuing from the previous line, the treatment of a greater yáng disease pattern in which, after the inappropriate use of precipitation, the exterior pattern is unresolved and chest yáng is damaged.

Commentary

The three characters that begin this line have generated a great deal of controversy amongst scholars. The phrase 若微寒 *ruò wēi hán* is literally taken to mean "if [the patient] is slightly cold," i.e., suffering from slight aversion to cold, and this interpretation has been offered. Shěn Míng-Zōng (沈明宗) considers this line to be a continuation of the previous line and writes, "If the pulse is skipping and [there is] fullness in the chest and slight aversion to cold, this indicates vacuity and [the yáng qì] is hampered and about to desert... Remove peony (*sháo yào*) and add aconite (*fù zǐ*) to protect and secure the true yáng."

Nevertheless, it is difficult to rationalize the use of aconite (*fù zǐ*) with a patient whose only sign is mild aversion to cold. Chén Niàn-Zǔ also makes a connection between these two lines, but comes to a different conclusion based on the interpretation of 微寒 *wēi hán* as a pulse that is faint and aversion to cold: "After erroneous precipitation in greater yáng disease, the yáng qì is debilitated and cannot move inward or outward... if the pulse is not skipping, [but] is faint and [there is] aversion to cold, it means yáng vacuity is already extreme... [There is] fear that the strength of cinnamon [twig] and [fresh] ginger is [too] mild and one must assist with aconite (*fù zǐ*)."

According to Chén Niàn-Zǔ, after erroneous precipitation of greater yáng disease, the pulse is faint and aversion to cold and fullness in the chest are present, indicating extreme vacuity of yáng; therefore, aconite (*fù zǐ*) is used. Comparing Cinnamon Twig Decoction Minus Peony (*guì zhī qù sháo yào tāng*) from the previous line with Cinnamon Twig Decoction Minus Peony Plus Aconite (*guì zhī qù sháo yào jiā fù zǐ tāng*) in this line, one finds that although both formulae resolve the fleshy exterior and dispel wind, the previous formula emphasizes freeing the chest yáng, while the current formula emphasizes restoring yáng. The previous formula is used when the chest yáng is depressed and stagnant, while the current formula is used when the yáng qì is insufficient. A comparison of these two formulae illustrates that a difference of even one ingredient can completely alter the main action of a formula.

All three interpretations rest on the notion that the vacuity of yáng qì is severe, even if 微寒 *wēi hán* is taken to mean slight aversion to cold, since aconite (*fù zǐ*) is used. However, the authors of the *Gāo Děng Cóng Shū* believe that 微寒 *wēi hán* should be interpreted as "a pulse that is faint and aversion to cold," and suggests that the original may have read 脉微恶寒 *mài wēi wù hán*.

Line 62

发汗后，身疼痛，脉沉迟者，桂枝加芍药生姜各一两人参三两新加汤主之。

Fā hàn hòu, shēn téng tòng, mài chén chí zhě, guì zhī jiā sháo yào shēng jiāng gè yì liǎng rén shēn sān liǎng xīn jiā tāng zhǔ zhī.

When after the promotion of sweating, [there is] generalized pain, and a pulse that is sunken and slow, Cinnamon Twig Decoction Newly Supplemented with One Liǎng Each of Peony and Fresh Ginger and Three Liǎng of Ginseng (*guì zhī jiā sháo yào shēng jiāng gè yī liǎng rén shēn sān liǎng xīn jiā tāng*) governs.

Formula

Cinnamon Twig Decoction Newly Supplemented with One Liǎng Each of Peony and Fresh Ginger and Three Liǎng of Ginseng (*guì zhī jiā sháo yào shēng jiāng gè yī liǎng rén shēn sān liǎng xīn jiā tāng*)

∘ Harmonize construction and defense; boost qì and harmonize construction.

桂枝三两（去皮） 芍药四两 甘草二两（炙） 人参三两 大枣十二枚（擘） 生姜四两

㈠ 右六味，以水一斗二升，煮取三升，去滓，温服一升。㈡ 本云，桂枝汤，今加芍药、生姜、人参。

Guì zhī sān liǎng (qù pí) sháo yào sì liǎng gān cǎo èr liǎng (zhì) rén shēn sān liǎng dà zǎo shí èr méi (bò) shēng jiāng sì liǎng (qiē)

(1) *Yòu liù wèi, yǐ shuǐ yī dǒu èr shēng, zhǔ qǔ sān shēng, qù zǐ, wēn fú yī shēng.* (2) *Běn yún: guì zhī tāng, jīn jiā sháo yào、shēng jiāng、rén shēn.*

cinnamon twig (桂枝 *guì zhī*, Cinnamomi Ramulus) 3 liǎng (remove bark)
peony (芍药 *sháo yào*, Paeoniae Radix) 4 liǎng
mix-fried licorice (甘草 *gān cǎo*, Glycyrrhizae Radix) 2 liǎng
ginseng (人参 *rén shēn*, Ginseng Radix) 3 liǎng
jujube (大枣 *dà zǎo*, Ziziphi Fructus) 12 pieces (broken)
fresh ginger (生姜 *shēng jiāng*, Zingiberis Rhizoma Recens) 4 liǎng (cut)

(1) [For] the above six ingredients use one dǒu and two shēng of water. Boil to get three shēng, remove the dregs and take one shēng, warm. (2) This is Cinnamon Twig Decoction (*guì zhī tāng*) with extra peony (*sháo yào*), fresh ginger (*shēng jiāng*), and ginseng (*rén shēn*).

Synopsis

The distinguishing features and treatment of generalized pain that is the result of damage to the qì and construction, following the issuing of sweat.

Commentary

This apparently simple line conveys important information about disease transmutation and treatment. Generalized pain is a primary sign of exterior diseases, which are generally resolved through the promotion of sweating. Here, sweating has been promoted, but the generalized pain is still present, suggesting that this sign no longer simply indicates exterior disease. It means that the construction qì has been damaged through the promotion of sweating and is unable to nourish the sinews. Furthermore, the pulse has changed and is no longer floating. A pulse that is sunken and slow here indicates insufficiency of qì and blood. By analyzing the formula, the signs, and the pulse, one can infer that sweating was promoted excessively and both yáng qì and yīn humor have been damaged. The construction and defense are in disharmony, the exterior disease has not resolved and the yáng qì and yīn humor are insufficient.

This pattern is simultaneous exterior-interior disease, but the internal damage is more severe than the exterior evil, so treatment involves supporting right and dispelling evil simultaneously, with emphasis on the former, using Cinnamon Twig Decoction Newly Supplemented with One Liǎng Each of Peony and Fresh Ginger and Three Liǎng of Ginseng (*guì zhī jiā sháo yào shēng jiāng gè yī liǎng rén shēn sān liǎng xīn jiā tāng*). This formula is Cinnamon Twig Decoction (*guì zhī tāng*) with ginseng (*rén shēn*). Ginseng (*rén shēn*) supplements the qì and engenders fluids. It supports right qì so that harmony may be restored and is often used when excessive sweating has damaged the yáng qì and yīn humor. Cinnamon Twig Decoction (*guì zhī tāng*) restores harmony to the defense and construction, mildly promotes sweating, and will resolve the exterior disease. A larger dose of peony (*sháo yào*) is used to supplement the damaged yīn and nourish blood. Fresh ginger (*shēng jiāng*) is also used in a larger dose to diffuse and free the yáng qì.

3.2 Cold Damage Exterior Repletion Patterns

The primary signs and pulse of cold damage exterior repletion are heat effusion (which may or may not be present in the early stages of the illness), aversion to cold, generalized pain, absence of sweating, panting, and a pulse that is floating and tight. In the *Shāng Hán Lùn* these patterns are referred to simply as cold damage.

The distinguishing feature of the pathomechanism of cold damage is that a cold evil fetters the exterior, blocking the defense and depressing the construction. Obstruction of the defense yáng causes aversion to cold and the struggle between defense yáng and exterior evil causes heat effusion; therefore, it is common for these two signs to occur simultaneously. When heat effusion does not occur, it is a sign that defense yáng has been severely obstructed and cannot yet struggle with the cold evil. This is temporary and should quickly give way to heat effusion. It should be noted that aversion to cold and aversion to wind are not criteria for differentiating wind strike and cold damage. These two signs differ primarily in degree of severity, with aversion to cold being more severe, and can both appear in either of the patterns. When defense yáng is blocked and construction-yīn is depressed, the sinews and bones are not warmed and moistened; consequently, the patient experiences generalized and joint pain. The interstices are blocked by the cold evil and no sweat can issue. When right qì rises to the exterior to combat the evil, the pulse becomes floating and tight. Because the lungs are in charge of breathing and the opening and closing of the interstices, when an evil fetters the exterior, the interstices are unable to diffuse properly and the lung qì becomes inhibited, giving rise to panting. In cold damage, the interstices of the flesh are blocked, there is absence of sweating, and right qì is relatively strong; therefore, this pattern is also called an "exterior repletion pattern." In greater yáng exterior repletion patterns, treatment focuses on the promotion of sweating in order to open the interstices of the flesh, and Ephedra Decoction (*má huáng tāng*) is the representative formula.

3.2.1 Ephedra Decoction Pattern

This section describes the characteristic signs of Ephedra Decoction (*má huáng tāng*) patterns. The main signs are aversion to wind and cold, heat effusion, stiffness and pain of the head and nape, generalized pain, lumbar pain, joint pain, absence of sweating, a floating tight or floating rapid pulse, and possibly panting or retching counterflow. In these patterns, right qì is generally strong and able to contend with the evil. After contraction of an external wind-cold evil that fetters the exterior, the defensive yáng is restrained, the construction-yīn is depressed and stagnant, the channel qì is inhibited, and right qì contends with evil qì. The evil may interfere with the lungs and stomach. The treatment method is to resolve the exterior with acridity and warmth, promote sweating, diffuse the lung, and stabilize panting. The main formula is Ephedra Decoction (*má huáng tāng*).

Ephedra Decoction (*má huáng tāng*) is appropriate for the treatment of the following conditions:

a) enduring greater yáng cold damage with unresolved exterior repletion;
b) greater yáng cold damage in which sweating has not yet been promoted and as a result nosebleed occurs and the exterior signs are still present; and
c) greater yáng and yáng brightness combination disease in which the greater yáng signs are more severe, with panting and chest fullness as the main manifestations.

Line 35

太阳病，头痛发热，身疼腰痛，骨节疼痛，恶风，无汗而喘者，麻黄汤主之。

Tài yáng bìng, tóu tòng fā rè, shēn téng yāo tòng, gǔ jié téng tòng, wù fēng, wú hàn ér chuǎn zhě, má huáng tāng zhǔ zhī.

When in greater yáng disease [there is] headache, heat effusion, generalized pain,* lumbar pain, joint pain, aversion to wind, absence of sweating, and panting, Ephedra Decoction (*má huáng tāng*) governs.

Text Note

* Generalized pain, 身疼 *shēn téng*: This term can mean the whole body or only the trunk. The translation "generalized pain" is intended to cover both these ideas. Terms like "body pain" seem to suggest the trunk, as opposed to the

limbs. Clearly, in some cases, a distinction can be drawn between different body areas. Unfortunately, this is often unclear and 身 *shēn* may include the limbs.

Formula

Ephedra Decoction (*má huáng tāng*)

∘ Promote sweating with acridity and warmth; diffuse the lung and stabilize panting.

麻黄三两（去节） 桂枝二两（去皮） 甘草一两（炙） 杏仁七十个（去皮尖）

(一) 右四味，以水九升，先煮麻黄，减二升，去上沫，内诸药，煮取二升半，去滓，温服八合。(二) 覆取微似汗，不须歠粥。(三) 余如桂枝法将息。

Má huáng sān liǎng (qù jié) guì zhī èr liáng (qù pí) gān cǎo yī liǎng (zhì) xìng rén qī shí gè (qù pí jiān)

(1) *Yòu sì wèi, yǐ shuǐ jiǔ shēng, xiān zhǔ má huang, jiǎn èr sheng, qù shàng mò, nà zhū yào, zhǔ qǔ èr shēng bàn, qù zǐ, wēn fú bā gě.* (2) *Fù qǔ wēi sì hàn, bù xū chuò zhōu.* (3) *Yú rú guì zhī fǎ jiāng xī.*

ephedra (麻黄 *má huáng*, Ephedrae Herba) 3 liǎng (remove nodes*)
cinnamon twig (桂枝 *guì zhī*, Cinnamomi Ramulus) 2 liǎng (remove bark)
mix-fried licorice (甘草 *gān cǎo*, Glycyrrhizae Radix) 1 liǎng
apricot kernel (杏仁 *xìng rén*, Armeniacae Semen) 70 pieces (remove skin and tips)

(1) [For] the above four ingredients use nine shēng of water. First boil ephedra (*má huáng*) to reduce [the water] by two shēng. Remove the foam [collecting] on top and add all the ingredients. Boil to get two and a half shēng, remove the dregs and take eight gě warm. (2) Cover [with bedclothes] to obtain mild sweating. It is not necessary to eat rice gruel [with the decoction]. (3) [One should] rest and [follow] the remainder of the directions as for Cinnamon Twig Decoction (*guì zhī tāng*).

Formula Note

* Ephedra (*má huáng*): According to the traditional understanding, for which laboratory tests have found no supporting evidence, the nodes of ephedra (*má huáng*) can check sweating and are therefore removed when this medicinal is used to promote sweating. The foam produced when ephedra (*má huáng*) is boiled is traditionally removed because it is thought to cause vexation.

Synopsis

The distinguishing features and treatment of greater yáng cold damage patterns.

Commentary

This line discusses greater yáng cold damage. Although the term "cold damage" does not appear in the text, we know that this is cold damage because Ephedra Decoction (*má huáng tāng*) is suggested. From this line and lines 1 and 3, the signs of greater yáng cold damage are seen to include heat effusion or as yet no heat effusion, aversion to wind or cold, absence of sweating, and headache, as well as pain and stiffness in the back of the neck, generalized pain, lumbar pain, joint pain, panting, and a pulse that is floating and tight. Of all these, the key sign is absence of sweating since, by indicating exterior repletion, it is the chief sign differentiating greater yáng cold damage from greater yáng wind strike. Sweating fails to occur when evil qì is strong and the patient's right qì is also strong. The right and evil qì contend and right qì cannot push out evil qì, which becomes lodged in the exterior and obstructs the outward movement of sweat. Headache, and pain and stiffness in the back of the neck, generalized pain, lumbar pain, and joint pain, occur when the evil, which is lodged in the exterior, inhibits the greater yáng channel qì. Panting occurs when the evil interferes with the lung, impairing lung diffusion and downbearing.

The basic pulse of greater yáng cold damage is tight and floating. However, this pulse is not generally considered absolutely essential for the identification of cold damage, and, in fact, it is not mentioned in this line. The following two lines describe patterns treated with Ephedra Decoction (*má huáng tāng*), in which the pulse is floating but not tight.

Ephedra Decoction (*má huáng tāng*) contains acrid, warm ephedra (*má huáng*), which promotes sweating, diffuses the lung, and stabilizes panting. Cinnamon twig (*guì zhī*) resolves and dissipates wind and cold and assists ephedra (*má huáng*) in the promotion of sweating. Apricot kernel (*xìng rén*) diffuses and downbears lung qì, thereby increasing the panting-stabilizing strength of ephedra (*má huáng*). Licorice (*gān cǎo*) harmonizes all the ingredients. Two aspects of the preparation method illustrate important points. Ephedra (*má huáng*) is cooked for a long time, moderating its ability to promote sweating and aiding in the prevention of excess sweating. The patient is not advised to eat rice gruel with the formula, although he/she is still advised to cover up with bedclothes. By contrast, Cinnamon Twig Decoction (*guì zhī tāng*) is designed for patients with weakness in construction and strength in defense; therefore eating rice gruel helps the formula to produce sweating, to boost the source of sweat, and to prevent excessive damage to right. In patients taking Ephedra Decoction (*má huáng tāng*) defense qì is obstructed, construction-yīn is depressed, and right is struggling with evil; there is no weakness in construction and therefore supplementation with rice gruel is unnecessary. Note that even in repletion patients, one can still damage the yáng qì by promoting sweating too harshly.

This line speaks not of "aversion to cold," which one would expect in a pattern treated with Ephedra Decoction (*má huáng tāng*), but of "aversion to wind" (see line 2, p. 41).

LINE 51

脉浮者，病在表，可发汗，宜麻黄汤。

Mài fú zhě, bìng zài biǎo, kě fā hàn, yí má huáng tāng.

When the pulse is floating, the disease is in the exterior, [and if] one can promote sweating, Ephedra Decoction (*má huáng tāng*) is appropriate.

SYNOPSIS

Using the pulse to represent the pattern, when disease is in the greater yáng and the promotion of sweating is appropriate, one can choose Ephedra Decoction (*má huáng tāng*).

COMMENTARY

A pulse that is floating as an indication of exterior disease is one that can be easily felt with light pressure and that is felt less distinctly, but not empty, when heavy pressure is applied. A pulse that is floating may also occur in internal damage miscellaneous disease manifesting in vacuity patterns, but in such cases, it feels empty when heavy pressure is applied.

This line tells us that a pulse that is floating indicates disease of the exterior, which is treated by promoting sweating with Ephedra Decoction (*má huáng tāng*). From our understanding of other lines of the *Shāng Hán Lùn*, however, we know that not all exterior patterns are treated by promoting sweating with this formula. Ephedra Decoction (*má huáng tāng*) is only used for greater yáng cold damage, which is characterized by absence of sweating with other greater yáng signs and usually a pulse that is floating and tight. As Chéng Yìng-Máo says, "If [there is] absence of sweating, sweating can be promoted, and Ephedra Decoction (*má huáng tāng*) is appropriate."

For more information about Ephedra Decoction (*má huáng tāng*) pattern, see line 3, p. 44, and line 35, p. 91.

LINE 52

脉浮而数者，可发汗，宜麻黄汤。

Mài fú ér shuò zhě, kě fā hàn, yí má huáng tāng.

When the pulse is floating and rapid, [if] one can promote sweating, Ephedra Decoction (*má huáng tāng*) is appropriate.

SYNOPSIS

In a greater yáng cold damage pattern, when the pulse is floating and rapid, it is still appropriate to use Ephedra Decoction (*má huáng tāng*).

COMMENTARY

This line is similar in structure to the previous line, describing an Ephedra Decoction (*má huáng tāng*) pattern with very little detail. However, unlike the previous line, it describes a specific pulse condition—floating and rapid. Because Ephedra Decoction (*má huáng tāng*) is prescribed, we conclude that this is greater yáng cold damage. In cold damage, a pulse that is floating and rapid is not normally expected. However, heat effusion can occur in cold damage, and when the body temperature rises, the pulse can become rapid. Thus, this line appears to be pointing out that a pulse that is floating and rapid may be observed in greater yáng cold damage. One must not be misled by only observing the pulse description that this is wind-warmth or a heat pattern; one should evaluate the signs as a whole.

LINE 37

(一) 太阳病，十日以去，脉浮细而嗜卧者，外已解也。(二) 设胸满胁痛者，与小柴胡汤；脉但浮者，与麻黄汤。

(1) *Tài yáng bìng, shí rì yǐ qù, mài fú xì ér shì wò zhě, wài yǐ jiě yě.* (2) *Shè xiōng mǎn xié tòng zhě, yǔ xiǎo chái hú tāng; mài dàn fú zhě, yǔ má huáng tāng.*

(1) When in greater yáng disease, after ten days have passed, the pulse is floating and fine, and [there is] somnolence,* the outer body has already resolved. (2) If [there is] fullness in the chest and rib-side pain, give Minor Bupleurum Decoction (*xiǎo chái hú tāng*); if the pulse is floating only, give Ephedra Decoction (*má huáng tāng*).

TEXT NOTE

* Somnolence, 嗜卧 *shì wò*: The Chinese term literally means "to like sleeping." In this context, the implication is that the patient tends to rest quietly and sleep, in order to regain his physical strength.

SYNOPSIS

Three possible scenarios that can occur in a patient with enduring greater yáng disease.

COMMENTARY

When a greater yáng disease has lasted for ten days or more and signs of exterior repletion are still observed, Ephedra Decoction (*má huáng tāng*) is still appropriate. In this line, a pulse that is described as "only floating" indicates an exterior repletion pattern, as in line 51, p. 93. This line emphasizes that no matter how long the disease has lasted, one can still use Ephedra Decoction (*má huáng tāng*). If the pattern has not changed, the treatment need not change. Only when the pattern has changed must one adjust the treatment accordingly.

Three developments are described in this line. In the first, which is described above, the exterior repletion pattern is still present.

The second is that the patient, after ten days or more of a greater yáng disease, has a tendency to sleep. This sign indicates recovery and should not be interpreted as a sign of vacuity. Because Zhāng Jī states that the exterior has resolved, we know that somnolence, here, indicates the evil has been eliminated, and right qì is not struggling with the evil any longer but has not yet been restored. In this situation, the patient tends to sleep in order to regain his or her strength. Whenever somnolence appears, one must investigate the pulse and all signs, since it does not necessarily mean that the patient is recovering. (See, for example, desire only to sleep as a manifestation of yáng vacuity in lesser yīn disease, line 282, p. 471.) A pulse that is floating and fine accords with this, since a pulse that is floating indicates that the evil has not entered the interior, and a pulse that is fine means that evil qì has abated, but right qì has not yet been restored.

The third development is that the evil has shifted into the lesser yáng. This transmutation is indicated by the presence of fullness in the chest and rib-side pain. Minor Bupleurum Decoction (*xiǎo chái hú tāng*) constitutes appropriate treatment. The pulse and accompanying signs should be considered, but one need not see all of the lesser yáng signs to conclude that it is a lesser yáng disease. See line 96, p. 410, for a complete discussion of Minor Bupleurum Decoction (*xiǎo chái hú tāng*).

LINE 46

㈠ 太阳病，脉浮紧，无汗发热，身疼痛，八九日不解，表证仍在，此当发其汗。㈡ 服药已，微除，其人发烦目瞑，剧者必衄，衄乃解。㈢ 所以然者，阳气重故也。㈣ 麻黄汤主之。

(1) *Tài yáng bìng, mài fú jǐn, wú hàn fā rè, shēn téng tòng, bā jiǔ rì bù jiě, biǎo zhèng réng zài, cǐ dāng fā qí hàn.* (2) *Fú yào yǐ, wēi chú, qí rén fā fán mù míng, jù zhě bì nǜ, nǜ nǎi jiě.* (3) *Suǒ yǐ rán zhě, yáng qì zhòng gù yě.* (4) *Má huáng tāng zhǔ zhī.*

(1) In greater yáng disease, when a pulse that is floating and tight, absence of sweating, heat effusion, and generalized pain are unresolved after eight or nine days, the exterior pattern is still present and one should promote sweating. (2) (After taking medicine, [the condition] is slightly relieved, and the person is vexed and the eyes are heavy.[1] If it is acute, there will be spontaneous external bleeding,[2] which will bring about resolution. (3) Why [this] is so is because the yáng qì is weighted.[3]) (4) Ephedra Decoction (*má huáng tāng*) governs.[4]

TEXT NOTES

1. Heavy eyes, 目瞑 *mù míng*: A tendency to close the eyes and a reluctance to open them, with aversion to the stimulation of strong light. 瞑 means to close the eyes.
2. Spontaneous external bleeding, 衄 *nǜ*: Bleeding from the nose, ears, flesh, gums, tongue, or breast not due to injury. Often, as here, it specifically denotes nosebleed, the most common form of this sign.
3. Yáng qì is weighted: 阳气重 *yáng qì zhòng*: Different interpretations of this term are offered. The yáng qì can be interpreted as either the patient's yáng qì or a yáng evil qì.
   a) A severe evil qì in yáng. Yóu Yí states, "In severe [patterns], the blood contends with the heat [and] the dynamic must cause spontaneous external bleeding.... This is because the yáng qì is too heavy [and] the construction and defense are both replete.... Yáng qì means an evil qì in yáng."

b) An exuberant heat evil. Chéng Wú-Jǐ states, "In severe [patterns], [there is] exuberant heat in the channels.... 'The yáng qì is weighted' means that the heat qì is weighted...."

c) Severe depression and obstruction of the yáng qì. Huáng Yuán-Yù (黄元御) states, "This is because in enduring illness that fails to resolve, the depression and obstruction of the yáng qì is very heavy."

4. Ephedra Decoction governs, 麻黄汤主之 *má huáng tāng zhǔ zhī*: Zhāng Jiān-Shàn (张兼善) writes that the phrase, "Ephedra Decoction (*má huáng tāng*) governs" should be placed directly after "one should promote sweating."

Synopsis

A supplementary discussion of the primary pulse in greater yáng cold damage patterns and possible reactions that may appear following the ingestion of Ephedra Decoction (*má huáng tāng*).

Commentary

The reader is presented with the signs of a typical case of cold damage exterior repletion. The only remarkable feature is that the disease has continued for a protracted period of time. Because of this fact, a more complicated picture emerges. Yóu Yí writes:

> A pulse that is floating and tight, absence of sweating, heat effusion, and generalized pain [indicate] a greater yáng Ephedra Decoction (*má huáng tāng*) pattern. For eight or nine days, there has been no resolution, the exterior signs are still present and Ephedra Decoction (*má huáng tāng*) is still appropriate. In the treatment of cold damage, one cannot be restricted by the number of days. If there are exterior signs and a floating pulse, even though it has been many days, [the promotion of] sweating is appropriate. Although the medicinals have been taken and the disease has been partially eliminated, the patient experiences vexation and heavy eyes. [This means] the evil in the defense has been eliminated and the heat in the construction has not yet been eliminated. In severe [patterns], the blood contends with the heat and this dynamic results in spontaneous external bleeding. [After] bleeding, the heat in the construction is eliminated and the disease resolves. It is so because the yáng qì is too heavy. The construction and defense are both replete, so there must be outward movement of both blood and sweat, followed by the resolution of evil qì. "Yáng qì" means an evil qì in yáng aspect.

According to this interpretation, enduring illness results in depression of a yáng evil which, in severe cases, is only fully resolved through the outward movement of both sweat and blood. Chéng Wú-Jǐ, however, presents another possibility:

> A pulse that is floating and tight, absence of sweating, heat effusion, and generalized pain [indicates] greater yáng cold damage. Even though it has been eight or nine days, the exterior signs are still present. One should promote sweating. [The patient] has taken warm, moderate, effusing medicinals and although there has been no great sweating, [the disease] has been partially eliminated. Vexation means generalized heat. Evil qì, not resolved

> through sweating, becomes depressed and transmutes into heat. It steams the channels and network vessels, effusing in the fleshy exterior and engendering heat vexation. The liver receives the blood; hence [there is] vision. At the start, the [evil] qì damages the construction, and as the cold transmutes into heat, it contends with the blood, and liver qì becomes disorderly; consequently, the eyes are heavy. In severe [cases], [there is] exuberant heat in the channels, causing frenetic movement of the blood, which means spontaneous external bleeding. [After] [there is] bleeding then the heat follows the blood and dissipates and [the disease] resolves. "The yáng qì is weighted" means that the heat qì is weighted. Give Ephedra Decoction (*má huáng tāng*) to resolve the evil previously [mentioned in the case of] greater yáng cold damage.

These two authors present two pathomechanisms that are fairly similar. The basic ideas can be summarized as follows. To treat this disease, Ephedra Decoction (*má huáng tāng*) is the appropriate formula. Nevertheless, because this is an enduring disease, after the formula is given, there are two possible outcomes. The first is that the disease is partially eliminated, but the exterior evil is blocked and depressed. In the opinion of Chéng Wú-Jǐ, the evil is depressed in the fleshy exterior and the channels, whereas Yóu Yí explains it as being depressed in the construction. Vexation and heavy eyes are indications of this depressed evil. In severe cases, the heat contends with the blood and causes frenetic movement and spontaneous external bleeding. The heat follows the blood out and the disease resolves.

While in the first two interpretations, "yáng qì is weighted" refers to the prevalence of evil qì, a contrasting idea is offered by Huáng Yuán-Yù, who interprets it in terms of the yáng qì of the body. In enduring illness, the yáng qì becomes depressed or "weighted" and is unable to outthrust evil qì.

Line 47

太阳病，脉浮紧，发热，身无汗， 自衄者愈。

Tài yáng bìng, mài fú jǐn, fā rè, shēn wú hàn, zì nǜ zhě yù.

When in greater yáng disease, the pulse is floating and tight, [and there is] heat effusion and absence of sweating, spontaneous external bleeding will bring about recovery.

Synopsis

The mechanism of recovery through spontaneous external bleeding in greater yáng cold damage patterns.

Commentary

In greater yáng disease, a pulse that is floating and tight and absence of sweating indicate cold damage exterior repletion. Both evil qì and right qì are strong and the contention between them results in heat effusion. In such cases, the evil may become depressed in the exterior and transform into heat. The heat damages the blood network vessels and may cause spontaneous bleeding. If it does, the heat will follow the blood out and the disease will resolve.

Like the previous line, this line describes the resolution of disease by spontaneous external bleeding. In this line, bleeding is due to failure to apply treatment in time, whereas in the previous line it occurs after taking Ephedra Decoction (*má huáng tāng*).

Line 55

伤寒脉浮紧，不发汗，因致衄者，麻黄汤主之。

Shāng hán mài fú jǐn, bù fā hàn, yīn zhì nǜ zhě, má huáng tāng zhǔ zhī.

When, in cold damage with pulse that is floating and tight, sweating is not promoted and this gives rise to spontaneous external bleeding, Ephedra Decoction (*má huáng tāng*) governs.

Synopsis

If sweating is not promoted in a greater yáng cold damage pattern and, as a result, there is spontaneous external bleeding, one must still promote sweating to resolve the exterior and should use Ephedra Decoction (*má huáng tāng*).

Commentary

This line is similar to line 47, p. 98, in that it refers to greater yáng cold damage in which failure to apply treatment in time causes spontaneous external bleeding. In this line, the disease does not resolve after bleeding occurs and it is necessary to treat with Ephedra Decoction (*má huáng tāng*). The pathomechanism of spontaneous external bleeding in these two lines is the same.

Line 36

太阳与阳明合病，喘而胸满者，不可下，宜麻黄汤。

Tài yáng yǔ yáng míng hé bìng, chuǎn ér xiōng mǎn zhě, bù kě xià, yí má huáng tāng.

When in greater yáng and yáng brightness combination disease* [there is] panting and fullness in the chest, [one] cannot use precipitation, [but instead] Ephedra Decoction (*má huáng tāng*) is appropriate.

Text Note

* Combination disease, 合病 *hé bìng*: In combination disease, signs of two or three channels appear at the same time. The *Shāng Hán Lùn* describes combination disease of the greater yáng and yáng brightness, greater yáng and lesser yáng, and yáng brightness and lesser yáng. Combination disease should be differentiated from dragover disease, 并病 *bìng bìng*, in which the signs of one channel have not yet ceased and signs of another channel appear. Dragover

disease occurs in greater yáng and yáng brightness and greater yáng and lesser yáng disease.

SYNOPSIS

In greater yáng and yáng brightness combination disease, when greater yáng disease is primary, the appropriate treatment method is first to resolve the exterior.

COMMENTARY

The description of this pattern as a combination disease implies that signs of both greater yáng and yáng brightness disease are present, even though these are not explicitly stated. However, by mentioning only panting and fullness in the chest, the text suggests that these are focal signs in this particular case, indicating that the exterior has been fettered by cold evil and the lung qì is obstructed. Although this is combination disease, the main signs involve the lung; therefore the exterior disease is more urgent than the interior. Precipitation, which would be appropriate if the yáng brightness interior repletion were urgent, is contraindicated. The promotion of sweating is the correct treatment and Ephedra Decoction (*má huáng tāng*) is suggested, indicating that the main pattern is greater yáng cold damage. When there are primary and secondary patterns, the primary pattern should be treated before the secondary one. In this case, the primary and secondary patterns are quite distinct, so that the principle of "treating the exterior before the interior" can be applied without any reservation. Precipitation would only be used first if the yáng brightness disease were more urgent than the greater yáng disease. See line 35, p. 91, for a complete discussion of Ephedra Decoction (*má huáng tāng*).

3.2.2 Contraindications for Ephedra Decoction

This section describes the contraindications for Ephedra Decoction (*má huáng tāng*). This formula is contraindicated in the following conditions:

a) debilitation of fluids and vacuity of blood;
b) insufficiency of fluids and lower burner heat;
c) debilitation of the qì and blood; and
d) yáng qì vacuity or yáng vacuity and yīn damage.

LINE 83

咽喉干燥者，不可发汗。

Yān hóu gān zào zhě, bù kě fā hàn.

When the throat is dry, [one] cannot promote sweating.

SYNOPSIS

This line points out that the promotion of sweating is contraindicated in insufficiency of yīn liquid, as manifest in a dry throat.

COMMENTARY

When the throat is dry, yīn liquid is insufficient and failing to bear upward to nourish and moisten the throat. Because the promotion of sweating would further deplete yīn liquid, the promotion of sweating is contraindicated. This line should not be taken to mean that the promotion of sweating is contraindicated only in cases of dry throat. In wind-cold exterior patterns, whenever signs of yīn liquid insufficiency are observed, acrid, warm exterior-resolving formulae should not be used unless they are modified so as not to damage yīn further.

LINE 84

淋家，不可发汗，发汗必便血。

Lín jiā, bù kě fā hàn, fā hàn bì biàn xuè.

[With] strangury patients,[1] one cannot promote sweating [because if] sweating is promoted there will be bloody excretions.[2]

TEXT NOTES

1. Strangury patients, 淋家 *lín jiā*: Patients who have a history of or frequently suffer from strangury (frequent, painful urination).
2. Bloody excretions, 便血 *biàn xuè*: The term 便血 *biàn xuè* has, in modern usage, come to be almost synonymous with bloody stool, but in the *Shāng Hán Lùn* this is not the case, and in this line, "bloody urine" is the accepted interpretation. 小便 *xiǎo biàn*, literally "lesser convenience," means urine or urination; 大便 *dà biàn*, literally "greater convenience," means stool. 便 *biàn* by itself can be interpreted as either urine or stool, depending on the context; we use the term "excretions" here to cover both possibilities. (See line 293, p. 513, for another example of 便血 *biàn xuè* as "bloody urine" and line 339, p. 544, for the only example in the *Shāng Hán Lùn* where 便血 *biàn xuè* refers to "bloody stool.")

SYNOPSIS

Using strangury patients as an example, this line points out that when yīn is depleted and heat amasses in the lower burner, the promotion of sweating is contraindicated.

COMMENTARY

This line suggests that care should be taken in treating patients for external contractions when they suffer from enduring and abiding diseases. Whereas a patient who presents with greater yáng cold damage signs accompanied by internal heat signs is usually treated according to the principle of first resolving the exterior and then treating the interior, patients with enduring disease cannot be treated the same way; both the internal contraction and the enduring disease have to be carefully considered. Strangury patients, who suffer from frequent, painful urination, often have depletion of yīn liquid and heat amassed in the lower burner. Even in greater yáng cold damage, one must not apply the method of promoting sweating with warmth and acridity, since it will cause further damage to yīn liquid that will exacerbate the evil heat, thereby causing bloody urine. Formulae given for exterior resolution in strangury patients or patients with yīn depletion and lower burner heat amassment must be modified to safeguard yīn.

LINE 85

疮家，虽身疼痛， 不可发汗，汗出则痓。

Chuāng jiā, suī shēn téng tòng, bù kě fā hàn, hàn chū zé cì.

[With] sores patients,[1] although they have generalized pain, [one] cannot promote sweating; if they sweat, there will be tetany.[2]

TEXT NOTES

1. Sores patients, 疮家 *chuāng jiā*: Patients with a history of sores on the body, typically over an extended period of time.
2. Tetany, 痓 *cì, cè*: Severe spasm or convulsion as observed in lockjaw. 痓 *cì, cè* is a synonym of 痉 *jìng*.

SYNOPSIS

Using sores patients as an example, this line points out that when both qì and blood are vacuous, although there is an exterior pattern, the promotion of sweating is contraindicated.

COMMENTARY

Patients with a long history of body sores are considered to have dual vacuity of qì and blood. When they suffer a new contraction of externally contracted disease, the promotion of sweating with warmth and acridity will further damage both the yáng qì and the yīn blood, and since this constitutes the error of "evacuating vacuity" (虚虚 *xū xū*, i.e., exacerbating vacuity), such a treatment is contraindicated. If promotion of sweating with warmth and acridity is applied in sores patients or other patients suffering from dual vacuity of qì and blood, it will wear yáng qì and further damage construction-blood, so that qì will be unable to warm and nourish the channels and the blood will be unable to moisten the sinews, resulting in tetany.

LINE 86

衄家，不可发汗， 汗出必额上陷脉急紧，直视不能眴，不得眠。

Nǜ jiā, bù kě fā hàn, hàn chū bì é shàng xiàn mài jí jǐn, zhí shì bù néng xuàn, bù dé mián.

[With] spontaneous external bleeding patients,[1] one cannot promote sweating; [if] sweat issues, the pulse in the depressions of the forehead will be tense and tight,[2] [the eyes will] be staring straight and unable to move, and there will be inability to sleep.

TEXT NOTES

1. Spontaneous external bleeding patients, 衄家 *nǜ jiā*: Patients with a history of bleeding not due to any physical damage. The most common form of spon-

taneous external bleeding is nosebleed and, in this context, it is taken to refer specifically to nosebleed.

2. The pulse in the depressions of the forehead will be tense and tight, 额上陷脉急紧 *é shàng xiàn mài jí jǐn*: There are differing interpretations of this clause.
   a) Yóu Yí and Chén Niàn-Zǔ agree that this means that the pulse felt in the depression near the temples is tense and tight.
   b) Yù Chāng (喻昌, style 嘉言 Jiā-Yán) explains that 额上陷 *é shàng xiàn* means that an abnormal depression on the forehead (abnormal depression of the temples), and that 脉急紧 *mài jí jǐn* means the sinews (of the eyes) are tense and tight, 脉 *mài* here being taken to mean 筋脉 *jīn mài*, sinews. Yù Chāng believes that this is a critical indicator of exhaustion of upper burner yīn essence. The authors of the *Gāo Děng Cóng Shū* do not accept this explanation. All these explanations may be considered, depending on the clinical presentation.

Synopsis

Using spontaneous external bleeding patients as an example, this line points out that when yīn and blood are depleted, the promotion of sweating is contraindicated.

Commentary

People with a long history of spontaneous external bleeding (especially nosebleed) generally suffer from yīn blood depletion. Yóu Yí, Chén Niàn-Zǔ, and Yù Chāng agree that promotion of sweating with warmth and acridity should not be applied to spontaneous external bleeding patients or those who suffer from yīn blood depletion even in the case of an external contraction, because it will further deplete yīn blood. Chén Niàn-Zǔ explains:

> People who habitually suffer from spontaneous external bleeding are called spontaneous external bleeding patients. The blood in the three yáng channels is vacuous; therefore, one cannot promote sweating. [If] sweat issues, there will be yīn collapse..... The blood of the three yáng [channels] cannot nourish the vessels; consequently, the pulse in the depressions of the forehead is tense and tight. The blood of the three yáng does not pass into the eyes; consequently, the eyes are staring straight and unable to move. The yáng blood is vacuous and scant, so the defensive qì cannot move into yīn [at night]; hence [there is] sleeplessness. This is a critical pattern of the three yáng [channels].

Because sweat and blood are of the same source, following the promotion of sweating in patients suffering from yīn blood depletion, yīn and blood will be further damaged, resulting in many different possible transmutations. Depleted yīn and blood are unable to nourish the channels and the pulse on the forehead becomes tense and tight.

Depleted blood is unable to nourish the eyes, which stare straight ahead and do not move normally. It is also unable to nourish the heart, so that the heart spirit is not contained and the patient cannot sleep normally.

LINE 87

亡血家，不可发汗，发汗则寒栗而振。

Wáng xuè jiā, bù kě fā hàn, fā hàn zé hán lì ér zhèn.

[With] blood collapse patients,[1] one cannot promote sweating, [because] the promotion of sweating will lead to cold shuddering and quivering.[2]

TEXT NOTES

1. Blood collapse patients, 亡血家 *wáng xuè jiā*: Patients who suffer frequent loss of blood and consequently have blood vacuity. In the *Shāng Hán Lùn*, blood collapse does not have the modern definition of critical blood vacuity. A blood collapse patient is a patient who for constitutional reasons frequently suffers from blood collapse. In this line, it is usually explained as specifically meaning a patient who has blood vacuity due to frequent loss of blood.
2. Cold shuddering and quivering, 寒栗而振 *hán lì ér zhèn*: Cold qì stirring in the interior with generalized cold, aversion to cold, and uncontrollable trembling.

SYNOPSIS

Using blood collapse patients as an example, this line points out that when blood is vacuous and qì is debilitated, the promotion of sweating is contraindicated.

COMMENTARY

The preceding line presented the negative outcome of promoting sweating in a patient who has vacuity of yīn and blood. This line takes that idea one step further and presents a similar situation, but here the result of the mistreatment manifests in both yáng qì and yīn blood. Blood collapse patients are known to have blood vacuity and qì debilitation; therefore, when such a patient suffers from an external contraction, promotion of sweating with warmth and acridity cannot be used since this will wear yīn blood and discharge yáng qì, not only exacerbating the vacuity, but also preventing the evil from being dispelled. When the yáng qì vacuity is thus exacerbated, yáng qì will lose its warming function and will fail to defend the exterior, so that there will be shivering. When the yīn blood is exacerbated, the sinews will be deprived of nourishment so there will be shaking. This latter development is an example of blood vacuity engendering wind.

Yīn blood and yáng qì are mutually dependent; consequently, when yīn becomes vacuous, yáng loses harmony. If sweating is employed, yīn will be damaged and yáng will be disharmonious. When the yáng is unable to warm the exterior, the patient feels cold and shudders. Quivering is a result of the loss of nourishment to the sinews because of yīn vacuity. This is a pattern of dual vacuity of the yīn blood and yáng qì.

LINE 88

汗家，重发汗，必恍惚心乱，小便已阴疼，与禹余粮丸。

Hàn jiā, chóng fā hàn, bì huǎng hū xīn luàn, xiǎo biàn yǐ yīn téng, yǔ yǔ yú liáng wán.

[When] a person who suffers from excessive sweating[1] is again[2] made to sweat, there will be abstraction and derangement[3] and yīn pain after urination.[4] Give Limonite Pill (*yǔ yú liáng wán*).

Text Notes

1. A person who suffers from excessive sweating, 汗家 *hàn jiā*: Patients who frequently sweat without physical exertion or warm temperatures.
2. Again, 重 *chóng*: This character can be read as *chóng* meaning "again" or as *zhòng* meaning "heavy" or "severe." In this line, 重发汗 *chóng fā hàn* means a mistreatment. It is a mistreatment because the patient is already sweating and sweating is promoted again, not because sweating is promoted too heavily. The promotion of heavy sweating is always inappropriate, regardless of the patient's constitution.
3. Abstraction and derangement, 恍惚心乱 *huǎng hū xīn luàn*: Abstraction is a condition in which the spirit is unstable and the patient is incapable of self-control. Derangement is inability to think coherently and act decisively due to vacuity of the spirit.
4. Yīn pain after urination, 小便已阴疼 *xiǎo biàn yǐ yīn téng*: Pain in the urethra following urination. "Yīn" often refers to the "private parts" and here it refers specifically to the urethra.

Formula

Limonite Pill (*yǔ yú liáng wán*)

This formula has been lost.

Synopsis

Using patients who suffer from excessive sweating as an example, this line points out that when yáng is vacuous, the promotion of sweating is contraindicated.

Commentary

Frequent sweating (night sweating or especially spontaneous sweating) is associated with constitutional dual vacuity of yīn and yáng. It is associated with yáng vacuity because sweating wears yáng qì and causes insecurity of the exterior, and with yīn vacuity since sweating allows yīn humor to discharge causing damage to yīn blood. However, yáng qì vacuity is the more important element because yáng qì vacuity is both a cause and a result of excessive sweating, so it creates a vicious circle, while yīn vacuity is merely a consequence. In this type of patient, even in external contractions, the further promotion of sweating with warmth and acridity is contraindicated. If sweating is promoted, further damage to yīn and yáng will occur. Exacerbated dual vacuity of yīn and yáng will deprive the heart of nourishment and cause the heart spirit to float astray, giving rise to abstraction and derangement. Furthermore, when liquid and humor are further damaged, they are unable to moisten the urinary orifice, which becomes rough and dry, causing pain following urination.

The formula is unknown to any *Shāng Hán Lùn* commentator. However, its name suggests that the chief ingredient is limonite (*yǔ yú liáng*), which promotes astriction and checks sweating. Furthermore, judging by the problem that it addresses, the formula seems to be used to supplement vacuity and address an emergency.

LINE 89

病人有寒，复发汗，胃中冷，必吐蚘。

Bìng rén yǒu hán, fù fā hàn, wèi zhōng lěng, bì tù huí.

A patient who has cold[1] and yet[2] is made to sweat has cold in the stomach[3] and will vomit roundworms.[4]

TEXT NOTES

1. A patient who has cold, 病人有寒 *bìng rén yǒu hán*: This phrase can be interpreted in several ways. *Gāo Děng Cóng Shū* interprets this phrase as yáng vacuity cold. Zhāng Xī-Jū writes, "'A patient who has cold' means that the stomach qì [of the patient] is usually cold." Zhāng Zhì-Cōng comments that this phrase means stomach qì vacuity.
2. Yet 复 *fù*: Fāng Yǒu-Zhí writes that 复 *fù* should be read as "but instead," 反 *fǎn*, implying that the treatment is erroneous.
3. Cold in the stomach, 胃中冷 *wèi zhōng lěng*: Cold may be the result of mistreatment or a restatement of the patient's original condition. Fāng Yǒu-Zhí, Zhāng Xī-Jū, and Zhāng Zhì-Cōng emphasize that the use of an inappropriate treatment method exacerbated the original cold condition.
4. Vomit roundworms, 吐蚘 *tù huí*: Because of vomiting and stomach counterflow, the contents of the intestines may move into the stomach. If there are parasites present, they will then be vomited out. However, in modern clinical practice, this phenomenon is rarely seen. Note that 蚘 *huí* is the same as 蛔 *huí*.

SYNOPSIS

When there is yáng vacuity and cold, the promotion of sweating is contraindicated.

COMMENTARY

The presence of cold suggests that the patient has yáng vacuity, stomach qì vacuity, or stomach cold. Although there is an exterior pattern, one should not promote sweating, since this treatment will further damage the yáng qì and exacerbate the cold. If the patient originally has vacuity cold in the stomach, further damage to the yáng qì incurred during sweating will exacerbate the condition. If, originally, there is yáng vacuity cold, further damage to the yáng qì can cause stomach cold and stomach qì counterflow. In either case, cold in the stomach causes the loss of normal stomach downbearing so that there is retching or vomiting.

LINE 50

㈠ 脉浮紧者，法当身疼痛，宜以汗解之。假令尺中迟者，不可发汗。㈡ 何以知然？以荣气不足，血少故也。

(1) *Mài fú jǐn zhě, fǎ dāng shēn téng tòng, yí yǐ hàn jiě zhī.* (2) *Jiǎ lìng chǐ zhōng chí zhě, bù kě fā hàn.* (3) *Hé yǐ zhī rán? Yǐ róng qì bù zú, xuè shǎo gù yě.*

(1) When the pulse is floating and tight, as a rule there should be generalized pain and [therefore,] it is appropriate to resolve [the illness] by sweating. (2) [However,] if the pulse at the cubit is slow,* [one] cannot promote sweating. (3) How does one know this? Because the construction qì is insufficient and the blood is scant.

TEXT NOTE

* The pulse at the cubit is slow, 尺中迟 *chǐ zhōng chí*: 尺中 *chǐ zhōng* means the cubit position.

SYNOPSIS

When construction and blood are insufficient, although there is an exterior pattern, the promotion of sweating is contraindicated.

COMMENTARY

A pulse that is floating and tight is a characteristic pulse felt in greater yáng cold damage. Furthermore, in this pattern, generalized pain is usually present and the promotion of sweating is the appropriate treatment. If the pulse at the cubit position is slow, one should not promote sweating. When the pulse at the cubit position is slow, it means that the construction qì and the blood are insufficient. The promotion of sweating would further damage the construction directly and the blood indirectly through the fluids; therefore it is contraindicated.

LINE 49

㈠ 脉浮数者，法当汗出而愈。㈡ 若下之，身重心悸者，不可发汗，当自汗出乃解。㈢ 所以然者，尺中脉微，此里虚，须表里实，津液自和，便自汗出愈。

(1) *Mài fú shuò zhě, fǎ dāng hàn chū ér yù.* (2) *Ruò xià zhī, shēn zhòng xīn jì zhě, bù kě fā hàn, dāng zì hàn chū nǎi jiě.* (3) *Suǒ yǐ rán zhě, chǐ zhōng mài wēi, cǐ lǐ xū, xū biǎo lǐ shí, jīn yè zì hé, biàn zì hàn chū yù.*

(1) When the pulse is floating and rapid, as a rule there should be sweating and [then] recovery. (2) If precipitation [is used], and [there is] generalized heaviness and heart palpitations, [one] cannot promote

sweating; [the person] must sweat spontaneously so that [the illness] is resolved. (3) Why [this] is so is because the pulse at the cubit is faint, which indicates interior vacuity. Exterior and interior need to be made replete,[1] [so that] liquid and humor[2] naturally become harmonious [and] then spontaneous sweating [will bring about] recovery.

TEXT NOTES

1. Replete, 实 *shí*: In a healthy state.
2. Liquid and humor, 津液 *jīn yè*: "Liquid," 津 *jīn*, is any of the thinner fluids of the human body. "Humor," 液 *yè*, is any of the thicker fluids. Since compound nouns in Chinese are made from near synonyms, it is possible to translate *jīn yè* loosely as "fluids." Here, we have used both terms to reflect the original Chinese.

SYNOPSIS

When the inappropriate use of precipitation has led to interior vacuity, the treatment should be to supplement vacuity and support the right, and the promotion of sweating is contraindicated.

COMMENTARY

The promotion of sweating is appropriate for the treatment of greater yáng disease with a pulse that is floating and rapid. If, however, precipitation is used, pathological transmutations will occur. The new signs of generalized heaviness and palpitations are explained in the text. The reader is told that the pulse at the cubit is faint and this indicates interior vacuity. Therefore, one knows that erroneous precipitation has resulted in interior vacuity. One should not promote sweating, but must wait for spontaneous sweating to occur. In order for spontaneous sweating to occur, one must supplement the vacuity. So although one should not promote sweating, treatment is still possible by strengthening the exterior and interior, so that the fluids become harmonized. In this way, the patient will be able to sweat and the disease will resolve.

3.2.3 Concurrent Patterns

The four concurrent patterns in greater yáng cold damage are represented by the following formulae: Pueraria Decoction (*gé gēn tāng*), Pueraria Decoction Plus Pinellia (*gé gēn jiā bàn xià tāng*), Major Green-Blue Dragon Decoction (*dà qīng lóng tāng*) and Minor Green-Blue Dragon Decoction (*xiǎo qīng lóng tāng*).

a) Pueraria Decoction (*gé gēn tāng*) pattern: Greater yáng cold damage signs plus marked hypertonicity and discomfort of the nape and back. The process is one in which wind-cold fetters the exterior, the defense and construction are blocked and depressed, the greater yáng channel qì is inhibited, the fluids are unable to ascend and the channel is not nourished and moistened. The appropriate treatment is to promote sweating and resolve the exterior and to engender liquid and moisten the channels.

b) Pueraria Decoction Plus Pinellia (*gé gēn jiā bàn xià tāng*) pattern: Greater yáng cold damage signs with diarrhea, or with retching and vomiting. In this pattern, wind-cold fetters the exterior, the defense and construction are blocked and depressed, and the exterior evil moves inward. It may distress the yáng brightness, causing the loss of normal large intestine function and diarrhea, or it may attack the stomach causing qì counterflow and retching and vomiting. The appropriate treatment is to promote sweating and resolve the exterior, to raise liquid and check diarrhea, or to downbear counterflow and check retching.

c) Major Green-Blue Dragon Decoction (*dà qīng lóng tāng*) pattern: Greater yáng cold damage signs plus vexation and agitation. The pulse is floating and tight, and no generalized pain exists, only heaviness which occasionally lightens. The process is one in which wind-cold fetters the exterior, the defense and construction are blocked and depressed, and depressed heat in the interior cannot be diffused and discharged. The appropriate treatment is to resolve the exterior with warmth and acridity and to clear interior heat.

d) Minor Green-Blue Dragon Decoction (*xiǎo qīng lóng tāng*) pattern: Greater yáng cold damage signs plus cough, panting, and retching counterflow. Thirst, diarrhea, dysphagia, inhibited urination, and fullness in the smaller abdomen may also be observed. In this pattern, wind-cold fetters the exterior, the defense and construction are blocked and depressed, and water-rheum collects in the interior. The fluids are not transformed and the rheum seeps into the bowels and viscera. The appropriate treatment is to resolve the exterior with warmth and acridity, and to flush and transform water-rheum.

LINE 31

太阳病，项背强几几，无汗恶风， 葛根汤主之。

Tài yáng bìng, xiàng bèi jiàng shū shū, wú hàn wù fēng, gé gēn tāng zhǔ zhī.

[In] greater yáng disease with a stretched stiff nape and back,* absence of sweating, and aversion to cold, Pueraria Decoction (*gé gēn tāng*) governs.

TEXT NOTE

* Stretched stiff nape and back, 项背强几几 *xiàng bèi jiàng shū shū*: This is the same expression as that used earlier in line 14, p. 79. In this line, however, the disease is cold damage exterior repletion, whereas in line 14, p. 79, it is wind strike exterior vacuity. Thus, this formula includes ephedra (*má huáng*), whereas Cinnamon Twig Decoction Plus Pueraria (*guì zhī jiā gé gēn tāng*), which is used in line 14, p. 79, does not. Note that both formulae below contain pueraria (*gé gēn*).

FORMULA

Pueraria Decoction (*gé gēn tāng*)

○ Promote sweating and resolve the exterior; engender liquid and soothe channels.

葛根四两　麻黄三两（去节）　桂枝二两（去皮）　生姜三两（切）　甘草二两（炙）　芍药二两　大枣十二枚（擘）

㈠ 右七味，以水一斗，先煮麻黄、葛根，减二升，去白沫，内诸药，煮取三升，去滓，温服一升。㈡ 覆取微似汗。㈢ 余如桂枝法将息及禁忌。㈣ 诸汤皆仿此。

Gé gēn sì liǎng má huáng sān liǎng (qù jié) guì zhī èr liǎng (qù pí) shēng jiāng sān liǎng (qiē) gān cǎo èr liǎng (zhì) sháo yào èr liǎng dà zǎo shí èr méi (bò)

(1) *Yòu qī wèi, yǐ shuǐ yī dǒu, xiān zhǔ má huáng、gé gēn, jiǎn èr shēng, qù bái mò, nà zhū yào, zhǔ qǔ sān shēng, qù zǐ, wēn fú yī shēng.* (2) *Fù qǔ wēi sì hàn.* (3) *Yú rú guì zhī fǎ jiāng xī jí jìn jì.* (4) *Zhū tāng jiē fǎng cǐ.*

pueraria (葛根 *gé gēn*, Puerariae Radix) 4 liǎng
ephedra (麻黄 *má huáng*, Ephedrae Herba) 3 liǎng (remove nodes)
cinnamon twig (桂枝 *guì zhī*, Cinnamomi Ramulus) 2 liǎng (remove bark)
fresh ginger (生姜 *shēng jiāng*, Zingiberis Rhizoma Recens) 3 liǎng (slice)
mix-fried licorice (甘草 *gān cǎo*, Glycyrrhizae Radix) 2 liǎng
peony (芍药 *sháo yào*, Paeoniae Radix) 2 liǎng
jujube (大枣 *dà zǎo*, Ziziphi Fructus) 12 pieces (broken)

(1) [For] the above seven ingredients, use one dǒu of water. First boil ephedra (*má huáng*) and pueraria (*gé gēn*) to reduce [the water] by two shēng. Remove the white foam and add all the ingredients. Boil to get three shēng, remove the dregs, and take one shēng, warm. (2) Cover [with bedclothes] to obtain mild sweating. (3) The remainder is as for Cinnamon Twig Decoction (*guì zhī tāng*) [with regard to] rest and contraindications. (4) [In fact,] all formulae based on Cinnamon Twig Decoction (*guì zhī tāng*) should be used according to this method.

SYNOPSIS

The distinguishing features and treatment of greater yáng cold damage with greater yáng channel qì constraint.

COMMENTARY

The author tells us that this is greater yáng disease, but does not explicitly state if it is wind strike or cold damage. Absence of sweating is indicative of cold damage, but aversion to wind is more indicative of wind strike. Generally, in such situations, the condition is inferred from the formula. One can better understand a poorly described disease pattern by looking at the prescribed treatment.

This formula is Cinnamon Twig Decoction (*guì zhī tāng*) plus ephedra (*má huáng*) and pueraria (*gé gēn*). The addition of ephedra (*má huáng*) promotes sweating and dispels evil. It is this addition which tells the reader that this pattern belongs to cold damage. Sweet and balanced pueraria (*gé gēn*) engenders liquid and soothes the channels. It is able to raise the clear yáng qì and check diarrhea.

It also reinforces the action of ephedra (*má huáng*) and cinnamon twig (*guì zhī*) in promoting sweating and resolving the exterior.

One may ask why a formula based on Cinnamon Twig Decoction (*guì zhī tāng*) is chosen if this is greater yáng cold damage. The answer sheds light on the author's view of the pathomechanism and his therapeutic approach. We already know that in cold damage, wind-cold evil fetters the exterior, resulting in the depression and stagnation of the construction and defense. In this pattern, normal diffusion of fluids through the greater yáng channel may be impaired. The fluids are insufficient to moisten and nourish the channel; hence stiffness and discomfort are felt in the nape and back along the channel pathway. In choosing a formula, one must be aware that although the exterior must be resolved, normal fluid movement has already been disrupted and normal moistening along the channel has been lost. Therefore, it is wise to promote sweating moderately, not harshly, and to harmonize construction and defense with Cinnamon Twig Decoction (*guì zhī tāng*). Nevertheless, absence of sweating is observed, so ephedra (*má huáng*) is also given, as in other cold damage situations. As above, pueraria (*gé gēn*) has the important action of engendering fluids and raising the clear qì from the lower burner. In this way, it soothes the channels that have been deprived of fluid nourishment.

Line 32

太阳与阳明合病者，必自下利，葛根汤主之。

Tài yáng yǔ yáng míng hé bìng zhě, bì zì xià lì, gé gēn tāng zhǔ zhī.

In greater yáng and yáng brightness combination disease, there will be[1] spontaneous diarrhea,[2] and [therefore,] Pueraria Decoction (*gé gēn tāng*) governs.

Text Notes

1. Will be, 必 *bì*: If 必 *bì* is assumed to have its normal meaning of "must" or "certainly," the present line means that diarrhea will definitely occur in greater yáng and yáng brightness combination disease. This statement would nevertheless contradict the following line (line 33), which describes the same disease pattern without diarrhea. In an attempt to reconcile the apparent contradiction, some commentators have interpreted *bì* here as meaning "might."
2. Spontaneous diarrhea, 自下利 *zì xià lì*: Loose stool that occurs without any known natural or iatrogenic cause, such as inappropriate precipitation.

Synopsis

The treatment of diarrhea in greater yáng and yáng brightness combination disease.

Commentary

This line and the one that follows provide another example of apparent inconsistencies in the text. This line presents greater yáng and yáng brightness disease that "must" include diarrhea, while the following line presents the same disease pattern, without diarrhea. See the Introduction for further discussion of this issue.

This pattern is simultaneous disease of the exterior and the interior. The interior disease, however, is considered secondary to the exterior one. We can infer this through an analysis of the formula. Pueraria Decoction (*gé gēn tāng*) is based on Ephedra Decoction (*má huáng tāng*), which has the primary action of promoting sweating and resolving the exterior. In this line, the presence of diarrhea indicates an interior condition, yet Pueraria Decoction (*gé gēn tāng*) is still used because once the exterior is resolved, the interior will spontaneously harmonize. Pueraria (*gé gēn*) is particularly appropriate here because it not only has mild exterior-resolving properties, but it also raises yáng and checks diarrhea.

LINE 33

太阳与阳明合病，不下利，但呕者，葛根加半夏汤主之。
Tài yáng yǔ yáng míng hé bìng, bù xià lì, dàn ǒu zhě, gé gēn jiā bàn xià tāng zhǔ zhī.

When in greater yáng and yáng brightness combination disease, diarrhea is absent, [and] only retching [is present], Pueraria Decoction Plus Pinellia (*gé gēn jiā bàn xià tāng*) governs.

FORMULA
Pueraria Decoction Plus Pinellia (*gé gēn jiā bàn xià tāng*)

∘ Promote sweating and resolve the exterior; downbear counterflow and stanch vomiting.

葛根四两 麻黄三两（去节） 甘草二两（炙） 芍药二两 桂枝二两（去皮） 生姜二两（切） 半夏半升（洗） 大枣十二枚（擘）

(一) 右八味，以水一斗，先煮葛根、麻黄，减二升，去白沫，内诸药，煮取三升，去滓，温服一升。(二) 覆取微似汗。

Gé gēn sì liǎng má huáng sān liǎng (qù jié) gān cǎo èr liǎng (zhì) sháo yào èr liǎng guì zhī èr liǎng (qù pí) shēng jiāng èr liǎng (qiē) bàn xià bàn shēng (xǐ) dà zǎo shí èr méi (bò)

(1) *Yòu bā wèi, yǐ shuǐ yī dǒu, xiān zhǔ gé gēn、má huáng, jiǎn èr shēng, qù bái mò, nà zhū yào, zhǔ qǔ sān shēng, qù zǐ, wēn fú yī shēng.* (2) *Fù qǔ wēi sì hàn.*

pueraria (葛根 *gé gēn*, Puerariae Radix) 4 liǎng
ephedra (麻黄 *má huáng*, Ephedrae Herba) 3 liǎng (remove nodes)
mix-fried licorice (甘草 *gān cǎo*, Glycyrrhizae Radix) 2 liǎng
peony (芍药 *sháo yào*, Paeoniae Radix)[1] 2 liǎng
cinnamon twig (桂枝 *guì zhī*, Cinnamomi Ramulus) 2 liǎng (remove bark)
fresh ginger (生姜 *shēng jiāng*, Zingiberis Rhizoma Recens) 2 liǎng (slice)
pinellia (半夏 *bàn xià*, Pinelliae Tuber) half shēng (washed)[2]
jujube (大枣 *dà zǎo*, Ziziphi Fructus) 12 pieces (broken)

(1) [For] the above eight ingredients use one dǒu of water. First boil pueraria (*gé gēn*) and ephedra (*má huáng*) to reduce [the water] by two shēng. Remove the white foam and add all the ingredients. Boil to get three shēng, remove the dregs, and take one shēng, warm. (2) Cover [with bedclothes] to obtain mild sweating.

FORMULA NOTES

1. Peony: Raw white peony (生白芍药 *shēng bái sháo yào*, Paeoniae Radix Alba Cruda).
2. Washed, 洗 *xǐ*: Because of the known toxicity of pinellia (半夏 *bàn xià*, Pinelliae Tuber), we can speculate that some procedure was possibly used to reduce the toxic effects. Precisely what procedure was used at the time when the *Shāng Hán Lùn* was written is now unknown. It is likely that this medicinal was washed until its ability to make the tongue numb was reduced or eliminated.

SYNOPSIS

The treatment of retching counterflow in greater yáng and yáng brightness combination disease.

COMMENTARY

In combination disease of the greater yáng and the yáng brightness, the exterior evil enters the interior and distresses the yáng brightness. The stomach and intestines are both part of the yáng brightness, and either may be affected by the evil. In the previous line, intestinal function is impaired, giving rise to diarrhea. In this line, it is the stomach that is affected and disharmony of the stomach qì gives rise to retching. Again, the treatment addresses the root; therefore, the focus is on resolving the exterior.

This formula is Pueraria Decoction (*gé gēn tāng*) plus pinellia (*bàn xià*). Acrid, warm pinellia (*bàn xià*) is added to downbear counterflow and stanch retching.

LINE 38

㈠ 太阳中风，脉浮紧，发热恶寒，身疼痛，不汗出而烦躁者，大青龙汤主之。㈡ 若脉微弱，汗出恶风者，不可服之。㈢ 服之则厥逆，筋惕肉瞤，此为逆也。

(1) *Tài yáng zhòng fēng, mài fú jǐn, fā rè wù hán, shēn téng tòng, bù hàn chū ér fán zào zhě, dà qīng lóng tāng zhǔ zhī.* (2) *Ruò mài wēi ruò, hàn chū wù fēng zhě, bù kě fú zhī.* (3) *Fú zhī zé jué nì, jīn tì ròu rún, cǐ wéi nì yě.*

(1) When in greater yáng wind strike the pulse is floating and tight, and [there is] heat effusion, aversion to cold, generalized pain, absence of sweating, and vexation and agitation, Major Green-Blue Dragon Decoction (*dà qīng lóng tāng*) governs. (2) If the pulse is faint and weak and [there is] sweating and aversion to wind, [the person] cannot take

this [formula]. (3) If [he] takes it there will be reverse-flow[1] and jerking sinews and twitching flesh,[2] indicating an adverse [treatment].

TEXT NOTES

1. Reverse-flow, 厥逆 *jué nì*: Cold in the extremities. In the *Shāng Hán Lùn*, but not necessarily in other texts, "reverse-flow" is taken to be synonymous with "reversal-cold of the limbs," 四肢厥冷 *sì zhī jué lěng*.
2. Jerking sinews and twitching flesh, 筋惕肉瞤 *jīn tì ròu shùn (rún)*: Mild jerking of the sinews, which can be due to blood or fluid insufficiency, cold-damp, or yáng vacuity. Here, it is due to yáng collapse, which stems from the inappropriate promotion of sweating.

FORMULA

Major Green-Blue Dragon Decoction (*dà qīng lóng tāng*).

◦ Resolve the exterior with warmth and acridity; clear interior heat.

麻黄六两（去节） 桂枝二两（去皮） 甘草二两（炙） 杏仁四十枚（去皮尖） 生姜三两（切） 大枣十枚（擘） 石膏如鸡子大（碎）

㈠ 右七味，以水九升，先煮麻黄，减二升，去上沫，内诸药，煮取三升，去滓，温服一升。㈡ 取微似汗。㈢ 汗出多者，温粉粉之。㈣ 一服汗者，停后服。㈤ 若复服，汗多亡阳遂虚，恶风，烦躁，不得眠也。

Má huáng liù liǎng (qù jié) guì zhī èr liǎng (qù pí) gān cǎo èr liǎng (zhì) xìng rén sì shí méi (qù pí jiān) shēng jiāng sān liǎng (qiē) dà zǎo shí méi (bò) shí gāo rú jī zǐ dà (suì)

(1) *Yòu qī wèi, yǐ shuǐ jiǔ shēng, xiān zhǔ má huáng, jiǎn èr shēng, qù shàng mò, nà zhū yào, zhǔ qǔ sān shēng, qù zǐ, wēn fú yī shēng.* (2) *Qǔ wēi sì hàn.* (3) *Hàn chū duō zhě, wēn fěn fěn zhī.* (4) *Yī fú hàn zhě, tíng hòu fú.* (5) *Ruò fù fú, hàn duō wáng yáng suì xū, wù fēng, fán zào, bù dé mián yě.*

ephedra (麻黄 *má huáng*, Ephedrae Herba) 6 liǎng (remove nodes)
cinnamon twig (桂枝 *guì zhī*, Cinnamomi Ramulus) 2 liǎng (remove bark)
mix-fried licorice (甘草 *gān cǎo*, Glycyrrhizae Radix) 2 liǎng
apricot kernel (杏仁 *xìng rén*, Armeniacae Semen) 40 pieces (remove skin and tip)
fresh ginger (生姜 *shēng jiāng*, Zingiberis Rhizoma Recens) 3 liǎng (cut)
jujube (大枣 *dà zǎo*, Ziziphi Fructus) 10 pieces (broken)
gypsum (石膏 *shí gāo*, Gypsum) a piece the size of a chicken's egg (crushed)

(1) [For] the above seven ingredients use nine shēng of water. First boil ephedra (*má huáng*) to reduce [the water] by two shēng. Remove the foam [collecting] on top and add all the ingredients. Boil to get three shēng, remove the dregs, and take one shēng, warm. (2) Obtain mild sweating. (3) If [there is] copious sweating, [apply] warm [rice] powder.* (4) As soon as [there is] sweating, stop taking the decoction. (5) [After sweating,] if the formula is taken again, there will be copious sweating and yáng collapse, and then vacuity, aversion to wind, vexation and agitation, and inability to sleep.

FORMULA NOTE

* [Apply] warm [rice] powder, 温粉粉之 *wēn fěn fěn zhī*: The application of warm rice powder to the outside of the body was a method used to check copious sweating. Commentators disagree about the exact ingredients to be used, as well as the exact method.

SYNOPSIS

a) The signs and treatment of greater yáng cold damage with interior heat.

b) Contraindications for the use of Major Green-Blue Dragon Decoction (*dà qīng lóng tāng*).

COMMENTARY

The interpretation of this line is problematic because Zhāng Jī states that this pattern belongs to greater yáng wind strike. In greater yáng wind strike, we expect a pulse that is floating and moderate, not floating and tight. A pulse that is floating and tight is the basic pulse in cold damage pattern. Furthermore, all the other signs—heat effusion, aversion to cold, generalized pain, and absence of sweating—are all typically seen in greater yáng cold damage. Previously an analysis of the formula has been used to clarify issues of this sort. In this line, the use of Major Green-Blue Dragon Decoction (*dà qīng lóng tāng*) is suggestive of cold damage because a large amount of ephedra (*má huáng*) is used. Ultimately it is impossible to resolve this issue because the text is unclear. Some commentators have asserted that Zhāng Jī meant not wind strike but a general exterior condition. If this assertion is true, however, it is not clear why he did not simply write greater yáng disease, as in other lines.

The pattern presented is a representative greater yáng cold damage pattern, with the addition of vexation and agitation. The presence of vexation and agitation cannot be explained through the pathomechanism of wind-cold evil fettering the exterior alone, and suggests that another disease process is also operant. We assume this to be interior heat because the formula suggested includes gypsum (*shí gāo*), which clears interior heat. When the exterior is fettered by wind-cold, no outward pathway exists for the interior heat; consequently, vexation and agitation arise. Both the exterior cold and the interior heat are repletion patterns. Major Green-Blue Dragon Decoction (*dà qīng lóng tāng*) contains Ephedra Decoction (*má huáng tāng*) in order to resolve the exterior. Fresh ginger (*shēng jiāng*) is added and, in combination with cinnamon twig (*guì zhī*) and a large dose of ephedra (*má huáng*), promotes sweating and dispels cold. These actions are offset by sweet, acrid, very cold gypsum (*shí gāo*), which clears interior heat, drains fire, and eliminates vexation. Mix-fried licorice (*gān cǎo*) and jujube (*dà zǎo*) are added to harmonize and protect the center and the fluids. This is a strong formula for the promotion of sweating, yet Zhāng Jī writes that "mild sweating" should be obtained. Why is this formula used to obtain mild sweating? The presence of vexation and agitation means that the exterior is fettered and depressed, leaving no outward pathway for the sweat. Therefore, a strong formula is needed to obtain even a mild sweat. Zhāng Jī cautions against the promotion of excessive sweating. As soon as mild sweat issues, ingestion of the formula should stop. Furthermore, if copious sweat issues, one is advised to apply warm rice powder to the exterior of the body to check the sweating. This is another indication of the importance of controlling the degree to which sweating is promoted.

In the second part of the line, the pulse is weak and faint, and sweating and aversion to wind are observed, which means that both the interior and exterior are vacuous and Major Green-Blue Dragon Decoction (*dà qīng lóng tāng*) must not be given. To give this formula would be to use a strong formula for the promotion of sweating with a vacuous patient. This constitutes an adverse treatment, since the loss of sweat will exacerbate the vacuity. In this case, the loss of sweat causes yáng collapse. The yáng qì is unable to warm and nourish the flesh and channels, giving rise to reverse-flow and to jerking sinews and twitching flesh.

Line 39

伤寒脉浮缓，身不疼，但重，乍有轻时，无少阴证者，大青龙汤发之。

Shāng hán mài fú huǎn, shēn bù téng, dàn zhòng, zhà yǒu qīng shí, wú shào yīn zhèng zhě, dà qīng lóng tāng fā zhī.

When in cold damage, the pulse is floating and moderate, and [there is] no generalized pain, only [generalized] heaviness, with sudden periods of lightness, and [there is] no lesser yīn disease, Major Green-Blue Dragon Decoction (*dà qīng lóng tāng*) will promote [sweating and resolve the disease].

Synopsis

A further discussion of the pattern of greater yáng cold damage with interior heat, its transmutations and treatment, on the basis of the previous line.

Commentary

As the previous line, this line poses some apparent contradictions. In cold damage, one expects a floating, tight pulse and generalized pain, yet in this line cold damage disease is described with a pulse that is floating and moderate, and no generalized pain. As before, an analysis of the formula can shed light on the disease. The use of Major Green-Blue Dragon Decoction (*dà qīng lóng tāng*) appears to indicate exterior repletion. If this is so, then how is one to explain the absence of generalized pain and the presence of heaviness with periods of lightness? According to the *Yī Zōng Jīn Jiàn*, "In cold damage, there should be generalized pain, [but] now [there is] no pain. This is a cold damage disease which simultaneously has wind strike signs. [When] the body [feels] light, the evil is in yáng. [When] the body [feels] heavy, the evil is in yīn."

The signs of cold damage, as they are seen in clinical practice, often vary from the presentation in the text. This pattern belongs to cold damage, but the signs are not typical. Exterior wind-cold may be mild or it may be severe, so the pulse may vary. The pulse is also influenced by the constitution of the patient. In line 38, p. 113, the severe evil and fierce contention between right qì and evil qì give rise to a pulse that is tight and to generalized pain. In the present line, a milder evil and more moderate struggle between right qì and evil qì manifest in a pulse that is floating and moderate, and in heaviness only, without generalized pain. The heaviness occasionally lightens because the disease is in the exterior and the yáng qì is temporarily able to push it out. When the heaviness returns, it is because the yáng qì retreats and the evil falls back into the construction-yīn.

This line illustrates that one must not equate individual signs or pulse qualities with a given pattern. Generalized heaviness may occur in lesser yīn disease; consequently, we are reminded in this line that "there are no lesser yīn signs." Heaviness that occurs in lesser yīn disease is unceasing and accompanied by reversal cold of the limbs, no heat effusion or aversion to cold, and a faint, fine pulse. In this pattern, the generalized heaviness is not unceasing; therefore, this is not a lesser yīn pattern. The heaviness in this line is the result of an evil fettering the exterior and obstructing the outward movement of sweat. Major Green-Blue Dragon Decoction (*dà qīng lóng tāng*) is used because heat is harassing the interior, producing vexation and agitation. In cold damage patterns with generalized heaviness, but without lesser yīn signs, one may use this formula. If vexation and agitation occur without greater yáng cold damage signs, this formula should not be used.

Line 40

伤寒表不解，心下有水气，干呕发热而咳，或渴，或利，或噎，或小便不利，少腹满，或喘者，小青龙汤主之。

Shāng hán biǎo bù jiě, xīn xià yǒu shuǐ qì, gān ǒu fā rè ér ké, huò kě, huò lì, huò yē, huò xiǎo biàn bù lì, shào fù mǎn, huò chuǎn zhě, xiǎo qīng lóng tāng zhǔ zhī.

When in cold damage the exterior has not resolved and [there is] water qì below the heart,[1] with dry retching, heat effusion and cough, and possibly thirst or diarrhea, or dysphagia,[2] or inhibited urination and lesser abdominal fullness,[3] or panting, Minor Green-Blue Dragon Decoction (*xiǎo qīng lóng tāng*) governs.

Text Notes

1. Water qì below the heart, 心下有水气 *xīn xià yǒu shuǐ qì*: "Below the heart" means the upper abdomen and stomach duct region. "Water qì" refers to water swelling or water-rheum, depending on the context. When understood as water swelling, it means pathological excesses of water in the body and, specifically, the swelling provoked by it. The main cause is impairment of movement and transformation of water due to spleen-kidney yáng vacuity. "Qì" in the term "water qì" reflects the notion of water in this context as a pervasive (pathological) phenomenon. When understood as water-rheum, it means fluid exuded by diseased organs. Clear thin fluid is known as "water" whereas thin sticky fluid is known as "rheum." These differ in name and form, but are in essence the same; hence the compound term.

a) According to the *Shāng Hán Lùn Yán Jiū Dà Cí Diǎn*, "water qì" refers to water-humor collecting in the interior of the body and all the pathological changes that occur as a result of the collected fluid.

b) According to the *Shí Yòng Zhōng Yī Cí Diǎn*, "water qì" can refer to water swelling, water-rheum, and/or phlegm-rheum.

2. Dysphagia, 噎 *yē*: A feeling of blockage in the throat.

3. Lesser abdominal fullness, 少腹满 *shào fù mǎn*: A subjective sensation of expansion and pressure, which may or may not be associated with objectively perceptible distention felt in the region of the abdomen below the umbilicus.

The term "lesser abdomen" (少腹 *shào fù*) refers to the part of the abdomen below the umbilicus (called lower abdomen in Western medicine), as opposed to the "greater abdomen" (大腹 *dà fù*), which refers to the part above the umbilicus (epigastrium). The lesser abdomen is also called 小腹 *xiǎo fù*, smaller abdomen. However, according to some, "lesser abdomen" specifically denotes the two lateral regions of the abdomen below the umbilicus.

FORMULA

Minor Green-Blue Dragon Decoction (*xiǎo qīng lóng tāng*)

○ Resolve the exterior with acridity and warmth; warm and transform water-rheum.

麻黄（去节） 芍药 细辛 干姜 甘草（炙） 桂枝（去皮）各三两 五味子半升 半夏（洗）半升

(一) 右八味，以水一斗，先煮麻黄，减二升，去上沫，内诸药，煮取三升，去滓，温服一升。(二) 若渴，去半夏，加栝楼根三两。(三) 若微利，去麻黄，加荛花，如一鸡子，熬令赤色。(四) 若噎者，去麻黄，加附子一枚，炮。(五) 若小便不利，少腹满者，去麻黄，加茯苓四两。(六) 若喘，去麻黄，加杏仁半升，去皮尖。(七) 且荛花不治利，麻黄主喘，今此语反之，疑非仲景意。

Má huáng (qù jié) sháo yào xì xīn gān jiāng gān cǎo (zhì) guì zhī (qù pí) gè sān liǎng wǔ wèi zǐ bàn shēng bàn xià (xǐ) bàn shēng

(1) *Yòu bā wèi, yǐ shuǐ yī dǒu, xiān zhǔ má huáng, jiǎn èr shēng, qù shàng mò, nà zhū yào, zhǔ qǔ sān shēng, qù zǐ, wēn fú yī shēng.* (2) *Ruò kě, qù bàn xià, jiā guā lóu gēn sān liǎng.* (3) *Ruò wēi lì, qù má huáng, jiā ráo huā, rú yī jī zǐ, áo lìng chì sè.* (4) *Ruò yē zhě, qù má huáng, jiā fù zǐ yī méi, pào.* (5) *Ruò xiǎo biàn bù lì, shǎo fù mǎn zhě, qù má huáng, jiā fú líng sì liǎng.* (6) *Ruò chuǎn, qù má huáng, jiā xìng rén bàn shēng, qù pí jiān.* (7) *Qiě ráo huā bù zhì lì, má huáng zhǔ chuǎn, jīn cǐ yǔ fǎn zhī, yí fēi zhòng jǐng yì.*

ephedra (麻黄 *má huáng*, Ephedrae Herba) 3 liǎng (remove nodes)
peony (芍药 *sháo yào*, Paeoniae Radix) 3 liǎng
asarum (细辛 *xì xīn*, Asiasari Herba cum Radice) 3 liǎng
dried ginger (干姜 *gān jiāng*, Zingiberis Rhizoma Exsiccatum) 3 liǎng
mix-fried licorice (甘草 *gān cǎo*, Glycyrrhizae Radix) 3 liǎng

cinnamon twig (桂枝 *guì zhī*, Cinnamomi Ramulus) 3 liǎng (remove bark)
schisandra (五味子 *wǔ wèi zǐ*, Schisandrae Fructus) half shēng
pinellia (半夏 *bàn xià*, Pinelliae Tuber) half shēng (washed)

(1) [For] the above eight ingredients use one dǒu of water. First boil ephedra (*má huáng*) to reduce [the water] by two shēng. Remove the foam [collecting] on top and add all the ingredients. Boil to get three shēng, remove the dregs, and take one shēng, warm. (2) If [there is] thirst, remove pinellia (*bàn xià*) and add 3 liǎng of trichosanthes root (*guā lóu gēn*). (3) If [there is] mild diarrhea, remove ephedra (*má huáng*), add a piece of gray wikstroemia flower (*ráo huā*) the size of a chicken's egg, and dry-fry until it is a red color. (4) If [there is] dysphagia, remove ephedra (*má huáng*) and add one piece of blast-fried aconite (*fù zǐ*). (5) If urination is inhibited and [there is] fullness in the lesser abdomen, remove ephedra (*má huáng*) and add 4 liǎng of poria (*fú líng*). (6) If [there is] panting, remove ephedra (*má huáng*) and add half a shēng of apricot kernel (*xìng rén*), without the skin and tips. (7) Actually, gray wikstroemia flower (*ráo huā*) does not treat diarrhea and ephedra (*má huáng*) treats panting. [As the text] now [stands], these statements are reversed and it is [therefore] doubted that this was Zhòng Jing's intention.*

FORMULA NOTE

* The final section of text is clearly an addition by a later editor pointing out an obvious transcription error.

SYNOPSIS

The pathology, clinical manifestations, and treatment of greater yáng disease with water-rheum collecting in the interior.

COMMENTARY

In this line, a patient who has water-rheum collecting in the interior contracts greater yáng cold damage disease. The exterior signs have not resolved, so although it is not written, one would expect to see signs including aversion to cold, absence of sweating, and heat effusion. This condition, however, is modified by the presence of water-rheum in the interior. The basic signs associated with this pattern and with Minor Green-Blue Dragon Decoction (*xiǎo qīng lóng tāng*) are dry retching and cough. The cough results from water-rheum assailing the lung and causing the loss of normal diffusion and downbearing. The retching results from water-rheum assailing the stomach and causing counterflow of stomach qì. This type of retching is dry and occurs in the presence of water-rheum because the regulation of water movement is impaired. Although water-rhuem collects in the interior, its presence does not imply excess fluid throughout the body, and the other signs in this line support this conclusion. Thirst, inhibited urination, diarrhea, and lesser abdominal fullness indicate the presence of fluid where it should not be and a lack of fluid where it should be. It should be noted that modern physicians often use this formula to treat what Western medicine calls asthma.

A comparison with two other related formulae is instructive. Major Green-Blue Dragon Decoction (*dà qīng lóng tāng*) is used in greater yáng cold damage patterns with interior heat manifesting as agitation and vexation. Minor Green-Blue Dragon Decoction (*xiǎo qīng lóng tāng*) is used for greater yáng cold damage patterns with water-rheum collected in the interior, which manifests as cough, panting, and dry retching. For cough and panting, Cinnamon Twig Decoction Plus Magnolia Bark and Apricot Kernel (*guì zhī jiā hòu pò xìng zǐ tāng*) may be considered, but it should be used for greater yáng wind strike (a condition of exterior vacuity), not for exterior repletion.

LINE 41

伤寒心下有水气，咳而微喘，发热不渴；服汤已，渴者，此寒去欲解也；小青龙汤主之。

Shāng hán xīn xià yǒu shuǐ qì, ké ér wēi chuǎn, fā rè bù kě; fú tāng yǐ, kě zhě, cǐ hán qù yù jiě yě; xiǎo qīng lóng tāng zhǔ zhī.

When in cold damage, [there is] water qì[1] below the heart, cough, mild panting, and heat effusion without thirst, (thirst, after taking the decoction,[2] means the cold is going and [the disease] is about to resolve) Minor Green-Blue Dragon Decoction (*xiǎo qīng lóng tāng*) governs.

TEXT NOTES

1. Water qì, 水气 *shuǐ qì*: Here, water-rheum.
2. After taking the decoction, 服汤已 *fú tāng yǐ*: Minor Green-Blue Dragon Decoction (*xiǎo qīng lóng tāng*) has already been taken.

SYNOPSIS

A further discussion of the primary distinguishing features and treatment of greater yáng disease with collected water-rheum and evidence that can be used to evaluate the efficacy of the treatment following the ingestion of medicinals.

COMMENTARY

The combination of water-rheum and cold damage exterior repletion may produce variable patterns, but cough and panting are commonly observed. The absence of thirst may indicate a slightly different water-rheum pattern, but in the preceding line the reader was alerted that thirst may or may not be present in these patterns. As in the previous line, cold damage with interior water-rheum is treated with Minor Green-Blue Dragon Decoction (*xiǎo qīng lóng tāng*). The significance of thirst following the ingestion of the formula has been interpreted in slightly different ways.

According to the *Yī Zōng Jīn Jiàn*, it is a positive sign and no further treatment is necessary. "Thirst that occurs after taking the decoction and the resolution [of the disease] through sweating is the thirst that follows sweating [observed when] the cold has gone and the interior is dry. It is not the thirst [with] absence of sweating [observed when] water-rheum impairs [fluid] transformation.... One should give a small amount of water to nourish dryness and allow the stomach to harmonize, thereby allowing recovery." This perspective is also held by Kē Qín who adds, "The decoction is taken, yet there is thirst. The interior water qì is dissipated and the exterior cold evil is also dissipated. This line aims to clarify that this thirst is a sign that [the disease] has resolved. [The author] feared that medicinals to allay thirst would be taken, which would nourish the water qì." In short, after taking the decoction, thirst is a positive result that means the treatment was correct. The patient should not be given medicinals for thirst, but should be instructed to drink a small amount of water.

Nevertheless, Wāng Hǔ (汪琥, style 苓友 Líng-Yǒu) offers a second interpretation and he writes: "The "thirst" in the previous line (line 40) is thirst before taking the decoction [which means] the fluids are not moving. The "thirst" in this line occurs after taking the decoction and [it means] fluid collapse after sweating." According to this interpretation, further medicinal treatment is indicated to replenish the fluids that have been lost through sweating; drinking water would be insufficient and ineffective.

3.3 MILD PATTERNS OF EXTERIOR DEPRESSION

Cinnamon Twig Decoction (*guì zhī tāng*), which harmonizes the construction and defense, is the primary formula for treating exterior vacuity patterns, while Ephedra Decoction (*má huáng tāng*), which promotes sweating and diffuses the lungs, is used to treat exterior repletion patterns. When disharmony of the construction and defense occurs simultaneously with a mild evil depressed in the exterior, neither of these formulae can be used individually. Combinations of these two formulae are used to treat these patterns, as described below.

a) Cinnamon Twig and Ephedra Half-and-Half Decoction (*guì zhī má huáng gè bàn tāng*) is used for patients who have had a greater yáng exterior pattern for an extended period of time. The main sign is alternating aversion to cold and heat effusion, in which the heat is more pronounced than the cold, and which occurs two or three times per day. The patient's face may be red, and generalized itching may be observed. No lesser yáng or yáng brightness signs should be observed. In these patterns, wind-cold fetters the exterior for an extended period of time, and an evil becomes depressed in the exterior. This formula, which is acrid, warm, and mild, promotes mild sweating.

b) Two Parts Cinnamon Twig One Part Ephedra Decoction (*guì zhī èr má huáng yī tāng*) patterns are characterized by alternating aversion to cold and heat effusion, in which the heat is more pronounced than the cold, and which occurs two times per day. This pattern is similar to the one above, but milder. The formula is a mild warm acrid one that promotes mild sweating.

c) In Two Parts Cinnamon Twig and One Part Spleen-Effusing Decoction (*guì zhī èr yuè bì yī tāng*) patterns, alternating aversion to cold and heat effusion, in which the heat is more pronounced than the cold, is accompanied by thirst and heart vexation. In this pattern, wind-cold fetters the exterior and mild interior heat is present. This formula promotes mild sweating and clears interior heat.

LINE 23

(一) 太阳病，得之八九日，如疟状，发热恶寒，热多寒少，其人不呕，清便欲自可，一日二三度发。(二) 脉微缓者，为欲愈也；脉微而恶寒者，此阴阳俱虚，不可更发汗、更下、更吐也；面色反有热色者，未欲解也，以其不能得小汗出，身必痒，宜桂枝麻黄各半汤。

(1) *Tài yáng bìng, dé zhī bā jiǔ rì, rú nüè zhuàng, fā rè wù hán, rè duō hán shǎo, qí rén bù ǒu, qīng biàn yù zì kě, yí rì èr sān dù fā.* (2) *Mài wēi huǎn zhě, wéi yù yù yě; mài wēi ér wù hán zhě, cǐ yīn yáng jù xū, bù kě gèng fā hàn, gèng xià, gèng tù yè; miàn sè fǎn yǒu rè sè zhě, wèi yù jiě yě, yǐ qí bù néng dé xiǎo hàn chū, shēn bì yǎng, yí guì zhī má huáng gè bàn tāng.*

(1) [In] greater yáng disease [lasting] eight or nine days and resembling malaria,[1] in which [there is] heat effusion and aversion to cold (with the heat effusion more pronounced than the aversion to cold), and in which the person does not retch, the excretions are still normal,[2] and [episodes] occur two or three times per day, then [the following applies]: (2) If the pulse is slightly moderate[3] this means [that there is] about to be recovery. If the pulse is faint and [there is] aversion to cold, this means that both yīn and yáng are vacuous[4] and one cannot further promote sweating, further precipitate, or further [cause] vomiting. However, a facial complexion with the color of heat[5] means [that the disease] is not about to resolve; and because the person cannot get up a light sweat, there will be generalized itching; [therefore,] Cinnamon Twig and Ephedra Half-and-Half Decoction (*guì zhī má huáng gè bàn tāng*) is appropriate.

TEXT NOTES

1. Resembling malaria, 如疟状 *rú nüè zhuàng*: Periodic occurrence of heat effusion and aversion to cold, without a set periodicity. It is not considered true malaria, because of the lack of set periodicity.
2. The excretions are still normal, 清便欲自可 *qīng biàn yù zì kě*: No abnormality in the stool and urine. 清 *qīng* is understood as 圊 *qīng*, which means toilet. The phrase 清便 *qīng biàn*, rendered here as "excretions," means stool and/or urine. The character 欲 *yù*, which means "about to," is here interpreted as "still" by the authors of both *Shāng Hán Lùn Yán Jiū Dà Cí Diǎn* and *Gāo Děng Zhōng Yī Yán Jiū Cān Kǎo Cóng Shū.*
3. The pulse is slightly moderate, 脉微缓 *mài wēi huǎn*: It is possible to interpret this as the "pulse is faint and moderate," but here 微 *wēi* is taken to mean

"slightly" because the pulse means that the disease is about to resolve. If the pulse were faint, one would not expect imminent resolution, since a faint pulse is an indication of severe vacuity.

4. Both yīn and yáng are vacuous, 阴阳俱虚 *yīn yǎng jù xū*: Vacuity of the interior and the exterior. Chéng Wú-Jǐ writes, "[With] a pulse that is faint and aversion to cold, the exterior and interior are vacuous; yáng means the exterior, yīn means the interior. A pulse that is faint indicates interior vacuity, and aversion to cold indicates exterior vacuity."

5. The color of heat, 热色 *rè sè*: The color of heat is red. Chéng Wú-Jǐ writes, "[The term] 'heat color' means red."

FORMULA

Cinnamon Twig and Ephedra Half-and-Half Decoction (*guì zhī má huáng gè bàn tāng*)

○ A mild acrid warm formula [that] promotes slight sweating.

桂枝一两十六铢（去皮） 芍药 生姜（切） 甘草（炙） 麻黄（去节）各一两 大枣四枚（擘） 杏仁二十四枚（汤浸，去皮尖及两仁者）

(一) 右七味，以水五升，先煮麻黄一二沸，去上沫，内诸药，煮取一升八合，去滓，温服六合。(二) 本云，桂枝汤三合，麻黄汤三合，并为六合，顿服。(三) 将息如上法。

Guì zhī yī liǎng shí liù zhū (qù pí) sháo yào, shēng jiāng (qiē), gān cǎo (zhì), má huáng (qù jié) gè yī liǎng dà zǎo sì méi (bò) xìng rén èr shí sì méi (tāng jìn, qù pí jiān jí liǎng rén zhě)

(1) *Yòu qī wèi, yǐ shuǐ wǔ shēng, xiān zhǔ má huáng yī èr fèi, qù shàng mò, nà zhū yào, zhǔ qǔ yī shēng bā gě, qù zǐ, wēn fú liù gě.* (2) *Běn yún guì zhī tāng sān gě, má huáng tāng sān gě, bìng wéi liù gě, dùn fú.* (3) *Jiāng xī rú shàng fǎ.*

cinnamon twig (桂枝 *guì zhī*, Cinnamomi Ramulus) 1 liǎng 16 zhū (remove bark)
peony (芍药 *sháo yào*, Paeoniae Radix) 1 liǎng
fresh ginger (生姜 *shēng jiāng*, Zingiberis Rhizoma Recens) 1 liǎng (cut)
mix-fried licorice (甘草 *gān cǎo*, Glycyrrhizae Radix) 1 liǎng
ephedra (麻黄 *má huáng*, Ephedrae Herba) 1 liǎng (remove nodes)
jujube (大枣 *dà zǎo*, Ziziphi Fructus) 4 pieces (broken)
apricot kernel (杏仁 *xìng rén*, Armeniacae Semen) 24 pieces (scald in hot water, and remove the skin, the tips, and the two kernels)*

(1) [For] the above seven ingredients use five shēng of water. First boil ephedra (*má huáng*) once or twice and remove the foam [collecting] on top. Add all [the other] ingredients and boil to get one shēng eight gě. Remove the dregs and take six gě warm. (2) This is three gě of Cinnamon Twig Decoction (*guì zhī tāng*) and three gě of Ephedra Decoction (*má huáng tāng*) combined to make six gě and taken as a single dose. (3) [One should] rest, as in the previous method [for Cinnamon Twig Decoction (*guì zhī tāng*)].

FORMULA NOTE

* Scald in hot water, and remove the skin, the tips, and the two kernels, 汤浸，去皮尖及两仁者 *tāng jìn, qù pí jiān jí liǎng rén zhě*: We do not know what the meaning of the phrase, "two kernels" is in this context.

SYNOPSIS

a) Three possible scenarios that may appear in unresolved greater yáng disease.

b) The distinguishing clinical features and treatment of greater yáng mild exterior depression patterns.

COMMENTARY

Eight or nine days is considered to be a long course for greater yáng disease. Heat effusion and aversion to cold, with the heat effusion predominant, is said to be similar to but not the same as malaria. It is not the same as malaria because it does not have the same set periodicity typical of malaria. It is not clear whether this means heat effusion and aversion to cold occurring simultaneously or whether it means alternating aversion to cold and heat effusion, as is seen in malaria. Regardless of which is the correct interpretation, it is clearly stated that the patient does not retch and the urine and stool are normal. This information is provided because after a protracted disease course, particularly when malaria-like signs are observed, one may be concerned that the disease has shifted to the lesser yáng. That the patient does not retch is one indication—although not an absolute assurance—that the disease has not shifted to the lesser yáng. Another possibility is that the disease has shifted to the yáng brightness, but since the heat and cold signs are not characteristic of a yáng brightness pattern and the stool and urine are normal, this is unlikely. On the basis of the information in the text, one can infer that the disease is still in the exterior and an unresolved evil is depressed in the exterior.

At this point, the reader is presented with three possible transmutations. The first is that the pulse is slightly moderate. If this pulse appears, one knows that the disease is about to resolve and no treatment is necessary. In the second, the pulse is faint, the heat effusion ceases, and aversion to cold continues, indicating that both the interior and the exterior have become vacuous. As a result, one cannot use sweating, precipitation, or vomiting to treat this patient, but must supplement the vacuity, so that right qì can expel the depressed evil. The third, in which the disease is not about to resolve, is characterized by red facial complexion and generalized itching, which occur because the patient is not able to sweat and the evil remains depressed in the exterior. Yóu Yí explains the itching as follows: "[When] an exuberant [exterior] evil attacks the channels and sinews, [there is] pain. [When] a mild evil moves in the skin, [there is] itching." According to Yóu Yí, this last condition occurs because the patient cannot get up a light sweat. The exterior is not obstructed by a repletion evil, for which the strong promotion of sweating with Ephedra Decoction (*má huáng tāng*) would be appropriate. Here, a mild evil is depressed in the exterior and the patient is unable to sweat normally. The defense and construction must be harmonized through the use of Cinnamon Twig Decoction (*guì zhī tāng*) and light sweating must be promoted through the use of Ephedra Decoction (*má huáng tāng*). As Yóu Yí writes:

> Seeing that [the patient] has not yet been able to sweat, this is not [a disease] Cinnamon Twig Decoction (*guì zhī tāng*) can resolve. Also, the evil

is mild, so Ephedra Decoction (*má huáng tāng*) cannot [be used] to promote sweating. Thus the two formulae are combined into one formula.

Cinnamon Twig and Ephedra Half-and-Half Decoction (*guì zhī má huáng gè bàn tāng*) contains equal proportions of the two formulae and the dosage of all ingredients is one-third of the original. This formula promotes sweating more strongly than Cinnamon Twig Decoction (*guì zhī tāng*) but less strongly than Ephedra Decoction (*má huáng tāng*). It resolves the exterior, mildly promotes sweating, and will not damage right qì.

LINE 25

㈠ 服桂枝汤，大汗出，脉洪大者，与桂枝汤，如前法。㈡ 若形似疟，一日再发者，汗出必解，宜桂枝二麻黄一汤。

(1) *Fú guì zhī tāng, dà hàn chū, mài hóng dà zhě, yǔ guì zhī tāng, rú qián fǎ.* (2) *Ruò xíng sì nüè, yí rì zài fā zhě, hàn chū bì jiě, yí guì zhī èr má huáng yī tāng.*

(1) When after taking Cinnamon Twig Decoction (*guì zhī tāng*), [there is] great sweating and the pulse is surging and large, use Cinnamon Twig Decoction (*guì zhī tāng*) as before. (2) If [the disease] resembles malaria, occurring twice a day,* sweating will resolve [the disease] and [therefore,] Two Parts Cinnamon Twig One Part Ephedra Decoction (*guì zhī èr má huáng yī tāng*) is appropriate.

TEXT NOTE

* Occurring twice a day, 一日再发 *yī rì zài fā*: Two occurrences each day. 再 *zài* means a second occurrence.

FORMULA

Two Parts Cinnamon Twig One Part Ephedra Decoction (*guì zhī èr má huáng yī tāng*)

∘ A mild acrid warm formula [that] promotes slight sweating.

桂枝一两十七铢（去皮） 芍药一两六铢 麻黄十六铢（去节） 生姜一两六铢（切） 杏仁十六个（去皮尖） 甘草一两二铢（炙） 大枣五枚（擘）

㈠ 右七味，以水五升，先煮麻黄一二沸，去上沫，内诸药，煮取二升，去滓，温服一升，日再服。㈡ 本云，桂枝汤二分，麻黄汤一分，合为二升，分再服。㈢ 今合为一方，将息如前法。

Guì zhī yī liǎng shí qī zhū (qù pí) sháo yào yī liǎng liù zhū má huáng shí liù zhū (qù jié) shēng jiāng yī liǎng liù zhū (qiē) xìng rén shí liù ge (qù pí jiān) gān cǎo yī liǎng èr zhū (zhì) dà zǎo wǔ méi (bò)

(1) *Yòu qī wèi, yǐ shuǐ wǔ shēng, xiān zhǔ má huáng yī èr fèi, qù shàng mò, nà zhū yào, zhǔ qǔ èr shēng, qù zǐ, wēn fú yī shēng, rì zài fú.* (2) *Běn yún guì zhī tāng èr fēn, má huáng tāng yī fēn, hé wéi èr shēng, fēn zài fú.* (3) *Jīn hé wéi yī fāng, jiāng xī rú qián fǎ.*

cinnamon twig (桂枝 *guì zhī*, Cinnamomi Ramulus) 1 liǎng 17 zhū (remove bark)
peony (芍药 *sháo yào*, Paeoniae Radix) 1 liǎng 6 zhū
ephedra (麻黄 *má huáng*, Ephedrae Herba) 16 zhū (remove nodes)
fresh ginger (生姜 *shēng jiāng*, Zingiberis Rhizoma Recens) 1 liǎng 6 zhū (cut)
apricot kernel (杏仁 *xìng rén*, Armeniacae Semen) 16 pieces (remove skin and tips)
mix-fried licorice (甘草 *gān cǎo*, Glycyrrhizae Radix) 1 liǎng 2 zhū
jujube (大枣 *dà zǎo*, Ziziphi Fructus) 5 pieces (broken)

(1) [For] the above seven ingredients use five shēng of water. First boil ephedra (*má huáng*) once or twice and remove the foam [collecting] on top. Add all [the other] ingredients and boil to get two shēng. Remove the dregs and take one shēng warm, then take again [the same] day. (2) This is two parts Cinnamon Twig Decoction (*guì zhī tāng*) and one part Ephedra Decoction (*má huáng tāng*) combined [to make] two shēng. Separate [into two parts], [take one] then take again. (3) Nowadays, [these two formula] are combined into one formula, and [one should] rest, as in the previous method [for Cinnamon Twig Decoction (*guì zhī tāng*)].

Synopsis

a) Three possible scenarios that may appear in unresolved greater yáng patterns.

b) The distinguishing clinical features and treatment of greater yáng mild exterior depression patterns.

Commentary

When Cinnamon Twig Decoction (*guì zhī tāng*) is given, the patient should sweat lightly so that the body just becomes moist. Above, following the ingestion of Cinnamon Twig Decoction (*guì zhī tāng*), copious sweat issues. This type of sweating is inappropriate and as Zhāng Jī writes in line 12, p. 60, "One cannot allow [the sweat] to flow like water, since the disease will not be eliminated [in this way]." The disease does not resolve and in the line above, the reader is presented with two possible transmutations. The first is that the pulse becomes surging and large. It might be inferred that the disease has shifted to the yáng brightness, but this does not appear to be the case since none of the signs generally associated with yáng brightness disease, like vexing thirst and great heat, are present. Furthermore, Cinnamon Twig Decoction (*guì zhī tāng*) is prescribed as it was given before. Although treated inappropriately, the disease has not transmuted and a greater yáng exterior pattern still exists. The other possibility is that the disease condition changes and gives the appearance of malaria. As in the previous line, this suggests periodic occurrences of heat effusion and aversion to cold and is indicative of an evil depressed in the exterior. The treatment in both lines is similar, although here the formula is two parts Cinnamon Twig Decoction (*guì zhī tāng*) to one part Ephedra Decoction (*má huáng tāng*), while in the previous line equal parts of both are given. Xú Dà Chūn comments, "The meaning of this [formula and that of] Cinnamon Twig and Ephedra Half-and-Half Decoction (*guì zhī má huáng gè bàn tāng*) is similar, but because great sweating has occurred, [the dose] of Cinnamon

Twig Decoction (*guì zhī tāng*) is slightly more and [the dose] of Ephedra Decoction (*má huáng tāng*) is slightly less."

One question that unfortunately remains unanswered is why, in a case of profuse sweating, a formula containing ephedra (*má huáng*) is suggested. A possible answer to this question is that whenever Zhāng Jī encountered a disease with the appearance of malaria, but which was not malaria, he used a combination of Cinnamon Twig Decoction (*guì zhī tāng*) and Ephedra Decoction (*má huáng tāng*), even if sweating had already occurred.

LINE 27

太阳病，发热恶寒，热多寒少，脉微弱者，此无阳也，不可发汗，宜桂枝二越婢一汤。

Tài yáng bìng, fā rè wù hán, rè duō hán shǎo, mài wēi ruò zhě, cǐ wú yáng yě, bù kě fā hàn, yí guì zhī èr yuè bì yī tāng.

When in greater yáng disease [there is] heat effusion and aversion to cold [with] more heat and less cold (a pulse that is faint and weak means that yáng is absent* and one cannot promote sweating), Two Parts Cinnamon Twig and One Part Spleen-Effusing Decoction (*guì zhī èr yuè bì yī tāng*) is appropriate.

TEXT NOTE

* Yáng is absent, 无阳 *wú yǎng*: Great vacuity of yáng qì.

FORMULA

Two Parts Cinnamon Twig and One Part Spleen-Effusing Decoction (*guì zhī èr yuè bì yī tāng*)

○ Promote sweating mildly; clear interior heat.

桂枝（去皮） 芍药 麻黄 甘草（炙）各十八铢 大枣四枚（擘） 生姜一两二铢（切） 石膏二十四铢（碎，绵裹）

(一) 右七味，以水五升，煮麻黄一二沸，去上沫，内诸药，煮取二升，去滓，温服一升。(二) 本云，当裁为越婢汤、桂枝汤合之，饮一升。(三) 今合为一方，桂枝汤二分，越婢汤一分。

Guì zhī (qù pí), sháo yào, má huáng, gān cǎo (zhì) gè shí bā zhū dà zǎo sì méi (bò) shēng jiāng yī liǎng èr zhū (qiē) shí gāo èr shí sì zhū (suì, mián guǒ)

(1) *Yòu qī wèi, yǐ shuǐ wǔ shēng, zhǔ má huáng yī èr fèi, qù shàng mò, nà zhū yào, zhǔ qǔ èr shēng, qù zǐ, wēn fú yī shēng.* (2) *Běn yún dāng cái wéi yuè bì tāng、guì zhī tāng hé zhī, yǐn yī shēng.* (3) *Jīn hé wéi yī fāng, guì zhī tāng èr fēn, yuè bì tāng yī fēn.*

cinnamon twig (桂枝 *guì zhī*, Cinnamomi Ramulus) (remove bark) 18 zhū

peony (芍药 *sháo yào*, Paeoniae Radix) 18 zhū
ephedra (麻黄 *má huáng*, Ephedrae Herba) 18 zhū
mix-fried licorice (甘草 *gān cǎo*, Glycyrrhizae Radix) 18 zhū
jujube (大枣 *dà zǎo*, Ziziphi Fructus) 4 pieces (broken)
fresh ginger (生姜 *shēng jiāng*, Zingiberis Rhizoma Recens) 1 liǎng 2 zhū (= 32 grams) (cut)
gypsum (石膏 *shí gāo*, Gypsum) 24 zhū (= 16 grams) (crushed, cotton-wrapped)

(1) [For] the above seven ingredients use five shēng of water. First boil ephedra (*má huáng*) once or twice, then remove the foam [collecting] on top. Add all the ingredients and boil to get two shēng. (2) Remove the dregs and take one shēng, warm. (3) This should be considered to be a combination of Cinnamon Twig Decoction (*guì zhī tāng*) and Spleen-Effusing Decoction (*yuè bì tāng*) taken in a one-shēng [dose]. (4) Nowadays, they are combined into one formula, with two parts of Cinnamon Twig Decoction (*guì zhī tāng*) to one part of Spleen-Effusing Decoction (*yuè bì tāng*).

SYNOPSIS

a) The distinguishing clinical features and treatment of a mild pattern of an exterior evil depressed in the greater yáng with interior heat.

b) An example of a contraindication for the use of Two Parts Cinnamon Twig and One Part Spleen-Effusing Decoction (*guì zhī èr yuè bì yī tāng*).

COMMENTARY

In greater yáng disease, heat effusion and aversion to cold are often present. The phrase "more heat and less cold" occurs only twice in the *Shāng Hán Lùn*, here and in line 23, p. 122. The situation described in this line is similar but not identical to that of line 23. In that line, the signs are periodic, whereas in this line, there is no indication of periodicity. Given the conditions described in the lines above, one would consider this pattern to be one of an evil depressed in the exterior and would expect a combination of Cinnamon Twig Decoction (*guì zhī tāng*) and Ephedra Decoction (*má huáng tāng*) to be used. In fact, Two Parts Cinnamon Twig and One Part Spleen-Effusing Decoction (*guì zhī èr yuè bì yī tāng*) contains elements of these two formulae, but it also includes gypsum (*shí gāo*). Because this ingredient clears interior heat, the authors of *Gāo Děng Cóng Shū* write that interior heat is also present in this pattern.

The middle section of this line has been explained in two ways. The first is that this line presents only one pattern and the phrase, "one cannot promote sweating," 不可发汗 *bù kě fā hàn*, means that because the pulse is faint and weak, one cannot promote great sweating. As Wāng Hǔ writes, "The four words 'one cannot promote sweating' mean that one should not again promote great sweating, because this patient's pulse is faint and weak, [there is] no yáng, and the fluids are scant. This formula, compared to the previous one, which lightly promoted sweating, is even milder."

Another possibility, as suggested by Zhāng Nán (章楠, style 虚谷 Xū-Gǔ), is that this line contains a grammatical inversion and in actual fact, describes two patterns. "This line is appropriately seen as two [lines]. [The section] "Two Parts Cinnamon Twig and One Part Spleen-Effusing Decoction (*guì zhī èr yuè bì yī tāng*) is appropriate" should be placed after "more heat and less cold." If the pulse is faint and weak, and this means that there is no yáng, how can one promote sweating again? Therefore, Zhāng Jī is stating a contraindication, that one cannot promote sweating."

Of the two interpretations presented above, the second is the more reasonable because of the general contraindication against the promotion of sweating. That is, even if the patient's pulse is not faint and weak, great sweating is generally not appropriate.

Line 48

㈠ 二阳并病，太阳初得病时，发其汗，汗先出不彻，因转属阳明，续自微汗出，不恶寒。㈡ 若太阳病证不罢者，不可下，下之为逆，如此可小发汗。㈢ 设面色缘缘正赤者，阳气怫郁在表，当解之、熏之。㈣ 若发汗不彻，不足言，阳气怫郁不得越，当汗不汗，其人躁烦，不知痛处，乍在腹中，乍在四肢，按之不可得，其人短气但坐，以汗出不彻故也，更发汗则愈。㈤ 何以知汗出不彻，以脉濇故知也。

(1) *Èr yáng bìng bìng, tài yáng chū dé bìng shí, fā qí hàn, hàn xiān chū bù chè, yīn zhuǎn shǔ yáng míng, xù zì wēi hàn chū, bù wù hán.* (2) *Ruò tài yáng bìng zhèng bù bà zhě, bù kě xià, xià zhī wéi nì, rú cǐ kě xiǎo fā hàn.* (3) *Shè miàn sè yuán yuán zhèng chì zhě, yáng qì fú yù zài biǎo, dāng jiě zhī、xūn zhī.* (4) *Ruò fā hàn bù chè, bù zú yán, yáng qì fú yù bù dé yuè, dāng hàn bù hàn, qí rén zào fán, bù zhī tòng chù, zhá zài fù zhōng, zhá zài sì zhī, àn zhī bù kě dé, qí rèn duǎn qì dàn zuò, yǐ hàn chū bù chè gù yě, gèng fā hàn zé yù.* (5) *Hé yǐ zhī hàn chū bù chè, yǐ mài sè gù zhī yě.*

(1) In dragover disease of the two yáng,[1] the disease begins in the greater yáng; sweating is promoted and the sweating is incomplete, which causes the disease to shift to the yáng brightness and [there is] continuous slight spontaneous sweating and absence of aversion to cold. (2) If the greater yáng disease pattern has not ceased, one cannot precipitate, because precipitation [would be] an adverse [treatment] and in this case, one can promote sweating mildly. (3) If the facial complexion is continuously full red,[2] the yáng qì[3] is depressed in the exterior and [one] should resolve [the exterior and] fume.[4] (4) If sweating is promoted incompletely, [that is to say] insufficiently to speak of,[5] the yáng qì is depressed and cannot pass out so there should be sweating but [there is] not. The person is agitated and vexed and does not know where the

pain is located; now it is in the abdomen, now it is in the extremities, and [when] pressing, one cannot find it.[6] The person is short of breath and can only sit.[7] This is because sweating was incomplete and further promotion of sweating will lead to recovery. (5) How can one know that the sweating was incomplete? One knows because the pulse is rough.

TEXT NOTES

1. Dragover disease of the two yáng, 二阳并病 *ér yáng bìng bìng*: Dragover disease of the greater yáng and yáng brightness channels. As in the *Yī Zōng Jīn Jiàn*, "... the two yáng means greater yáng and yáng brightness...." Dragover disease is differentiated from combination disease in terms of temporal appearance of signs. In both dragover disease and combination disease, signs of more than one channel appear. In dragover disease, disease of one channel has not yet ceased when signs of another channel appear. In combination disease, signs belonging to more than one channel appear simultaneously. See also line 36, p. 99.
2. The facial complexion is continuously full red, 面色缘缘正赤 *miàn sè yuán yuán zhèng chì*: 缘缘 *yuán yuán* means unceasing; 正赤 *zhèng chì* means a full red color.
3. Yáng qì, 阳气 *yáng qì*: Evil qì, not the defensive yáng of the patient.
4. [One] should resolve [the exterior and] fume, 当解之，熏之 *dāng jiě zhī, xūn zhī*: The promotion of sweating to resolve the exterior, and fuming the exterior. Although in many places in the text Zhāng Jī describes fuming as a mistreatment, he appears to regard it as appropriate in this situation.
5. [That is to say] insufficiently to speak of, 不足言 *bù zú yán*: Three different interpretations are offered for this phrase.
   a) The first interpretation, which we have used in the translation, is that the amount of sweat is so small that it is not worth mentioning. The authors of *Shāng Hán Lùn Yì Shì* state, "Sweating is promoted, [but the sweat] does not outthrust; [therefore,] although there is sweating, it is not worth mentioning."
   b) The second interpretation is that it refers to the phrase that follows, and means that it goes without saying that when there is incomplete sweating, the yáng qì must be depressed; it is unnecessary to state this point. Wāng Hǔ writes, "[Describing] this situation, sweating is promoted incompletely, and this person's yáng qì is depressed and cannot pass out; it is insufficient to speak of. 'Insufficient to speak of' means that it (incomplete sweating) follows as a matter of course (when yáng qì is depressed); [therefore,] it is unnecessary to state this."
   c) The final interpretation is that it relates to the phrase that follows and means that incomplete sweating is insufficient to produce a condition of yáng qì depression. Chéng Wú-Jǐ writes, "If the promotion of sweating is incomplete, this is insufficient to then say that yáng qì is depressed. [One can] only [say] that there should have been [an appropriate amount of] sweating and there was not [this amount of] sweating. [It is true that] the

yáng qì cannot pass out; the evil has no exit and is severely congested in the channel; therefore [there is] vexation and agitation."

6. [When] pressing, one cannot find it, 按之不可得 *àn zhī bù kě dé*: No pain when the area is palpated. Zhōu Yáng-Jùn writes, "[There is] no real pain, that is why it says, 'when pressing, one cannot find it'."
7. Short of breath and can only sit, 短气但坐 *duǎn qì dàn zuò*: The patient's breathing is short, rapid, and shallow and may be discontinuous. The patient is not comfortable lying down and can only sit up.

SYNOPSIS

The distinguishing clinical features and treatment of two scenarios that can occur following the incomplete promotion of sweating in a greater yáng disease.

COMMENTARY

In dragover disease of the greater yáng and yáng brightness channels, the greater yáng signs have not yet ceased and yáng brightness signs appear. This occurs because the promotion of sweating was incomplete. That is, the sweating was insufficient to expel the evil and it shifts into the yáng brightness. Aversion to cold ceases and aversion to heat and continuous slight sweating may be observed, indicating a shift to the yáng brightness. Although the evil is shifting into the yáng brightness, if the greater yáng signs have not completely ceased, one cannot precipitate the interior. This treatment would cause any residual exterior evil to fall inward and it is described by Zhāng Jī as an adverse [treatment], 逆 *nì*. One may promote sweating, but only mild sweating, since sweat has already been lost.

If the face appears continuously red, it means that the evil is depressed in the exterior and one should promote sweating and fume the exterior.

The section of text starting from "if sweating is promoted incompletely" refers back to the beginning of the line. Sweating has been promoted incompletely, but the disease has not shifted to the yáng brightness. The signs in this section indicate an evil depressed in the exterior. Sweating was promoted to expel the evil, but because of the method used or the patient's constitution, the evil has not resolved and blocks the exterior. Movement of the yáng qì is impaired, resulting in vexation and agitation. The patient feels discomfort, but cannot identify the exact location. When the exterior is blocked, lung qì becomes inhibited, resulting in shortness of breath and ability to feel comfortable only when sitting up. Zhāng Jī explains that this is all the result of incomplete sweating and that sweating should be promoted again in order to bring about resolution.

In the final section, Zhāng Jī suggests that the pulse provides a basis for determining whether the sweating is incomplete. He explains that if the pulse is rough, it means that sweating is incomplete. When sweating is incomplete, evil qì becomes depressed in the exterior and blocks the flow of yáng qì.

4 TRANSMUTED PATTERNS OF GREATER YÁNG DISEASE

Transmuted patterns can occur either as a result of inappropriate treatment, when an extremely severe exterior evil is contracted, or as a result of factors related to the constitution of the patient. Many of the transmuted patterns presented here are the result of inappropriate treatment, including sweating, precipitation, vomiting, and fire. These transmuted patterns are not the only outcomes of inappropriate treatment; by reading further we can understand the pathomechanism of the pattern, the method of identifying the pattern and differentiating further treatments, and the principles for choosing formulae and individual medicinals. Looking at these transmuted patterns, we will see that many are commonly encountered in clinical practice and that the suggested formulae are commonly used in the treatment of these patterns. These treatment principles and accompanying formulae can, therefore, be used not only in greater yáng transmuted patterns, but if they are well understood, in a wide range of clinical applications. In greater yáng disease, transmuted patterns are classified into patterns of heat, vacuity cold, yīn-yáng dual vacuity, water amassment, blood amassment, chest bind, storehouse bind, glomus, heat above and cold below, adverse treatment with fire, and those that are about to resolve.

4.1 TREATMENT PRINCIPLES FOR TRANSMUTED PATTERNS

LINE 16A

㈠太阳病三日，已发汗，若吐、若下、若温针，仍不解者，此为坏病，桂枝不中与之也。㈡观其脉证，知犯何逆，随证治之。...

(1) *Tài yáng bìng sān rì, yǐ fā hàn, ruò tù、 ruò xià、 ruò wēn zhēn, réng bù jiě zhě, cǐ wéi huài bìng, guì zhī bù zhōng yǔ zhī yě.* (2) *Guān qí mài zhèng, zhī fàn hé nì, suí zhèng zhì zhī....*

(1) When greater yáng disease [has lasted for] three days [and] sweating has already been promoted, if vomiting, [or] if precipitation, [or] if warm needling[1] [has been used] and still [there is] no resolution,[2] this is an aggravated disease[3] [in which] Cinnamon Twig [Decoction] (*guì zhī [tāng]*)[4] should not be given. (2) Observe the pulse and signs, know what error [you] have committed,[5] [and then] treat according to the signs....

TEXT NOTES

1. Warm needling, 温针 *wēn zhēn*: After the needle is inserted, moxa floss is placed on the handle and lit in order to warm the needle and the local area. This technique is used to warm the channels and free the vessels and to move the qì and quicken the blood.
2. Still [there is] no resolution, 仍不解者 *rěng bù jiě zhě*: The disease has not resolved, but the exterior evil is no longer present. Exterior signs are absent, but the patient has not recovered and a negative transmutation has taken place.
3. This is an aggravated disease, 此为坏病 *cǐ wéi huài bìng*: A negative change in the disease course following inappropriate treatment.

4. Cinnamon Twig [Decoction] (*guì zhī* [*tāng*]) 桂枝 *guì zhī*: The full name is not written in the text, but this is assumed to mean the formula, not the single medicinal cinnamon twig (*guì zhī*).

Synopsis

The treatment principles for transmuted patterns that occur following the mistreatment of a greater yáng disease.

Commentary

In greater yáng disease, the standard treatment is the promotion of sweating. Here, sweating has been promoted, but apparently it was unsuccessful and consequently, other treatments were used. The disease has not resolved and has instead transformed into what Zhāng Jī refers to as an aggravated disease, 坏病 *huài bìng*. One may observe many different transmutations depending upon what treatments have been given. The reader is advised not to give Cinnamon Twig Decoction (*guì zhī tāng*), but to investigate the patient's current condition and treat accordingly. This line expresses an important element of the spirit of the text. The *Shāng Hán Lùn* was arguably the first text to explicitly suggest the principle that much later in history came to be called "determining treatment by the patterns identified," 辨症论治 *biàn zhèng lùn zhì*. That is, it is not simply a matter of which formula to use for the treatment of which sign, but also one of understanding the pathomechanism and any transmutations. The result of this approach is that different patterns may be treated with the same formula and that different formulae may be used to treat the same pattern. One must use the diagnostic tools of inspection, listening and smelling, inquiry, and palpation to identify the pattern. Once the pattern is clearly understood, the choice of the correct treatment can then be made. The suggestion of this approach is important, of course, not only in the treatment of aggravated diseases, but in the physician's general approach to treatment.

4.2 Differentiation of Vacuity and Repletion Patterns

Line 70

㈠ 发汗后恶寒者，虚故也。㈡ 不恶寒，但热者，实也。㈢ 当和胃气，与调胃承气汤。

(1) *Fā hàn hòu wù hán zhě, xū gù yě.* (2) *Bù wù hán, dàn rè zhě, shí yě.* (3) *Dāng hé wèi qì, yǔ tiáo wèi chéng qì tāng.*

(1) After sweating is promoted, if [there is] aversion to cold, [this] is because of vacuity. (2) If aversion to cold is absent, and only heat [effusion]* [is present], this indicates repletion. (3) One should harmonize the stomach qì with Stomach-Regulating Qì-Coordinating Decoction (*tiáo wèi chéng qì tāng*).

Text Note

* Heat [effusion], 热 *rè*: The term translated as "heat effusion" is usually 发热 *fā rè*, but here this single character, 热 *rè*, is considered equivalent.

Formula

Stomach-Regulating Qì-Coordinating Decoction (*tiáo wèi chéng qì tāng*). See line 248, p. 327, for a full discussion of this formula.

Synopsis

The differentiation of vacuity and repletion scenarios after the promotion of sweating.

Commentary

This line presents two scenarios which may occur when a disease fails to resolve after the promotion of sweating. The first is characterized by aversion to cold and the second by heat effusion. The promotion of sweating does, in fact, cause some damage to the body, but Zhāng Jī recognized that the presence of an evil also damages the body. The use of a mildly harmful treatment method will ultimately benefit the patient.

This line specifies the damage that may result from of the promotion of sweating. Aversion to cold is the result of an inability of vacuous yáng qì to warm the exterior, following damage to right qì. Heat effusion without aversion to cold is the result of damage to the fluids and transformation to heat repletion. The patient's constitution also plays a role in the development of disease; consequently, in patients who are already vacuous, treatment may exacerbate the vacuity and in patients with exuberant yáng, treatment may damage yīn humor. An examination of the formula reveals that it is used for yáng brightness disease with dryness, heat, and internal bind and is appropriate for repletion patterns. The repletion pattern in the second part of this line is one of internal dryness and heat that is the result of damage to the fluids caused by the promotion of sweating. This type of transmutation, following the promotion of sweating, is most likely to occur in a patient with a preexisting condition of yáng exuberance and yīn vacuity.

Line 60

㈠ 下之后，复发汗，必振寒，脉微细。㈡ 所以然者，以内外俱虚故也。

(1) *Xià zhī hòu, fù fā hàn, bì zhèn hán, mài wēi xì.* (2) *Suǒ yǐ rán zhě, yǐ nèi wài jù xū gù yě.*

(1) After precipitation, [if] sweating is promoted, there will be quivering with cold[1] and a pulse that is faint and fine.[2] (2) Why [this] is so is because both the interior and the exterior are vacuous.[3]

Text Notes

1. Quivering with cold, 振寒 *zhèn hán*: A subjective feeling of cold with trembling and aversion to cold.

2. A pulse that is faint and fine, 脉微细 *mài wēi xì*: A pulse that feels indistinct and that is as thin as a thread. Readers should be careful to avoid associating with this pulse description the definitions given to pulse terms after Zhāng Jī's time, according to which "fine" is taken to mean not only thin and thread-like, but also clearly defined, and hence cannot be used to describe a pulse that is described as "faint." For other examples, see the discussion in the Introduction, p. 20.
3. Interior and exterior vacuity, 内外俱虚 *nèi wài jū xū*: When precipitation is used, the interior yīn fluids are damaged and when sweating is promoted, the exterior yáng qì is damaged. This results in dual vacuity of the interior yīn humor and the exterior yáng qì.

Synopsis

A transmuted pattern that occurs when, after precipitation, sweating is promoted, resulting in vacuity of interior, exterior, yīn, and yáng.

Commentary

In general, precipitation is not a method often recommended in the *Shāng Hán Lùn* and even more rare is its use prior to the promotion of sweating to resolve an existing exterior pattern. Precipitation followed by the promotion of sweating is used when, in a simultaneous interior-exterior pattern, the treatment of the interior pattern is considered urgent due to its severity and the exterior pattern is mild. Therefore, precipitation in an existing exterior pattern is usually a mistreatment. Quivering with cold occurs when the yáng is damaged and unable to warm the exterior. The damage to the yáng qì is also reflected in a faint pulse. A pulse that is fine indicates damage to yīn humor.

The causal relationship between the different parts of this line should be noted. The pattern described in the first sentence is not the only possible pattern resulting from this type of erroneous treatment. In line 59, p. 259, the same mistreatment results in inhibited urination and fluid collapse. In this line, Zhāng Jī emphasizes that if the result of mistreatment is dual vacuity of the interior and exterior, one will see certain signs. If the result of the mistreatment is another pattern, perhaps because of constitutional differences or slightly different treatment methodology, these particular signs probably will not appear.

4.3 Cold and Heat: Differentiation of True and False Patterns

Line 11

病人身大热，反欲得衣者，热在皮肤，寒在骨髓也；身大寒，反不欲近衣者，寒在皮肤，热在骨髓也。

Bìng rén shēn dà rè, fǎn yù dé yī zhě, rè zài pí fū, hán zài gǔ suǐ yě; shēn dà hán, fǎn bù yù jìn yī zhě, hán zài pí fū, rè zài gǔ suǐ yě.

When the patient has great generalized heat,* but desires to put [more] clothes on, the heat is in the skin and the cold is in the bone marrow;

when [there is] great generalized cold,* but [the patient] has no desire for clothes, the cold is in the skin and the heat is in the bone marrow.

TEXT NOTE

* Great generalized heat, 身大热 *shēn dà rè*; great generalized cold, 身大寒 *shēn dà hán*: Differences of opinion exist on how to interpret these terms. It is possible to argue for an interpretation as heat effusion, 发热 *fā rè*, and aversion to cold, 恶寒 *wù hán*, as Zhāng Jī sometimes uses simply heat, 热 *rè*, and cold, 寒 *hán*, to represent these concepts. Nevertheless, these terms may only mean a subjective feeling of heat or cold on the part of the patient. This heat or cold may or may not be palpable upon examination. The authors of the *Shāng Hán Lùn Yán Jiū Dà Cí Diǎn* interpret these terms as heat or cold that is palpable upon examination.

SYNOPSIS

From the patient's desire for or aversion to putting on more clothes, one can identify true and false signs.

COMMENTARY

In this line, the skin represents the exterior and the bone marrow represents the interior. This distinction may be used to determine true and false signs. When the patient feels hot, subjectively or objectively, yet has a fear of the cold and wants to wear more clothing, it indicates false heat and true cold. Exuberant yīn cold in the interior and vacuous yáng floating to the exterior give a false impression of heat. Conversely, when the patient feels cold but fears heat and wants to remove layers of clothing, it indicates false cold and true heat. Exuberant heat is depressed in the interior and obstructs the passage of yáng qì to the exterior. The vacuous yáng qì is unable to warm the exterior and gives a false impression of cold. According to yīn-yáng theory, extreme cold resembles heat and extreme heat resembles cold. In fact, extreme heat or cold can convert into its opposite. Because false signs occur in severe conditions and their misidentification as true signs can lead to a critical exacerbation of the condition method based on false signs may be damaging to the patient, considerable importance is given to identifying them correctly.

LINE 120

㈠ 太阳病，当恶寒发热，今汗自出，反不恶寒发热，关上脉细数者，以医吐之过也。㈡ 一、二日吐之者，腹中饥，口不能食；三、四日吐之者，不喜糜粥，欲食冷食，朝食暮吐，以医吐之所致也，此为小逆。

(1) *Tài yáng bìng, dāng wù hán fā rè, jīn hàn zì chū, fǎn bù wù hán fā rè, guān shàng mài xì shuò zhě, yǐ yī tù zhī guò yě.* (2) *Yī、èr rì tù zhī zhě, fù zhōng jī, kǒu bù néng shí; sān、sì rì tù zhī zhě, bù xǐ mí zhōu, yù shí lěng shí, zhāo shí mù tù, yǐ yī tù zhī suǒ zhì yě, cǐ wéi xiǎo nì.*

(1) In greater yáng disease, [when] there should be aversion to cold and heat effusion, [there is] now spontaneous sweating, but aversion to cold and heat effusion are absent and the bar pulse is fine and rapid,[1] [it is] because vomiting [treatment] was used [incorrectly].[2] (2) If vomiting [is used] on the first or second day of [greater yáng disease], [there is a feeling of] hunger in the abdomen, but [the person] cannot eat. If vomiting [is used] on the third or fourth day of [greater yáng disease], the person dislikes gruel, desires to eat cold food, and vomits in the evening food eaten in the morning. This is the result of vomiting [treatment], [which] means this is a minor adverse [treatment].

TEXT NOTES

1. Used incorrectly, 过 *guò*: A therapeutic error. 过, literally "to cross," is here used in the extended sense of "transgression."
2. The bar pulse is fine and rapid, 关上脉细数 *guān shàng mài xì shuò*: The bar pulse is specified because it gives information about the center burner. Qián Huáng (钱潢, style 天来 Tiān-Lái) writes, "'Above the bar' (关上 *guān shàng*) means the bar pulse."

SYNOPSIS

a) A transmuted pattern of vacuity cold in the stomach that is the result of mistreatment of a greater yáng disease.

b) The differentiation of vacuity heat and vacuity cold in the stomach.

COMMENTARY

The patient in this line originally contracted greater yáng disease. But at this point the absence of heat effusion and aversion to cold and the presence of a pulse that is fine and rapid indicate that the exterior disease has already transformed, as a result of the misuse of vomiting treatment. Vomiting is suggested as appropriate treatment generally only in cases of heat evil depressed in the chest. Vomiting treatment has the action of effusing and dissipating, but it cannot be used as a replacement for exterior resolution. Furthermore, as suggested by the presence of spontaneous sweating and a fine, rapid pulse, the use of this type of treatment has damaged the qì, particularly the stomach qì.

The specification of the number of days is probably not to be taken literally, but rather as an approximation of the length of the illness. In the beginning, the evil is mild and the damage to the stomach qì from the use of vomiting is also relatively mild. The patient still feels hungry, but is not able to eat. After a longer course of disease, the evil is deeper and more severe; hence the damage to the stomach qì is more serious. Even a desire for easily digestible foods like gruel is lacking. In fact, one of the results of the presence of an exterior evil is that the stomach becomes both vacuous and dry. Dryness easily engenders heat; consequently the patient desires cold foods. A vacuous-cold stomach does not digest food well, so the food collects in the stomach and is vomited up at night. This therapeutic error is considered minor because the pathological changes are restricted primarily to the local region of the stomach and recovery is still possible.

LINE 122

(一) 病人脉数，数为热，当消谷引食，而反吐者，此以发汗，令阳气微，膈气虚，脉乃数也。(二) 数为客热，不能消谷，以胃中虚冷，故吐也。

(1) *Bìng rén mài shuò, shuò wéi rè, dāng xiāo gǔ yǐn shí, ér fǎn tù zhě, cǐ yǐ fā hàn, lìng yáng qì wēi, gé qì xū, mài nǎi shuò yě.* (2) *Shuò wéi kè rè, bù néng xiāo gǔ, yǐ wèi zhōng xū lěng, gù tù yě.*

(1) When the patient's pulse is rapid, rapidity means heat, [so] there should be rapid hungering and [large] food intake,[1] but if instead [there is] vomiting, this is because the promotion of sweating caused yáng qì debilitation and diaphragm qì vacuity[2] [and therefore] the pulse is rapid. (2) [A pulse that is] rapid means visiting heat[3] and [the person] cannot digest food. Because [there is] vacuity cold in the stomach, [there is] vomiting.

TEXT NOTES

1. Rapid hungering and [large] food intake, 消谷引食 *xiāo gǔ yǐn shí*: Excessive appetite and ability to consume large amounts of food, which is generally associated with stomach repletion heat.
2. Diaphragm qì vacuity, 膈气虚 *gé qì xū*: Here, the indication is that the stomach qì has become vacuous. The diaphragm separates the lung and heart from the center burner and the area below the diaphragm is considered the region of the stomach. Qián Huáng explains, "If the yáng qì of the stomach and stomach duct is exuberant, then [the patient] is able to digest [food] swiftly and to drink. This type [of pattern] is not exuberant heat qì in the stomach. Following erroneous sweating, the yáng qì is debilitated; the diaphragm region is empty and vacuous. [These signs are] the result of vacuous yáng straying to the outer body."
3. Visiting heat, 客热 *kè rè*: False heat or vacuity heat. The term "visiting," 客 *kè*, is generally used in descriptions of exterior evils invading the body. In this line, however, "visiting" refers to the the ephemeral, insubstantial nature of false or vacuity heat.

SYNOPSIS

a) Inappropriate promotion of sweating may lead to a pattern of vacuity cold in the stomach.

b) A differentiation between true and false, cold and heat patterns that may occur when the pulse is rapid.

COMMENTARY

Following the use of sweating, the yáng qì is damaged and vacuity cold is present in the stomach. Because Zhāng Jī is discussing damage following the promotion of sweating, we know that the use of this method was either inappropriate for the disease or it was used excessively. Digestion is impaired, giving rise to counterflow vomiting. Although a rapid pulse often occurs in heat patterns, if true stomach heat existed, one would expect rapid hungering and increased food intake. These signs are absent and instead vomiting is observed. Looking again at the pulse, a true stomach heat pulse should not only be rapid, but also forceful. We may surmise that the pulse is rapid and forceless because the yáng qì has been damaged. This pattern is true cold and false heat. Here, Zhāng Jī emphasizes that a rapid pulse does not always mean true heat.

4.4 Identifying the Order of the Promotion of Sweating and Use of Precipitation

Line 90

㈠本发汗，而复下之，此为逆也；若先发汗，治不为逆。㈡本先下之，而反汗之，为逆；若先下之，治不为逆。

(1) *Běn fā hàn, ér fù xià zhī, cǐ wéi nì yě; ruò xiān fā hàn, zhì bù wéi nì.* (2) *Běn xiān xià zhī, ér fǎn hàn zhī, wéi nì; ruò xiān xià zhī, zhì bù wéi nì.*

(1) When sweating [should have been] promoted originally, yet precipitation [was used],* this is an adverse [treatment]. If sweating is first promoted, it is not adverse treatment. (2) When precipitation [should have been] used originally, but sweating is promoted, this is an adverse [treatment]. If precipitation is first used, it is not an adverse treatment.

Text Note

* Yet precipitation [was used], 而复下之 *ér fù xià zhī*: The promotion of sweating is the correct treatment, yet precipitation was used instead. In this context, 复 *fù* implies that one is acting counter to the correct treatment strategy.

Synopsis

In simultaneous interior-exterior disease, the order of promotion of sweating and use of precipitation is described.

Commentary

To treat greater yáng disease, the promotion of sweating is the correct treatment. It allows the evil to be resolved through sweating. If precipitation is used, the evil may fall into the interior. In simultaneous disease of the exterior and interior, one must choose the treatment according to the severity and urgency of the two diseases. One may first treat the exterior and then treat the interior, or first treat the interior and then treat the exterior, or simultaneously treat both. These principles are presented in this line. The first section explains that it is an adverse treatment if one first uses precipitation, when the promotion of sweating is appropriate. It is also an adverse treatment if one first promotes sweating when precipitation is appropriate. To illustrate these principles, we will refer to two lines from the text, line 36, p. 99, and line 124, p. 205.

Line 36 is an example of simultaneous interior-exterior disease in which sweating is promoted appropriately.

Line 124 is an example of using precipitation first, even though the exterior disease is still present. The simultaneous promotion of sweating and use of precipitation may be appropriate when the exterior and interior patterns are equally severe.

Line 91

㈠ 伤寒，医下之，续得下利，清谷不止，身疼痛者，急当救里。㈡ 后身疼痛，清便自调者，急当救表。㈢ 救里宜四逆汤，救表宜桂枝汤。

(1) *Shāng hán, yī xià zhī, xù dé xià lì, qīng gǔ bù zhǐ, shēn téng tòng zhě, jí dāng jiù lǐ.* (2) *Hòu shēn téng tòng, qīng biàn zì tiáo zhě, jí dāng jiù biǎo.* (3) *Jiù lǐ yí sì nì tāng, jiù biǎo yí guì zhī tāng.*

(1) When cold damage is treated with precipitation, and [this is] followed by incessant clear-food diarrhea[1] and generalized pain, one should urgently relieve the interior [disease]. (2) After [treating the interior], [if there is] generalized pain, and the excretions become regulated,[2] one should urgently relieve the exterior [disease]. (3) For relieving the interior [disease], Counterflow Cold Decoction (*sì nì tāng*) is appropriate; for relieving the exterior [disease], Cinnamon Twig Decoction (*guì zhī tāng*) is appropriate.

Text Notes

1. Incessant clear-food diarrhea, 下利清谷不止 *xià lì qīng gǔ bù zhǐ*: Incessant diarrhea that is watery and contains undigested food.
2. The excretions become regulated, 清便自调 *qīng biàn zì tiáo*: Earlier in the line, a reference is made to the stool; therefore, both the *Shāng Hán Lùn Yán Jiū Dà Cí Diǎn* ("*Shāng Hán Lùn* Studies Dictionary") and the *Gāo Děng Cóng Shū* ("Advanced Reference Series") explain this phrase as meaning that the stool becomes normal. Nevertheless, according to Yù Chāng the phrase above means that the urine is clear and the stool is regular, indicating that the interior yáng has been restored.

Synopsis

a) A pattern that occurs following the inappropriate use of precipitation in an exterior pattern.

b) Identifies the order and urgency of interior and exterior treatment.

Commentary

In greater yáng cold damage, the use of precipitation is an adverse treatment, as is stated in line 44, p. 69: "Greater yáng disease in which the exterior pattern has not resolved cannot be precipitated [since] precipitation would be an adverse [treatment]. When [one] desires to resolve the exterior, Cinnamon Twig Decoction (*guì zhī tāng*) is appropriate." The results of this mistreatment vary depending on the particular circumstances of the case. As Yóu Yí writes, "The disease [course] depends on the heat and cold of the patient's qì and evil qì, [as well as] yīn and yáng of the viscera qì." In the situation described above, incessant clear-food diarrhea and generalized pain result from erroneous precipitation. According to Chéng Wú-Jǐ, these signs indicate that the interior qì is insufficient. He does not ascribe the signs to any one organ system. Yù Chāng ascribes these signs to the spleen, writing, "Clear-food diarrhea indicates debilitation of the spleen yáng and inability [of the spleen] to transform food and drink. Generalized pain indicates there is exuberant yīn evil in the interior, obstructing the sinews and channels."

This type of diarrhea may also be considered a sign of the kidney, as described in *Gāo Děng Cóng Shū*. Incessant clear-food diarrhea, as a sign of damage to the kidney yáng, is considered an indication of more severe damage to yáng from the misuse of precipitation, and is thought to be different from the diarrhea resulting from damage to the spleen and stomach. Generalized pain indicates that the exterior disease has not yet resolved; hence an interior and an exterior disease are both present. No matter how one explains these signs, it is clear from the text that incessant clear-food diarrhea is a serious sign and should be treated first. The exterior signs can only be treated after resolving the urgent interior signs. If one considers that the original disease is the root and later diseases are the tips, this is an example of first treating the tip, then treating the root. It can also be said that in a situation where the yáng qì is vacuous, one should not use medicinals that resolve the exterior, even mild ones, since the promotion of sweating may further damage the yáng qì. One must first restore yáng with a formula such as Counterflow Cold Decoction (*sì nì tāng*) and only then can one resolve the exterior. See line 323, p. 475, for a comprehensive discussion of Counterflow Cold Decoction (*sì nì tāng*).

LINE 92

㈠ 病发热头痛，脉反沉，若不差，身体疼痛，当救其里。㈡ 四逆汤方。

(1) *Bìng fā rè tóu tòng, mài fǎn chén, ruò bù chài, shēn tǐ téng tòng, dāng jiù qí lǐ.* (2) *Sì nì tāng fāng.*

(1) [When] in illness [there is] heat effusion and headache, but the pulse is sunken, and if (after taking Ephedra, Asarum, and Aconite Decoction (*má huáng xì xīn fù zǐ tāng*))[1] [there is] no recovery[2] and [there is] generalized pain, one should relieve the interior. (2) Counterflow Cold Decoction (*sì nì tāng*) [is appropriate].[3]

TEXT NOTES

1. After taking Ephedra, Asarum, and Aconite Decoction (*má huáng xì xīn fù zǐ tāng*): This clause does not appear in the original text. See the commentary below for a complete discussion.
2. If [there is] no recovery, 若不差 *ruò bù chài*: In this phrase, 差 *chài* means 瘥 *chài*, "to recover."
3. Counterflow Cold Decoction (*sì nì tāng*) [is appropriate], 四逆汤方 *sì nì tāng fāng*: The style of this clause does not conform to the rest of the text. Nonetheless, it is taken to mean that the formula is appropriate.

SYNOPSIS

In simultaneous interior-exterior disease, one may have to reject the signs and follow the pulse; treat the interior first and then the exterior.

COMMENTARY

A disease in which the main signs are heat effusion and headache is usually an exterior disease. In exterior patterns the pulse is generally floating, but here it is sunken. Zhāng Jī uses the word "but" 反 *fǎn*, to mean that this is not the pulse characteristic that is expected; consequently this may be not an exterior pattern, but an interior one. Line 301, p. 506, describes a lesser yīn disease with heat effusion and a pulse that is sunken. In that situation, Ephedra, Asarum, and Aconite Decoction (*má huáng xì xīn fù zǐ tāng*) is used. The rationale for the formula's inclusion here is that the text reads, "If [there is] no recovery...." This phrase implies that treatment was attempted and was unsuccessful. Clearly, this pattern is similar to that presented in line 301, p. 506, and that is why the formula is included here. This pattern can be seen as simultaneous disease of the greater yáng and the lesser yīn. Ephedra, Asarum, and Aconite Decoction (*má huáng xì xīn fù zǐ tāng*) has been given, but generalized pain, an exterior sign, is still present. The pulse is sunken, though, so the first step is to warm the interior and invigorate yáng, lest by further promoting sweating one should cause yáng collapse. Once the yáng is strengthened, the body should be able to expel any remaining exterior evil. If not, once the patient's condition is stabilized, additional treatment can be attempted.

4.5 HEAT PATTERNS

In greater yáng disease, a transmuted pattern of heat can occur as the result of inappropriate precipitation or vomiting, when early in the disease an exterior evil moves quickly from the exterior into the interior owing to the strength of the evil or weakness of right qì, or when late in the disease residual heat remains in the interior. One basic pattern, referred to as "vacuity vexation," is characterized by heart vexation, inability to sleep, and anguish in the heart, and it is treated with Gardenia and Fermented Soybean Decoction (*zhī zǐ chǐ tāng*), which clears and diffuses depressed heat. When vacuity vexation is accompanied by shortage of qì, it is treated with Gardenia, Licorice, and Fermented Soybean Decoction (*zhī zǐ gān cǎo chǐ tāng*), which also supplements the qì. When vacuity vexation is accompanied by retching, it is treated with Gardenia, Fresh Ginger, and Fermented Soybean Decoction (*zhī zǐ shēng jiāng chǐ tāng*), which also harmonizes the stomach and checks retching. When depressed fire in the chest influences the qì dynamic of the stomach, resulting in not only heart vexation but also abdominal fullness, the appropriate formula is Gardenia and Magnolia Bark Decoction (*zhī zǐ hòu pò tāng*), which clears heat and dissipates fullness. When a pill medicine is used to precipitate and this damages the center so that there is heat in the upper body and cold in the center, the appropriate formula is Gardenia and Dried Ginger Decoction (*zhī zǐ gān jiāng tāng*), which clears heat from the upper burner and warms the center burner. It should be noted that in patterns of spleen and/or kidney yáng vacuity with enduring sloppy stool, the original formula is contraindicated.

In a greater yáng disease, when as a result of inappropriate promotion of sweating or the use of precipitation, an exterior evil falls into the interior, transforms to heat, and distresses the lungs, causing congestion of the lung qì and panting, the appropriate formula is Ephedra, Apricot Kernel, Licorice, and Gypsum Decoction (*má huáng xìng rén gān cǎo shí gāo tāng*), which clears heat and diffuses the lung. White Tiger Decoction Plus Ginseng (*bái hǔ jiā rén shēn tāng*), which clears heat, boosts the qì, and engenders liquid, is used when sweating is promoted and copious sweat issues, with the result that the qì and yīn are damaged and evil qì shifts into the yáng brightness, giving rise to signs such as vexation thirst and a pulse that is surging and large. If precipitation is used inappropriately in a greater yáng disease, the evil can enter the interior, transform to heat, and distress the large intestine, causing incessant diarrhea. This pattern is treated with Pueraria, Scutellaria, and Coptis Decoction (*gé gēn huáng qín huáng lián tāng*), which clears heat and checks diarrhea. Scutellaria Decoction (*huáng qín tāng*) and Scutellaria Decoction Plus Pinellia and Fresh Ginger (*huáng qín jiā bàn xià shēng jiāng tāng*) can both be used in greater yáng and lesser yáng combination disease. The former is used when heat in the interior distresses the lower burner, causing diarrhea, and the latter is used when heat in the interior distresses the stomach, causing counterflow ascent of the stomach qì, which manifests as retching.

4.5.1 Gardenia and Fermented Soybean Decoction Patterns

The pattern treated with Gardenia and Fermented Soybean Decoction (*zhī zǐ chǐ tāng*) is known as vacuity vexation. If heat evil falls inward and becomes depressed in the chest and diaphragm, it will harass the heart and the chest region. Vacuity vexation is the result either of treatment or of residual heat from a heat disease. It is not the result of repletion heat evil invading the body. There are three main pathomechanisms associated with vacuity vexation.

a) Heat evil falling inward and collecting in the chest and diaphragm following the inappropriate use of vomiting or precipitation.

b) Heat evil directly entering the interior and becoming depressed in the chest in the early stage of an externally contracted disease.

c) In a protracted illness, a heat evil which has not been completely expelled becomes depressed in the chest.

Heart vexation and inability to sleep, which in severe cases becomes tossing and turning, and anguish in the heart, are commonly associated with these patterns. Gardenia and Fermented Soybean Decoction (*zhī zǐ chǐ tāng*) clears and diffuses heat evils, resolves depression, and eliminates vacuity vexation. If vacuity vexation occurs with shortage of qì, one should add mix-fried licorice (*gān cǎo*), which supplements vacuity. If the stomach qì loses harmony, add fresh ginger (*shēng jiāng*) to check retching. For fire depressed in the chest which influences the qì dynamic and results in stuffiness in the chest and/or pain, the basic formula may be used. If irregularity of the qì dynamic results in heart vexation, abdominal fullness, and disquiet lying and sitting, use Gardenia and Magnolia Bark Decoction (*zhī zǐ hòu pò tāng*) to clear heat and dissipate fullness. If inappropriate use of precipitation results in diarrhea with a pattern of heat in the upper burner, cold in the center burner, generalized heat effusion, and mild heart vexation, use Gardenia and Dried Ginger Decoction (*zhī zǐ gān jiāng tāng*) to clear heat in the upper burner and warm the center burner. Gardenia and Fermented Soybean Decoction (*zhī zǐ chǐ tāng*) should not be used if the patient usually has sloppy stool, since this may indicate yáng qì vacuity and use of this formula would cause further damage.

LINE 76B

发汗吐下后，虚烦不得眠，若剧者，必反覆颠倒，心中懊侬，栀子豉汤主之；若少气者，栀子甘草豉汤主之；若呕者，栀子生姜豉汤主之。

Fā hàn tù xià hòu, xū fán bù dé mián, ruò jù zhě, bì fǎn fù diān dǎo, xīn zhōng ào nóng, zhī zǐ chǐ tāng zhǔ zhī; ruò shào qì zhě, zhī zǐ gān cǎo chǐ tāng zhǔ zhī; ruò ǒu zhě, zhī zǐ shēng jiāng chǐ tāng zhǔ zhī.

[When] after the promotion of sweating, the use of vomiting, or the use of precipitation, [there is] vacuity vexation[1] and inability to sleep, and if [the condition] is severe, [with] tossing and turning[2] and anguish in the heart,[3] Gardenia and Fermented Soybean Decoction (*zhī zǐ chǐ tāng*) governs. If [there is] shortage of qì,[4] Gardenia, Licorice, and Fermented Soybean Decoction (*zhī zǐ gān cǎo chǐ tāng*) governs. If [there is] retching, Gardenia, Fresh Ginger, and Fermented Soybean Decoction (*zhī zǐ shēng jiāng chǐ tāng*) governs.

TEXT NOTES

1. Vacuity vexation, 虚烦 *xū fán*: Heat depressed in the chest, harassing the chest and diaphragm. The question that arises is why the term "vacuity vexation" is used.

   Yóu Yí explains that "[The use] of vomiting, precipitation, or sweating repeatedly damages the fluids and evil qì falls inward; this is vacuity vexation. Vacuity vexation means the right [qì] is insufficient and evil qì harasses, so [there is] vexation."

   The authors of *Yī Zōng Jīn Jiàn* state, "Most vexation [that occurs] without precipitation, vomiting, or sweating belongs to heat; hence it is called heat vexation. Most vexation [that occurs] following precipitation, vomiting, or sweating belongs to vacuity; hence it is called vacuity vexation." Any of the methods described above may damage right qì. Evil qì is then able to exploit the vacuity and sink inward to the chest. From this point of view, vacuity vexation is a result of vacuity of the right qì, with evil falling into the chest.

Kē Qín offers another explanation: "If one wants to know yáng brightness vacuity vexation, it is the opposite of repletion heat in the stomach domain. That is, it is the vacuity of emptiness and vacuity, not the vacuity of weakness and vacuity." In other words, vacuity vexation means vexation due to vacuity heat as distinct from vexation due to repletion heat. It does not mean vexation due to vacuity of right qì.

One may also consider the opinion of Shěn Míng-Zōng, who writes, "Sweating, precipitation, and vomiting damage the qì of the chest and stomach. A formless evil falls inward and harasses the chest, and [there is] no phlegm-rheum bind. Thus [there is] vacuity vexation." In this explanation, which is a combination of the two previous ones, a formless or empty heat evil harasses the interior and the treatment results in vacuity of right qì.

2. Tossing and turning, 反复颠倒 *fǎn fù diān dào*: Inability to fall asleep with repeated turning and tossing in bed.
3. Anguish in the heart, 心中懊侬 *xīn zhōng ào nóng*: A subjective feeling of severe vexing depression in the heart. The patient feels harassed, even to the point of derangement, and cannot calm down.
4. Shortage of qì, 少气 *shǎo qì*: Weak, short, hasty breathing, a weak voice, and a tendency to take deep breaths in order to continue speaking.

FORMULAE

Gardenia and Fermented Soybean Decoction (*zhī zǐ chǐ tāng*)

◦ Clear and diffuse depressed heat.

栀子十四个（擘） 香豉四合（绵裹）

右二味，以水四升，先煮栀子，得二升半，内豉，煮取一升半，去滓，分为二服，温进一服，得吐者，止后服。

zhī zǐ shí sì ge (bò) xiāng chǐ sì gě (mián guǒ)

Yòu èr wèi, yǐ shuǐ sì shēng, xiān zhǔ zhī zǐ, dé èr shēng bàn, nà chǐ, zhǔ qǔ yī shēng bàn, qù zǐ, fēn wéi èr fú, wēn jìn yī fú, dé tù zhě, zhǐ hòu fú.

gardenia (栀子 *zhī zǐ*, Gardeniae Fructus) 14 pieces (broken)

fermented soybean (香豉 *xiāng chǐ*, Glycines Semen Fermentatum)[1] 4 gě (cotton-wrapped)

[For] the above two ingredients use four shēng of water. First boil gardenia (*zhī zǐ*) to get two and a half shēng. Add fermented soybean (*xiāng chǐ*) and boil to get one and a half shēng. Remove the dregs. Divide into two doses and take one warm. (If vomiting occurs, stop giving [doses].[2])

FORMULA NOTES

1. Fermented soybean (*xiāng chǐ*) is now referred to as 淡豆豉 *dàn dòu chǐ*.

2. If vomiting occurs, stop giving [doses], 得吐者，止后服 *dé tù zhě, zhǐ hòu fú*: The significance of this phrase is controversial, and different commentators have offered many varied opinions.

   Chéng Wú-Jǐ represents the school of thought that this is a vomiting formula. This point of view is based on three main points:

   a) Zhāng Jī wrote this phrase to explain that after giving this formula, the patient should vomit, after which time no more doses should be given. This confirms that it is a vomiting formula.

   b) This formula and Melon Stalk Powder (*guā dì sǎn*) contain fermented soybean (*xiāng chǐ*). The latter formula is known to be a vomiting formula; therefore this confirms that the former has the same use.

   c) The disease position in the original pattern is in the upper body. After taking the medicinals, depressed heat will be loosened and able to move. The right qì takes advantage of this opportunity to expel the evil. Following the principle of "bring up and out what is high," we can understand that this formula is used to induce vomiting, thereby bringing out the evil in the chest.

   Chén Yuán-Xī (陈元犀) represents the school of thought that this is not a vomiting formula. This point of view is based on four main points:

   a) The formula is only composed of two ingredients and neither clearly induces vomiting.

   b) In the original pattern, following the use of sweating, vomiting, and precipitation, a heat evil remains and harasses the chest and diaphragm. If one again uses vomiting, this will increase the vacuity, and goes against the intention of the line.

   c) This line contains the suggestion that if the patient vomits, one can add fresh ginger (*shēng jiāng*). How can one add a medicinal that checks retching to a formula used to induce vomiting?

   d) In clinical practice, after giving this formula, it is rare to have a patient vomit.

   In our opinion, this formula is not intended to induce vomiting.

Gardenia, Licorice, and Fermented Soybean Decoction (*zhī zǐ gān cǎo chǐ tāng*)

栀子十四个（擘） 甘草二两（炙） 香豉四合（绵裹）

右三味，以水四升，先煮栀子、甘草取二升半，内豉，煮取一升半，去滓，分二服，温进一服，得吐者，止后服。

zhī zǐ shí sì ge (bò) gān cǎo èr liǎng (zhì) xiāng chǐ sì gě (mián guǒ)

Yòu sān wèi, yǐ shuǐ sì shēng, xiān zhǔ zhī zǐ 、 gān cǎo, qǔ èr shēng bàn, nà chǐ, zhǔ qǔ yī shēng bàn, qù zǐ, fēn èr fú, wēn jìn yī fú, dé tù zhě, zhǐ hòu fú.

gardenia (栀子 *zhī zǐ*, Gardeniae Fructus) 14 pieces (broken)
mix-fried licorice (甘草 *gān cǎo*, Glycyrrhizae Radix) 2 liǎng

fermented soybean (香豉 *xiāng chǐ*, Glycines Semen Fermentatum) 4 gě (cotton-wrapped)

For the above three ingredients, use four shēng of water. First boil gardenia (*zhī zǐ*) and mix-fried licorice (*gān cǎo*) to get two and a half shēng, [then] add fermented soybean (*xiāng chǐ*) and boil to get one and a half shēng. Remove the dregs and divide into two doses. Take one dose warm. If [the patient] vomits, cease taking [the formula].

Gardenia, Fresh Ginger, and Fermented Soybean Decoction (*zhī zǐ shēng jiāng chǐ tāng*)

栀子十四个（擘） 生姜五两 香豉四合（绵裹）

右三味，以水四升，先煮栀子、生姜，取二升半，内豉，煮取一升半，去滓，分二服，温进一服，得吐者，止后服。

zhī zǐ shí sì ge (bò) shēng jiāng wǔ liǎng xiāng chǐ sì gě (mián guǒ)

Yòu sān wèi, yǐ shuǐ sì shēng, xiān zhǔ zhī zǐ 、 shēng jiāng, qǔ èr shēng bàn, nà chǐ, zhǔ qǔ yī shēng bàn, qù zǐ, fēn èr fú, wēn jìn yī fú, dé tù zhě, zhǐ hòu fú.

gardenia (栀子 *zhī zǐ*, Gardeniae Fructus) 14 pieces (broken)

fresh ginger (生姜 *shēng jiāng*, Zingiberis Rhizoma Recens) 5 liǎng

fermented soybean (香豉 *xiāng chǐ*, Glycines Semen Fermentatum) 4 gě (cotton-wrapped)

For the above three ingredients, use four shēng of water. First boil gardenia (*zhī zǐ*) and fresh ginger (*shēng jiāng*) to get two and a half shēng, [then] add fermented soybean (*xiāng chǐ*) and boil to get one and a half shēng. Remove the dregs and divide into two doses. Take one dose warm. If [the patient] vomits, cease taking [the formula].

Synopsis

The identification and treatment of vacuity vexation that is the result of heat harassing the chest and diaphragm.

Commentary

Three main pathomechanisms are associated with depressed heat harassing the chest and diaphragm. One is that following inappropriate treatment of cold damage, unresolved heat becomes depressed in the chest. The second is that an external evil transforms to heat and becomes depressed in the chest. The third is that following a heat disease, residual heat becomes depressed in the chest. In this line, the formed heat is eliminated through the treatment, but residual heat becomes depressed in the chest. The signs of this condition are vacuity vexation, inability to sleep, tossing and turning, and anguish in the heart.

An analysis of the formula makes the meaning of the line clearer. There are only two ingredients in the formula, gardenia (*zhī zǐ*) and fermented soybean (*xiāng chǐ*). Bitter, cold gardenia (*zhī zǐ*) clears heat in all three burners. It also resolves heat depression and eliminates vexation. Fermented soybean (*xiāng chǐ*) resolves the exterior and diffuses heat. Combined, these two ingredients clear heat, eliminate vexation, and do not have any supplementing qualities, reinforcing the idea that vacuity vexation is not right qì vacuity, but vexation that is the result of residual heat, not replete heat, depressed in the chest. If vacuity vexation were the result of right qì vacuity, one would expect the formula to contain medicinals that supplement vacuity. Therefore, as Kē Qín suggests, vacuity vexation probably does not mean vacuity of right qì. Here, the term "vacuity" seems to suggest that vexation is the result of the treatment, not the result of a repletion heat evil falling into the chest. Therefore, it is termed vacuity vexation by contrast to vexation that is the result of repletion heat. The heat evil in the chest is formless; therefore, mass and a glomus lump are absent.

The other two formulae included in line 76B above are straightforward modifications of the initial formula. In the first, sweet licorice (*gān cǎo*) is added to supplement qì shortage, because it supplements the spleen, boosts qì, and has mild heat-clearing ability. In the second, fresh ginger (*shēng jiāng*), which downbears counterflow and checks retching, is added to treat retching.

LINE 77

发汗，若下之，而烦热，胸中窒者，栀子豉汤主之。

Fā hàn, ruò xià zhī, ér fán rè, xiōng zhōng zhì zhě, zhī zǐ chǐ tāng zhǔ zhī.

[After] sweating is promoted, if precipitation is used and [there is] heat vexation[1] and stuffiness in the chest,[2] Gardenia and Fermented Soybean Decoction (*zhī zǐ chǐ tāng*) governs.

TEXT NOTES

1. Heat vexation, 烦热 *fán rè*: This term has been interpreted in two slightly different ways: heart vexation accompanied by heat effusion, or agitation with a subjective feeling of heat and oppression. Chéng Yìng-Máo writes, "Vexation and heat: the two words are connected. Vexation is in the interior and heat is in the exterior. Fire depressed in the chest exploits this vacuity and settles [in the chest]."

   In the line above, heat vexation appears following the use of precipitation in an exterior pattern; therefore it is likely that it is the result of an exterior evil falling into the interior and becoming depressed in the chest. In line 240, p. 400, the same term is thought to be evidence of an unresolved exterior pattern. Zhāng Lù writes, "Heat vexation is depression, oppression and disquiet, and a manifestation of heat that has not effused. When vexation occurs in the absence of sweating, vomiting, or precipitation, it indicates a greater yáng exterior pattern. In the *Nèi Jīng*, [it is written,] '[For] a patient with heat vexation, [when] sweat issues, [there will] then be resolution."'

2. Stuffiness in the chest, 胸中窒 *xiōng zhōng zhì*: A feeling of blockage and inhibited movement in the chest.

SYNOPSIS

The signs and treatment of heat depressed in the chest, congesting the qì dynamic.

COMMENTARY

This line is an extension of the previous line, in which Gardenia and Fermented Soybean Decoction (*zhī zǐ chǐ tāng*) was introduced. Following the promotion of sweating and the use of precipitation, residual heat becomes depressed in the chest, giving rise to agitation with a subjective feeling of heat and stuffiness in the chest. Depressed heat in the chest inhibits lung function, which causes the qì dynamic to lose regulation. The qì does not move smoothly and a feeling of blockage and oppression in the chest arises. A comparison of this line with the previous one reveals slight differences in the presenting signs, but a great similarity in the basic pathomechanism; therefore the formula is the same.

LINE 78

伤寒五六日，大下之后，身热不去，心中结痛者，未欲解也，栀子豉汤主之。

Shāng hán wǔ liù rì, dà xià zhī hòu, shēn rè bù qù, xīn zhōng jié tòng zhě, wèi yù jiě yě, zhī zǐ chǐ tāng zhǔ zhī.

When in cold damage [that has lasted for] five or six days, [if] after great precipitation, the generalized heat has not gone[1] and [there is] binding pain in the heart,[2] the disease is not about to resolve and Gardenia and Fermented Soybean Decoction (*zhī zǐ chǐ tāng*) governs.

TEXT NOTES

1. Generalized heat has not gone, 身热不去 *shēn rè bù qù*: There are different interpretations of this phrase.
   a) According to Zhāng Zhì-Cōng, Wáng Kěn-Táng (王肯堂, style 宇泰 Yù-Tài), and Chéng Yìng-Máo, this phrase means an unresolved exterior heat evil.
   b) According to Kē Qín, this phrase means heat bound in the chest.
2. Binding pain in the heart, 心中结痛 *xīn zhōng jié tòng*: Pain in the chest due to binding depression of qì.

SYNOPSIS

The signs and treatment of heat depressed in the chest, inhibiting the qì and blood, with binding pain in the heart.

COMMENTARY

The use of precipitation is inappropriate in cold damage patterns and as in the previous two lines, following treatment, residual heat becomes depressed in the chest. It congests the qì dynamic and in mild cases can cause stuffiness in the chest, and in severe cases, binding pain in the heart. Both these chest signs are the result of depressed heat; therefore, both may be treated with Gardenia and Fermented Soybean Decoction (*zhī zǐ chǐ tāng*), which clears heat and diffuses depression. Although depressed heat in the chest influences the movement of qì and blood, no medicinals are added to move the qì or quicken the blood because the root is depressed heat. Once the root is resolved the signs will resolve.

To avoid confusion later, it will be helpful to discuss some of the differences between binding pain in the heart, 心中结痛 *xīn zhōng jié tòng*, and chest bind, 结胸 *jié xiōng*. Pain in the chest occurs in both conditions, but it differs in intensity and sensitivity to palpation. Binding pain in the heart is characterized by a chest that is soft when palpated and pain that is not severe, whereas chest bind is marked by hardness upon palpation that may extend into the lesser abdomen, and severe pain that is exacerbated by pressure. The pathomechanism and the treatment of chest bind are discussed further in line 128, p. 211.

LINE 79

伤寒下后，心烦腹满，卧起不安者，栀子厚朴汤主之。

Shāng hán xià hòu, xīn fán fù mǎn, wò qǐ bù ān zhě, zhī zǐ hòu pò tāng zhǔ zhī.

When, after precipitation has been used in cold damage, [there is] heart vexation,[1] abdominal fullness, and fidgetiness whether lying or sitting,[2] Gardenia and Magnolia Bark Decoction (*zhī zǐ hòu pò tāng*) governs.

TEXT NOTES

1. Heart vexation, 心烦 *xīn fán*: This sign is considered milder than, but similar to, vexation and agitation 烦燥 *fán zào*.
2. Fidgetiness whether lying or sitting, 卧起不安 *wò qǐ bù ān*: Inability to find a comfortable resting position, accompanied by fidgeting.

FORMULA

Gardenia and Magnolia Bark Decoction (*zhī zǐ hòu pò tāng*).

∘ Clear heat and eliminate vexation; loosen the center and disperse fullness.

栀子十四个（擘） 厚朴四两（炙，去皮） 枳实四枚（水浸，炙令黄）

右三味，以水三升半，煮取一升半，去滓，分二服，温进一服，得吐者，止后服。

Zhī zǐ shí sì ge (bò) hòu pò sì liǎng (zhì, qù pí) zhǐ shí sì méi (shuǐ jìn, zhì lìng huáng)

Yòu sān wèi, yǐ shuǐ sān shēng bàn, zhǔ qǔ yī shēng bàn, qù zǐ, fēn èr fú, wēn jìn yī fú, dé tù zhě, zhǐ hòu fú.

gardenia (栀子 *zhī zǐ*, Gardeniae Fructus) 14 pieces (broken)
magnolia bark (厚朴 *hòu pò*, Magnoliae Cortex) 4 liǎng (remove bark, mix-fry)
unripe bitter orange (枳实 *zhǐ shí*, Aurantii Fructus Immaturus) 4 pieces (soaked in water and mix-fried until yellow*)

[For] the above three ingredients use three and a half shēng of water. Boil to get one and a half shēng and remove the dregs. Divide into two doses and take one, warm. (If vomiting occurs, stop giving [doses].)

FORMULA NOTE

* Unripe bitter orange (*zhǐ shí*): This medicinal is steeped in water and then mix-fried until it turns a deep yellow color. The goal of mix-frying the fruit is to moderate the bitter, cold nature of the raw agent. In modern practice, unripe bitter orange (*zhǐ shí*) is primarily used stir-fried. When processed in this way it dissipates accumulation and disperses glomus. Used raw, it has a stronger ability to break qì and transform phlegm. In modern practice, mix-frying specifically refers to stir-frying with liquid adjuvants, but at the time of the *Shāng Hán Lùn*, it is not clear what specific processing method was used and it may refer simply to stir-frying. In the modern method the adjuvant and materials are first blended, covered, and left to stand for a short time before frying, so that the adjuvant soaks well into the materials. The most commonly used adjuvants are honey, vinegar, wine, and brine.

SYNOPSIS

The signs and treatment of heat harassing the chest and diaphragm, with heart vexation and abdominal fullness.

COMMENTARY

Following inappropriate precipitation in a cold damage disease, the exterior evil falls inward to the chest. In this pattern, the evil becomes depressed in the chest and accumulates in the stomach, resulting in not only heart vexation, but also abdominal fullness. Discomfort in the chest region and the stomach results in the patient's inability to find a comfortable resting position. Heart vexation and abdominal fullness may also be seen in yáng brightness bowel repletion, but here the absence of any signs of stool bind suggests that yáng brightness disease is unlikely. This pattern is depression of a formless evil heat in the chest and abdomen. The evil heat is described as formless because neither abdominal pain nor stool bind is present.

Gardenia and Magnolia Bark Decoction (*zhī zǐ hòu pò tāng*) is used to treat this disease. In this variation of Gardenia and Fermented Soybean Decoction (*zhī zǐ chǐ tāng*), fermented soybean (*xiāng chǐ*), which resolves the exterior and diffuses heat, is replaced by magnolia bark (*hòu pò*) and unripe bitter orange (*zhǐ shí*). Here, the heat diffusing properties of fermented soybean (*xiāng chǐ*) are not considered important, whereas the ability of magnolia bark (*hòu pò*) and unripe bitter orange (*zhǐ shí*) to move the qì and dissipate accumulation is crucial.

One may want to compare this formula with the Qì-Coordinating Decoctions. If one substitutes rhubarb (*dà huáng*) for gardenia (*zhī zǐ*), the formula becomes Minor Qì-Coordinating Decoction (*xiǎo chéng qì tāng*). The addition of mirabilite (*máng xiāo*) to Minor Qì-Coordinating Decoction (*xiǎo chéng qì tāng*) creates Major Qì-Coordinating Decoction (*dà chéng qì tāng*) and the substitution of licorice (*gān cǎo*) for the magnolia bark (*hòu pò*) and unripe bitter orange (*zhǐ shí*) in Major Qì-Coordinating Decoction (*dà chéng qì tāng*) creates Stomach-Regulating Qì-Coordinating Decoction (*tiáo wèi chéng qì tāng*). Apart from being helpful in terms of remembering the formulae, this comparison illustrates the differences between the signs described here and those associated with yáng brightness bowel repletion.

Line 80

伤寒，医以丸药大下之，身热不去，微烦者，栀子干姜汤主之。

Shāng hán, yī yǐ wán yào dà xià zhī, shēn rè bù qù, wēi fán zhě, zhī zǐ gān jiāng tāng zhǔ zhī.

When in cold damage great precipitation is performed with a pill medicine,* the generalized heat is not gone and [there is] mild vexation; [therefore,] Gardenia and Dried Ginger Decoction (*zhī zǐ gān jiāng tāng*) governs.

Text Note

* Pill medicine, 丸药 *wán yào*: A powerful draining precipitant medicine sold in pill form and popular during the Hàn Dynasty. There were two types of pill medicine: a hot-natured one based on croton (*bā dòu*) and a cold-natured one based on kansui (*gān suì*).

Formula

Gardenia and Dried Ginger Decoction (*zhī zǐ gān jiāng tāng*)

◦ Clear upper [burner] heat; warm center [burner] cold.

栀子十四个（擘） 干姜二两

右二味，以水三升半，煮取一升半，去滓，分二服，温进一服，得吐者，止后服。

Zhī zǐ shí sì ge (bò) gān jiāng èr liǎng

Yòu èr wèi, yǐ shuǐ sān shēng bàn, zhǔ qǔ yī shēng bàn, qù zǐ, fēn èr fú, wēn jìn yī fú, dé tù zhě, zhǐ hòu fú.

gardenia (栀子 *zhī zǐ*, Gardeniae Fructus) 14 pieces (broken)
dried ginger (干姜 *gān jiāng*, Zingiberis Rhizoma Exsiccatum) 2 liǎng

[For] the above two ingredients use three shēng of water. Boil to get one and a half shēng and remove the dregs. Divide into two doses and take one, warm. (If vomiting occurs, stop giving [doses].)

Synopsis

The signs and treatment of heat harassing the chest and diaphragm with diarrhea from cold in the center burner.

Commentary

This is a further refinement of the patterns already presented. Inappropriate treatment of cold damage causes an exterior evil to fall inwards and become depressed in the chest. The generalized heat does not resolve and mild vexation arises. In addition, the treatment used here is strong draining precipitation. Draining precipitation easily damages the qì of the spleen and stomach. One may surmise that vacuity in the center burner results from this type of treatment and an analysis of the formula supports this supposition. This is a pattern of heat in the upper burner and cold in the center burner. Gardenia (*zhī zǐ*) clears heat from all three burners and eliminates vexation, while dried ginger (*gān jiāng*) warms the center burner. Later in the text, Coptis Decoction (*huáng lián tāng*) is also used in the treatment of upper heat and lower cold. The difference is that this pattern is characterized by generalized heat effusion and mild vexation, while in that case the main sign is vomiting. See line 173, p. 247, for a further discussion of Coptis Decoction (*huáng lián tāng*).

Line 81

凡用栀子汤， 病人旧微溏者，不可与服之。

Fán yòng zhī zǐ tāng, bìng rén jiù wēi táng zhě, bù kě yǔ fú zhī.

In all applications[1] of Gardenia Decoction (*zhī zǐ tāng*),[2] if the person usually has slightly sloppy stool,[3] one cannot give [this formula].

Text Notes

1. In all applications, 凡用 *fán yòng*: All patterns that have been described in which Gardenia and Fermented Soybean Decoction (*zhī zǐ chǐ tāng*) is appropriate.
2. Gardenia Decoction (*zhī zǐ tāng*) is taken to mean Gardenia and Fermented Soybean Decoction (*zhī zǐ chǐ tāng*) or its variants.
3. Usually has slightly sloppy stool, 旧微溏 *jiù wēi táng*: A person who, prior to the onset of illness, has thin, watery stool.

Synopsis

Contraindications for the use of Gardenia and Fermented Soybean Decoction (*zhī zǐ chǐ tāng*).

Commentary

Sloppy stool, generally an indication of weakness in the spleen and stomach or weakness in the spleen and kidney, may in some cases indicate heat, but in this case it indicates vacuity of the spleen yáng and/or kidney yáng. It is unnecessary to decide exactly which organ is vacuous. This formula should not be used in vacuity-type stool patterns; the key point being the presence of vacuity, not sloppy stool. A particular interdiction exists against its use in cases of enduring vacuity-type sloppy stool because, as in any enduring condition, right qì is weakened. Gardenia and Fermented Soybean Decoction (*zhī zǐ chǐ tāng*) is contraindicated because its main ingredient, gardenia (*zhī zǐ*), is cold and bitter. Use of this type of formula in a patient with center burner vacuity will further damage the qì of the center burner and result in an exacerbation of the sloppy stool. In a pattern of upper burner depressed heat, where this formula seems the most appropriate, with sloppy stool, the dosage of gardenia (*zhī zǐ*) should be reduced and/or additional ingredients that supplement and warm the center burner should be included, as in Gardenia and Dried Ginger Decoction (*zhī zǐ gān jiāng tāng*). This contraindication may be extended to include a wide spectrum of cases. When the qì of the center burner is insufficient, cold and bitter formulae should be used cautiously or avoided altogether.

4.5.2 Ephedra, Apricot Kernel, Licorice, and Gypsum Decoction Patterns

Line 63, 162

发汗后，不可更行桂枝汤，汗出而喘，无大热者，可与麻黄杏仁甘草石膏汤。

Fā hàn hòu, bù kě gèng xíng guì zhī tāng, hàn chū ér chuǎn, wú dà rè zhě, kě yǔ má huáng xìng rén gān cǎo shí gāo tāng.

After the promotion of sweating, ([one] cannot again use Cinnamon Twig Decoction (*guì zhī tāng*)[1]) if sweat issues, and [there is] panting[2] and great heat is absent, one can use Ephedra, Apricot Kernel, Licorice, and Gypsum Decoction (*má huáng xìng rén gān cǎo shí gāo tāng*).

下后，不可更行桂枝汤，若汗出而喘，无大热者，可与麻黄杏子甘草石膏汤。

Xià hòu bù kě gèng xíng guì zhī tāng, ruò hàn chū ér chuǎn, wú dà rè zhě, kě yǔ má huáng xìng zǐ gān cǎo shí gāo tāng.

After precipitation, ([one cannot again use Cinnamon Twig Decoction (*guì zhī tāng*)][1]) if sweat issues, and [there is] panting,[2] and great heat is absent, one can use Ephedra, Apricot Kernel, Licorice, and Gypsum Decoction (*má huáng xìng zǐ gān cǎo shí gāo tāng*).

Text Notes

1. Two of the Sòng lines are treated here together because they are identical except that one begins with "after the promotion of sweating" and the other with "after precipitation." This and the following note apply to both lines. Some commentators suggest that this is an example of grammatical inversion and that this clause could be moved ahead so that the line reads: "After promoting sweating, [if] sweat issues, and [there is] panting, and great heat [effusion] is absent, one cannot again use Cinnamon Twig Decoction (*guì zhī tāng*). One can use Ephedra, Apricot Kernel, Licorice, and Gypsum Decoction (*má huáng xìng rén gān cǎo shí gāo tāng*)."
2. Panting, 喘 *chuǎn*: Urgent, hasty, and difficult breathing. When severe, it may be accompanied by gaping mouth, raised shoulders, flaring nostrils, and inability to lie flat.

FORMULA

Ephedra, Apricot Kernel, Licorice, and Gypsum Decoction (*má huáng xìng rén gān cǎo shí gāo tāng*).

∘ Clear heat and diffuse the lung.

麻黄四两（去节） 杏仁五十个（去皮尖） 甘草二两（炙） 石膏半斤（碎、绵裹）

(一) 右四味，以水七升，先煮麻黄，减二升，去上沫，内诸药，煮取二升，去滓，温服一升。(二) 本云，黄耳杯。

Má huáng sì liǎng (qù jié) xìng rén wǔ shí ge (qù pí jiān) gān cǎo èr liǎng (zhì) shí gāo bàn jīn (suì, mián guǒ)

(1) *Yòu sì wèi, yǐ shuǐ qī shēng, xiān zhǔ má huáng, jiǎn èr shēng, qù shàng mò, nà zhū yào, zhǔ qǔ èr shēng, qù zǐ, wēn fú yī shēng.* (2) *Běn yún, huáng ěr pēi.*

ephedra (麻黄 *má huáng*, Ephedrae Herba) 4 liǎng (remove nodes)
apricot kernel (杏仁 *xìng rén*, Armeniacae Semen) 50 pieces (remove skin and tips)
mix-fried licorice (甘草 *gān cǎo*, Glycyrrhizae Radix) 2 liǎng
gypsum (石膏 *shí gāo*, Gypsum) half jīn (crushed and cotton-wrapped)

(1) [For] the above four ingredients, use seven shēng of water. First boil ephedra (*má huáng*) to reduce [the water] by two shēng. Remove the foam [collecting] on top and add all the ingredients. Boil to get two shēng, remove the dregs, and take one shēng warm. (2) This [formula] is [to be put in] a yellow-eared cup.*

FORMULA NOTE

* A yellow-eared cup, 黄耳杯 *huáng ěr pēi*: A Hàn Dynasty drinking vessel that is yellow and has loop handles (the "ears"). In this phrase 杯 *pēi* is read as 杯 *bēi*. The significance of this cup is unknown to modern commentators.

SYNOPSIS

The signs and treatment of panting that is the result of evil heat congested in the lungs after the promotion of sweating.

COMMENTARY

Greater yáng disease is properly treated through the promotion of sweating. In this line, because the disease has not resolved following the use of this method, one knows that the formula was inappropriate for the patient or not strong enough to expel the evil. Also, it is clear that precipitation is an inappropriate method for use in greater yáng disease. In both cases the evil, instead of being resolved, falls inward and becomes congested in the lung, causing qì counterflow. The loss of normal diffusing and downbearing causes panting. Heat congesting in the lung also steams the fluids in the lung, forcing them out through the surface of the body in the form of sweat.

An analysis of the formula reinforces the idea that "great heat is absent" means that there is no great heat in the exterior, despite the presence of exuberant heat congestion in the lung. The combination of ephedra (*má huáng*) and gypsum (*shí gāo*) clears and diffuses lung heat and stabilizes panting. Furthermore, when a large dose of gypsum (*shí gāo*) is given with a smaller dose of ephedra (*má huáng*), the two diffuse the lung without drying and clear lung heat without causing stagnation, because the cold, sweet nature of gypsum (*shí gāo*) moderates the warm, acrid nature of ephedra (*má huáng*). Apricot kernel (*xìng rén*) diffuses and downbears lung qì. It increases the formula's ability to stabilize panting. Licorice (*gān cǎo*) harmonizes all the ingredients, as well as harmonizing the center and mildly supplementing the qì.

Three other formulae are also used to treat sweating and panting: a) Cinnamon Twig Decoction Plus Magnolia Bark and Apricot Kernel (*guì zhī jiā hòu pò xìng zǐ tāng*), which can be used when exterior-resolution is required; b) Ephedra Decoction (*má huáng tāng*), which can be used when sweating is absent; and c) White Tiger Decoction (*bái hǔ tāng*), which can be used to treat yáng brightness interior heat.

4.5.3 White Tiger Decoction Plus Ginseng Patterns

LINE 26

服桂枝汤，大汗出后，大烦渴不解，脉洪大者，白虎加人参汤主之。

Fú guì zhī tāng, dà hàn chū hòu, dà fán kě bù jiě, mài hóng dà zhě, bái hǔ jiā rén shēn tāng zhǔ zhī.

When, after Cinnamon Twig Decoction (*guì zhī tāng*) is taken and a great sweat has issued, [there is] great vexation and thirst, and [the disease] is unresolved* and the pulse is surging and large, White Tiger Decoction Plus Ginseng (*bái hǔ jiā rén shēn tāng*) governs.

TEXT NOTE

* Great vexation and thirst, and [the disease] is unresolved, 大烦渴不解 *dà fán kě bù jiě*: This phrase can be interpreted in several ways, depending upon where one chooses to break the phrase. The most likely interpretation, as reflected in our translation, is that there is great vexation, great thirst, and an unresolved disease. Some commentators, however, have interpreted this phrase as meaning that there is great vexation and unresolved thirst.

FORMULA

White Tiger Decoction Plus Ginseng (*bái hǔ jiā rén shēn tāng*).

○ Clear qì [aspect] and discharge heat; boost qì and engender liquid.

知母六两　石膏一斤（碎，绵裹）　甘草二两（炙）　粳米六合　人参三两

右五味，以水一斗，煮米熟，汤成，去滓，温服一升，日三服。

Zhī mǔ liù liǎng　shí gāo yī jīn (suì, mián guǒ)　gān cǎo èr liǎng (zhì)　gēng mǐ liù gě　rén shēn sān liǎng

Yòu wŭ wèi, yĭ shuĭ yī dŏu, zhŭ mĭ shú, tāng chéng, qù zĭ, wēn fú yī shēng, rì sān fú.

anemarrhena (知母 *zhī mŭ*, Anemarrhenae Rhizoma) 6 liăng
gypsum (石膏 *shí gāo*, Gypsum) 1 jin = 16 liăng (crushed and cotton-wrapped)
mix-fried licorice (甘草 *gān căo*, Glycyrrhizae Radix) 2 liăng
rice (粳米 *gēng mĭ*, Oryzae Semen) 6 gě
ginseng (人参 *rén shēn*, Ginseng Radix) 3 liăng

[For] the above five ingredients use one dŏu of water. Boil [until] the rice is cooked and it becomes a soup. Remove the dregs and take one shēng, warm, three times a day.

Synopsis

The signs and treatment of damage to the qì and yīn that is the result of exuberant yáng brightness heat after the ingestion of Cinnamon Twig Decoction (*guì zhī tāng*).

Commentary

Recalling previous lines in which Cinnamon Twig Decoction (*guì zhī tāng*) was given, it is clear that the problem this line presents originates in "great sweating." When Cinnamon Twig Decoction (*guì zhī tāng*) is given, sweat should issue mildly, so that the body becomes damp. One is cautioned against causing profuse sweating or continuing to use the formula after the initial sweating. The yáng qì steams the fluids to produce sweat, so when sweating is excessive, it damages both the yáng qì and yīn liquid. When yīn liquid is damaged, the heat is reinforced and may transfer to the yáng brightness. The key signs in this pattern are great vexation and unquenchable thirst. Vexation and thirst result from damage to the qì and liquid and belong to a pattern of yáng brightness exuberant heat. A pulse that is surging and large indicates heat steaming in the yáng brightness and causing the ascension of qì and blood.

This disease is considered a yáng brightness stomach heat pattern and one may ask why White Tiger Decoction (*bái hŭ tāng*) is not used. In this disease stomach heat damages the fluid. The fluid damage is serious, as indicated by the presence of great vexation and unquenchable thirst. Thus, although one must clear heat, it is also necessary to engender liquid and boost the qì, as both have been damaged. Anemarrhena (*zhī mŭ*) and gypsum (*shí gāo*) both clear heat and nourish yīn. Gypsum (*shí gāo*) also eliminates vexation and allays thirst. Mix-fried licorice (*gān căo*) and rice (*gēng mĭ*) nourish the stomach and harmonize the center. These four ingredients constitute White Tiger Decoction (*bái hŭ tāng*). The addition of ginseng (*rén shēn*) is necessary because of the damage to the fluid and the qì. Ginseng (*rén shēn*) supplements the qì and engenders fluid. The heat-clearing action of White Tiger Decoction (*bái hŭ tāng*) is not sufficient to resolve the disease, so it is used in combination with the liquid-engendering, qì-supplementing properties of ginseng (*rén shēn*). Great sweating following the ingestion of Cinnamon Twig Decoction (*guì zhī tāng*) and a pulse that is surging and large is also mentioned in line 25, p. 125. In line 25, however, "great vexation and unquenchable thirst" is absent; therefore, the evil is still in the exterior and the suggested treatment is another dose of Cinnamon Twig Decoction (*guì zhī tāng*).

4.5.4 Pueraria, Scutellaria, and Coptis Decoction Patterns

LINE 34

太阳病，桂枝证，医反下之，利遂不止，脉促者，表未解也；喘而汗出者，葛根黄芩黄连汤主之。

Tài yáng bìng, guì zhī zhèng, yī fǎn xià zhī, lì suì bù zhǐ, mài cù zhě, biǎo wèi jiě yě; chuǎn ér hàn chū zhě, gé gēn huáng qín huáng lián tāng zhǔ zhī.

When in a greater yáng disease [the condition is a] Cinnamon Twig [Decoction] (*guì zhī* [*tāng*]) pattern, but the physician precipitates, [causing] incessant diarrhea and a pulse that is skipping, it means that the exterior has not resolved; when [there is] panting and sweating, Pueraria, Scutellaria, and Coptis Decoction (*gé gēn huáng qín huáng lián tāng*) governs.

FORMULA
Pueraria, Scutellaria, and Coptis Decoction (*gé gēn huáng qín huáng lián tāng*).

◦ Clear heat and check diarrhea; resolve interior and exterior [patterns].

葛根半斤　甘草二两（炙）　黄芩三两　黄连三两

右四味，以水八升，先煮葛根，减二升，内诸药，煮取二升，去滓，分温再服。

Gé gēn bàn jīn　gān cǎo èr liǎng (zhì)　huáng qín sān liǎng　huáng lián sān liǎng

Yòu sì wèi, yǐ shuǐ bā shēng, xiān zhǔ gé gēn, jiǎn èr shēng, nà zhū yào, zhǔ qǔ èr shēng, qù zǐ, fēn wēn zài fú.

pueraria (葛根 *gé gēn*, Puerariae Radix) half jīn (8 liǎng)
mix-fried licorice (甘草 *gān cǎo*, Glycyrrhizae Radix) 2 liǎng
scutellaria (黄芩 *huáng qín*, Scutellariae Radix) 3 liǎng
coptis (黄连 *huáng lián*, Coptidis Rhizoma) 3 liǎng

[For] the above four ingredients, use eight shēng of water. First boil pueraria (*gé gēn*) to reduce [the water] by two shēng. Add all the ingredients. Boil to get two shēng and remove the dregs. Divide [into two parts], and take warm twice a day.

SYNOPSIS
A discussion of the signs and treatment of diarrhea from interior heat complicated by an exterior evil.

COMMENTARY
When precipitation is used in cases of an exterior evil, the evil falls inward

resulting in chest bind or, as in this case, diarrhea. The action of precipitation, by causing downward movement in the body, actually drags the evil into the body and down into the lower burner. On the basis of the formula one can infer that evil qì has transformed into heat and harassed the intestines, causing incessant diarrhea. Nevertheless, the patient's yáng qì is exuberant and still has strength to contend with the evil in the exterior, as indicated by a pulse that is skipping. This pulse also indicates that the exterior has not yet resolved and heat is harassing the lung. Panting means that the lungs have lost the ability to depurate and downbear. The heat evil steams the fluids and forces them to stray to the exterior, so sweat issues.

Pueraria (*gé gēn*) is the most important ingredient in the formula. It resolves the fleshy exterior, raises the clear yáng, and checks diarrhea. Also important to treat diarrhea are scutellaria (*huáng qín*) and coptis (*huáng lián*), which clear interior heat, thicken the intestines and stomach, and check diarrhea. "Thickening" refers to strengthening and fortifying stomach and intestinal function. Licorice (*gān cǎo*) harmonizes the center, boosts the qì, and moderates the actions of the other ingredients. Although this formula is thought to resolve both the exterior and the interior conditions, it is primarily a formula to clear interior heat and resolve diarrhea. It may also be used for incessant diarrhea without exterior signs.

4.5.5 Scutellaria Decoction and Scutellaria Decoction Plus Pinellia and Fresh Ginger Patterns

LINE 172

太阳与少阳合病，自下利者，与黄芩汤；若呕者，黄芩加半夏生姜汤主之。

Tài yáng yǔ shào yáng hé bìng, zì xià lì zhě, yǔ huáng qín tāng; ruò ǒu zhě, huáng qín jiā bàn xià shēng jiāng tāng zhǔ zhī.

When in greater yáng and lesser yáng combination disease [there is] spontaneous diarrhea,* give Scutellaria Decoction (*huáng qín tāng*); if [there is] retching, Scutellaria Decoction Plus Pinellia and Fresh Ginger (*huáng qín jiā bàn xià shēng jiāng tāng*) governs.

TEXT NOTE

* Spontaneous diarrhea, 自下利 *zì xià lì*: Loose stool that occurs without any known cause, such as inappropriate precipitation.

FORMULAE

Scutellaria Decoction (*huáng qín tāng*).

∘ Clear heat and check diarrhea.

黄芩三两　芍药二两　甘草二两（炙）　大枣十二枚（擘）

右四味，以水一斗，煮取三升，去滓，温服一升，日再、夜一服。

huáng qín sān liǎng sháo yào èr liǎng gān cǎo èr liǎng (zhì) dà zǎo shí èr méi (bò)

Yòu sì wèi, yǐ shuǐ yī dǒu, zhǔ qǔ sān shēng, qù zǐ, wēn fú yī shēng, rì zài 、 yè yī fú.

scutellaria (黄芩 *huáng qín*, Scutellariae Radix) 3 liǎng
peony (芍药 *sháo yào*, Paeoniae Radix) 2 liǎng
mix-fried licorice (甘草 *gān cǎo*, Glycyrrhizae Radix) 2 liǎng
jujube (大枣 *dà zǎo*, Ziziphi Fructus) 12 pieces (broken)

[For] the above four ingredients use one dǒu of water. Boil to get three shēng and remove the dregs. Take one shēng warm, [then] once [during] the day and again at night.*

Scutellaria Decoction Plus Pinellia and Fresh Ginger (*huáng qín jiā bàn xià shēng jiāng tāng*).

◦ Downbear counterflow and check retching.

黄芩三两 芍药二两 甘草二两（炙） 大枣十二枚（擘） 半夏半升（洗） 生姜一两半（一方三两，切）

右六味，以水一斗，煮取三升，去滓，温服一升，日再、夜一服。

Huáng qín sān liǎng sháo yào èr liǎng gān cǎo èr liǎng (zhì) dà zǎo shí èr méi (bò) bàn xià bàn shēng (xǐ) shēng jiāng yī liǎng bàn (yī fāng sān liǎng, qiē)

Yòu liù wèi, yǐ shuǐ yī dǒu, zhǔ qǔ sān shēng, qù zǐ, wēn fú yī shēng, rì zài 、 yè yī fú.

scutellaria (黄芩 *huáng qín*, Scutellariae Radix) 3 liǎng
peony (芍药 *sháo yào*, Paeoniae Radix) 2 liǎng
mix-fried licorice (甘草 *gān cǎo*, Glycyrrhizae Radix) 2 liǎng
jujube (大枣 *dà zǎo*, Ziziphi Fructus) 12 pieces (broken)
pinellia (半夏 *bàn xià*, Pinelliae Tuber) half shēng (washed)
fresh ginger (生姜 *shēng jiāng*, Zingiberis Rhizoma Recens) 1 liǎng (cut)

[For] the above six ingredients use one dǒu of water. Boil to get three shēng and remove the dregs. Take one shēng warm, [then] once [during] the day and again at night.*

FORMULA NOTE

* Take one shēng warm, [then] once [during] the day and again at night, 日再、夜一服 *rì zài、 yè yī fú*: One shēng of the three shēng decoction is taken immediately, then one shēng is taken during the day, and the final shēng is taken in the evening.

SYNOPSIS

The signs and treatment of diarrhea and retching or vomiting that may occur in greater yáng and lesser yáng combination disease.

COMMENTARY

As in previous lines, when the pattern is referred to as a combination disease one may assume that signs of both channels are present. Nevertheless, any particular sign that is explicitly mentioned in the text should be given more significance. In this pattern signs of both greater yáng disease and lesser yáng disease are present, but spontaneous diarrhea is highlighted by its inclusion in the text. This line presents a lesser yáng disease, rather than a greater yáng pattern, since spontaneous diarrhea is more common in lesser yáng patterns. Heat evil depressed in the lesser yáng may move inward and harass the yáng brightness, causing heat diarrhea.

An analysis of the formula reinforces this idea. Scutellaria Decoction (*huáng qín tāng*) is suggested for this pattern. Scutellaria (*huáng qín*), after which the formula is named and which is used in the highest dosage, is bitter and cold. It clears liver and gallbladder heat and checks diarrhea. Peony (*sháo yào*) nourishes liver yīn and quells the liver. It can control liver and gallbladder qì which counterflow transversely, overwhelming the spleen and stomach, and causing diarrhea. This combination is important for the treatment of heat diarrhea.

Another possibility suggested by this line is that when heat evil becomes depressed in the lesser yáng, it may invade the stomach and cause retching. In this event, the same basic formula is used, but pinellia (*bàn xià*) and fresh ginger (*shēng jiāng*) are added. These two ingredients harmonize the stomach, downbear counterflow, and suppress retching.

4.6 VACUITY COLD PATTERNS

Inappropriate treatment of a greater yáng disease can result in a transmuted pattern of vacuity cold. These patterns can be divided into heart yáng vacuity, yáng vacuity with water qì, spleen vacuity, and kidney yáng vacuity.

4.6.1 Heart Yáng Vacuity Patterns

In the patterns below, excessive promotion of sweating or the use of fire methods to force sweating damages the heart yáng and causes conditions such as heart palpitations and fright mania. These are patterns of heart yáng vacuity, but because the process of damaging the heart yáng varies, the signs also vary. If the heart yáng is damaged through excessive sweating, giving rise to signs such as heart palpitations with a liking for pressure, the appropriate formula is Cinnamon Twig and Licorice Decoction (*guì zhī gān cǎo tāng*), which warms and frees the heart yáng. If a fire method is used and then precipitation is also used, it can cause heart yáng vacuity. The heart spirit strays, giving rise principally to vexation and agitation. This pattern is a more severe vacuity than the previous one and is treated with Cinnamon Twig, Licorice, Dragon Bone, and Oyster Shell Decoction (*guì zhī gān cǎo lóng gǔ mǔ lì tāng*), which warms and frees the heart yáng, and quiets the spirit by subduing and settling. If the damage to the heart yáng is even more severe and yáng collapses, signs such as fright mania may result. In this case, the appropriate formula is Cinnamon Twig Minus Peony Plus Dichroa Leaf, Dragon Bone, and Oyster Shell Counterflow-Stemming Decoction (*guì zhī qù sháo yào jiā shǔ qī mǔ lì lóng gǔ jiù nì tāng*), which warms and frees the heart yáng, settles fright and quiets the spirit, and constrains floating yáng. If the use of red-hot needling damages the heart yáng and lower burner cold qì ascends counterflow, giving rise to running piglet, the appropriate formula is Cinnamon Twig Decoction Plus Extra Cinnamon (*guì zhī jiā guì tāng*), which warms and frees the heart yáng, and calms upsurge and downbears counterflow.

4.6.1.1 Cinnamon Twig and Licorice Decoction Patterns

Line 64

发汗过多，其人叉手自冒心，心下悸，欲得按者，桂枝甘草汤主之。

Fā hàn guò duō, qí rén chā shǒu zì mào xīn, xīn xià jì, yù dé àn zhě, guì zhī gān cǎo tāng zhǔ zhī.

When copious sweating has been promoted and the person's hands are crossed over the heart[1] and there are palpitations below the heart,[2] with a desire for pressure, Cinnamon Twig and Licorice Decoction (*guì zhī gān cǎo tāng*) governs.

Text Notes

1. Hands crossed over the heart, 叉手自冒心 *chā shǒu zì mào xīn*: The hands are crossed and covering the chest in the area where the movement from the palpitations is felt.
2. Palpitations below the heart, 心下悸 *xīn xià jì*: A feeling of light pounding in the upper stomach region, just below the tip of the breast bone, not in the heart.

Formula

Cinnamon Twig and Licorice Decoction (*guì zhī gān cǎo tāng*)

∘ Supplement heart yáng.

桂枝四两（去皮） 甘草二两（炙）

右二味，以水三升，煮取一升，去滓，顿服。

Guì zhī sì liǎng (qù pí) gān cǎo èr liǎng (zhì)
Yòu èr wèi, yǐ shuǐ sān shēng, zhǔ qǔ yī shēng, qù zǐ, dùn fú.

cinnamon twig (桂枝 *guì zhī*, Cinnamomi Ramulus) (remove bark) 4 liǎng
mix-fried licorice (甘草 *gān cǎo*, Glycyrrhizae Radix) 2 liǎng

[For] the above two ingredients use three shēng of water. Boil to get one shēng. Remove the dregs and take in one single dose.

Synopsis

The signs and treatment of heart palpitations that occur after sweating is promoted excessively and damages the heart yáng.

Commentary

Sweat is the humor of the heart and is produced through the steaming action of the heart yáng. When copious sweating is promoted, it may damage the heart yáng. Damage to the heart yáng results in a loss of the normal defense and protection of the heart and produces palpitations. A desire for pressure means that the palpitations are vacuous in nature. The indication of vacuity is further suggested by the patient's posture. The patient covers the heart in order to quiet the palpitations and protect from the outside what cannot be protected from the inside. The heart cannot protect itself because the heart yáng has been damaged.

Cinnamon Twig and Licorice Decoction (*guì zhī gān cǎo tāng*) supplements and boosts the heart yáng. Acrid, sweet, and warm, cinnamon twig (*guì zhī*) enters the heart, warming the channels, freeing yáng, and assisting yáng. Mix-fried licorice (*gān cǎo*) is sweet and warm. It supplements the center and boosts the qì. The combination of these two medicinals engenders the yáng qì and returns the heart yáng, thereby relieving palpitations.

4.6.1.2 Cinnamon Twig, Licorice, Dragon Bone, and Oyster Shell Decoction Patterns

Line 118

火逆下之，因烧针烦躁者，桂枝甘草龙骨牡蛎汤主之。

Huǒ nì xià zhī, yīn shāo zhēn fán zào zhě, guì zhī gān cǎo lóng gǔ mǔ lì tāng zhǔ zhī.

If adverse [treatment] by fire[1] [is followed by] precipitation, and because of red-hot needling[2] [there is] vexation and agitation, Cinnamon Twig, Licorice, Dragon Bone, and Oyster Shell Decoction (*guì zhī gān cǎo lóng gǔ mǔ lì tāng*) governs.

Text Notes

1. Adverse [treatment] by fire, 火逆 *huǒ nì*: Inappropriate use of a fire treatment.
2. Red-hot needling, 烧针 *shāo zhēn*: In *Gāo Děng Cóng Shū* this method is referred to as warm needling. The *Shāng Hán Lùn Yán Jiū Dà Cí Diǎn*, however, explains that this technique, also referred to as fire needling (火针 *huǒ zhēn*), involves heating the tip of the needle until it is red hot, quickly inserting it, and then massaging the needle site after removal. This method warms the channels and frees the vessels, and moves qì and quickens blood. It is appropriate for cold-damp impediment (寒湿痹 *hán shī bì*) pain and other similar patterns. Red-hot needling is to be clearly distinguished from warm needling (温针 *wēn zhēn*), which involves the placing of moxa floss, 艾绒 *ài róng*, on the handle of the needle and burning it to warm the needle and the local area. See line 16A, p. 132, and line 119, p. 277, for warm needling.

Formula

Cinnamon Twig, Licorice, Dragon Bone, and Oyster Shell Decoction (*guì zhī gān cǎo lóng gǔ mǔ lì tāng*)

- Supplement heart yáng; subdue, settle, and pacify the spirit.

桂枝一两（去皮） 甘草二两（炙） 牡蛎二两（熬） 龙骨二两

右四味，以水五升，煮取二升半，去滓，温服八合，日三服。

Guì zhī yī liǎng (qù pí) gān cǎo èr liǎng (zhì) mǔ lì èr liǎng (áo) lóng gǔ èr liǎng

Yòu sì wèi, yǐ shuǐ wǔ shēng, zhǔ qǔ èr shēng bàn, qù zǐ, wēn fú bā gě, rì sān fú.

cinnamon twig (桂枝 *guì zhī*, Cinnamomi Ramulus) 1 liǎng (remove bark)
mix-fried licorice (甘草 *gān cǎo*, Glycyrrhizae Radix) 2 liǎng
oyster shell (牡蛎 *mǔ lì*, Ostreae Concha) 2 liǎng (dry-fry)
dragon bone (龙骨 *lóng gǔ*, Mastodi Ossis Fossilia) 2 liǎng

[For] the above four ingredients use five shēng of water. Boil to get two and a half shēng. Remove the dregs and take eight gě warm, three times a day.

SYNOPSIS

The signs and treatment of heart yáng vacuity vexation and agitation.

COMMENTARY

Two ambiguities arise in this line. The first ambiguity concerns the nature of the red-hot needling method discussed in the note above. The second concerns the number of erroneous treatments the patient has received. The first mistreatment is the inappropriate use of an unspecified fire method. The second is the inappropriate use of precipitation. The ambiguity lies in whether "red-hot needling," mentioned after precipitation, is a third mistreatment or whether it refers to the first mistreatment, adverse treatment by fire. Zhāng Zhì-Cōng and Chéng Wú-Jǐ agree that the red-hot needling constitutes a third mistreatment, whereas Yù Chāng and Qián Huáng believe that only two mistreatments occurred and that red-hot needling is the fire method.

Despite these differences of interpretation, all the commentators agree that the use of fire methods to force sweating damages the heart yáng. Not only that, but because fire methods are generally uncomfortable for the patient, they also easily disquiet the heart spirit. After damage to the heart yáng it loses warmth and nourishment and the heart spirit cannot be contained. The result of this treatment is vexation and agitation; hence Cinnamon Twig, Licorice, Dragon Bone, and Oyster Shell Decoction (*guì zhī gān cǎo lóng gǔ mǔ lì tāng*) is used. Dragon bone (*lóng gǔ*) and oyster shell (*mǔ lì*) subdue and settle and quiet the spirit. Cinnamon twig (*guì zhī*) and mix-fried licorice (*gān cǎo*) warm and free the heart yáng.

4.6.1.3 Cinnamon Twig Minus Peony Plus Dichroa, Dragon Bone, and Oyster Shell Counterflow-Stemming Decoction Patterns

Line 112

伤寒脉浮，医以火迫劫之，亡阳，必惊狂，卧起不安者，桂枝去芍药加蜀漆牡蛎龙骨救逆汤主之。

Shāng hán mài fú, yī yǐ huǒ pò jié zhī, wáng yáng, bì jīng kuáng, wò qǐ bù ān zhě, guì zhī qù sháo yào jiā shǔ qī mǔ lì lóng gǔ jiù nì tāng zhǔ zhī.

When in cold damage the pulse is floating and the physician uses fire [treatment] to force [sweating],[1] and [as a result] yáng collapses,[2] [then] there will be fright mania[3] and fidgetiness whether lying or sitting; Cinnamon Twig Minus Peony Plus Dichroa Leaf, Dragon Bone, and Oyster Shell Counterflow-Stemming Decoction (*guì zhī qù sháo yào jiā shǔ qī mǔ lì lóng gǔ jiù nì tāng*) governs.

Text Notes

1. Fire [treatment] is used to force [sweating], 火迫劫之 *huǒ pò jié zhī*: Using a fire method (red-hot needling, fire fuming, moxibustion) to force sweating.
2. Yáng collapse, 亡阳 *wáng yáng*: Critical vacuity of yáng qì. Here yáng collapse is understood to mean collapse of the heart yáng. Sweat is the humor of the heart and is produced through the steaming action of the heart yáng. When sweating is forced or promoted improperly, it may damage the heart yáng.
3. Fright mania, 惊狂 *jīng kuáng*: Apprehension and manic derangement.

Formula

Cinnamon Twig Minus Peony Plus Dichroa Leaf, Dragon Bone, and Oyster Shell Counterflow-Stemming Decoction (*guì zhī qù sháo yào jiā shǔ qī mǔ lì lóng gǔ jiù nì tāng*)

∘ Supplement heart yáng; settle fright and quiet the spirit.

桂枝三两（去皮） 甘草二两（炙） 生姜三两（切） 大枣十二枚（擘） 牡蛎五两（熬） 蜀漆三两（洗去腥） 龙骨四两

㈠ 右七味，以水一斗二升，先煮蜀漆，减二升，内诸药，煮取三升，去滓，温服一升。㈡ 本云，桂枝汤，今去芍药，加蜀漆、牡蛎、龙骨。

Guì zhī sān liǎng (qù pí) gān cǎo èr liǎng (zhì) shēng jiāng sān liǎng (qiē) dà zǎo shí èr méi (bò) mǔ lì wǔ liǎng (áo) shǔ qī sān liǎng (xǐ qù xīng) lóng gǔ sì liǎng

(1) *Yòu qī wèi, yǐ shuǐ yī dǒu èr shēng, xiān zhǔ shǔ qī, jiǎn èr shēng, nà zhū yào, zhǔ qǔ sān shēng, qù zǐ, wēn fú yī shēng.* (2) *Běn yún guì zhī tāng, jīn qù sháo yào, jiā shǔ qī、 mǔ lì、 lóng gǔ.*

cinnamon twig (桂枝 *guì zhī*, Cinnamomi Ramulus) 3 liǎng (remove bark)
mix-fried licorice (甘草 *gān cǎo*, Glycyrrhizae Radix) 2 liǎng
fresh ginger (生姜 *shēng jiāng*, Zingiberis Rhizoma Recens) 3 liǎng (cut)
jujube (大枣 *dà zǎo*, Ziziphi Fructus) 12 pieces (broken)
oyster shell (牡蛎 *mǔ lì*, Ostreae Concha) 5 liǎng (dry-fry)
dichroa leaf (蜀漆 *shǔ qī*, Dichroae Folium)* 3 liǎng (wash to remove fishy smell)
dragon bone (龙骨 *lóng gǔ*, Mastodi Ossis Fossilia) 4 liǎng

(1) [For] the above seven ingredients use one dǒu and two shēng of water. First boil dichroa leaf (*shǔ qī*) and reduce by two shēng. Add all [the other] ingredients and boil to get three shēng. Remove the dregs and take one shēng warm. (2) This is Cinnamon Twig Decoction (*guì zhī tāng*) without peony (*sháo yào*), and with dichroa leaf (*shǔ qī*), oyster shell (*mǔ lì*), and dragon bone (*lóng gǔ*).

FORMULA NOTE

* Dichroa leaf (*shǔ qī*): The leaves of dichroa (*cháng shān*).

SYNOPSIS

The signs and treatment of fright mania from collapse of the heart yáng caused by inappropriate use of a fire method.

COMMENTARY

When in cold damage the pulse is floating, one should promote sweating. Nevertheless, heavy sweating is contraindicated. Here a fire method is used which causes excessive sweating, yáng collapse, and the heart spirit to float astray. Yáng collapse may take the form of collapse of kidney yáng, heart yáng, or defensive yáng. Kidney yáng collapse is treated by warming the kidney and returning yáng with formulae such as Counterflow Cold Decoction (*sì nì tāng*). Cinnamon Twig Decoction Plus Aconite (*guì zhī jiā fù zǐ tāng*), which secures the exterior and protects yáng, is appropriate to treat collapse of the defensive yáng. The signs above, however, clearly indicate collapse of the heart yáng. When the heart yáng collapses, the heart spirit cannot be contained and subdued, so it floats outward. Mild patterns may include palpitations or agitation and vexation, whereas more severe patterns may include fright mania.

Cinnamon Twig Minus Peony Plus Dichroa Leaf, Dragon Bone, and Oyster Shell Counterflow-Stemming Decoction (*guì zhī qù sháo yào jiā shǔ qī mǔ lì lóng gǔ jiù nì tāng*) contains cinnamon twig (*guì zhī*) and licorice (*gān cǎo*), which engender, warm, and free the yáng qì, so that it returns to the heart. Fresh ginger (*shēng jiāng*) and jujube (*dà zǎo*) boost the center and harmonize. Oyster shell (*mǔ lì*) and dragon bone (*lóng gǔ*) are heavy settlers that pacify the heart spirit by subduing and restraining yáng. The use of dichroa leaf (*shǔ qī*) has been explained in two ways. Zhāng Xī-Jū, Chéng Wú-Jǐ, and Fāng Yǒu-Zhí explain that the adverse use of fire treatment gives rise to fire evil, which acrid dichroa leaf (*shǔ qī*) dissipates and discharges. Wáng Zǐ-Jiē (王子接, style 晋三 Jìn-Sān) and Zēng Yǐng-Fǔ (曾颖甫) offer the explanation that by dispelling phlegm-rheum, dichroa leaf (*shǔ qī*) is able to resolve fright mania and other disorders of the spirit. Although this formula is very similar to that used in the previous line, the dosages are all increased, indicating the increased severity of this pattern.

Lines 64, 118, and 112 deal with disorders of the heart yáng. These patterns vary in degree of severity, sign pattern, and treatment. A simple comparison of the three lines will be illustrative. The pattern in line 64, p. 162, can be described as heart yáng insufficiency or mild heart yáng vacuity and is characterized by palpitations and a desire for pressure on the chest in the region of the heart. Line 118, p. 163, describes mild heart yáng vacuity characterized by vexation and agitation. Damaged heart yáng or severe heart yáng vacuity is the pattern in line 112, p. 165. Fright mania and generalized discomfort characterize severe heart yáng vacuity. All the formulae include cinnamon twig (*guì zhī*) and licorice (*gān cǎo*), which supplement and free the heart yáng. In the mild case, these medicinals are sufficient, but in the case of moderate heart yáng vacuity, dragon bone (*lóng gǔ*) and oyster shell (*mǔ lì*) are added to subdue and settle, and thus quiet spirit. Fresh ginger (*shēng jiāng*) and jujube (*dà zǎo*), which boost the center and harmonize, and dichroa leaf (*shǔ qī*), which dispels turbid phlegm and dissipates fire, are included in the formula for the treatment of severe heart yáng vacuity.

4.6.1.4 Cinnamon Twig Decoction Plus Extra Cinnamon Patterns

LINE 117

(一) 烧针令其汗，针处被寒，核起而赤者，必发奔豚。(二) 气从少腹上冲心者，灸其核上各一壮，与桂枝加桂汤，更加桂二两也。

(1) *Shāo zhēn lìng qí hàn, zhēn chù bèi hán, hé qǐ ér chì zhě, bì fā bēn tún.* (2) *Qì cóng shào fù shàng chōng xīn zhě, jiǔ qí hé shàng gè yí zhuàng, yǔ guì zhī jiā guì tāng, gèng jiā guì èr liǎng yě.*

(1) When red-hot needling [is used to] cause sweating,[1] the needling site contracts cold,[2] and if a red node forms, [the person] will develop running piglet.[3] (2) When qì from the lesser abdomen surges upward to the heart, use one cone of moxa on each node and give Cinnamon Twig Decoction Plus Extra Cinnamon (*guì zhī jiā guì tāng*), adding 2 liǎng of cinnamon (*guì*).[4]

TEXT NOTES

1. Red-hot needling [is used to] cause sweating, 烧针令其汗 *shāo zhēn lìng qí hàn*: Red-hot needling is generally said to force sweating, that is, it is a harsh way to promote sweating.

2. The needling site contracts cold, 针处被寒 *zhēn chù bèi hán*: Following the use of a red-hot needle, the needling site is not properly protected and cold evil invades and blocks the area.
3. Running piglet, 奔豚 *bēn tún*: The sensation of qì surging upward from the lesser abdomen into the chest and heart.
4. Cinnamon (*guì*): According to Fāng Yǒu-Zhí, this refers to cinnamon bark (*ròu guì*), but according to Xú Dà Chūn and the authors of *Gāo Děng Cóng Shū*, this refers to cinnamon twig (*guì zhī*).

FORMULA

Cinnamon Twig Decoction Plus Extra Cinnamon (*guì zhī jiā guì tāng*)

◦ Warm and free the heart yáng; calm [upward] surging and downbear counterflow.

桂枝五两（去皮） 芍药三两 生姜三两（切） 甘草二两（炙） 大枣十二枚（擘）

(一) 右五味，以水七升，煮取三升，去滓，温服一升。(二) 本云，桂枝汤，今加桂满五两，所以加桂者，以能泄奔豚气也。

Guì zhī wǔ liǎng (qù pí) sháo yào sān liǎng shēng jiāng sān liǎng (qiē) gān cǎo èr liǎng (zhì) dà zǎo shí èr méi (bò)

(1) *Yòu wǔ wèi, yǐ shuǐ qī shēng, zhǔ qǔ sān shēng, qù zǐ, wēn fú yī shēng.* (2) *Běn yún guì zhī tāng, jīn jiā guì mǎn wǔ liǎng, suǒ yǐ jiā guì zhě, yǐ néng xiè bēn tún qì yě.*

cinnamon twig (桂枝 *guì zhī*, Cinnamomi Ramulus) 5 liǎng (remove bark)
peony (芍药 *sháo yào*, Paeoniae Radix) 3 liǎng
fresh ginger (生姜 *shēng jiāng*, Zingiberis Rhizoma Recens) 3 liǎng (cut)
mix-fried licorice (甘草 *gān cǎo*, Glycyrrhizae Radix) 2 liǎng
jujube (大枣 *dà zǎo*, Ziziphi Fructus) 12 pieces (broken)

(1) [For] the above five ingredients use seven shēng of water. Boil to get three shēng, remove the dregs and take one shēng warm. (2) This is Cinnamon Twig Decoction (*guì zhī tāng*) with cinnamon [twig] (*guì zhī*) added to a full five liǎng. Cinnamon [twig] (*guì zhī*) is added in order to discharge running piglet qì.

SYNOPSIS

The signs and treatment of running piglet caused by heart yáng vacuity.

COMMENTARY

Red-hot needling is used to force sweating. When a red-hot needle is applied the interstices open and allow sweat to issue. If appropriate care is not taken, the opening of the interstices may allow an evil to enter the body, as it does in the present line. Cold evil lodges in the needle site and causes a node to form. Another result of red-hot needling is that forced sweating damages the heart yáng. When the heart yáng is damaged, it cannot warm the kidney yīn. Running piglet occurs when kidney yīn cold exploits heart yáng vacuity and qì surges upward. Running piglet may be caused by different factors. In *Jīn Guì Yào Lüè* it is said to be caused by fright. In the line above, it is the result of yīn cold exploiting yáng vacuity and surging upward.

Moxibustion is used on the surface of the body to warm and dissipate the congealed cold. Cinnamon Twig Decoction Plus Extra Cinnamon (*guì zhī jiā guì tāng*) is Cinnamon Twig Decoction (*guì zhī tāng*) with an increased dosage of cinnamon twig (*guì zhī*). It harmonizes the construction and defense and, because of the additional cinnamon twig (*guì zhī*), it also warms and frees the heart yáng. The formula calms upsurge and downbears counterflow. The action of the formula is different, however, if "add cinnamon" is taken to mean cinnamon bark (*ròu guì*) rather than cinnamon twig (*guì zhī*). Zhāng Nán mentions this ambiguity and offers a rational solution to it:

> As handed down [traditionally, did] the formula add cinnamon twig (*guì zhī*) or cinnamon bark (*ròu guì*)? If calming a kidney evil, adding cinnamon bark (*ròu guì*) is appropriate. If resolving a greater yáng evil, cinnamon twig (*guì zhī*) is appropriate.

4.6.2 Yáng Vacuity and Water Qì Patterns

In greater yáng disease the promotion of sweating or use of vomiting or precipitation can damage yáng qì, causing yáng vacuity. In some patients, constitutional factors can cause the development of water qì patterns or acute conditions. When in yáng vacuity with water qì, the patient experiences palpitations in the abdomen and running piglet is about to occur, the appropriate formula is Poria (Hoelen), Cinnamon Twig, Licorice, and Jujube Decoction (*fú líng guì zhī gān cǎo dà zǎo tāng*), which warms and frees the yáng, and moves water qì. Poria (Hoelen), Cinnamon Twig, Ovate Atractylodes, and Licorice Decoction (*fú líng guì zhī bái zhú gān cǎo tāng*) is used when the inappropriate use of vomiting or precipitation damages the yáng, giving rise to signs such as fullness below the heart and qì surging up to the chest. If following the promotion of sweating water qì collects in the interior and the greater yáng channel qì is inhibited, resulting in signs such as headache, nape and neck pain, and fullness and pain below the heart, the appropriate formula is Cinnamon Twig Decoction Minus Cinnamon Twig Plus Poria (Hoelen) and Ovate Atractylodes (*guì zhī qù guì jiā fú líng bái zhú tāng*), which fortifies the spleen and moves water.

4.6.2.1 Poria (Hoelen), Cinnamon Twig, Licorice, and Jujube Decoction Patterns

LINE 65

发汗后，其人脐下悸者，欲作奔豚，茯苓桂枝甘草大枣汤主之。

Fā hàn hòu, qí rén qí xià jì zhě, yù zuò bēn tún, fú líng guì zhī gān cǎo dà zǎo tāng zhǔ zhī.

When, after sweating has been promoted, the person has palpitations below the umbilicus about to become running piglet, Poria (Hoelen), Cinnamon Twig, Licorice, and Jujube Decoction (*fú líng guì zhī gān cǎo dà zǎo tāng*) governs.

FORMULA

Poria (Hoelen), Cinnamon Twig, Licorice, and Jujube Decoction (*fú líng guì zhī gān cǎo dà zǎo tāng*)

○ Warm and free the heart yáng; transform qì and move water.

茯苓半斤　桂枝四两（去皮）　甘草二两（炙）　大枣十五枚（擘）。

(一) 右四味，以甘澜水一斗，先煮茯苓，减二升，内诸药，煮取三升，去滓，温服一升，日三服。(二) 作甘澜水法：取水二斗，置大盆内，以杓扬之，水上有珠子五六千颗相逐，取用之。

Fú líng bàn jīn guì zhī sì liǎng (qù pí) gān cǎo èr liǎng (zhì) dà zǎo shí wǔ méi (bò)

(1) *Yòu sì wèi, yǐ gān lán shuǐ yī dǒu, xiān zhǔ fú líng, jiǎn èr shēng, nà zhū yào, zhǔ qǔ sān shēng, qù zǐ, wēn fú yī shēng, rì sān fú.* (2) *Zuò gān lán shuǐ fǎ: qǔ shuǐ èr dǒu, zhì dà pén nèi, yǐ sháo yáng zhī, shuǐ shàng yǒu zhū zǐ wǔ liù qiān kē xiāng zhú, qǔ yòng zhī.*

poria (茯苓 *fú líng*, Poria) half shēng

cinnamon twig (桂枝 *guì zhī*, Cinnamomi Ramulus) 4 liǎng (remove bark)

mix-fried licorice (甘草 *gān cǎo*, Glycyrrhizae Radix) 2 liǎng

jujube (大枣 *dà zǎo*, Ziziphi Fructus) 15 pieces (broken)

(1) [For] the above four ingredients use one dǒu of worked water.* First boil poria (*fú líng*) and reduce by two shēng. Add all [the other] ingredients, boil to get three shēng, and remove the dregs. Take one shēng warm, three times a day. (2) Method for making worked water: Take two shēng of water and put it in a large basin. [Repeatedly] scoop [and pour] using a ladle, until there are five or six thousand water droplets on the surface, [which can then] be used.

TEXT NOTE

* Worked water, 甘澜水 *gān lán shuǐ*: This method first appears in the *Huáng Dì Nèi Jīng*, and is thought to prevent the cooking water from assisting the water evil in the body. Furthermore, water's original nature is said to be salty, and by preparing it in this way, it is changed to a sweet nature; therefore, it does not assist the kidney, but instead boosts the spleen and stomach.

SYNOPSIS

The signs and treatment of running piglet that is about to occur caused by heart yáng vacuity.

COMMENTARY

The heart above serves as a cover governing fire, while the kidney below governs water. When the heart yáng is sufficient, it settles and contains the kidney water, preventing it from flooding. If the heart yáng is damaged, it is unable to control the kidney water, which begins to move. Movement of the kidney water is felt as palpitations below the umbilicus and it may be followed by running piglet. These preliminary palpitations, felt when the kidney water begins to move, are very mild in comparison with those felt in running piglet. Poria (Hoelen), Cinnamon Twig, Licorice, and Jujube Decoction (*fú líng guì zhī gān cǎo dà zǎo tāng*) is based on Cinnamon Twig and Licorice Decoction (*guì zhī gān cǎo tāng*); hence an important action is to warm and free the heart yáng. The base formula also downbears counterflow and calms upward surging. Jujube (*dà zǎo*) fortifies the spleen and banks up earth, in order to disinhibit water. Poria (*fú líng*), the sovereign ingredient, is precooked, thereby increasing its ability to disinhibit the urine. Poria (*fú líng*), which quiets the heart, is useful in cases of heart yáng vacuity and related spirit disorders. Worked water, which is sweet and moderate, is used to prepare the formula, because it is believed not to assist the water evil, but instead to boost the spleen and stomach.

4.6.2.2 Poria (Hoelen), Cinnamon Twig, Ovate Atractylodes, and Licorice Decoction Patterns

Line 67

伤寒，若吐若下后，心下逆满，气上冲胸，起则头眩，脉沉紧，发汗则动经，身为振振摇者，茯苓桂枝白术甘草汤主之。

Shāng hán, ruò tù ruò xià hòu, xīn xià nì mǎn, qì shàng chōng xiōng, qǐ zé tóu xuàn, mài chén jǐn, fā hàn zé dòng jīng, shēn wéi zhèn zhèn yáo zhě, fú líng guì zhī bái zhú gān cǎo tāng zhǔ zhī.

When, in cold damage, after vomiting or precipitation, [there is] counterflow fullness below the heart,[1] the qì surges upward to the chest, [the person experiences] dizzy head upon standing, and the pulse is sunken and tight, ([if] sweating is promoted, the channels will be stirred[2] and there will be quivering and trembling[3]) then Poria (Hoelen), Cinnamon Twig, Ovate Atractylodes, and Licorice Decoction (*fú líng guì zhī bái zhú gān cǎo tāng*) governs.

Text Notes

1. Counterflow fullness below the heart, 心下逆满 *xīn xià nì mǎn*: A feeling of distention and fullness in the region of the stomach and stomach duct, with qì rising up into the chest.
2. The channels are stirred, 动经 *dòng jīng*: Damage to the channels that is the result of a loss of fluid nourishment, following fluid damage from the inappropriate promotion of sweating.

3. Quivering and trembling, 振振摇 *zhèn zhèn yáo*: Involuntary spasmodic movements of the body related to channel damage.

FORMULA

Poria (Hoelen), Cinnamon Twig, Ovate Atractylodes, and Licorice Decoction (*fú líng guì zhī bái zhú gān cǎo tāng*)

∘ Warm yáng and fortify the spleen; disinhibit water and downbear [upward] surging [qì].

茯苓四两　桂枝三两（去皮）　白术　甘草各二两（炙）

右四味，以水六升，煮取三升，去滓，分温三服。

Fú líng sì liǎng　guì zhī sān liǎng (qù pí)　bái zhú　gān cǎo gè èr liǎng (zhì)
Yòu sì wèi, yǐ shuǐ liù shēng, zhǔ qǔ sān shēng, qù zǐ, fēn wēn sān fú.

poria (茯苓 *fú líng*, Poria) 4 liǎng
cinnamon twig (桂枝 *guì zhī*, Cinnamomi Ramulus) 3 liǎng (remove bark)
ovate atractylodes (白术 *bái zhú*, Atractylodis Ovatae Rhizoma) 2 liǎng
mix-fried licorice (甘草 *gān cǎo*, Glycyrrhizae Radix) 2 liǎng

[For] the above four ingredients use six shēng of water. Boil to get three shēng and remove the dregs. Divide into three [doses] and take warm.

SYNOPSIS

The signs and treatment of water qì surging upward.

COMMENTARY

The inappropriate use of precipitation or vomiting can damage the spleen and stomach, leading to center qì vacuity. When this damage occurs, movement and transformation of fluids is impaired, which here results in water-rheum amassment. Water qì then ascends counterflow, intimidating the region below the heart and invading the chest. Water qì collecting below the heart causes a feeling of fullness and that invasion of the chest causes dizziness, since water qì, which should move downward, instead rises. (While the terms "water-rheum" and "water qì" both refer to pathological fluids, water-rheum is generally stationary and localized, while water qì is active and pervasive.) A pulse that is sunken and tight further supports the suggestion of water-rheum. Zhāng Jī writes in *Jīn Guì Yào Lüè*, "[With] pulses [that are] sunken, there should be water." A pulse that is sunken indicates water and a pulse that is tight indicates cold. Poria (Hoelen), Cinnamon Twig, Ovate Atractylodes, and Licorice Decoction (*fú líng guì zhī bái zhú gān cǎo tāng*) is used to warm yáng and disinhibit water when cold-rheum collects in the center burner.

Possible grammatical inversion allows this line to be interpreted in two ways. If we assume that "[If] sweating is promoted, the channels will be stirred and there will be generalized quivering and trembling" belongs after the formula name, we may conclude that this formula treats the pattern presented in the first part of the line and that the promotion of sweating constitutes an adverse treatment, as it will damage the channels. The authors of *Gāo Děng Cóng Shū* use this rationale to divide this line into two parts. The section up to and including the pulse is the first part, and the promotion of sweating is the second. They suggest that this line contains grammatical inversion and that the formula should be used to treat the original condition, but if sweating is erroneously promoted, severely damaging the yáng qì and giving rise to generalized quivering and trembling, they suggest True Warrior Decoction (*zhēn wǔ tāng*), which contains aconite (*fù zǐ*) and strongly warms yáng. (For a complete discussion of True Warrior Decoction (*zhēn wǔ tāng*), see line 316, p. 483.)

According to a second interpretation put forward by *Yī Zōng Jīn Jiàn*, one should read the line as it stands since the formula treats damage to the channels from promotion of sweating.

> ... [there is] erroneous precipitation or vomiting, so the chest [yáng] is vacuous and the evil falls [inward]. Thus, [there is] counterflow fullness below the heart and qì surges upward to the chest. If the pulse is floating and tight, the exterior has still not resolved and [if] sweating is absent, one should use Ephedra Decoction (*má huáng tāng*). Here the pulse is sunken and tight, so this patient must usually have intermingling cold and rheum. Dizziness upon standing means the yáng qì of the chest is already vacuous, so one cannot [use] vomiting or [promote] sweating. If one instead [assumes] that the pulse being sunken and tight indicates repletion, does not consider that dizziness [means] vacuity, and erroneously promotes sweating, this is without reason. The exterior channels will be stirred, the defensive yáng will [become] more vacuous, the whole body will [be unable] to depend [on the defensive yáng], and there will be generalized quivering and trembling. This is governed by Poria (Hoelen), Cinnamon Twig, Ovate Atractylodes, and Licorice Decoction (*fú líng guì zhī bái zhú gān cǎo tāng*), which on the one hand flushes rheum and supports yáng, and on the other regulates the defense and harmonizes the construction.

One criticism of the view expressed in *Yī Zōng Jīn Jiàn* is that Poria (Hoelen), Cinnamon Twig, Ovate Atractylodes, and Licorice Decoction (*fú líng guì zhī bái zhú gān cǎo tāng*) does not contain ingredients that strongly support yáng. In the original condition, mild yáng vacuity already existed as a result of the previous mistreatment. If one then promotes sweating, further damaging yáng qì that is already vacuous, one would expect that the formula would contain ingredients that more strongly support the yáng qì.

4.6.2.3 Cinnamon Twig Decoction Minus Cinnamon Twig Plus Poria (Hoelen) and Ovate Atractylodes Patterns

Line 28

服桂枝汤，或下之，仍头项强痛，翕翕发热，无汗，心下满微痛，小便不利者，桂枝去桂加茯苓白术汤主之。

Fú guì zhī tāng, huò xià zhī, réng tóu xiàng jiàng tòng, xì xì fā rè, wú hàn, xīn xià mǎn wēi tòng, xiǎo biàn bù lì zhě, guì zhī qù guì jiā fú líng bái zhú tāng zhǔ zhī.

When Cinnamon Twig Decoction (*guì zhī tāng*) is taken, or precipitation [is used] and [there is] still stiffness and pain of the head and nape, feather-warm heat effusion, absence of sweating, fullness below the heart with slight pain, and inhibited urination, Cinnamon Twig Decoction Minus Cinnamon Twig Plus Poria (Hoelen) and Ovate Atractylodes (*guì zhī qù guì jiā fú líng bái zhú tāng*) governs.

FORMULA

Cinnamon Twig Decoction Minus Cinnamon Twig Plus Poria (Hoelen) and Ovate Atractylodes (*guì zhī qù guì jiā fú líng bái zhú tāng*)

∘ Fortify the spleen and disinhibit water in order to free yáng qì.

芍药三两　甘草二两（炙）　生姜（切）、白术、茯苓各三两　大枣十二枚（擘）

(一) 右六味，以水八升，煮取三升，去滓，温服一升。(二) 小便利则愈。(三) 本云，桂枝汤，今去桂枝加茯苓、白术。

Sháo yào sān liǎng　gān cǎo èr liǎng (zhì)　shēng jiāng (qiē)　bái zhú　fú líng gè sān liǎng　dà zǎo shí èr méi (bò)

(1) *Yòu liù wèi, yǐ shuǐ bā shēng, zhǔ qǔ sān shēng, qù zǐ, wēn fú yī shēng.* (2) *Xiǎo biàn lì zé yù.* (3) *Běn yún guì zhī tāng, jīn qù guì zhī jiā fú líng、bái zhú.*

peony (芍药 *sháo yào*, Paeoniae Radix) 3 liǎng
mix-fried licorice (甘草 *gān cǎo*, Glycyrrhizae Radix) 2 liǎng
fresh ginger (生姜 *shēng jiāng*, Zingiberis Rhizoma Recens) 3 liǎng (cut)
ovate atractylodes (白术 *bái zhú*, Atractylodis Ovatae Rhizoma) 3 liǎng
poria (茯苓 *fú líng*, Poria) 3 liǎng
jujube (大枣 *dà zǎo*, Ziziphi Fructus) 12 pieces (broken)

(1) [For] the above six ingredients use eight shēng of water. Boil to get three shēng, remove the dregs and take one shēng warm. (2) [After] urination is uninhibited, then [there will be] recovery. (3) This is Cinnamon Twig Decoction (*guì zhī tāng*) without cinnamon [twig] (*guì [zhī]*) and with poria (*fú líng*) and ovate atractylodes (*bái zhú*).

SYNOPSIS

The signs and treatment of the pattern in which, after the promotion of sweating and the use of precipitation, water qì collects in the interior and the greater yáng channel qì is inhibited.

COMMENTARY

One can imagine that the physician whose actions are described in this line, upon seeing a patient with stiffness and pain in the head and nape, feather-warm heat effusion, and absence of sweating, may have thought of an exterior disease for which Cinnamon Twig Decoction (*guì zhī tāng*) would be appropriate. It is also possible that, on encountering slight pain and fullness below the heart and inhibited urination, the physician felt that this indicated interior repletion, which would be relieved by precipitation. Nevertheless, following the use of these treatments, the original signs are still present and one may assume that this is neither a Cinnamon Twig Decoction (*guì zhī tāng*) pattern, nor a pattern for which precipitation is appropriate. How, then, should one interpret this pattern? According to Chéng Wú-Jǐ and *Yī Zōng Jīn Jiàn*, these signs indicate an unresolved exterior pattern and rheum collecting in the interior. Nonetheless, Kē Qín writes that this is not an exterior pattern, but water qì congesting and binding below the heart. He emphasizes that "... the root of the disease is below the heart and the pathomechanism involves the bladder." Furthermore, Chén Niàn-Zǔ and Táng Zōng-Hǎi (唐宗海, style 容川 Róng-Chuān) suggest that the critical point for the understanding of this line is the abnormal movement of water in the greater yáng, by which they mean the bladder, not the channel.

Diseases of the interior may manifest in exterior signs and vice-versa. Water evil in the interior can inhibit bladder qì and disrupt qì transformation, resulting in inhibited urination. When the qì of the bladder becomes inhibited, it may affect both the organ and the channel. Bladder channel qì stagnates, giving rise to stiffness and pain in the head and nape. Qì transformation in the bladder becomes impaired, giving rise to inhibited urination. The presence of water qì in the interior may also congest the qì dynamic, as indicated by the presence of fullness below the heart.

An analysis of the formula is normally used to help explain a line which is unclear. Such an analysis does not shed much light on this line since the formula itself is interpreted in three different ways. The focus of the disagreement is whether or not one should remove cinnamon twig (*guì zhī*) from the formula.

a) The first interpretation, represented by the opinions of Fāng Yǒu-Zhí, Chén Niàn-Zǔ, and Táng Zōng-Hǎi, is that one should remove cinnamon twig (*guì zhī*). Sweating is absent, so these authors do not think that cinnamon twig (*guì zhī*) is appropriate. Furthermore, although simultaneous disease of the exterior and interior is present, the most important aspect is water-rheum, so one should not use cinnamon twig (*guì zhī*) to resolve the exterior. Instead, one should use poria (*fú líng*), ovate atractylodes (*bái zhú*), and peony (*sháo yào*) to treat the interior condition. According to this interpretation, the evil is primarily in the bladder organ, not the channel, and the treatment principle of resolving the fleshy exterior, appropriate for an evil in the channel, should be changed to one of disinhibiting water.

b) A second interpretation, represented by the *Yī Zōng Jīn Jiàn*, is that the ingredient to be removed from this formula is not cinnamon twig (*guì zhī*), but peony (*sháo yào*). The rationale for this point of view is explained as follows. First, if one removes cinnamon twig (*guì zhī*), no medicinals to treat the exterior disease remain and the exterior disease should be treated. Second, in some versions of the text, directions are given indicating that the formula should be prepared and taken just as Cinnamon Twig Decoction (*guì zhī tāng*). If cinnamon twig (*guì zhī*) is removed from the formula, the actions of the formula are significantly altered and this preparation method might not be appropriate. Third, the pattern of fullness and slight pain below the heart is the same as the chest fullness pattern for which Cinnamon Twig Decoction Minus Peony (*guì zhī qù sháo yào tāng*) is used. These three points, however, are problematic. The first, that without cinnamon twig (*guì zhī*) the formula contains nothing to treat the exterior disease, is problematic because cinnamon twig (*guì zhī*), though used to treat exterior patterns, is generally not used alone for conditions without sweating. Regarding the directions for the use of the formula, the line referring to Cinnamon Twig Decoction (*guì zhī tāng*) does not appear in all versions of the text and its inclusion is open to question. The final point, regarding the similarity with chest fullness, is problematic simply because of differences between the two conditions with regard to disease location and pathomechanism.

c) Finally, a third interpretation is represented by Chéng Wú-Jǐ, who writes that neither cinnamon twig (*guì zhī*) nor peony (*sháo yào*) should be removed. In his opinion, Cinnamon Twig Decoction (*guì zhī tāng*) is used to treat the exterior condition, and poria (*fú líng*) and ovate atractylodes (*bái zhú*) are used to disinhibit the urine and move the collecting rheum. The criticism of this point of view is that Cinnamon Twig Decoction (*guì zhī tāng*) is not generally used to treat diseases without sweating.

4.6.3 Spleen Vacuity Patterns

Spleen vacuity transmuted patterns can be the result of inappropriate treatment or occur due to the constitution of the patient. When sweating is promoted excessively, or the patient has a constitutional tendency toward spleen vacuity, and signs such as abdominal fullness and distention appear, the appropriate formula is Magnolia Bark, Fresh Ginger, Pinellia, Licorice, and Ginseng Decoction (*hòu pò shēng jiāng bàn xià gān cǎo rén shēn tāng*), which fortifies the spleen and eliminates fullness. When following contraction of cold damage no treatment is given and after a short period of time the patient develops signs of interior vacuity such as heart palpitations and vexation, the appropriate formula is Minor Center-Fortifying Decoction (*xiǎo jiàn zhōng tāng*), which supplements the spleen and harmonizes qì and blood. Cinnamon Twig and Ginseng Decoction (*guì zhī rén shēn tāng*) is used in patterns when the inappropriate use of precipitation causes vacuity cold and diarrhea because it warms the center and resolves the exterior.

4.6.3.1 Magnolia Bark, Fresh Ginger, Pinellia, Licorice, and Ginseng Decoction Patterns

LINE 66

发汗后，腹胀满者，厚朴生姜半夏甘草人参汤主之。

Fā hàn hòu, fù zhàng mǎn zhě, hòu pò shēng jiāng bàn xià gān cǎo rén shēn tāng zhǔ zhī.

When, after the promotion of sweating, [there is] abdominal distention and fullness, Magnolia Bark, Fresh Ginger, Pinellia, Licorice, and Ginseng Decoction (*hòu pò shēng jiāng bàn xià gān cǎo rén shēn tāng*) governs.

FORMULA

Magnolia Bark, Fresh Ginger, Pinellia, Licorice, and Ginseng Decoction (*hòu pò shēng jiāng bàn xià gān cǎo rén shēn tāng*)

∘ Fortify the spleen and warm and move; loosen the center and eliminate fullness.

厚朴半斤（炙，去皮） 生姜十斤（切） 半夏半升（洗） 甘草二两 人参一两

右五味，以水一斗，煮取三升，去滓，温服一升，日三服。

Hòu pò bàn jīn (zhì, qù pí) shēng jiāng shí jīn (qiē) bàn xià bàn shēng (xǐ) gān cǎo èr liǎng rén shēn yī liǎng

Yòu wǔ wèi, yǐ shuǐ yī dǒu, zhǔ qǔ sān shēng, qù zǐ, wēn fú yī shēng, rì sān fú.

magnolia bark (厚朴 *hòu pò*, Magnoliae Cortex) half jīn (mix-fry, remove bark)
fresh ginger (生姜 *shēng jiāng*, Zingiberis Rhizoma Recens) 10 jīn (cut)
pinellia (半夏 *bàn xià*, Pinelliae Tuber) half shēng (washed)
licorice (甘草 *gān cǎo*, Glycyrrhizae Radix) 2 liǎng
ginseng (人参 *rén shēn*, Ginseng Radix) 1 liǎng

[For] the above five ingredients use one dǒu of water. Boil to get three shēng and remove the dregs. Take one shēng warm, three times a day.

SYNOPSIS

The signs and treatment of abdominal distention from spleen vacuity with qì stagnation.

COMMENTARY

The promotion of sweating damages the yáng qì. Previously it has been emphasized that heart yáng may be damaged, but spleen yáng may also be damaged. This damage may occur if sweating is promoted excessively or if sweating is promoted in a patient with spleen vacuity. The spleen manages movement and transformation and governs the abdominal region. When the spleen is vacuous, movement and transformation are impaired, giving rise to damp turbidity. The qì stagnates, a problem that can be considered a direct result of abnormal movement and transformation or the result of damp turbidity congesting the qì dynamic. In view of the formula chosen, the abdominal fullness in this pattern is understood to be a mixture of repletion and vacuity. Licorice (*gān cǎo*) and ginseng (*rén shēn*) are used to supplement the spleen and stomach, and assist movement and transformation. The dosage, however, is relatively small compared to the other ingredients because repletion is also present. Magnolia bark (*hòu pò*), which disperses distention and eliminates fullness, is used with fresh ginger (*shēng jiāng*) and pinellia (*bàn xià*). Fresh ginger (*shēng jiāng*) fortifies the spleen in order to dissipate fullness. Pinellia (*bàn xià*) harmonizes the stomach, downbears counterflow, opens binds, and flushes phlegm. The formula strongly moves qì and disperses distention, while mildly supplementing the spleen and assisting transformation.

Abdominal distention and fullness is a sign that is frequently seen in clinic practice. It can be differentiated into repletion and vacuity. The presence of persistent abdominal distention and fullness that the patient refuses to allow one to palpate, accompanied by dry and bound stool, suggests a pattern in which the yáng brightness stomach domain is replete. Intermittent abdominal distention and fullness that likes pressure and is accompanied by diarrhea, indicates a greater yīn spleen vacuity cold pattern.

4.6.3.2 Minor Center-Fortifying Decoction Patterns

LINE 102

伤寒二三日，心中悸而烦者，小建中汤主之。

Shāng hán èr sān rì, xīn zhōng jì ér fán zhě, xiǎo jiàn zhōng tāng zhǔ zhī.

When in cold damage [that has lasted for] two or three days, [there are] palpitations and vexation in the heart,* Minor Center-Fortifying Decoction (*xiǎo jiàn zhōng tāng*) governs.

TEXT NOTE

* Palpitations and vexation, 心中悸而烦 *xīn zhōng jì ér fán*: Here the palpitations are described as being "in" the heart, i.e., not below the heart or in the abdomen. The palpitations are accompanied by a subjective feeling of vexation.

FORMULA

Minor Center-Fortifying Decoction (*xiǎo jiàn zhōng tāng*)

∘ Fortify the center and supplement the spleen; harmonize qì and blood.

桂枝三两（去皮） 芍药六两 生姜三两（切） 甘草二两（炙） 大枣十二枚（擘） 胶饴一升

㈠ 右六味，以水七升，煮取三升，去滓，温服一升，日三服。㈡ 呕家不可用小建中汤，以甜故也。

Guì zhī sān liǎng (qù pí) sháo yào liù liǎng shēng jiāng sān liǎng (qiē) gān cǎo èr liǎng (zhì) dà zǎo shí èr méi (bò) jiāo yí yī shēng

(1) *Yòu liù wèi, yǐ shuǐ qī shēng, zhǔ qǔ sān shēng, qù zǐ, wēn fú yī shēng, rì sān fú.* (2) *Oǔ jiā bù kě yòng xiǎo jiàn zhōng tāng, yǐ tián gù yě.*

cinnamon twig (桂枝 *guì zhī*, Cinnamomi Ramulus) 3 liǎng (remove bark)
peony (芍药 *sháo yào*, Paeoniae Radix) 6 liǎng
fresh ginger (生姜 *shēng jiāng*, Zingiberis Rhizoma Recens) 3 liǎng (cut)
mix-fried licorice (甘草 *gān cǎo*, Glycyrrhizae Radix) 2 liǎng
jujube (大枣 *dà zǎo*, Ziziphi Fructus) 12 pieces (broken)
malt sugar (胶饴 *jiāo yí*, Granorum Saccharon) 1 shēng

[For] the above six ingredients use seven shēng of water. Boil to get three shēng, remove the dregs and take one shēng warm three times a day. Persons who are frequently nauseous cannot use Minor Center-Fortifying Decoction (*xiǎo jiàn zhōng tāng*) because it is sweet.

SYNOPSIS

The signs and treatment of heart palpitations and vexation in cold damage complicated by interior vacuity.

COMMENTARY

The patient has only been ill for several days and no inappropriate treatment has been given; therefore, the appearance of palpitations and vexation is a sign of interior vacuity, reflecting the patient's constitution. These signs indicate depletion of the qì and blood and dual vacuity of the heart and spleen. Palpitations occur because when the qì and blood are insufficient, the heart lacks what it normally governs (i.e., the blood) and is harassed by the exterior evil. Harassment by an evil disquiets the heart spirit and produces vexation, but not the more severe sign of "vexation and agitation" that indicates a heat evil harassing deeper in the interior. An analysis of Minor Center-Fortifying Decoction (*xiǎo jiàn zhōng tāng*) reinforces these conclusions. This formula is Cinnamon Twig Decoction (*guì zhī tāng*) plus malt sugar (*jiāo yí*). Malt sugar (*jiāo yí*) warms and supplements the center, regulates and nourishes the spleen and stomach, and relaxes tension and relieves pain. The original formula, Cinnamon Twig Decoction (*guì zhī tāng*), harmonizes the construction and defense, while the variation harmonizes both the exterior and the interior. The large dose of peony (*sháo yào*) enriches yīn and nourishes blood, resolving the root of this disorder.

4.6.3.3 Cinnamon Twig and Ginseng Decoction Patterns

LINE 163

太阳病，外证未除，而数下之，遂协热而利，利下不止，心下痞硬，表里不解者，桂枝人参汤主之。

Tài yáng bìng, wài zhèng wèi chú, ér shuò xià zhī, suì xié rè ér lì, lì xià bù zhǐ, xīn xià pǐ yìng, biǎo lǐ bù jiě zhě, guì zhī rén shēn tāng zhǔ zhī.

When in greater yáng disease, the exterior pattern has not yet been eliminated, and precipitation has been used repeatedly, [and consequently, there is] incessant complex diarrhea,[1] a hard glomus below the heart,[2] and [both] the exterior and the interior are not resolved, Cinnamon Twig and Ginseng Decoction (*guì zhī rén shēn tāng*) governs.

TEXT NOTES

1. Incessant complex diarrhea, 协热而利，利下不止 *xié rè ér lì, lì xià bù zhǐ*: Severe diarrhea that occurs in a mixed pattern of vacuity cold in the interior

and unresolved heat in the exterior. This type of diarrhea is often the result of using precipitation when an unresolved exterior evil is still present. Precipitation causes vacuity cold in the interior, which the exterior evil exploits. It harasses the interior and causes diarrhea. "Complex" refers to the complex pattern of interior cold and exterior heat.

2. A hard glomus below the heart, 心下痞硬 *xīn xià pǐ yìng*: Hardness in the region of the stomach and upper stomach duct that is the result of an impairment of the qì dynamic in the upper stomach duct area.

FORMULA

Cinnamon Twig and Ginseng Decoction (*guì zhī rén shēn tāng*)

◦ Warm the center and resolve the exterior.

桂枝四两（别切） 甘草四两（炙） 白术三两 人参三两 干姜三两

右五味，以水九升，右煮四味，取五升，内桂，更煮取三升，去滓，温服一升，日再、夜一服。

Guì zhī sì liǎng (bié qiē) gān cǎo sì liǎng (zhì) bái zhú sān liǎng rén shēn sān liǎng gān jiāng sān liǎng

Yòu wǔ wèi, yǐ shuǐ jiǔ shēng, yòu zhǔ sì wèi, qǔ wǔ shēng, nà guì, gèng zhǔ qǔ sān shēng, qù zǐ, wēn fú yī shēng, rì zài、 yè yī fú.

cinnamon twig (桂枝 *guì zhī*, Cinnamomi Ramulus) 4 liǎng (cut separately)*
mix-fried licorice (甘草 *gān cǎo*, Glycyrrhizae Radix) 4 liǎng
ovate atractylodes (白术 *bái zhú*, Atractylodis Ovatae Rhizoma) 3 liǎng
ginseng (人参 *rén shēn*, Ginseng Radix) 3 liǎng
dried ginger (干姜 *gān jiāng*, Zingiberis Rhizoma Exsiccatum) 3 liǎng

[For] the above five ingredients use nine shēng of water. First boil [the last four ingredients] to get five shēng. Add cinnamon twig (*guì zhī*) and boil again to get three shēng. Remove the dregs. Take one shēng warm, once [during] the day and again at night.

FORMULA NOTE

* Cut separately, 别切 *bié qiē*: In the *Zhù Jiě Shāng Hán Lùn*, it says "remove the bark" (去皮 *qù pí*) instead.

SYNOPSIS

The signs and treatment of cold-heat complex diarrhea from greater yīn spleen qì vacuity following inappropriate precipitation.

COMMENTARY

In greater yáng disease, if precipitation is used instead of the promotion of sweating, the disease not only fails to resolve, but may fall inward. In the present line, precipitation is used repeatedly, damaging the spleen and stomach and causing the evil to fall inward. The interior becomes cold and vacuous and the exterior heat is still present; consequently, incessant complex diarrhea is observed. Hard glomus is the result of cold congealing in the interior. Because the diarrhea is severe, the emphasis of the treatment is to warm the interior in order to check the diarrhea and to dissipate congealed cold. Cinnamon Twig and Ginseng Decoction (*guì zhī rén shēn tāng*) is Center-Rectifying Decoction (*lǐ zhōng tāng*) plus cinnamon twig (*guì zhī*). Ginseng (*rén shēn*), ovate atractylodes (*bái zhú*), licorice (*gān cǎo*), and dried ginger (*gān jiāng*) warm the center, dissipate cold, supplement the spleen and stomach, and check diarrhea. The addition of cinnamon twig (*guì zhī*) resolves the exterior and dissipates residual evil from the exterior.

One may compare Cinnamon Twig and Ginseng Decoction (*guì zhī rén shēn tāng*) with Pueraria, Scutellaria, and Coptis Decoction (*gé gēn huáng qín huáng lián tāng*) to illustrate the important differences between these two formulae. Both are used to treat diarrhea resulting from inappropriate precipitation in greater yáng disease. The former is used when the evil enters the interior and transforms to cold, while the latter is used for an evil which transforms to heat. Heat signs that may accompany diarrhea in a Pueraria, Scutellaria, and Coptis Decoction (*gé gēn huáng qín huáng lián tāng*) pattern include generalized heat, panting, and sweating.

4.6.4 Kidney Yáng Vacuity Patterns

Inappropriate promotion of sweating and use of precipitation can damage yáng, and in certain patients this can cause transmuted patterns of kidney yáng vacuity. When exuberant yīn distresses vacuous yáng, resulting in vexation and agitation, the appropriate formula is Dried Ginger and Aconite Decoction (*gān jiāng fù zǐ tāng*), which warms and returns yáng. When vexation and agitation is the result of yīn-yáng dual vacuity following inappropriate promotion of sweating and use of precipitation, the appropriate formula is Poria (Hoelen) Counterflow Cold Decoction (*fú líng sì nì tāng*), which returns yáng and boosts yīn. True Warrior Decoction (*zhēn wǔ tāng*) is used when excessive sweating damages yáng and gives rise to yáng vacuity water flooding because of its ability to warm yáng and disinhibit water.

4.6.4.1 Dried Ginger and Aconite Decoction Patterns

LINE 61

下之后，复发汗，昼日烦躁不得眠，夜而安静，不呕不渴，无表证，脉沉微，身无大热者， 干姜附子汤主之。

Xià zhī hòu, fù fā hàn, zhòu rì fán zào bù dé mián, yè ér ān jìng, bù ǒu bù kě, wú biǎo zhèng, mài chén wēi, shēn wú dà rè zhě, gān jiāng fù zǐ tāng zhǔ zhī.

When precipitation [has been used], yet sweating is then promoted so that [the person] in the daytime is vexed, agitated, and sleepless, but by night time becomes peaceful and retching, thirst, exterior signs, and great generalized heat are [all] absent, and the pulse is sunken and faint, then Dried Ginger and Aconite Decoction (*gān jiāng fù zǐ tāng*) governs.

FORMULA

Dried Ginger and Aconite Decoction (*gān jiāng fù zǐ tāng*)

◦ Warm urgently and return yáng.

干姜一两　附子一枚（生用，去皮，切八片）

右二味，以水三升，煮取一升，去滓，顿服。

Gān jiāng yī liǎng fù zǐ yī méi (shēng yòng, qù pí, qiē bā piàn)

Yòu èr wèi, yǐ shuǐ sān shēng, zhǔ qǔ yī shēng, qù zǐ, dùn fú.

dried ginger (干姜 *gān jiāng*, Zingiberis Rhizoma Exsiccatum) 1 liǎng

aconite (附子 *fù zǐ*, Aconiti Tuber Laterale) 1 piece (use raw, remove skin, cut into eight slices)

[For] the above two ingredients use three shēng of water. Boil to get one shēng, remove the dregs and take in one single dose.

SYNOPSIS

The signs and treatment for the pattern of yáng vacuity and yīn exuberance in which yīn distresses yáng and causes vexation and agitation.

COMMENTARY

The use of precipitation easily damages the yáng qì and if sweating is then promoted it will cause further damage, here leading to yáng vacuity and yīn exuberance. The same inappropriate treatment in different patients may result in different patterns, depending on the strength or weakness of the original evil, the potency of the formula that is used, the constitution of the patient, and the patient's living environment. In a cold climate it is likely that many patients have weakened yáng. In these patients mistreatment may have easily resulted in yáng vacuity. In a warm climate, where many patients already exhibit signs of fluid insufficiency, mistreatment may more likely result in yīn depletion.

Vexation and agitation occur in greater yáng disease, yáng brightness disease, and lesser yáng disease. In greater yáng disease, it can occur when an external evil fetters the exterior and heat is depressed in the interior. In lesser yáng disease, this sign manifests as heart vexation with retching. If accompanied by great thirst, agitation and vexation is indicative of yáng brightness disease. In the present line, exterior signs are absent; therefore this is not greater yáng disease. Retching and thirst are absent; hence this pattern of vexation and agitation belongs to a category that is different from the three above. The pulse is sunken and faint. The sunken quality indicates exuberant yīn in the interior and the faint quality indicates debilitated yáng. Exuberant yīn harasses yáng and yáng is unable to match the strength of yīn. Yáng should be effulgent during the daytime and yīn should enter yáng, but when yáng is vacuous, it is unable to overcome yīn and this struggle results in vexation and agitation during the daytime. Normally, at night, the yáng qì recedes and yīn becomes exuberant. In this situation, yáng is debilitated and yīn overly exuberant, so at night the patient is tranquil because vacuous yáng easily enters exuberant yīn.

The phrase "no great generalized heat" has been interpreted in several ways. Chéng Wú-Jǐ states, "'great generalized heat... absent' means no heat [effusion] in the exterior...." He and the authors of *Yī Zōng Jīn Jiàn* agree that this phrase means the absence of heat effusion, which would indicate an exterior pattern. Another interpretation is provided by the authors of *Gāo Děng Cóng Shū* who explain that it refers not to the heat effusion seen in exterior conditions, but to false heat from vacuous yáng straying to the exterior. If great generalized heat were present it would mean that yīn and yáng were about to separate and the situation would be extremely critical. This condition has not reached the critical stage; therefore, this interpretation is perhaps more difficult to substantiate in the text, but it may still be considered.

The formula, Dried Ginger and Aconite Decoction (*gān jiāng fù zǐ tāng*), is Counterflow Cold Decoction (*sì nì tāng*) without licorice (*gān cǎo*). It treats only yáng and is used in cases of great vacuity of the yáng qì and exuberant yīn in the interior. Dried ginger (*gān jiāng*) warms the spleen yáng, and aconite (*fù zǐ*) supports the kidney yáng. When yáng is increased, the yīn will dissipate. The yáng qì will return to the root and yīn qì will then be restrained. Raw aconite (*fù zǐ*) is used for maximum effect and the moderating effects of licorice (*gān cǎo*) are not considered appropriate, so it is removed.

4.6.4.2 Poria (Hoelen) Counterflow Cold Decoction Patterns

LINE 69

发汗，若下之，病仍不解，烦躁者，茯苓四逆汤主之。

Fā hàn, ruò xià zhī, bìng réng bù jiě, fán zào zhě, fú líng sì nì tāng zhǔ zhī.

After the promotion of sweating, if precipitation [is used] and the disease still does not resolve, and [there is] vexation and agitation, Poria (Hoelen) Counterflow Cold Decoction (*fú líng sì nì tāng*) governs.

FORMULA

Poria (Hoelen) Counterflow Cold Decoction (*fú líng sì nì tāng*)

∘ Return yáng and boost yīn.

茯苓四两　人参一两　附子一枚（生用，去皮，破八片）　甘草二两（炙）　干姜一两半

右五味，以水五升，煮取三升，去滓，温服七合，日二服。

Fú líng sì liǎng　rén shēn yī liǎng　fù zǐ yī méi (shēng yòng, qù pí, pò bā piàn) gān cǎo èr liǎng (zhì)　gān jiāng yī liǎng bàn

Yòu wǔ wèi, yǐ shuǐ wǔ shēng, zhǔ qǔ sān shēng, qù zǐ, wēn fú qī gě, rì èr fú.

poria (茯苓 *fú líng*, Poria) 4 liǎng
ginseng (人参 *rén shēn*, Ginseng Radix) 1 liǎng

aconite (附子 *fù zǐ*, Aconiti Tuber Laterale) 1 piece (use raw, remove skin, break into eight pieces)

mix-fried licorice (甘草 *gān cǎo*, Glycyrrhizae Radix) 2 liǎng

dried ginger (干姜 *gān jiāng*, Zingiberis Rhizoma Exsiccatum) 1.5 liǎng

[For] the above five ingredients use five shēng of water. Boil to get three shēng, remove the dregs, and take seven gě warm twice a day.

SYNOPSIS

The signs and treatment of vexation and agitation from dual vacuity of yīn and yáng that occurs following the promotion of sweating and use of precipitation.

COMMENTARY

This line is similar to the previous one in that sweating is promoted, precipitation is used, and vexation and agitation result from the treatment. It differs in that it prescribes a different formula. From the differences between the formulae one may infer that the vexation and agitation in the previous line is the result of yáng vacuity and exuberant yīn, whereas in this line it is the result of dual vacuity of yīn and yáng. It is possible that one would also see such signs as reverse-flow, fatigue, and a pulse that is sunken.

This example reinforces the concept that the same treatment or mistreatment, used in different patients, may have a different result. In the previous line, exterior signs are absent, whereas in this line, we are told that the disease has not resolved. The meaning of this line is not that signs of greater yáng disease are still present, but that a disease pattern still exists. Although this idea is not explicit in the text, it can be deduced from the formula. Poria (Hoelen) Counterflow Cold Decoction (*fú líng sì nì tāng*) contains aconite (*fù zǐ*) and dried ginger (*gān jiāng*), which return yáng and stem counterflow. It does not contain any ingredients for resolving exterior disease. Aconite (*fù zǐ*) and dried ginger (*gān jiāng*) were also used in the formula in the previous line. Ginseng (*rén shēn*), which supplements the original qì, boosts fluids, and quiets the spirit, is added. Ginseng (*rén shēn*) is the main ingredient for boosting the fluids. Licorice (*gān cǎo*) boosts the qì and harmonizes the center, further supporting yáng. The inclusion of poria (*fú líng*), as the sovereign, is perhaps more problematic since disinhibiting urination in patients with yīn vacuity is generally contraindicated. One explanation for its inclusion is that poria (*fú líng*), which fortifies the spleen, nourishes the heart, and quiets the spirit, disinhibits the urine without damaging yīn and is considered to boost the spleen yīn. The term "spleen yīn" means both the fluid component of the spleen, which includes blood, humor, and fluids, and the relative yīn nature of the spleen in comparison to the stomach yáng. One can, by fortifying the spleen, boost spleen yīn. In other words, one fortifies the spleen without causing dryness.

4.6.4.3 True Warrior Decoction Patterns

Line 82

太阳病发汗，汗出不解，其人仍发热，心下悸，头眩，身瞤动，振振欲擗地者，真武汤主之。

Tài yáng bìng fā hàn, hàn chū bù jiě, qí rén réng fā rè, xīn xià jì, tóu xuán, shēn shùn (rún) dòng, zhèn zhèn yù pì dì zhě, zhēn wǔ tāng zhǔ zhī.

When in greater yáng disease, sweating has been promoted and sweat issues [but the disease] does not resolve, the person still has heat effusion, and [there are] palpitations below the heart, dizzy head, generalized twitching,[1] and [the person is] quivering and about to fall,[2] True Warrior Decoction (*zhēn wǔ tāng*) governs.

Text Notes

1. Generalized twitching, 身瞤动 *shēn shùn (rún) dòng*: Jerking and jumping of the body's sinews.
2. [The person is] quivering and about to fall, 振振欲擗地 *zhèn zhèn yù pì dì*: The patient is trembling and is unstable on his/her feet, as if about to fall. He/she feels uneasy, flustered, and dizzy and wants to sit down. When this sign occurs with generalized twitching it is considered more severe than either one appearing individually. Yù Chāng writes, "Palpitations mean interior vacuity, dizzy head means upper body vacuity, and generalized twitching where the patient is quivering and about to fall means channel vacuity."

   Kē Qín states, "... [the phrase] 'the patient is quivering and about to fall' qualifies generalized twitching."

Formula

True Warrior Decoction (*zhēn wǔ tāng*)

∘ Warm yáng and disinhibit water.

茯苓　芍药　生姜各三两（切）　白术二两　附子一枚（炮，去皮，破八片）

右五味，以水八升，煮取三升，去滓，温服七合，日三服。

Fú líng　sháo yào　shēng jiāng gè sān liǎng (qiē)　bái zhú èr liǎng　fù zǐ yī méi (pào, qù pí, pò bā piàn)

Yòu wǔ wèi, yǐ shuǐ bā shēng, zhǔ qǔ sān shēng, qù zǐ, wēn fú qī gě, rì sān fú.

poria (茯苓 *fú líng*, Poria) 3 liǎng
peony (芍药 *sháo yào*, Paeoniae Radix) 3 liǎng
fresh ginger (生姜 *shēng jiāng*, Zingiberis Rhizoma Recens) 3 liǎng (cut)

ovate atractylodes (白术 *bái zhú*, Atractylodis Ovatae Rhizoma) 2 liǎng
aconite (附子 *fù zǐ*, Aconiti Tuber Laterale) 1 piece (blast-fry, remove skin, break into 8 pieces)

[For] the above five ingredients use eight shēng of water. Boil to get three shēng, remove the dregs, and take seven gě warm, three times a day.

SYNOPSIS

The signs and treatment of yáng vacuity water flooding caused by excessive promotion of sweating that damages yáng.

COMMENTARY

In greater yáng disease one should promote sweating, and if sweat issues but the disease does not resolve, it suggests that the original diagnosis was incorrect, the formula chosen was incorrect, or the patient was too weak for the promotion of sweating to be effective. One might infer from this line that because heat effusion continues, the exterior evil is still present, but this would be incorrect. This sign occurs after sweating and is due to vacuous yáng qì floating to the exterior. One can deduce this from the formula True Warrior Decoction (*zhēn wǔ tāng*), which does not contain any ingredients for the treatment of exterior conditions. Furthermore, the other signs are also suggestive of yáng vacuity. When yáng is vacuous, it cannot control water, which exploits the weakness and rises up, causing palpitations below the heart. Yáng vacuity results in dizziness because normal movement of the clear yáng is impaired. If owing to vacuity, yáng qì fails to perform its function of nourishing and warming the sinews, generalized twitching may result. The pattern is one of water flood due to spleen and kidney yáng vacuity. True Warrior Decoction (*zhēn wǔ tāng*) contains poria (*fú líng*), which disinhibits water, and ovate atractylodes (*bái zhú*), which dries dampness; together they fortify the spleen and control water. It also contains aconite (*fù zǐ*) which invigorates the kidney yáng. For further discussion of True Warrior Decoction (*zhēn wǔ tāng*), see line 316, p. 483.

Poria (Hoelen), Cinnamon Twig, Ovate Atractylodes, and Licorice Decoction (*fú líng guì zhī bái zhú gān cǎo tāng*), discussed on line 67, p. 171, also treats vacuity with invasion of water. The difference between the patterns treated by the two formulae is one of severity. The pattern in line 67 involves water qì surging upward with vacuity of the spleen and heart. The pattern here is water flooding with spleen and kidney yáng vacuity.

This pattern may also be compared with the Poria (Hoelen) Five Powder (*wǔ líng sǎn*) pattern, in which water amasses internally (see line 71, p. 195). In that pattern, internal water amassment impairs qì transformation in the bladder, whereas here water floods as a result of yáng vacuity. Poria (Hoelen) Five Powder (*wǔ líng sǎn*) treats disorders of the bladder, the greater yáng, whereas True Warrior Decoction (*zhēn wǔ tāng*) treats the kidney, the lesser yīn. When comparing patterns one should pay attention to the dosages. Poria (Hoelen) Five Powder (*wǔ líng sǎn*) contains more ingredients for disinhibiting water and appears to be a stronger formula, even though it is used to treat a milder condition. This appearance is deceiving, though, because the amounts used in Poria (Hoelen) Five Powder (*wǔ líng sǎn*) are very small in comparison to those used in True Warrior Decoction (*zhēn wǔ tāng*).

4.7 YĪN AND YÁNG VACUITY PATTERNS

In greater yáng disease the promotion of sweating and use of precipitation can damage both yīn and yáng. When the inappropriate promotion of sweating damages both yīn and yáng, giving rise to vexation and agitation, and vomiting counterflow, the appropriate formula is Licorice and Dried Ginger Decoction (*gān cǎo gān jiāng tāng*), which warms the center and returns yáng. When damage to the yīn impairs the patient's ability to extend the limbs, Peony and Licorice Decoction (*sháo yào gān cǎo tāng*) is used to return yīn because of its sweet, sour nature. Following the promotion of sweating, if the disease does not resolve and aversion to cold is observed as a sign of yīn-yáng dual vacuity, Peony, Licorice, and Aconite Decoction (*sháo yào gān cǎo fù zǐ tāng*) is suggested because it supports yáng and boosts yīn. When, in the course of a greater yáng disease, heart yīn and yáng become vacuous and there are signs such as a pulse that is bound and intermittent and palpitations, the appropriate formula is Honey-Fried Licorice Decoction (*zhì gān cǎo tāng*), which frees yáng and opens the pulse, and enriches yīn and nourishes the blood.

4.7.1 Licorice and Dried Ginger Decoction Patterns and Peony and Licorice Decoction Patterns

LINE 29

㈠伤寒脉浮，自汗出，小便数，心烦，微恶寒，脚挛急，反与桂枝欲攻其表，此误也。㈡得之便厥，咽中干，烦躁吐逆者，作甘草干姜汤与之，以复其阳；若厥愈足温者，更作芍药甘草汤与之，其脚即伸；若胃气不和，谵语者，少与调胃承气汤；若重发汗，复加烧针者，四逆汤主之。

(1) *Shāng hán mài fú, zì hàn chū, xiǎo biàn shuò, xīn fán, wēi wù hán, jiǎo luán jí, fǎn yǔ guì zhī yù gōng qí biǎo, cǐ wù yě.* (2) *Dé zhī biàn jué, yān zhōng gān, fán zào tù nì zhě, zuò gān cǎo gān jiāng tāng yǔ zhī, yǐ fù qí yáng; ruò jué yù zú wēn zhě, gèng zuò sháo yào gān cǎo tāng yǔ zhī, qí jiǎo jí shēn; ruò wèi qì bù hé, zhān yǔ zhě, shǎo yǔ tiáo wèi chéng qì tāng; ruò chóng fā hàn, fù jiā shāo zhēn zhě, sì nì tāng zhǔ zhī.*

(1) When, in cold damage, the pulse is floating and [there is] spontaneous sweating, frequent urination, heart vexation, mild aversion to cold, and hypertonicity of the feet, but Cinnamon Twig [Decoction] (*guì zhī* [*tāng*]) is given in order to attack the exterior, this is an error. (2) If [the person] is given this [formula], there will be reversal,[1] a dryness in the throat, vexation and agitation, and counterflow vomiting,[2] [so one should use] Licorice and Dried Ginger Decoction (*gān cǎo gān*

jiāng tāng) to restore yáng. If a counterflow [patient] recovers, and the feet become warm, one can then use Peony and Licorice Decoction (*sháo yào gān cǎo tāng*) and the feet will then [be able to] stretch. If the stomach qì is disharmonious and [there is] delirious speech, give a little[3] Stomach-Regulating Qì-Coordinating Decoction (*tiáo wèi chéng qì tāng*). If sweating has been promoted repeatedly, then red-hot needling is used, Counterflow Cold Decoction (*sì nì tāng*) governs.

TEXT NOTES

1. Reversal, 厥 *jué*: Reversal cold of the extremities.
2. Counterflow vomiting, 吐逆 *tù nì*: Vomiting is the external manifestation of this condition and counterflow refers to the underlying pathomechanism.
3. Give a little, 少与 *shǎo yǔ*: Give a smaller dosage than normal, not to precipitate, but to harmonize.

FORMULAE

Licorice and Dried Ginger Decoction (*gān cǎo gān jiāng tāng*)

◦ First, warm the center to restore yáng, then [use a] sour and sweet [decoction] to restore yīn.

甘草四两（炙）　干姜二两

右二味，以水三升，煮取一升五合，去滓，分温再服。

Gān cǎo sì liǎng (zhì)　gān jiāng èr liǎng

Yòu èr wèi, yǐ shuǐ sān shēng, zhǔ qǔ yī shēng wǔ gě, qù zǐ, fēn wēn zài fú.

mix-fried licorice (甘草 *gān cǎo*, Glycyrrhizae Radix) 4 liǎng

dried ginger (干姜 *gān jiāng*, Zingiberis Rhizoma Exsiccatum) 2 liǎng

[For] the above two ingredients use three shēng of water. Boil to get one shēng and five gě and remove the dregs. Divide [into two parts], and take warm, twice a day.

Peony and Licorice Decoction (*sháo yào gān cǎo tāng*)

白芍药、甘草（炙）各四两

右二味，以水三升，煮取一升五合，去滓，分温再服。

Bái sháo yào　gān cǎo (zhì) gè sì liǎng

Yòu èr wèi, yǐ shuǐ sān shēng, zhǔ qǔ yī shēng wǔ gě, qù zǐ, fēn wēn zài fú.

peony (芍药 *sháo yào*, Paeoniae Radix) 4 liǎng

mix-fried licorice (甘草 *gān cǎo*, Glycyrrhizae Radix) 4 liǎng

[For] the above two ingredients use three shēng of water. Boil to get one shēng five gě and remove the dregs. Divide [into two parts], and take warm, twice a day.

Synopsis

Transmuted patterns of cold damage complicated by vacuity that are inappropriately treated by the promotion of sweating, and their treatment according to signs.

Commentary

The disease pattern in this line is described as "cold damage," which is apparently used here in its broader sense since although the pulse is floating, sweat spontaneously issues. If the term were meant in the narrower sense of a cold damage pattern for which Ephedra Decoction (*má huáng tāng*) is appropriate, no spontaneous sweating would be present. A pulse that is floating, spontaneous sweating, and mild aversion to cold are suggestive of a Cinnamon Twig Decoction (*guì zhī tāng*) pattern, but the other signs must also be considered. Frequent urination indicates a pattern of vacuous yáng unable to contain the fluids. Heart vexation and hypertonicity of the feet here indicate insufficiency of yīn humor. When the yīn humor are insufficient, they cannot nourish the heart or moisten the sinews. This pattern is greater yáng exterior vacuity with dual vacuity of yīn and yáng. Cinnamon Twig Decoction (*guì zhī tāng*), which harmonizes the exterior by the promotion of mild sweating, is not appropriate. One must support yáng and resolve the exterior. The yīn need not be treated because once yáng is restored, the fluids will be contained and yīn replenished. This reflects the principle that it is easier to treat yáng than yīn. When yáng is secure, yīn will be preserved and when yáng is engendered, yīn will increase.

In this pattern if Cinnamon Twig Decoction (*guì zhī tāng*) is given, pathological transmutations will occur. Resolving the exterior will exacerbate the exterior vacuity and damage both yīn and yáng. Further damage to yáng results in reversal cold because the yáng qì is unable to warm the extremities. Reversal cold also indicates impairment of the qì dynamic, resulting from vacuity of the yáng qì. This impairment is further reflected in the presence of counterflow vomiting. The loss of sweat further damages yīn, and the throat becomes dry from lack of fluid nourishment. Vacuous yáng and debilitated fluids are unable to nourish the heart; hence the spirit is unquiet and vexation and agitation are observed. Licorice and Dried Ginger Decoction (*gān cǎo gān jiāng tāng*) is an acrid, sweet formula that restores yáng. Dried ginger (*gān jiāng*) warms the center and restores the yáng, while licorice (*gān cǎo*) harmonizes the center. By restoring yáng to the center burner, spleen qì is fortified and normal qì movement resumes. When this occurs the limbs become warm because the yáng qì is replete and flows normally. Peony and Licorice Decoction (*sháo yào gān cǎo tāng*) is a sour, sweet formula which boosts the yīn and restores the fluids. Peony (*sháo yào*) boosts yīn and nourishes the blood, while licorice (*gān cǎo*) supplements the center. These two ingredients resolve hypertonicity of the sinews, restoring the ability to stretch and move freely.

One aspect of this pattern is insufficiency of yīn humor. If warm medicinals to restore yáng are used excessively, it may further damage yīn and cause a loss of stomach harmony and delirious speech. This pattern is severe damage to yīn fluids and dryness-heat in the stomach; therefore, a small dose of Stomach-Regulating Qì-Coordinating Decoction (*tiáo wèi chéng qì tāng*) is given to clear heat and harmonize the stomach. See line 248, p. 327, for a further discussion of this formula.

If the pattern above is treated with repeated sweating, it will not resolve. If one then uses red-hot needling to force sweating, it will cause severe damage to the yáng qì. In that case, Counterflow Cold Decoction (*sì nì tāng*) may be used to return the yáng and eliminate counterflow. See line 323, p. 475, for a further discussion of this formula.

4.7.2 Peony, Licorice, and Aconite Decoction Patterns

LINE 68

发汗，病不解，反恶寒者，虚故也，芍药甘草附子汤主之。
Fā hàn, bìng bù jiě, fǎn wù hán zhě, xū gù yě, sháo yào gān cǎo fù zǐ tāng zhǔ zhī.

When sweating is promoted, [if] the disease does not resolve, and instead [there is] aversion to cold, [this is because of] vacuity; [hence] Peony, Licorice, and Aconite Decoction (*sháo yào gān cǎo fù zǐ tāng*) governs.

FORMULA
Peony, Licorice, and Aconite Decoction (*sháo yào gān cǎo fù zǐ tāng*)

∘ Support yáng and boost yīn.

芍药 甘草（炙）各三两 附子一枚（炮，去皮，破八片）

(一) 右三味，以水五升，煮取一升五合，去滓，分温三服。(二) 疑非仲景方。

Sháo yào gān cǎo (zhì) gè sān liǎng fù zǐ yī méi (pào, qù pí, pò bā piàn)

(1) *Yòu sān wèi, yǐ shuǐ wǔ shēng, zhǔ qǔ yī shēng wǔ gě, qù zǐ, fēn wēn sān fú.* (2) *Yí fēi zhòng jǐng fāng.*

peony (芍药 *sháo yào*, Paeoniae Radix) 3 liǎng
mix-fried licorice (甘草 *gān cǎo*, Glycyrrhizae Radix) 3 liǎng
aconite (附子 *fù zǐ*, Aconiti Tuber Laterale) 1 piece (blast fry, remove skin, break into 8 pieces)

(1) [For] the above three ingredients use five shēng of water. Boil to get one shēng and five gě and remove the dregs. Divide into three [parts] and take warm, three times [a day]. (2) It is doubted that this is [Zhāng] Zhòng Jǐng's formula.*

FORMULA NOTE

* It is doubted that this is [Zhāng] Zhòng Jǐng's formula, 疑非[张]仲景方 *yí fēi zhòng jǐng fāng*: This is an addition to the text by an unknown editor.

SYNOPSIS
The signs and treatment of yīn and yáng dual vacuity following the promotion of sweating.

COMMENTARY

In greater yáng disease, when sweating is promoted properly, the exterior evil should be eliminated and aversion to cold should cease. In this line, sweating is promoted and not only does the disease not resolve, but aversion to cold persists. Xú Bīn (徐彬, style 忠可 Zhōng-Kě) emphasizes that the aversion to cold has not resolved and it has increased in severity: "Sweat has [issued] and the disease has not resolved, so the pattern is still as before. "Instead" is only used with aversion to cold, [which means] it is increased in comparison to the earlier [condition]." That the disease has not resolved does not mean that the exterior has not resolved, but that a transmutation has occurred.

Zhāng Jī explains that the presence of aversion to cold indicates vacuity, and commentators have offered different interpretations of what type of vacuity this means. Chéng Wú-Jǐ explains this pattern as dual vacuity of construction and defense. Qián Huáng suggests that the signs indicate vacuity of the yáng qì. The yáng qì is unable to warm the exterior and engenders exterior cold. *Yī Zōng Jīn Jiàn* defines this pattern more narrowly as vacuity of the defense qì, which is unable to defend the exterior properly. Based primarily on the inclusion of aconite (*fù zǐ*) in the formula used in this line, the authors of *Gāo Děng Cóng Shū* conclude that this pattern is dual vacuity of yīn and yáng.

In attempting to reconcile these different viewpoints, one may also consider the statement of Chéng Wú-Jǐ that, "...Sweating is promoted, the disease is not resolved and instead, [there is] aversion to cold. The construction [yīn] and defensive [yáng] are both vacuous. Sweat issues and the construction [yīn becomes] vacuous. Aversion to cold [means] vacuity of the defensive [yáng]..." If one considers that defensive yáng and construction-yīn are simply specific types of yáng and yīn, one can grasp a wider range of explanations. Because aconite (*fù zǐ*) warms the channels and restores yáng, its use supports the indications of yáng vacuity. Peony (*sháo yào*) supplements the blood and contracts yīn, supporting the idea that yīn is also vacuous. Licorice (*gān cǎo*) supports the other two ingredients by warming and supplementing the center.

4.7.3 Honey-Fried Licorice Decoction Patterns

LINE 177

伤寒脉结代，心动悸，炙甘草汤主之。

Shāng hán mài jié dài, xīn dòng jì, zhì gān cǎo tāng zhǔ zhī.

[For] cold damage with a pulse that is bound and intermittent, and stirring heart palpitations,* Honey-Fried Licorice Decoction (*zhì gān cǎo tāng*) governs.

TEXT NOTE

* Stirring palpitations, 心动悸 *xīn dòng jì*: Severe palpitations in which the heart can be seen beating against the clothing.

FORMULA

Honey-Fried Licorice Decoction (*zhì gān cǎo tāng*)

○ Free yáng and restore the pulse; enrich yīn and nourish the blood.

甘草四两（炙） 生姜三两（切） 人参二两 生地黄一斤 桂枝三两（去皮） 阿胶二两 麦门冬半升（去心） 麻仁半升 大枣三十枚（擘）

㈠ 右九味，以清酒七升，水八升，右煮八味，取三升，去滓，内胶烊消尽，温服一升，日三服。㈡ 一名复脉汤。

Gān cǎo sì liǎng (zhì) shēng jiāng sān liǎng (qiē) rén shēn èr liǎng shēng dì huáng yī jīn guì zhī sān liǎng (qù pí) ē jiāo èr liǎng mài mén dōng bàn shēng (qù xīn) má rén bàn shēng dà zǎo sān shí méi (bò)

(1) *Yòu jiǔ wèi, yǐ qīng jiǔ qī shēng, shuǐ bā shēng, yòu zhǔ bā wèi, qǔ sān shēng, qù zǐ, nà jiāo yáng xiāo jìn, wēn fú yī shēng, rì sān fú.* (2) *Yī míng fù mài tāng.*

mix-fried licorice (甘草 *gān cǎo*, Glycyrrhizae Radix) 4 liǎng

fresh ginger (生姜 *shēng jiāng*, Zingiberis Rhizoma Recens) 3 liǎng (cut)

ginseng (人参 *rén shēn*, Ginseng Radix) 2 liǎng

dried/fresh rehmannia (生地黄 *shēng dì huáng*, Rehmanniae Radix Exsiccata seu Recens) 1 jīn

cinnamon twig (桂枝 *guì zhī*, Cinnamomi Ramulus) 3 liǎng (remove bark)

ass hide glue (阿胶 *ē jiāo*, Asini Corii Gelatinum) 2 liǎng

ophiopogon (麦门冬 *mài mén dōng*, Ophiopogonis Tuber) half shēng (remove hearts[1])

hemp seed (麻仁 *má rén*, Cannabis Semen) half shēng

jujube (大枣 *dà zǎo*, Ziziphi Fructus) 30 pieces (broken)

(1) [For] the above nine ingredients use seven shēng of clear wine[2] and eight shēng of water. First boil eight ingredients [excluding ass hide glue (*ē jiāo*)] to get three shēng and remove the dregs. Add ass hide glue (*ē jiāo*) and warm [until] completely dispersed. Take one shēng warm, three times a day. (2) Another name is Pulse-Restorative Decoction.

TEXT NOTES

1. Remove the hearts, 去心 *qù xīn*: The heart of ophiopogon (*mài mén dōng*) was considered to cause vexation and oppression, but this side-effect has not been validated by modern research.
2. Clear wine, 清酒 *qīng jiǔ*: A form of aged rice wine. It frees the channels, harmonizes the qì and blood, and dissipates congealed cold.

SYNOPSIS

The signs and treatment of heart yīn and yáng dual vacuity.

COMMENTARY

When a patient contracts an exterior evil, the presentation is influenced by the patient's constitution, the strength of the evil, and any treatments used. This line provides little information. It is possible that an exterior evil has entered the greater yáng channel and then shifted to the lesser yīn heart channel. This transmutation may have been the result of mistreatment, or a particularly strong evil or a weak patient. Because of constitutional weakness some patients may exhibit a pulse that becomes intermittent each time they contract an exterior evil.

The heart governs the blood vessels and relies on yīn, yáng, qì, and blood. If any of these elements is vacuous the heart loses nourishment and palpitations may occur. Furthermore, if qì and blood are vacuous, movement in the vessels may become abnormal. The vessels may lose fullness, which is felt as an intermittent quality. Palpitations may be caused by many different factors, including vacuity resulting from the promotion of sweating or the use of precipitation, heat evil harassing the heart, insufficiency of the center qì with internal rheum, and qì and blood debilitation. No treatment has been given, so one may rule out mistreatment as the cause. Heat evil, phlegm-rheum, and insufficiency of center qì are not mentioned and an analysis of the formula reveals no ingredients for the treatment of these patterns, so one can eliminate these possibilities. Therefore, one can conclude that this is probably a pattern of constitutional qì and blood debilitation.

Honey-Fried Licorice Decoction (*zhì gān cǎo tāng*) contains ingredients that address three different aspects of this pattern. Mix-fried licorice (*gān cǎo*), ginseng (*rén shēn*), and jujube (*dà zǎo*) supplement and warm the heart qì. Ophiopogon (*mài mén dōng*), hemp seed (*má rén*), dried/fresh rehmannia (*shēng dì huáng*), and ass hide glue (*ē jiāo*) nourish the heart yīn and blood. Fresh ginger (*shēng jiāng*), cinnamon twig (*guì zhī*), and clear wine (*qīng jiǔ*) rouse the heart yáng. In combination, these medicinals free yáng, restore the pulse, enrich yīn, and nourish the blood.

LINE 178

㈠ 脉按之来缓，时一止复来者，名曰结。㈡ 又脉来动而中止，更来小数，中有还者反动，名曰结，阴也。㈢ 脉来动而中止，不能自还，因而复动者，名曰代，阴也。㈣ 得此脉者，必难治。

(1) *Mài àn zhī lái huǎn, shí yī zhǐ fù lái zhě, míng yuē jié.* (2) *Yòu mài lái dòng ér zhōng zhǐ, gèng lái xiǎo shuò, zhōng yǒu huán zhě fǎn dòng, míng yuē jié, yīn yě.* (3) *Mài lái dòng ér zhōng zhǐ, bù néng zì huán, yīn ér fù dòng zhě, míng yuē dài, yīn yě.* (4) *Dé cǐ mài zhě, bì nán zhì.*

(1) When [one] presses the pulse, [and finds that] it arrives moderately, stops, and then arrives again, this is called bound. (2) Also, when the pulse arrives stirring* and then stops, again arriving small and rapid, returning [to normal] but stirring [again], this, [too], is called bound,

[which is a] yīn [pulse]. (3) When the pulse arrives stirring and stops, [but] is unable to return [to normal], because it is again stirring, this is called intermittent, [which is a] yīn [pulse]. (4) When [one] get these pulses, [the disease] is difficult to treat.

Text Note

* Stirring, 动 *dòng*: The pulse suddenly appears after a period in which it had stopped.

Synopsis

The special evidence and prognosis associated with bound pulses and intermittent pulses.

Commentary

Pulses that are bound or intermittent share the principal characteristic that the movement in the vessel can be felt to stop temporarily, but they differ in important ways. A pulse that is bound only stops for a short period, returns to normal spontaneously, and when it returns is felt to be slightly rapid. This pulse is associated with qì and blood stagnation and inhibition of the qì pathways. Here, stagnation is the result of vacuity, not of repletion. A pulse that is intermittent stops for a longer period of time, does not spontaneously return to normal, continues to exhibit a stirring quality, and is not rapid. This type of pulse is associated with severe debilitation of qì and qì-blood vacuity. A pulse that is intermittent is a more serious sign than a pulse that is bound.

These pulses are considered to be yīn pulses because they are generally associated with vacuity of yīn, yáng, qì, and blood. When such pulses are felt, one knows that the disease is probably of a serious nature and therefore difficult to treat.

4.8 Water Amassment Patterns

During greater yáng disease, if the spleen's ability to move and transform fluids, and the bladder's qì transformative function are impaired, excessive intake of fluids can cause water to collect in the interior. Water amassment patterns are characterized by inhibited urination, dissipation thirst, vexation thirst, and immediate vomiting of ingested fluids. Poria (Hoelen) Five Powder (*wǔ líng sǎn*) is used in these patterns because of its ability to transform qì and move water, and resolve the exterior. This pattern should be differentiated from stomach vacuity with water collecting, in which thirst is absent. For this pattern the appropriate formula is Poria (Hoelen) and Licorice Decoction (*fú líng gān cǎo tāng*), which warms the stomach and disinhibits water.

LINE 71

㈠ 太阳病，发汗后，大汗出，胃中干，烦躁不得眠，欲得饮水者，少少与饮之，令胃气和则愈。㈡ 若脉浮，小便不利，微热消渴者，五苓散主之。

(1) *Tài yáng bìng, fā hàn hòu, dà hàn chū, wèi zhōng gān, fán zào bù dé mián, yù dé yǐn shuǐ zhě, shǎo shǎo yǔ yǐn zhī, lìng wèi qì hé zé yù.* (2) *Ruò mài fú, xiǎo biàn bù lì, wēi rè xiāo kě zhě, wǔ líng sǎn zhǔ zhī.*

(1) When in greater yáng disease, after sweating is promoted and great sweat issues, [if there is] dryness in the stomach,[1] vexation and agitation with insomnia, and a desire to drink water, giving a small amount of water will harmonize the stomach qì so that recovery [will ensue]. (2) If the pulse is floating and [there is] inhibited urination, slight heat,[2] and dispersion-thirst,[3] Poria (Hoelen) Five Powder (*wǔ líng sǎn*) governs.

TEXT NOTES

1. Dryness in the stomach, 胃中干 *wèi zhōng gān*: Depletion of the fluids of the stomach.
2. Slight heat, 微热 *wēi rè*: A mild feeling of heat in the body, which may or may not be palpable.
3. Dispersion-thirst, 消渴 *xiāo kě*: Thirst unallayed by copious intake of water, accompanied by scant urination. The same term, often translated as "wasting thirst," is more commonly used outside the *Shāng Hán Lùn* as as the name of disease that is characterized by this sign, among others, and that partly corresponds to diabetes in Western medicine. Here, however, the term simply denotes a sign, not a disease.

FORMULA

Poria (Hoelen) Five Powder (*wǔ líng sǎn*)

∘ Transform qì and move water, in order to resolve the exterior.

猪苓十八铢（去皮） 泽泻一两六铢 白术十八铢 茯苓十八铢 桂枝半两（去皮）

㈠ 右五味，捣为散，以白饮和服方寸匕，日三服。㈡ 多饮暖水，汗出愈。㈢ 如法将息。

Zhū líng shí bā zhū (qù pí) zé xiè yī liǎng liù zhū bái zhú shí bā zhū fú líng shí bā zhū guì zhī bàn liǎng (qù pí)

(1) *Yòu wǔ wèi, dǎo wéi sǎn, yǐ bái yǐn huò fú fāng cùn bǐ, rì sān fú.* (2) *Duō yǐn nuǎn shuǐ, hàn chū yù.* (3) *Rú fǎ jiāng xī.*

polyporus (猪苓 *zhū líng*, Polyporus) 18 zhū[1] (remove skin)

alisma (泽泻 *zé xiè*, Alismatis Rhizoma) 1 liǎng 6 zhū
ovate atractylodes (白术 *bái zhú*, Atractylodis Ovatae Rhizoma) 18 zhū
poria (茯苓 *fú líng*, Poria) 18 zhū
cinnamon twig (桂枝 *guì zhī*, Cinnamomi Ramulus) half liǎng (remove bark)

(1) [For] the above five ingredients, pound to a powder. Mix into a white [rice] cool decoction.[2] Take the formula with a square-inch-spoon,[3] three times a day. (2) Drink copious amounts of warm water [and when] sweat issues, [there will be] recovery. (3) Follow the [previous] method [described for Cinnamon Twig Decoction (*guì zhī tāng*) with regard to] rest.

Formula Notes

1. Zhū, 铢 *zhū*: 1/24 of a liǎng.
2. Mix into a white [rice] cool decoction, 以白饮和 *yǐ bái yǐn huò*: One should make a soup with white rice and mix in the ingredients.
3. Take the formula with a square-inch-spoon, 服方寸匕 *fú fāng cùn bǐ*: An ancient method for measuring the amount of a decoction to be taken that involves using a square spoon, each side of which measures one cùn, to measure out the decoction. This amount is roughly equivalent to 6-9 grams.

Synopsis

a) The signs and treatment of water amassment.

b) Differentiation of this pattern from depletion of stomach liquid, following the promotion of sweating.

Commentary

Greater yáng disease is properly treated through the promotion of sweating, but as has been stated previously, only a very light sweat should issue. In this line, sweating has been promoted improperly because profuse sweat issues. The reader is presented with two possible transmutations following this mistreatment. The first is that the stomach becomes dry and the second is that the pulse is still floating and urination is inhibited.

The promotion of sweating, particularly in excess, easily damages the body fluids. In the present line, the damage primarily affects the fluids in the stomach. The stomach becomes dry and disharmonious, leading to vexation and agitation. Dryness in the stomach also causes the patient to desire fluids. One should not confuse the vexation and agitation in this pattern with that seen in yáng brightness disease. In yáng brightness patterns, the vexation is generally described as "great" and is accompanied by constipation or some other disruption of normal bowel function. Disharmony of the stomach easily causes insomnia. On the basis of these signs, one knows that the exterior disease has already resolved, but the fluids of the stomach have been damaged. The treatment consists in giving the patient frequent, small amounts of water to drink. Because stomach function is impaired, drinking of copious amounts of water may result in collecting rheum; therefore, the patient should not be allowed to drink large quantities of water. The frequent drinking of small amounts of water will restore stomach harmony and resolve the disease.

In the second situation, following copious sweating, the pulse is still floating and urination is inhibited. Mild heat and thirst that is difficult to resolve are also observed. A pulse that is floating and mild heat indicate that the exterior evil has not been eliminated, but the evil has also moved from the channel into the interior, entering the bladder and impairing bladder function. When the qì transformation of the bladder is impaired, the waterways are not regulated properly, the fluids do not move, and the evil binds with collecting water. Collecting water amasses in the lower burner, inhibiting urination; and because fluid movement is impaired, thirst arises.

Poria (Hoelen) Five Powder (*wǔ líng sǎn*) treats internal water amassment and exterior patterns, although it may also be used in the absence of an exterior evil. This formula is an example of simultaneously treating interior and exterior disease. Poria (*fú líng*), polyporus (*zhū líng*), and alisma (*zé xiè*) percolate and disinhibit water. Ovate atractylodes (*bái zhú*) fortifies the spleen and dispels dampness. Cinnamon twig (*guì zhī*) frees yáng, transforms qì, and resolves the exterior. The most important action of the formula is to disinhibit the urine, but in any disease where water collects, the spleen should be fortified. When the spleen is strong, the water can be controlled; therefore, the inclusion of ingredients to fortify the spleen is also important. The movement of water also depends on the qì transformation of the bladder. Cinnamon twig (*guì zhī*) warms and stimulates the bladder qì, so that normal movement is restored. Eating rice gruel with the decoction is suggested, as it is when giving Cinnamon Twig Decoction (*guì zhī tāng*). The fluids have already been damaged through excessive sweating and if one wants to disinhibit the urine, providing extra fluid nourishment will assist this process.

LINE 72

发汗已，脉浮数，烦渴者，五苓散主之。

Fā hàn yǐ, mài fú shuò, fán kě zhě, wǔ líng sǎn zhǔ zhī.

When sweating has already been promoted, the pulse is floating and rapid, and [there is] vexation and thirst,* Poria (Hoelen) Five Powder (*wǔ líng sǎn*) governs.

TEXT NOTE

* Vexation and thirst, 烦渴 *fán kě*: According to *Shāng Hán Lùn Yán Jiū Dà Cí Diǎn*, this can be interpreted as vexation and thirst, indicating two separate entities, or vexing thirst, indicating severe thirst.

SYNOPSIS

A supplementary description of the pulse and signs of the water amassment pattern.

COMMENTARY

In the previous line, following the promotion of sweating the pulse was floating. Here the pulse is floating and rapid, indicating that the exterior pattern has not yet resolved and that heat is present. In the previous line mild heat was present, and one may assume that in both cases an external evil has entered the bladder and transformed to heat. The exterior evil impairs the qì transformation of the bladder, which, in combination with the loss of fluids from sweating, results in abnormal fluid movement. The resultant internal dryness causes vexation. Likewise, abnormal fluid movement can cause severe thirst. Whether one interprets 烦渴 *fán kě* as vexation and thirst or vexing thirst, the clinical significance is the same. In either case, Poria (Hoelen) Five Powder (*wǔ líng sǎn*) can be used to restore normal function to the bladder and allow the fluids to move freely. Fāng Yǒu-Zhí writes of using: "... Poria Four, 四苓 *sì líng* [polyporus (*zhū líng*), alisma (*zé xiè*), ovate atractylodes (*bái zhú*), and poria (*fú líng*)], to moisten ... [and] cinnamon twig (*guì zhī*) in order to harmonize [the exterior]."

In the presence of internal dryness and mild heat one uses a formula whose ingredients disinhibit urine and dry dampness because the root is water amassment. The signs indicate dryness, but the pathomechanism involves abnormal movement of water. If the function of the bladder is restored, the water will move normally and be properly distributed; consequently, the dryness will resolve.

Vexation and thirst appear in three basic patterns following the promotion of sweating. In the previous line, the stomach fluids were damaged and frequently drinking small amounts of water was suggested to restore harmony. In the second part of that line and the line above, water amasses in the lower burner and an exterior pattern remains unresolved; therefore, Poria (Hoelen) Five Powder (*wǔ líng sǎn*) is used. The third pattern is exuberant qì-aspect heat damaging the fluids in yáng brightness disease. This pattern is treated with White Tiger Decoction Plus Ginseng (*bái hǔ jiā rén shēn tāng*). For a full discussion of White Tiger Decoction Plus Ginseng (*bái hǔ jiā rén shēn tāng*) see line 26, p. 156. The signs in these patterns are similar, but the pathomechanisms are different.

LINE 74

中风发热，六七日不解而烦，有表里证，渴欲饮水，水入则吐者，名曰水逆，五苓散主之。

Zhòng fēng fā rè, liù qī rì bù jiě ér fán, yǒu biǎo lǐ zhèng, kě yù yǐn shuǐ, shuǐ rù zé tù zhě, míng yuē shuǐ nì, wǔ líng sǎn zhǔ zhī.

When in wind strike [the person has] heat effusion unresolved after six or seven days and vexation, [so that] [there is] an exterior and an interior pattern[1] [marked by] thirst with a desire to drink water and immediate vomiting of ingested fluids, [this] is called water counterflow,[2] [for which] Poria (Hoelen) Five Powder (*wǔ líng sǎn*) governs.

TEXT NOTES

1. [There is] an exterior and interior pattern, 有表里证 *yǒu biǎo lǐ zhèng*: Wind strike and heat effusion are signs of greater yáng disease, which is an exterior disease. Thirst and vomiting of fluids are signs of water amassment, which is an interior disease. Both exterior and interior signs are present at the same time.
2. Water counterflow, 水逆 *shuǐ nì*: A condition in which the patient feels thirst and desires to drink, but immediately vomits ingested fluids. This sign is a

manifestation of severe water amassment, which arises when rheum evil collects in the interior and ingested water is not transformed into fluids ("fluids" here referring not to ingested fluids, but to bodily fluids.)

SYNOPSIS

The clinical manifestation and treatment of severe water amassment pattern.

COMMENTARY

This pattern is similar to those in the preceding lines with an unresolved exterior evil but signs of interior water amassment also exist. Known as water counterflow, this sign reflects a more severe water amassment pattern in water that is ingested is immediately regurgitated. In water counterflow the water evil attacks the stomach, impairing downbearing. Because fluid movement is disturbed, the patient feels thirsty; but the stomach cannot move the ingested fluids properly and vomiting immediately occurs. Although this sign is more severe, the pathomechanism is the same as in previous water amassment patterns and involves an unresolved exterior evil; hence one can still give Poria (Hoelen) Five Powder (*wǔ líng sǎn*).

LINE 73

伤寒汗出而渴者，五苓散主之；不渴者，茯苓甘草汤主之。

Shāng hán hàn chū ér kě zhě, wǔ líng sǎn zhǔ zhī; bù kě zhě, fú líng gān cǎo tāng zhǔ zhī.

When in cold damage [there is] sweating and thirst, Poria (Hoelen) Five Powder (*wǔ líng sǎn*) governs. [If] thirst is absent, Poria (Hoelen) and Licorice Decoction (*fú líng gān cǎo tāng*) governs.

FORMULA

Poria (Hoelen) and Licorice Decoction (*fú líng gān cǎo tāng*)

∘ Warm the stomach and transform rheum; free yáng and disinhibit water.

茯苓二两　桂枝二两（去皮）　甘草一两（炙）　生姜三两（切）

右四味，以水四升，煮取二升，去滓，分温三服。

Fú líng èr liǎng guì zhī èr liǎng (bié qiē) gān cǎo yī liǎng (zhì) shēng jiāng sān liǎng (qiē)

Yòu sì wèi, yǐ shuǐ sì shēng, zhǔ qǔ èr shēng, qù zǐ, fēn wēn sān fú.

poria (茯苓 *fú líng*, Poria) 2 liǎng
cinnamon twig (桂枝 *guì zhī*, Cinnamomi Ramulus) 2 liǎng (remove the bark)
mix-fried licorice (甘草 *gān cǎo*, Glycyrrhizae Radix) 1 liǎng
fresh ginger (生姜 *shēng jiāng*, Zingiberis Rhizoma Recens) 3 liǎng (cut)

[For] the above four ingredients use four shēng of water and boil to get two shēng. Remove the dregs, divide into three [doses] and take warm.

Synopsis

A differentiation between water amassment in the bladder and stomach vacuity collecting water, in terms of signs and treatment.

Commentary

In the previous lines sweating is promoted to resolve an exterior evil and causes thirst and inhibited urination. An exterior evil enters the greater yáng channel and the bladder, impairing the movement of water and causing thirst and inhibited urination. In those patterns water collects in the lower burner. In this line the reader is presented with two possibilities and must make the connection with the previous lines, since the key sign, inhibited urination, is not stated in the text. This line clarifies which formula to use from the location of the collecting water.

In the first pattern, following the promotion of sweating, the qì is damaged and bladder qì transformation becomes inhibited. Fluids are not properly distributed and cannot move upward. The mouth and tongue become dry and the patient is thirsty. This pattern, characterized by inhibited urination and thirst, is treated with Poria (Hoelen) Five Powder (*wŭ líng săn*), indicating water collecting in the lower burner.

In the second pattern, following the promotion of sweating it is not the bladder qì that is damaged but the yáng qì of the stomach. The stomach function of decomposition is impaired and water collects in the center burner. The second pattern, characterized by inhibited urination without thirst, is treated with Poria (Hoelen) and Licorice Decoction (*fú líng gān căo tāng*), indicating that the water is collecting in the center burner, not the lower.

Both patterns involve water collecting in the interior; consequently, both formulae warm yáng and transform water. The emphasis of Poria (Hoelen) Five Powder (*wŭ líng săn*) is opening yáng and disinhibiting water, whereas the emphasis of Poria (Hoelen) and Licorice Decoction (*fú líng gān căo tāng*) is warming the stomach and dissipating water.

Poria (Hoelen) and Licorice Decoction (*fú líng gān căo tāng*) warms the stomach and transforms water. Fresh ginger (*shēng jiāng*), which warms the stomach in order to dissipate water qì, is the sovereign. Poria (*fú líng*) fortifies the spleen and percolates and disinhibits water. Cinnamon twig (*guì zhī*) frees yáng and transforms qì. Licorice (*gān căo*) harmonizes the center. (Poria (Hoelen) Five Powder (*wŭ líng săn*) is discussed in line 71, p. 195.)

Line 127

太阳病，小便利者，以饮水多，必心下悸；小便少者，必苦里急也。

Tài yáng bìng, xiăo biàn lì zhĕ, yĭ yĭn shuĭ duō, bì xīn xià jì; xiăo biàn shăo zhĕ, bì kŭ lĭ jí yĕ.

When in greater yáng disease [if] urination is uninhibited, the drinking of copious [amounts of] water will result in palpitations below the heart; [if] urination is scant, [the person will] suffer from abdominal urgency.*

Text Note

* Abdominal urgency, 里急 *lǐ jí*: A feeling of distention and fullness in the small abdomen, accompanied by urgency to urinate and discomfort.

Synopsis

The location of collecting water can be identified according to whether urination is inhibited or uninhibited.

Commentary

This line may be read in two ways, leading to different interpretations. The basic question concerns the clause, "copious drinking of water," and whether it refers to both of the situations presented in this line or only the first.

Many commentators read this line as a discussion of two transmutations that occur in greater yáng disease following the drinking of large amounts of fluid. The *Yī Zōng Jīn Jiàn* and Chéng Wú-Jǐ suggest that "the drinking of copious [amounts of] water" should be placed directly after "greater yáng disease." Chéng Wú-Jǐ writes, "[When] copious water is ingested and urination is spontaneously uninhibited, water does not amass in the interior. Only in the abdomen is there copious water and it causes palpitations below the heart.... [When] copious water is ingested and urination is inhibited, water amasses in the interior and does not move; [the person] will suffer from abdominal urgency." In the first transmutation, urination is uninhibited and in the second, urination is scant. The *Yī Zōng Jīn Jiàn* clarifies that in this type of pattern, the state of the stomach qì will also affect the outcome: "In the onset of greater yáng disease, [there is] no desire to drink water. [When the disease] shifts to the yáng brightness, a desire to drink water [arises]. These [patterns] are normal. In the present line, at the beginning of greater yáng disease, the copious drinking of water suggests that the person has constitutional stomach dryness. If the stomach yáng is not debilitated, the ingested water can be distributed to the exterior, causing sweat [to issue] and [the disease] to resolve. Copious water is ingested and the stomach qì is not full. Since the urination is uninhibited, [water] will collect in the center burner and cause palpitations below the heart. If, further, urination is scant, water collects in the lower burner and [the patient] will suffer from abdominal urgency."

One may also consider that when urination is inhibited, one need not ingest large amounts of water for urination to be uncomfortable. It is possible that "suffer from abdominal urgency" is simply a clarification of what occurs when urination is scant. On the basis of this interpretation, abdominal urgency is a result of water collecting in the lower burner because urination is inhibited, regardless of whether or not copious amounts of water are ingested. During the course of a greater yáng disease, if the patient takes in an excessive amount of water, water qì may collect in the interior. This line describes signs that one can use to identify the location of the collecting water. When the urination is normal, the water collects in the center, not the lower burner, and impairs the movement and transformation functions of the spleen and stomach. This collecting water is not transformed and invades the heart, causing palpitations in the upper abdomen. When urination is inhibited, the amount becomes scant and water collects in the lower burner. Qì transformation in the bladder becomes impaired and water is not transformed. The lesser abdomen becomes distended and full, and a feeling of urinary urgency exists. Previous lines in the text suggest that for water collecting in the center burner, Poria (Hoelen) and Licorice Decoction (*fú líng gān cǎo tāng*) be given. Poria (Hoelen) Five Powder (*wǔ líng sǎn*) is suggested for water collecting in the lower burner.

4.9 Blood Amassment Patterns

In blood amassment transmuted patterns, spirit signs such as mania are commonly observed because static blood and heat evil bind in the lower burner and invade upward, affecting the spirit. Many of these patients develop hypertonicity, fullness, and hardness in the lesser abdomen, and the pulse is generally deep. Because the evil is in the blood, bladder qì transformation is unaffected and urination is usually normal in these patterns, which is an important difference between blood amassment and water amassment. If the exterior pattern has resolved and the blood amassment is mild, Peach Kernel Qì-Coordinating Decoction (*táo hé chéng qì tāng*), which expels stasis and discharges heat, is used. When blood amassment is severe, Dead-On Decoction (*dǐ dàng tāng*) is used because it breaks blood and expels stasis. When blood amassment is severe, but the disease dynamic is moderate, perhaps because the stasis is abiding and not acute, Dead-On Pill (*dǐ dàng wán*) is suggested because the harsh ingredients are moderated when prepared in pill form.

Line 106

㈠ 太阳病不解，热结膀胱，其人如狂，血自下，下者愈。㈡ 其外不解者，尚未可攻，当先解其外。㈢ 外解已，但少腹急结者，乃可攻之，宜桃核承气汤。

(1) *Tài yáng bìng bù jiě, rè jié páng guāng, qí rén rú kuáng, xuè zì xià, xià zhě yù.* (2) *Qí wài bù jiě zhě, shàng wèi kě gōng, dāng xiān jiě qí wài.* (3) *Wài jiě yǐ, dàn shào fù jí jié zhě, nǎi kě gōng zhī, yí táo hé chéng qì tāng.*

(1) When a greater yáng disease is unresolved and heat binds in the bladder,[1] the person is as if manic,[2] and spontaneous blood descent[3] will bring recovery. (2) If the exterior has not been resolved, [one should] not yet attack,[4] [but] should first resolve the exterior. (3) When the exterior has been resolved and [there is] only tense bound lesser abdomen, [one] can attack[5] and [therefore,] Peach Kernel Qì-Coordinating Decoction (*táo hé chéng qì tāng*) is appropriate.

Text Notes

1. Heat binds in the bladder, 热结膀胱 *rè jié pāng guāng*: Three slightly different explanations are offered for this phrase.
   a) Heat evil and blood stasis contending in the lower burner. Yóu Yí writes, "Heat evil enters the blood. This is a lower burner blood amassment pattern."
   b) Heat evil and blood stasis contending in the bladder. Chéng Wú-Jǐ writes, "The bladder channel [belongs] to the greater yáng. An unresolved greater yáng channel heat evil follows the channel and enters the mansion. This is what 'heat bound in the bladder' means." (Mansion refers to the bladder itself, as opposed to the bladder channel.)
   c) Heat evil and blood stasis contending in the interior of the body. Fāng Yǒu-Zhí writes, "Heat bound in the bladder [means]... heat [evil] and [blood] stasis following the greater yáng [channel] in the interior...."
2. As if manic, 如狂 *rú kuáng*: A mild abnormality of the spirit-mind, in which the patient has episodes of mania and periods of normalcy.
3. Spontaneous blood descent, 血自下 *xuè zì xià*: Blood in the urine or the stool.
4. Attack, 可攻 *kě gōng*: In this context, attacking means freeing stasis and discharging heat. This analysis is based on the formula used.
5. Tense bound lesser abdomen, 少腹急结 *shào fù jí jié*: Hypertonicity, distention, fullness, hardness, and pain in the lesser abdomen.

Formula

Peach Kernel Qì-Coordinating Decoction (*táo hé chéng qì tāng*)

∘ Expel stasis and discharge heat.

桃仁五十个（去皮尖） 大黄四两 桂枝二两（去皮） 甘草二两（炙） 芒消二两

(一) 右五味，以水七升，煮取二升半，去滓，内芒消，更上火微沸，下火，先食温服五合，日三服。(二) 当微利。

Táo rén wǔ shí ge (qù pí jiān) dà huáng sì liǎng guì zhī èr liǎng (qù pí) gān cǎo èr liǎng (zhì) máng xiāo èr liǎng

(1) *Yòu wǔ wèi, yǐ shuǐ qī shēng, zhǔ qǔ èr shēng bàn, qù zǐ, nà máng xiāo, gèng shàng huǒ wēi fèi, xià huǒ, xiān shí wēn fú wǔ gě, rì sān fú.* (2) *Dāng wēi lì.*

peach kernel (桃仁 *táo rén*, Persicae Semen) 50 pieces (remove skin and tips*)
rhubarb (大黄 *dà huáng*, Rhei Rhizoma) 4 liǎng
cinnamon twig (桂枝 *guì zhī*, Cinnamomi Ramulus) 2 liǎng (remove bark)
mix-fried licorice (甘草 *gān cǎo*, Glycyrrhizae Radix) 2 liǎng
mirabilite (芒硝 *máng xiāo*, Mirabilitum) 2 liǎng

(1) [For] the above five ingredients use seven shēng of water. Boil [the first four ingredients] to get two and a half shēng. Remove the dregs and add mirabilite (*máng xiāo*). Again place on the fire and boil slightly. Remove from the fire and before eating take five gě warm, three times a day. (2) [There] should be slight diarrhea.

FORMULA NOTE

* Remove the skin and tips, 去皮尖 *qù pí jiān*: It is not clear why Zhāng Jī suggests that the skin and tips of peach kernel (*táo rén*) be removed. It may reflect knowledge of the presence of toxic components concentrated in these two areas of the seed. Since Zhāng Jī uses peach kernel (*táo rén*) in this formula to quicken the blood, he could not have been acting in accordance with the notion arising in the Míng and Qīng Dynasties that the skin and tips of this medicinal should be removed when it is used to moisten the intestines, but that they should be retained when it is used to move the blood since these parts have the strongest blood-moving action.

SYNOPSIS

The signs and treatment of the mild blood amassment pattern.

COMMENTARY

When a greater yáng evil is unresolved it may transform to heat and follow the channel into the interior. "Interior" can be interpreted to mean the interior of the body, the lower burner, or the urinary bladder. The heat causes a manic-like state when it enters the blood. If the blood flows freely, the heat will cause frenetic movement of the blood. The blood will move into the stool or the urine and the heat will follow the blood and resolve. "[If there is] spontaneous blood descent, it will bring recovery."

If, however, the blood is not flowing freely because of a preexisting condition of blood stasis or because the heat damages the blood and causes blood stasis, the heat will contend with the blood stasis, causing blood amassment in the lower burner. The two clinical signs of blood amassment presented here are a mania-like condition and tense lesser abdominal bind. Lesser abdominal bind is a direct result of blood amassment in the lower burner. The mania-like condition is a result of blood heat and blood stasis in the lower burner. The heat evil cannot flow out below and because heat tends to rise upward, it harasses the upper body. The evil moves upward in the blood and the heart governs the blood vessels, so the heat affects the heart. Because the heart governs the spirit, a heat evil harassing the heart can cause a mania-like condition.

When one is treating a pattern of blood amassment following contraction of a greater yáng exterior evil, the exterior must be resolved before the interior can be treated. Zhāng Jī emphasizes this point because the treatment that he suggests for blood amassment, expelling stasis and discharging heat, would cause an unresolved exterior evil to fall inward and possibly exacerbate the condition. Once the exterior is resolved, one may precipitate the blood. This general principle can be applied not only to blood amassment patterns, but generally to any disease pattern with exterior signs.

Peach Kernel Qì-Coordinating Decoction (*táo hé chéng qì tāng*) is Stomach-Regulating Qì-Coordinating Decoction (*tiáo wèi chéng qì tāng*) with a smaller dose of mirabilite (*máng xiāo*) and with the addition of peach kernel (*táo rén*) and cinnamon twig (*guì zhī*). The addition of peach kernel (*táo rén*), which quickens the blood and expels stasis, and cinnamon twig (*guì zhī*), which warms and frees the blood vessels, increases the ability of the formula to precipitate heat and stasis.

Because the formula's most important action is expelling stasis, not freeing the stool, the dosage of mirabilite (*máng xiāo*) is reduced.

The location of blood amassment is in the lower burner. Peach Kernel Qì-Coordinating Decoction (*táo hé chéng qì tāng*) attacks and precipitates blood stasis. In order to speed the absorption of the decoction and maximize its efficacy, the decoction should be taken on an empty stomach; consequently, in the directions for the formula it is suggested that the decoction be taken before eating.

Line 124

㈠ 太阳病六七日，表证仍在，脉微而沉，反不结胸，其人发狂者，以热在下焦，少腹当硬满，小便自利者，下血乃愈。㈡ 所以然者，以太阳随经，瘀热在里故也，抵当汤主之。

(1) *Tài yáng bìng liù qī rì, biǎo zhèng réng zài, mài wēi ér chén, fǎn bù jié xiōng, qí rén fā kuáng zhě, yǐ rè zài xià jiāo, shào fù dāng yìng mǎn, xiǎo biàn zì lì zhě, xià xuè nǎi yù.* (2) *Suǒ yǐ rán zhě, yǐ tài yáng suí jīng, yū rè zài lǐ gù yě, dǐ dàng tāng zhǔ zhī.*

(1) When in greater yáng disease [that has lasted for] six or seven days, the exterior pattern is still present and the pulse is faint and sunken, but chest bind[1] is absent, and the person is manic,[2] it is because the heat is in the lower burner, so the lesser abdomen is hard and full, urination is spontaneously uninhibited and precipitating the blood [will bring] recovery. (2) Why [this] is so is because [the evil] followed the greater yáng channel, and [there is] stasis heat in the interior; [therefore,] Dead-On Decoction (*dǐ dàng tāng*) governs.

Text Notes

1. Chest bind, 结胸 *jié xiōng*: Pain with hardness and fullness in the area above the diaphragm and below the heart.
2. Manic, 发狂 *fā kuāng*: A severe spirit abnormality characterized by agitation and significant alterations in the patient's speech, behavior, and thought. Delirious speech, hallucinations, and inappropriate behavior may also be observed.

Formula

Dead-On Decoction (*dǐ dàng tāng*)

- Break blood and dispel stasis.

水蛭（熬） 虻虫各三十个（去翅足，熬） 桃仁二十个（去皮尖） 大黄三两（酒洗）

㈠ 右四味，以水五升，煮取三升，去滓，温服一升。㈡ 不下，更服。

Shuǐ zhì (áo) méng chóng gè sān shí ge (qù chì zú, áo) táo rén èr shí ge (qù pí jiān) dà huáng sān liǎng (jiǔ xǐ)

(1) *Yòu sì wèi, yǐ shuǐ wǔ shēng, zhǔ qǔ sān shēng, qù zǐ, wēn fú yī shēng.* (2) *Bù xià, gèng fú.*

leech (水蛭 *shuǐ zhì*, Hirudo seu Whitmania) 30 pieces (dry fry*)
tabanus (虻虫 *méng chóng*, Tabanus) 30 pieces (remove wings and legs, dry fry*)
peach kernel (桃仁 *táo rén*, Persicae Semen) 20 pieces (remove skin and tips)
rhubarb (大黄 *dà huáng*, Rhei Rhizoma) 3 liǎng (wash with wine)

(1) [For] the above four ingredients use five shēng of water and boil to get three shēng. Remove the dregs and take one shēng warm. (2) [If there is] no diarrhea, take again.

Formula Note

* Dry fry, 熬 *áo*: These two ingredients cannot be used raw so they are prepared through some cooking process in order to make them safe for internal use. This same Chinese term now usually refers to boiling over a low flame. In modern practice, these medicinals are usually stone baked.

Synopsis

The pulse, signs, and treatment of severe blood amassment pattern.

Commentary

Greater yáng disease that has failed to resolve in six or seven days is normally characterized by a pulse that is floating. In the pattern described in the present line, however, the pulse is faint and sunken, indicating that the evil has entered the interior and transformed into heat. In interior heat patterns, it is important to determine the precise location of the heat. In the present line, we are told that chest bind is absent. We may infer, therefore, that there is no hardness and pain below the heart or oppression in the chest that would indicate that the heat were located in the chest. Furthermore, this patient has a spirit disorder, mania, which Zhāng Jī attributes to heat in the lower burner. As in the previous line, an unresolved exterior evil has transformed to heat and entered the lower burner. It contends with the blood and the blood becomes static. In the previous line a mania-like condition and tense lesser abdominal bind are present, but in this line the same pathomechanism results in hardness and fullness in the lesser abdomen and mania. Blood heat and blood stasis causes blood amassment. This pattern is further suggested by the pulse, which is sunken and faint. A pulse that is sunken indicates interior disease. A pulse that is faint indicates severe congestion of the qì and blood. This condition is more severe than the one in the previous line, perhaps because of constitutional differences between the patients or differences in the strength of the evil. Although this pattern is more severe, the uninhibited urination suggests that the qì dynamic of the bladder is still normal. Because of the severity of this pattern no spontaneous resolution through bleeding is possible as in the previous line.

Dead-On Decoction (*dǐ dàng tāng*) is a harsh formula for attacking and expelling blood stasis. Leech (*shuǐ zhì*) and tabanus (*méng chóng*) expel malign blood and break blood accumulation. Rhubarb (*dà huáng*) flushes evil heat and moves stasis in a downward direction, reinforcing the lubrication and disinhibition provided by peach kernel (*táo rén*). This formula powerfully breaks blood and expels stasis; therefore, it should only be used for cases of blood stasis in repletion patterns. In elderly or weak patients or those with internal bleeding this formula can only be used with extreme caution, if at all. Its use is contraindicated for patients who are currently bleeding or pregnant.

LINE 125

太阳病，身黄，脉沉结，少腹硬，小便不利者，为无血也；小便自利，其人如狂者，血证谛也，抵当汤主之。

Tài yáng bìng, shēn huáng, mài chén jié, shào fù yìng, xiǎo biàn bù lì zhě, wéi wú xuè yě; xiǎo biàn zì lì, qí rén rú kuáng zhě, xuè zhèng dì yě, dǐ dàng tāng zhǔ zhī.

When in greater yáng disease, [there is] generalized yellowing,* a pulse that is sunken and bound, hardness in the lesser abdomen, and inhibited urination, [this] means that [there is] no blood [amassment]. [When] urination is uninhibited and the person is as if manic, [the previous signs indicate] a true blood pattern, [for which] Dead-On Decoction (*dǐ dàng tāng*) governs.

TEXT NOTE

* Generalized yellowing, 身黄 *shēn huáng*: The facial complexion, general skin color, eyes, and urine are all bright yellow. Also written as 发黄 *fā huáng*.

SYNOPSIS

a) Further discussion of the pulse and signs of the severe blood amassment pattern.

b) The essential features for identifying this pattern.

COMMENTARY

This line provides guidance for the reader when identifying blood amassment patterns. The key to this identification is whether or not urination is inhibited. The signs of generalized yellowing and hardness in the lesser abdomen do not indicate blood amassment if the urination is inhibited. When urination is inhibited, these signs indicate damp-heat steaming in the interior, which is not related to blood stasis or amassment.

These signs, however, do indicate blood amassment when urination is uninhibited. A pulse that is sunken means that the disease is in the interior, and a pulse that is bound means blood stasis. Hardness in the lesser abdomen is further indication of stasis in the lower burner. As described earlier, blood amassment can lead to a manic-like condition, as in this line. Blood amassment in the lower burner can give rise to blood heat and blood stasis, and lead to generalized yellowing.

Many modern commentators make reference to the liver and gallbladder in describing the pathomechanism of generalized yellowing, although Zhāng Jī did not understand it this way. Kē Qín provides an explanation that does not refer to the liver and gallbladder and is presumably closer to Zhāng Jī's original conception:

> Greater yáng disease with generalized yellowing and mania can be differentiated by blood and qì [aspect]. [When] urination is inhibited and generalized yellowing [occurs], the disease is in the qì aspect.... If urination is uninhibited and generalized yellowing [occurs], the disease is in the blood aspect. Damp-heat collects in the skin and generalized yellowing [occurs] because the defensive qì does not move. Dry blood binds in the bladder and generalized yellowing [occurs] because the construction qì is not distributed.

LINE 126

伤寒有热，少腹满，应小便不利，今反利者，为有血也，当下之，不可余药，宜抵当丸。

Shāng hán yǒu rè, shào fù mǎn, yīng xiǎo biàn bù lì, jīn fǎn lì zhě, wéi yǒu xuè yě, dāng xià zhī, bù kě yú yào, yí dǐ dàng wán.

In cold damage with heat[1] and lesser abdominal fullness, urination should be inhibited; but now urination is uninhibited, which means [there is] blood [amassment,] so one should precipitate [the blood]. [One] cannot spare [any or anything of the] medicinals [required][2] and [so] Dead-On Pill (*dǐ dàng wán*) is appropriate.

TEXT NOTES

1. Cold damage with heat, 伤寒有热 *shāng hán yǒu rè*: A cold damage pattern with generalized heat. Yóu Yí writes, "'With heat' means generalized heat." Kē Qín, however, interprets this phrase as indicating that the exterior evil has not resolved: "'With heat' means that the exterior pattern is still present."
2. Cannot spare [any or anything of the] medicinals [required], 不可余药 *bù kě yú yào*: Two meanings are suggested. One is that only this formula can be used, since any other formula would not be efficacious. The other, more likely, meaning is that when the medicinals are taken they must be taken with the dregs; therefore, the pill is used here, not the decoction. Although the preparation instructions do not specifically say so, it is generally held that the dregs should not be strained off.

FORMULA

Dead-On Pill (*dǐ dàng wán*)

- Break blood and expel stasis; use harsh medicinals moderately.

水蛭二十个（熬） 虻虫二十个（去翅足，熬） 桃仁二十五个（去皮尖） 大黄三两

㈠右四味，捣分四丸。㈡以水一升，煮一丸，取七合服之。㈢晬时当下血，若不下者，更服。

Shuǐ zhì èr shí ge (áo) méng chóng èr shí ge (qù chì zú, áo) táo rén èr shí wǔ ge (qù pí jiān) dà huáng sān liǎng

(1) *Yòu sì wèi, dǎo fēn sì wán.* (2) *Yǐ shuǐ yī shēng, zhǔ yī wán, qǔ qī gě fú zhī.* (3) *Zuì shí dāng xià xuè, ruò bù xià zhě, gèng fú.*

leech (水蛭 *shuǐ zhì*, Hirudo seu Whitmania) 20 pieces (dry-fry)
tabanus (虻虫 *méng chóng*, Tabanus) 20 pieces (remove wing and legs, dry-fry)
peach kernel (桃仁 *táo rén*, Persicae Semen) 25 pieces (remove skin and tip)
rhubarb (大黄 *dà huáng*, Rhei Rhizoma) 3 liǎng

(1) [For] the above four ingredients, pound, separate and [form] into four pills. (2) Use one shēng of water and boil one pill to get seven gě. Take [the decoction]. (3) Within one day,[1] there should be blood descent.[2] If [there is] no descent, take again.[3]

TEXT NOTES

1. One day, 晬时 *zuì shí*: A period of twenty-four hours; a night and a day.
2. Blood descent, 下血 *xià xuè*: Here, this term means blood appearing in the stool or the urine, but in other places it can refer to uterine bleeding. This term can be used to describe a treatment, as in "precipitating the blood," and it can also be used to describe the downward movement of blood, as in "blood descent."
3. If [there is] no descent, take again, 若不下者，更服 *ruò bù xì zhě, gèng fú*: Because pill forms are gentler and slower acting than decotions, precipitation using the pill form of Dead-On Pill (*dǐ dàng wán*) can be expected to take up to a day to occur. The formula be taken again only if precipitation does not occur within about one day.

SYNOPSIS

a) The essential features for distinguishing water amassment from blood amassment.

b) The treatment of the severe pattern of blood amassment when the disease dynamic is mild.

COMMENTARY

This line further emphasizes the importance of urination as a diagnostic indicator. The presence of an unresolved exterior pattern, "cold damage with heat" and lesser abdominal fullness, suggests that the evil has entered the urinary bladder and caused water amassment. In that case, however, urination should be inhibited, whereas in this line, urination is uninhibited. Therefore, these signs indicate blood amassment and should be treated by precipitating the blood.

Dead-On Pill (*dǐ dàng wán*) is a gentler version of Dead-On Decoction (*dǐ dàng tāng*). The dosages of leech (*shuǐ zhì*) and tabanus (*méng chóng*) are reduced, while the amount of peach kernel (*táo rén*) is slightly increased and rhubarb (*dà huáng*) remains the same. Furthermore, pill forms are gentler and slower acting than decoctions.

This formula is considered moderate by comparison on the one hand with the mild Peach Kernel Qì-Coordinating Decoction (*táo hé chéng qì tāng*) and on the other with the harsh Dead-On Decoction (*dǐ dàng tāng*). For mild cases of blood amassment with mania-like signs and mild lesser abdominal bind, Peach Kernel Qì-Coordinating Decoction (*táo hé chéng qì tāng*) may be used. For severe cases of blood amassment with mania and hardness in the lesser abdomen, Dead-On Decoction (*dǐ dàng tāng*) is necessary. When the signs are similar to those in which Dead-On Decoction (*dǐ dàng tāng*) is used but are less severe, or when the patient is in a weakened condition, one may instead choose Dead-On Pill (*dǐ dàng wán*).

4.10 Chest Bind Patterns

Chest bind patterns are the result of a heat evil falling inward and binding with water-rheum. They can be the result of inappropriate precipitation, but they can also occur in the absence of mistreatment. Chest bind patterns are divided into two main categories, heat repletion and cold repletion.

Heat repletion chest bind can be further subdivided into three categories on the basis of the formula used to treat the pattern.

a) Major Chest Bind Pill (*dà xiàn xiōng wán*) is used when the location of the chest bind is relatively high. Apart from hardness and pain in the chest region, this pattern is also characterized by stiffness of the nape that appears similar to soft tetany. This formula expels water and flushes repletion. Its use as a pill moderates the harshness of the ingredients.

b) In the Major Chest Bind Decoction (*dà xiàn xiōng tāng*) pattern, the chest bind is below the heart, in the rib-side. In severe patterns it may stretch down into the abdomen. This pattern is characterized by pain below the heart that is stone-like when pressed, or hardness, fullness, and pain from below the heart down into the lesser abdomen that the patient refuses to allow one to palpate. Accompanying signs that may be observed include a pulse that is sunken and tight, bound stool, and late afternoon tidal heat effusion. This formula drains heat and expels water, and flushes repletion and breaks binds. In this pattern if the pulse is floating one should not precipitate since this will cause death. Furthermore, if the main signs of chest bind are present, and vexation and agitation are observed, the patient will die.

c) Minor Chest Bind Decoction (*xiǎo xiàn xiōng tāng*) is used when phlegm heat gives rise to chest bind in a clearly circumscribed area directly below the heart. The hardness and pain in this pattern does not extend down into the abdomen. The area may be painful with or without pressure. The pulse is floating and slippery. This formula disperses phlegm and opens binds.

Cold repletion chest bind patterns occur when water-rheum and cold evil bind below the heart. This pattern is characterized by pain in the region of the chest and stomach duct. The stool may or may not be bound. This pattern is similar to heat repletion chest bind, but heat signs such as heat effusion and vexation are absent. Three Agents White Powder (*sān wù bái sǎn*) is used to attack cold and expel water and to break binds.

LINE 128

(一) 问曰：病有结胸，有藏结，其状何如？(二) 答曰：按之痛，寸脉浮，关脉沉，名曰结胸也。

(1) *Wèn yuē: bìng yǒu jié xiōng, yǒu zàng jié, qí zhuàng hé rú?* (2) *Dá yuē: àn zhī tòng, cùn mài fú, guān mài chén, míng yuē jié xiōng yě.*

Question: There is a disease [called] chest bind,[1] and there is [one called] storehouse bind.[2] What form does it take? Answer: [If there is] pain when pressure is applied, and the inch pulse is floating, and the bar pulse is sunken, this is called chest bind.

TEXT NOTES

1. Chest bind, 结胸 *jié xiōng*: The principal signs of chest bind are pain below the heart and palpable hardness and fullness. In major chest bind, these signs may extend down into the region of the stomach duct or further down into the lesser abdomen. In minor chest bind, the signs are localized to the region directly below the heart. The pathomechanism is that an exterior evil falls inward into the region of the chest and diaphragm. Chest bind is often, but not necessarily, the result of inappropriate precipitation. The exterior evil, once in the chest, binds with phlegm-rheum or water-rheum, which are tangible evils. Chest bind may be differentiated in terms of heat and cold, as well as severity.
2. Storehouse bind, 藏结 *zàng jié*: Visceral vacuity and yáng debilitation with bound yīn cold. Also called "visceral bind," 脏结 *zàng jié*.

SYNOPSIS

The primary pulse and signs of the chest bind pattern.

COMMENTARY

Zhāng Jī compares chest bind and storehouse bind because they are similar and must be clearly differentiated. This line describes some of the key signs associated with chest bind. In chest bind patterns, evil heat falls into the interior and becomes bound in the region of the chest and diaphragm with tangible phlegm or water evil. Chest bind is a repletion pattern; consequently, pressure on the area produces pain. An inch pulse that is floating indicates a yáng evil in the chest and diaphragm. A bar pulse that is sunken indicates bound and congealed water evil in the chest and diaphragm or the center. The center is important because phlegm and water evils are said to arise from there. The phlegm or water evil, from the center, contends with and becomes bound with heat evil in the region of the chest and diaphragm. Therefore, the region of the chest and diaphragm and the center should be considered in chest bind patterns.

4.10.1 Heat Repletion Chest Bind Patterns

4.10.1.1 Major Chest Bind Pill Patterns

Line 131

㈠ 病发于阳，而反下之，热入因作结胸，病发于阴，而反下之，因作痞也。㈡ 所以成结胸者，以下之太早故也。㈢ 结胸者，项亦强，如柔痓状，下之则和，宜大陷胸丸。

(1) *Bìng fā yú yáng, ér fǎn xià zhī, rè rù yīn zuò jié xiōng, bìng fā yú yīn, ér fǎn xià zhī, yīn zuò pǐ yě.* (2) *Suǒ yǐ chéng jié xiōng zhě, yǐ xià zhī tài zǎo gù yě.* (3) *Jié xiōng zhě, xiàng yì jiàng, rú róu cì zhuàng, xià zhī zé hé, yí dà xiàn xiōng wán.*

(1) [When] the disease springs from yáng, yet precipitation is used, the heat enters [the interior] and causes chest bind. [When] the disease springs from yīn, yet precipitation is used, [the evil] causes a glomus. (2) Why [the disease] becomes chest bind [is] because precipitation was used too early. (3) In chest bind, with nape stiffness as [in] soft tetany,* precipitate and then [there will be] harmony. Major Chest Bind Pill (*dà xiàn xiōng wán*) is appropriate.

Text Note

* Soft tetany, 柔痓 *róu cì*: Tetany is a disease characterized by neck and back stiffness and an arched back. When accompanied by sweating it is called soft tetany. If sweating is absent it is called hard tetany.

Formula
Major Chest Bind Pill (*dà xiàn xiōng wán*)

∘ Expel water and break binds; attack moderately with harsh medicinals.

大黄半斤　葶苈子半升（熬）　芒消半升　杏仁半升（去皮尖，熬黑）

㈠ 右四味，捣筛二味，内杏仁、芒消合研如脂，和散。㈡ 取如弹丸一枚，别捣甘遂末一钱匕，白蜜二合，水二升，煮取一升；温顿服之，一宿乃下；如不下，更服，取下为效。㈢ 禁如药法。

Dà huáng bàn jīn　tíng lì zǐ bàn shēng (áo)　máng xiāo bàn shēng　xìng rén bàn shēng (qù pí jiān, áo hēi)

(1) *Yòu sì wèi, dǎo shāi èr wèi, nà xìng rén、máng xiāo hé yán rú zhī, huò sǎn.* (2) *Qǔ rú dàn wán yī méi, bié dǎo gān suì mò yī qián bǐ, bái mì èr gě, shuǐ èr shēng, zhǔ qǔ yī shēng; wēn dùn fú zhī, yī xiǔ nǎi xià; rú bù xià, gèng fú, qǔ xià wéi xiào.* (3) *Jìn rú yào fǎ.*

rhubarb (大黄 *dà huáng*, Rhei Rhizoma) half jīn

tingli (葶苈子 *tíng lì zǐ*, Descurainiae seu Lepidii Semen) half shēng (dry-fry)

mirabilite (芒硝 *máng xiāo*, Mirabilitum) half shēng

apricot kernel (杏仁 *xìng rén*, Armeniacae Semen) half shēng (remove skin and tips, dry-fry till black)

(1) [For] the above four ingredients, pound and sieve the [first] two [rhubarb (*dà huáng*) and tingli (*tíng lì zǐ*)]. Grind mirabilite (*máng xiāo*) and apricot kernel (*xìng rén*) [to make a] fat-like [mixture] and mix in [the other two ingredients]. (2) Make pellet pills.[1] Separately pound 1 qián-spoonful[2] of kansui (*gān suì*) into powder and [combine with] two gě of honey and two shēng of water. Boil to get one shēng. Take warm as a single dose, and [the patient] will have diarrhea after a night. If [the patient] does not have diarrhea, take further doses until diarrhea shows that [the medication] has been effective. (3) Follow these instructions carefully.[3]

Formula Notes

1. Pellet pills, 弹丸 *dàn wán*: Pills approximately the size of a small ball, about 5–6 grams each.
2. Qián-spoonful, 钱匕 *qián bǐ*: The qián-spoon is a measuring device for powders used in the Hàn Dynasty. One qián-spoonful is equivalent to approximately 1.5–1.8 grams or 5–6 fēn.
3. Follow these instructions carefully, 禁如药法 *jìn rú yào fǎ*: The character 禁 *jìn*, normally meaning "forbid," is here understood to mean "carefully."

Synopsis

a) A differentiation between the causes of chest bind and of glomus.

b) The signs and treatment of chest bind when the evil is bound higher in the upper burner.

Commentary

In this line a comparison is made between disease springing from the yáng and disease springing from the yīn and between chest bind and glomus. Disease springing from the yáng and disease springing from the yīn can be interpreted in different ways, reflecting several viewpoints that may help the reader to understand the text. Yáng and yīn can be understood to denote the exterior and interior of the body, the defense and the construction, or different channels. The broadest perspective is offered by Kē Qín who writes, "Yáng means external and describes the body's [exterior]. Yīn means the interior and means the chest and below the heart." Shū Zhào (舒诏, style 驰远 Chí-Yuǎn) offers a slight variation by referring not to the exterior and the interior but to the defense and construction. "Disease springing from yáng means wind damaging the defense; disease springing from yīn means cold damaging the construction." From the interior and exterior, the construction and defense, Qián Huáng narrows his explanation to the channels: "... springing from yáng means an evil in the yáng channels... [and]... springing from yīn means an evil in the yīn channels." Zhāng Zhì-Cōng narrows this perspective further in his commentary: "Disease springing from yáng means disease springing from the greater yáng channel; disease springing from yīn means disease springing from the lesser yīn channel."

Disease springing from yáng means an exterior pattern, and in exterior patterns one should resolve the exterior. If precipitation is used, as it was in this case, the evil may fall inward. When the evil falls inward it can cause chest bind. This pattern is identified as major chest bind on the basis of the suggested formula, Major Chest Bind Pill (*dà xiàn xiōng wán*). In all the lines in this section, chest bind involves a repletion heat evil bound in the interior. Line 141B, p. 223, however, contains a reference to a cold repletion chest bind, although most chest bind patterns involve heat.

Disease springing from yīn means an interior pattern, but this is not a repletion pattern; therefore, precipitation should not be used. When it is, spleen and stomach qì is damaged. Damage to the qì of the center burner impairs upbearing and downbearing of qì and results in stagnation. This stagnation causes a glomus in the region of the center burner just below the heart.

The phrase, "heat enters" is used to describe the exterior evil falling inward and causing chest bind. No such phrase is used for the yīn pattern because the evil is already considered to be in the interior. In the yīn pattern the use of precipitation does not cause the evil to fall inward, it simply damages the stomach qì. Furthermore, we are told that precipitation was used too early in the yáng pattern and this mistreatment causes chest bind. No such indication of time is given for the glomus. Appropriate timing is important when considering the use of a treatment like precipitation in exterior diseases. Precipitation must not be used in exterior patterns, particularly in the early states. In the case of interior diseases, however, it is not the timeliness of precipitation that is important, but its suitability in terms of the presence of repletion or vacuity.

The final section describes chest bind with signs of soft tetany. Major chest bind occurs in the region of the chest, diaphragm, the center burner just below the heart, and the lesser abdomen. When water and heat become bound in this region they obstruct normal movement of fluids. Stiffness in the neck means that the channels have been deprived of normal nourishment and moistening as a result of the congestion.

Major Chest Bind Pill (*dà xiàn xiōng wán*) is Major Chest Bind Decoction (*dà xiàn xiōng tāng*) with mirabilite (*máng xiāo*), apricot kernel (*xìng rén*), and honey (*bái mì*). Rhubarb (*dà huáng*) and mirabilite (*máng xiāo*) drain heat, break binds, and flush phlegm. Kansui (*gān suì*) harshly expels water-rheum and breaks binds. These are the most important ingredients in the formula. Tingli (*tíng lì zǐ*) drains the lungs and apricot kernel (*xìng rén*) disinhibits the lungs. These two ingredients open and course the lungs. When the upper source of the water is free, the water bound in the chest will be able to flow down and out. This phenomenon is similar to what occurs if one punches a hole in a can and turns it upside down. The liquid will not flow out until a hole is opened in the top of the can. The lungs, water's upper source, must be open for the water to flow out through the lower burner. This method of treatment later became formally known as "lifting the pot and removing the lid" (提壶揭盖 *tí hú jiē gài*).

In the text the reader is told that both chest bind and glomus may result from the inappropriate use of precipitation. It should be noted that these two signs may also occur in the absence of mistreatment.

4.10.1.2 Major Chest Bind Decoction Patterns

LINE 134

(一) 太阳病，脉浮而动数，浮则为风，数则为热，动则为痛，数则为虚，头痛发热，微盗汗出，而反恶寒者，表未解也。(二) 医反下之，动数变迟，膈内拒痛，胃中空虚，客气动膈，短气躁烦，心中懊侬，阳气内陷，心下因硬，则为结胸，大陷胸汤主之。(三) 若不结胸，但头汗出，余处无汗，剂颈而还，小便不利，身必发黄。

(1) *Tài yáng bìng, mài fú ér dòng shuò, fú zé wéi fēng, shuò zé wéi rè, dòng zé wéi tòng, shuò zé wéi xū, tóu tòng fā rè, wēi dào hàn chū, ér fǎn wù hán zhě, biǎo wèi jiě yě.* (2) *Yī fǎn xià zhī, dòng shuò biàn chí, gé nèi jù tòng, wèi zhōng kōng xū, kè qì dòng gé, duǎn qì zào fán, xīn zhōng ào nóng, yáng qì nèi xiàn, xīn xià yīn yìng, zé wéi jié xiōng, dà xiàn xiōng tāng zhǔ zhī.* (3) *Ruò bù jié xiōng, dàn tóu hàn chū, yú chù wú hàn, jì jǐng ěr huán, xiǎo biàn bù lì, shēn bì fā huáng.*

(1) In greater yáng disease, when the pulse is floating, stirred,[1] and rapid, floating means wind, rapid means heat, stirred means pain, and rapid means vacuity. [There is] headache, heat effusion, mild night sweating, and yet aversion to cold, [because] the exterior has not yet resolved. (2) But the physician uses precipitation and the movement and rapidity [of the pulse] changes to slowness. In the diaphragm [there is] pain that refuses [pressure]. [With] empty vacuity in the stomach,[2] visiting qì[3] stirs the diaphragm and [there is] shortness of breath, vexation and agitation, and anguish in the heart. The yáng qì[4] falls inward and causes hardness below the heart, which means chest bind; [therefore,] Major Chest Bind Decoction (*dà xiàn xiōng tāng*) governs. (3) If [there is] no chest bind, only sweat issuing from the head—and without sweat elsewhere—that stops at the neck, and urination is inhibited, there will be generalized yellowing.

Text Notes

1. The pulse is ... stirred, 脉动 *mài dòng*: The pulse is moving irregularly. This pulse is not the same as the modern stirred pulse, 动脉 *dòng mài* (a pulse that is forceful, rapid, and slippery, like a bean that is bobbing).
2. Visiting qì, 客气 *kè qì*: A term for an exterior evil that emphasizes its entry into the body from the exterior.
3. Empty vacuity in the stomach, 胃中空虚 *wèi zhōng kōng xū*: Vacuity of the stomach qì resulting from inappropriate precipitation. When this term is used, it is followed by the term "visiting qì," indicating that damage to the center burner qì allows an exterior evil to invade the region of the diaphragm.
4. Yáng qì, 阳气 *yáng qì*: Here, an exterior evil that is yáng in nature.

Formula

Major Chest Bind Decoction (*dà xiàn xiōng tāng*)

∘ Harshly attack water-rheum; discharge heat and break binds.

大黄六两（去皮） 芒消一升 甘遂一钱匕

㈠ 右三味，以水六升，先煮大黄取二升，去滓，内芒消，煮一两沸，内甘遂末，温服一升。㈡ 得快利，止后服。

Dà huáng liù liǎng (qù pí) máng xiāo yī shēng gān suì yī qián bǐ

(1) *Yòu sān wèi, yǐ shuǐ liù shēng, xiān zhǔ dà huáng qǔ èr shēng, qù zǐ, nà máng xiāo, zhǔ yī liǎng fèi, nà gān suì mò, wēn fú yī shēng.* (2) *Dé kuài lì, zhǐ hòu fú.*

rhubarb (大黄 *dà huáng*, Rhei Rhizoma) 6 liǎng (remove skin)
mirabilite (芒硝 *máng xiāo*, Mirabilitum) 1 shēng
kansui (甘遂 *gān suì*, Kansui Radix) 1 qián-spoonful

(1) [For] the above three ingredients use six shēng of water. First boil rhubarb (*dà huáng*) to get two shēng. Remove the dregs and add mirabilite (*máng xiāo*). Bring to a boil once or twice. Add kansui (*gān suì*) powder and take one shēng warm. (2) As soon as diarrhea occurs, stop taking [the decoction].

Synopsis

The signs and treatment of the pattern in which the inappropriate use of precipitation in an exterior pattern causes chest bind and yellowing.

Commentary

In greater yáng disease one often finds a pulse that is floating, and as this line explains, a pulse that is floating indicates a wind evil. Furthermore, a pulse that is rapid indicates heat. Zhāng Jī explains that a pulse that is stirred indicates pain, which may refer to the generalized pain that commonly occurs in externally contracted diseases. He also states, "rapidity means vacuity." This clause, however, is omitted in the *Yī Zōng Jīn Jiàn* because of questions regarding its authorship and difficulty in understanding its meaning, since a pulse that is rapid generally indicates the presence of heat. Nonetheless, a pulse that is rapid can be found in vacuous patients or when a repletion evil is absent in the interior, as is suggested by the authors of *Gāo Děng Zhōng Yī Yán Jiū Cān Kǎo Cóng Shū*; therefore, this omission appears unnecessary.

It is clear that heat evil is present in the exterior and the appearance of headache and heat effusion reinforces this idea. Mild night sweating, however, is also present and is more indicative of an internal pattern in which yīn has been damaged. Zhāng Jī attempts to clarify this by adding "... yet aversion to cold." The presence of aversion to cold indicates an exterior condition. The night sweating can be understood to be the result of two factors: the constitution of the patient and the strength of the evil. At night, the defensive yáng should move into yīn. When the defensive yáng enters yīn, the exterior is less secure. If the defensive yáng is weak and/or the exterior evil is very strong, the decreased security of the exterior may result in sweating.

Precipitation should not normally be used when an exterior pattern exists and in this case inappropriate treatment causes the evil to fall inward, giving rise to chest bind in which heat evil binds with water evil in the chest and the center burner. This congestion impairs the qì dynamic, which causes the pulse to become slow. Here, the pulse is slow not because of internal cold but because of congestion. The impairment of the qì dynamic also results in pain in the region of the diaphragm. The diaphragm is invaded by visiting qì because it has become vacuous. This vacuity is the result of damage from inappropriate precipitation. This damage is indicated by the phrase, "empty vacuity in the stomach." Damage in the center burner impairs the movement of qì. When qì movement is impaired, the chest, which is the sea of qì, cannot receive and disperse qì normally and the breath becomes short. Agitation and vexation with anguish in the heart are the result of heat binding with water evil and harassing the heart. Finally, hardness below the heart is an important sign, commonly seen in cases of chest bind. It is a concrete indication that heat evil has fallen inward and become bound with a water or phlegm evil in the region of the chest, diaphragm, and center burner. Major Chest Bind Decoction (*dà xiàn xiōng tāng*) is the treatment of choice for chest bind.

If the evil falls inward but does not cause chest bind, it may combine with damp evil in the center burner. Because it is a heat evil, sweat would normally issue, as the heat moved outward, but when it combines with damp evil, the strength of the heat is reduced and sweat only issues from the head. The damp evil, normally discharged through the urine, combines with the heat and urination becomes inhibited. The damp-heat steams in the interior and produces generalized yellowing.

Major Chest Bind Decoction (*dà xiàn xiōng tāng*) is an extremely harsh and fierce formula. Rhubarb (*dà huáng*) drains heat and flushes repletion, and mirabilite (*máng xiāo*) breaks binds. These two ingredients drain bound heat from the chest and heart. Kansui (*gān suì*) is a harsh agent that drains water and expels rheum. This formula harshly attacks bound water-rheum evil. Since it can easily damage right qì, as soon as the patient experiences diarrhea ingestion of the formula should be stopped.

LINE 135

伤寒六七日，结胸热实，脉沉而紧，心下痛，按之石硬者，大陷胸汤主之。

Shāng hán liù qī rì, jié xiōng rè shí, mài chén ér jǐn, xīn xià tòng, àn zhī shí yìng zhě, dà xiàn xiōng tāng zhǔ zhī.

When in cold damage [that has lasted for] six or seven days, [there is] chest bind heat repletion,* in which the pulse is sunken and tight and [there is] pain below the heart, which is stone-hard when pressure is applied, Major Chest Bind Decoction (*dà xiàn xiōng tāng*) governs.

TEXT NOTE

* Chest bind heat repletion, 胸结热实 *xiōng jié rè shí*: Compare with cold repletion chest bind in line 141B, p. 223.

SYNOPSIS

The primary pulse and signs of major chest bind.

COMMENTARY

This pattern is an example of chest bind that occurs without inappropriate precipitation. The transmutation from cold damage to chest bind, over a period of six or seven days, may be the result of the patient's constitution or a strong exterior evil. In previous discussions of chest bind it has been mentioned that a distinction is made between heat and cold patterns. Here, Zhāng Jī explicitly tells the reader that this pattern is chest bind heat repletion. The three signs—a pulse that is sunken and tight, pain below the heart, and stonelike hardness—are the basic characteristics of chest bind. A pulse that is sunken indicates interior disease and congestion. A pulse that is tight indicates repletion and pain. Pain below the heart is the result of congestion in the local area. This congestion occurs because of the heat evil and the water or phlegm that become bound between the heart and the diaphragm. The area below the heart is stone-like when pressure is applied, reflecting the repletion present in this pattern. Major Chest Bind Decoction (*dà xiàn xiōng tāng*), which drains heat, expels water, and breaks binds, is the appropriate formula for this pattern.

LINE 136

伤寒十余日，热结在里，复往来寒热者，与大柴胡汤；但结胸，无大热者，此为水结在胸胁也，但头微汗出者，大陷胸汤主之。

Shāng hán shí yú rì, rè jié zài lǐ, fù wǎng lái hán rè zhě, yǔ dà chái hú tāng; dàn jié xiōng, wú dà rè zhě, cǐ wéi shuǐ jié zài xiōng xié yě, dàn tóu wēi hàn chū zhě, dà xiàn xiōng tāng zhǔ zhī.

When cold damage [has lasted for] more than ten days, [and] heat binds in the interior, yet [there is] alternating [aversion to] cold and heat [effusion],* give Major Bupleurum Decoction (*dà chái hú tāng*); if [there is] only chest bind and great heat [effusion] is absent, indicating water bind in the chest and rib-side, and slight sweat issuing only from the head, Major Chest Bind Decoction (*dà xiàn xiōng tāng*) governs.

Text Note

* Alternating [aversion to] cold and heat [effusion], 往来寒热 *wǎng lái hán rè*: Alternating appearance of aversion to cold and heat effusion. When one is present, the other is absent. In this pattern, the two signs are clearly differentiated, but do not exhibit a set periodicity. See line 96, p. 410, for further discussion of this sign in lesser yáng disease.

Synopsis

Comparing and distinguishing between the patterns of lesser yáng internal repletion and major chest bind.

Commentary

In cold damage that has persisted for more than ten days, it is possible that the evil will shift into the interior and transform into heat. In this line we are told that the heat binds in the interior, but alternating aversion to cold and heat effusion is also present; this combination of signs indicates yáng brightness and lesser yáng combination disease. It is possible that these signs would be accompanied by retching, glomus below the heart, or fullness under the rib-side. Major Bupleurum Decoction (*dà chái hú tāng*) resolves both yáng brightness and lesser yáng disease. (For a full discussion of this formula, see line 103, p. 431.)

In the second part of the line only chest bind is present; no other signs are observed. Great heat is absent and one may assume the absence of alternating aversion to cold and heat effusion. Chest bind is a pattern of heat and water evil bound together. In this case Zhāng Jī emphasizes that the water bind is the most important aspect. The binding together of water and heat impairs the movement of fluids. The fluids cannot outthrust, so no sweat issues over most of the body and sweat only issues slightly from the head. One should use Major Chest Bind Decoction (*dà xiàn xiōng tāng*) to clear heat, expel water, and break binds.

Line 137

太阳病，重发汗而复下之，不大便五六日，舌上燥而渴，日晡所小有潮热，从心下至少腹硬满而痛不可近者，大陷胸汤主之。

Tài yáng bìng, chóng fā hàn ér fù xià zhī, bù dà biàn wǔ liù rì, shé shàng zào ér kě, rì bū suǒ xiǎo yǒu cháo rè, cóng xīn xià zhì shào fù yìng mǎn ér tòng bù kě jìn zhě, dà xiàn xiōng tāng zhǔ zhī.

When in greater yáng disease, sweating is promoted repeatedly, yet precipitation is [also used] and [there is] inability to defecate for five or six days, a dry tongue and thirst, minor tidal heat effusion[1] in the late afternoon,[2] and hardness, fullness, and pain, [extending] from below the heart to the lesser abdomen and [which the person will] not allow [anyone even to get] near,[3] Major Chest Bind Decoction (*dà xiàn xiōng tāng*) governs.

TEXT NOTES

1. Tidal heat effusion, 潮热 *cháo rè*: A feeling of heat that occurs at set intervals and may or may not be accompanied by palpable heat effusion. See line 220, p. 336, for further explanation.
2. Late afternoon, 日晡所 *rì bū suǒ*: The period of time approaching the evening, which includes both the ninth and tenth earthly branches, approximately 3–7 P.M.
3. Pain ... [which the person will] not allow [anyone even to get] near, 痛不可近 *tòng bù kě jìn*: Severe pain that is exacerbated by pressure. The patient refuses any attempts to palpate the area.

SYNOPSIS

Distinguishing between the patterns of chest bind and yáng brightness bowel repletion.

COMMENTARY

Although the promotion of sweating is appropriate in greater yáng disease, repeated promotion of sweating is generally not appropriate. It is also clearly not appropriate to follow it with precipitation. Repeated promotion of sweating damages the fluids and precipitation causes the evil to fall inward. Water and heat bind in the interior and yáng brightness internal repletion is present. Damage to the fluids impairs normal fluid movement, as does the congestion present in chest bind. The stomach becomes dry, producing thirst, inability to defecate, and a dry tongue. Heat in the yáng brightness results in mild tidal heat effusion, which means that this pattern may be slightly different from a yáng brightness bowel repletion pattern. The presence of bound heat and water is demonstrated by hardness and fullness in the entire abdominal region. Major Chest Bind Decoction (*dà xiàn xiōng tāng*) expels water evils, clears heat, and breaks binds.

As was stated above, this pattern is similar to, but not the same as, a yáng brightness bowel repletion pattern. In the pattern above, chest bind is present in the region of the chest and diaphragm, whereas in bowel repletion, the repletion heat is in the stomach and intestines. Tidal heat effusion occurs in bowel repletion and it is not generally mild, as it is here. The area of fullness and hardness described above includes the entire region from just below the heart down to the lower abdomen; in bowel repletion the pain and fullness is around the umbilicus and in the abdomen. Furthermore, the pain described here is much more severe than that which is described in bowel repletion patterns.

Line 132

结胸证，其脉浮大者，不可下，下之则死。

Jié xiōng zhèng, qí mài fú dà zhě, bù kě xià, xià zhī zé sǐ.

When in chest bind patterns, the pulse is floating and large, one cannot precipitate, [because] precipitation will lead to death.

Synopsis

In chest bind patterns, when the pulse is floating and large, the use of offensive precipitation is contraindicated.

Commentary

The pulse in chest bind patterns is generally sunken, replete, and forceful, but here it is floating and large. The pulse may be large and forceful or large and forceless. In either case one should not precipitate. A pulse that is floating indicates the presence of an exterior evil even though an evil has also fallen inward causing the chest bind. If the pulse is floating, large, and forceless, it indicates vacuity of right qì and exuberance of evil qì. Fāng Yǒu-Zhí writes:

> Floating means [an evil] in the exterior. Large means vacuity. The contention between floating and vacuity means that an exterior [evil] is present and has not yet completely entered the interior. One knows that the interior [evil] is not yet completely replete. Precipitation will result in the vacuous interior qì deserting and the exterior evil that has not yet been eliminated falling inward.

If one precipitates, the vacuous right qì will be further damaged. When vacuous right qì is made more vacuous, it may result in death.

The other possibility is that the pulse is large and forceful, indicating internal repletion. If the pulse is floating, large, and forceful, one must first resolve the exterior and then precipitate the interior. If precipitation is used first, it will cause the exterior evil to fall inward and exacerbate the chest bind.

Line 133

结胸证悉具，烦躁者亦死。

Jié xiōng zhèng xī jù, fán zào zhě yì sǐ.

When all the signs of chest bind* are present, and [there is] vexation and agitation, [the patient will] die.

Text Note

* The signs of chest bind, 结胸证 *jié xiōng zhèng*: An area of pain below the heart that is hard when pressed. In severe cases, hardness, fullness, and pain in the area between the heart and the lesser abdomen, accompanied by no stool, dry tongue with thirst, and tidal heat effusion in the evening.

Synopsis

The identification of the prognosis in chest bind patterns.

Commentary

Previously, in line 134, p. 215, vexation and agitation is presented as a possible sign in cases of chest bind and it does not necessarily indicate a fatal condition. Here Zhāng Jī writes that if the major signs of chest bind are present and one also sees vexation and agitation, the patient will die. This apparent contradiction can be reconciled by considering mild and severe disease patterns. Here we are told that vexation and agitation is a critical sign of a fatal condition. This pattern is more serious than the one presented in line 134, p. 215. The bound evil is lodged deep within the chest and the right qì has been severely damaged. One hesitates to precipitate because right qì is already debilitated, but without treatment the bound evil will restrict the movement of qì and cause further damage. Neither option is acceptable and the situation will easily become critical.

4.10.1.3 Minor Chest Bind Decoction Patterns

Line 138

小结胸病，正在心下，按之则痛，脉浮滑者，小陷胸汤主之。

Xiǎo jié xiōng bìng, zhèng zài xīn xià, àn zhī zé tòng, mài fú huá zhě, xiǎo xiàn xiōng tāng zhǔ zhī.

When in minor chest bind disease, [the location is] directly below the heart* and painful when pressure is applied, and the pulse is floating and slippery, Minor Chest Bind Decoction (*xiǎo xiàn xiōng tāng*) governs.

Text Note

* Directly below the heart 正在心下 *zhèng zài xīn xià*: In minor chest bind, the disease is localized to the area directly below the heart, whereas in major chest bind, the location may be in the chest, below the heart, or extending from the chest down into the lesser abdomen.

Formula

Minor Chest Bind Decoction (*xiǎo xiàn xiōng tāng*)

- Clear heat, flush phlegm, and open binds.

黄连一两　半夏半升（洗）　栝楼实大者一枚

右三味，以水六升，先煮栝楼，取三升，去滓，内诸药，煮取二升，去滓，分温三服。

Huáng lián yī liǎng　bàn xià bàn shēng (xǐ)　guā lóu shí dà zhě yī méi

Yòu sān wèi, yǐ shuǐ liù shēng, xiān zhǔ guā lóu, qǔ sān shēng, qù zǐ, nà zhū yào, zhǔ qǔ èr shēng, qù zǐ, fēn wēn sān fú.

coptis (黄连 *huáng lián*, Coptidis Rhizoma) 1 liǎng
pinellia (半夏 *bàn xià*, Pinelliae Tuber) half shēng (washed)
trichosanthes fruit (栝楼实 *guā lóu shí*, Trichosanthis Fructus) 1 large fruit*

[For] the above three ingredients use six shēng of water. First boil trichosanthes (*guā lóu*) to get three shēng. Remove the dregs and add all [the other] ingredients. Boil to get two shēng and remove the dregs. Separate into three doses and take warm.

Formula Note

* One large fruit: The authors of *Gāo Děng Zhōng Yī Yán Jiū Cān Kǎo Cóng Shū* write that this is approximately 20 grams, but because of variety in the size of the fruit any exact gram measure can only be an approximation.

Synopsis

The signs and treatment of minor chest bind.

Commentary

Minor chest bind is similar to, but milder than, major chest bind. Like major chest bind it is the result of an exterior evil falling inward, either spontaneously or as the result of inappropriate treatment. In minor chest bind the affected area is smaller than in major chest bind, involving only the area directly below the heart. Whereas in major chest bind the pain is severe with or without pressure, in minor chest bind, pain only occurs when pressure is applied. The pulse in minor chest bind is floating and slippery. Floating means a yáng evil whose location is more superficial, when compared with a pulse that is sunken, as in major chest bind. Slippery means that whereas in major chest bind, water evil is present, in minor chest bind, heat and phlegm evil predominate.

Minor Chest Bind Decoction (*xiǎo xiàn xiōng tāng*) clears heat, flushes phlegm, and opens binds. This formula opens with acridity and downbears with bitterness. Bitter, cold coptis (*huáng lián*) drains heat bind from the region of the heart. Acrid, warm pinellia (*bàn xià*) flushes phlegm-rheum. Sweet, cold trichosanthes fruit (*guā lóu shí*) flushes heat and phlegm and conducts turbid phlegm downwards. It also assists coptis (*huáng lián*) in clearing heat and pinellia (*bàn xià*) in both transforming phlegm and opening binds.

4.10.2 Cold Repletion Chest Bind Patterns

Line 141B

...寒实结胸，无热证者，与三物小陷胸汤，白散亦可服。

... *Hán shí jié xiōng, wú rè zhèng zhě, yǔ sān wù xiǎo xiàn xiōng tāng, bái sàn yì kě fú.*

... When in cold repletion chest bind, heat signs [are] absent, give Three Agents Minor Chest Bind Decoction (*sān wù xiǎo xiàn xiōng tāng*). White Powder (*bái sǎn*) can also be taken.*

Text Note

* Give Three Agents Minor Chest Bind Decoction (*sān wù xiǎo xiàn xiōng tāng*). White Powder (*bái sǎn*) can also be taken, 与三物小陷胸汤，白散亦可服 *yǔ sān wù xiǎo xiàn xiōng tāng, bái sǎn yì kě fú*: According to the *Qiān Jīn Yì Fāng* and the *Jīn Guì Yù Hán Jīng* (金匮玉函经 "The Canon of the Golden Coffer and Jade Sheath"), this line should appear as "give Three Agents White Powder (*sān wù bái sǎn*). This opinion is generally accepted.

Formula

Three Agents White Powder (*sān wù bái sǎn*)

○ Warm and expel cold evil; flush phlegm and break binds.

桔梗三分　巴豆一分（去皮心，熬黑，研如脂）　贝母三分

(一) 右三味，为散，内巴豆，更于臼中杵之，以白饮和服，强人半钱匕，羸者减之。(二) 病在膈上必吐，在膈下必利。(三) 不利，进热粥一杯；利过不止，进冷粥一杯。

Jié gěng sān fēn　bā dòu yī fēn (qù pí xīn, áo hēi, yán rú zhī)　bèi mǔ sān fēn

(1) *Yòu sān wèi, wéi sǎn, nà bā dòu, gèng yú jiù zhōng chǔ zhī, yǐ bái yǐn huò fú, qiáng rén bàn qián bǐ, léi zhě jiǎn zhī.* (2) *Bìng zài gé shàng bì tù, zài gé xià bì lì.* (3) *Bù lì, jìn rè zhōu yī bēi; lì guò bù zhǐ, jìn lěng zhōu yī bēi.*

platycodon (桔梗 *jié gěng*, Platycodonis Radix) 3 fēn

croton frost (巴豆霜 *bā dòu shuāng*, Crotonis Seminis Pulvis) 1 fēn (remove skin and center, dry-fry [until] black, grind [to make] like fat)

fritillaria (贝母 *bèi mǔ*, Fritillariae Bulbus) 3 fēn

(1) [For] the above three ingredients, [make] into powder. Croton (*bā dòu*) [should] be pounded again in a mortar. Mix into a white [rice] decoction and take. Strong people [may take] a half qián-spoonful. For thin and weak [people], reduce [the dosage]. (2) [If] the disease is above the diaphragm, there will be vomiting. [If] it is below the diaphragm, there will be diarrhea. (3) [If there is] no diarrhea, drink one cup of hot gruel. [If there is] incessant diarrhea, drink one cup of cold gruel.

Synopsis

The signs and treatment of cold repletion chest bind.

Commentary

Cold repletion chest bind is the result of a cold evil falling into the chest and binding with phlegm-rheum. The signs are similar to those of heat repletion chest bind, except no signs of heat such as thirst, dry tongue, or vexation are present. The cold evil bound in the chest causes stagnation of the chest yáng, disinhibits the qì dynamic, and impairs the dissemination of fluids; consequently, one may also see signs such as fear of cold and liking warmth, cough, shortness of breath, or difficult defecation. Because cold repletion chest bind is a repletion pattern, the pulse is generally sunken, tight, and forceful.

Three Agents White Powder (*sān wù bái sǎn*) warms and expels cold evil, flushes phlegm, and breaks binds. The chief ingredient in the formula is acrid, hot, and toxic croton (*bā dòu*), which attacks and expels cold and water, drains cold accumulations downward, and breaks binds. Fritillaria (*bèi mǔ*) resolves depression, opens binds, and eliminates phlegm. Platycodon (*jié gěng*) opens the lung qì, disinhibits the lung, dissipates binds, and eliminates phlegm. It also conducts the other ingredients upward so the effect is strongest in the area of the bind. Because this is a harsh formula it is taken with a white rice soup in order to protect the stomach qì. Depending on the location of the chest bind, different reactions to the formula may be observed. If the location is higher, above the diaphragm, the evil will be expelled through vomiting. If the evil is located lower, below the diaphragm, it will be drained through diarrhea. This formula is hot, but if it is not hot enough to break the cold bind, hot gruel may be taken to strengthen the formula. On the other hand, if ingestion of the formula results in incessant diarrhea, cold gruel may be taken to reduce stomach and intestinal heat engendered by the formula.

4.11 STOREHOUSE BIND PATTERNS

Storehouse bind transmuted patterns belong to yīn, cold, and vacuity. They are characterized by hardness, fullness, and pain below the heart, diarrhea, and other signs of vacuity cold. These patterns are difficult to treat and the prognosis for patients is poor.

LINE 129

㈠ 何谓藏结？㈡ 答曰：如结胸状，饮食如故，时时下利，寸脉浮，关脉小细沉紧，名曰藏结。㈢ 舌上白胎滑者，难治。

(1) *Hé wèi zàng jié?* (2) *Dá yuē: rú jié xiōng zhuàng, yǐn shí rú gù, shí shí xià lì, cùn mài fú, guān mài xiǎo xì chén jǐn, míng yuē zàng jié.* (3) *Shé shàng bái tāi huá zhě, nán zhì.*

(1) What is storehouse bind? (2) Answer: [When there are] signs like chest bind, eating and drinking are normal,[1] [and there is] frequent diarrhea, an inch pulse that is floating, and a bar pulse that is small, fine, sunken, and tight, it is called storehouse bind. (3) When the tongue fur is white and glossy,[2] this [pattern] is difficult to treat.

TEXT NOTES

1. Eating and drinking are normal, 饮食如故 *yǐn shí rú gù*: The patient's intake of food and drink is normal.
2. The tongue fur is white and glossy, 舌上白胎滑 *shé shàng bái tāi huá*: In this phrase, the character 胎 *tāi*, which means fetus or birth, has been substituted for the standard character used for the tongue fur, 苔 *tāi*.

SYNOPSIS

The pulse, signs, and prognosis of storehouse bind.

COMMENTARY

Storehouse bind and chest bind share some common signs, so Zhāng Jī uses one to explain the other. In chest bind the pain and hardness below the heart may extend down into the abdomen. In storehouse bind the pain and fullness is under the rib-side and/or the abdomen, but the basic similarity between the two patterns ends there. Chest bind occurs when heat evil falls inward and binds with water and/or phlegm in the center and upper burners. In storehouse bind the viscera are vacuous and yáng is debilitated. A yīn cold evil exploits the vacuity and binds in the viscera.

A patient with storehouse bind is able to eat and drink normally, whereas with chest bind the feelings of congestion in the center and upper burners may lead to decreased food intake. Yīn cold bind in the viscera and yáng vacuity is reflected in frequent diarrhea, a sign of storehouse bind; in chest bind, however, if the stool is abnormal it will probably be bound or difficult. Cold in the center burner and debilitation of the yáng qì is also suggested by the bar pulse, which is small, fine, sunken, and tight. The inch pulse is floating, indicating that the evil entered the body from the exterior, another similarity with chest bind. This similarity also illustrates the importance of considering the patient's constitution. When an exterior evil falls inward in a patient who is strong, it may cause chest bind, but if an evil falls inward in a patient who has yáng vacuity, it may cause storehouse bind. Storehouse bind is much more difficult to treat. Bound cold and congealed yīn humor are reflected in the white and glossy tongue fur.

Storehouse bind is difficult to treat because one should attack the bound evil in the interior, but the patient is weak and yáng is vacuous. One cannot attack for fear of causing further debilitation, and one cannot supplement for fear of strengthening the bound evil.

LINE 130

藏结无阳证，不往来寒热，其人反静，舌上胎滑者，不可攻也。

Zàng jié wú yáng zhèng, bù wǎng lái hán rè, qí rén fǎn jìng, shé shàng tāi huá zhě, bù kě gōng yě.

When in storehouse bind, yáng signs[1] [are] absent, [and there is no] alternating [aversion to] cold and heat [effusion], but the person is tranquil and the tongue fur is glossy, one cannot attack.[2]

TEXT NOTES

1. Yáng signs, 阳证 *yáng zhèng*: Signs of heat and/or exterior disease.
2. Attack, 攻 *gōng*: Here, precipitation.

Synopsis

A further description of the signs and treatment contraindications of the storehouse bind pattern.

Commentary

Storehouse bind occurs when yīn cold binds in the viscera of patients whose yáng qì is debilitated. Yáng signs—including heat effusion alternating with aversion to cold, and vexation and agitation—are absent. The absence of yáng signs means the absence of a greater yáng pattern. Alternating aversion to cold and heat effusion are absent, suggesting that this pattern does not belong to the lesser yáng. The patient is tranquil, without vexation and agitation, indicating that this is not a yáng brightness pattern. A white, glossy tongue fur reflects the presence of bound yīn cold in the interior. As in the previous line, in a patient with yáng debilitation and bound yīn cold, one cannot attack.

Although Zhāng Jī does not suggest any formulae for treating storehouse bind, later commentators have suggested Center-Rectifying Decoction (*lǐ zhōng tāng*) plus unripe bitter orange (*zhǐ shí*). Center-Rectifying Decoction (*lǐ zhōng tāng*) warms the center and supplements yáng, while unripe bitter orange (*zhǐ shí*) breaks qì and dissipates binds.

Line 167

病胁下素有痞，连在脐傍，痛引少腹，入阴筋者，此名藏结，死。

Bìng xié xià sù yǒu pǐ, lián zài qí páng, tòng yǐn shào fù, rù yīn jīn zhě, cǐ míng zàng jié, sǐ.

An illness in which usually glomus under the rib-side extends to the side of the umbilicus, [but now] the pain stretches into the lesser abdomen and enters the yīn sinew* is called storehouse bind and [bodes] death.

Text Note

* Yīn sinew, 阴筋 *yīn jīn*: The penis.

Synopsis

The critical signs of storehouse bind.

Commentary

This line presents a variation of storehouse bind. Here, without mistreatment the patient has glomus under the rib-side, extending to the side of the umbilicus. This is an abiding ailment that should be viewed differently than a new external contraction. In abiding ailments, the original qì becomes vacuous and right qì cannot restrain invading evil. The invading evil exacerbates the original stagnation and a bind forms. The increased stagnation and bind produces pain that extends into the lesser abdomen, and that when severe, enters the yīn sinew (penis). At this point, yīn cold is extreme and yáng qì is expiring; therefore, this pattern cannot be treated.

4.12 GLOMUS PATTERNS

Glomus is a localized subjective feeling of fullness and blockage, and in the *Shāng Hán Lùn* it generally develops as a result of inappropriate precipitation causing heat evil to fall inward and bind with a formless evil in the interior, impairing the qì dynamic. A glomus pattern may also occur when vacuous stomach qì is exploited by a heat evil. The pathomechanism producing glomus can be seen as a direct result of an evil in the interior or the presence of an evil impairing the qì dynamic. Both processes probably play a role in the production of this sign pattern. These patterns involve a formless evil; therefore, the area of congestion below the heart is soft and pain is absent. Generally, one of the five Heart-Draining Decoctions (*xiè xīn tāng*) is used to treat these patterns. Any exterior pattern should be resolved before a glomus pattern is treated.

Glomus patterns are divided into category by the type of glomus and the appropriate formula. The main categories are heat glomus, cold-heat complex glomus, water glomus, and phlegm glomus.

a) Rhubarb and Coptis Heart-Draining Decoction (*dà huáng huáng lián xiè xīn tāng*) treats heat glomus in which heat evil congests the qì dynamic. This pattern is characterized by a glomus below the heart that is soft when pressed. The pulse may be floating and the tongue fur may be yellow. Heart vexation is also commonly present. This formula clears heat and drains glomus.

b) In Aconite Heart-Draining Decoction (*fù zǐ xiè xīn tāng*) patterns, a heat glomus is present and the exterior yáng is insufficient. In addition to glomus below the heart, there is aversion to cold and sweating. This formula supports yáng and drains glomus.

c) The glomus treated with Pinellia Heart-Draining Decoction (*bàn xià xiè xīn tāng*) is often the product of inappropriate precipitation used in lesser yáng disease, which not only causes a glomus, but also causes counterflow ascent of stomach qì. It is a cold-heat complex glomus pattern in which the glomus below the heart is soft, not painful, and accompanied by retching counterflow and diarrhea. This formula harmonizes the stomach and downbears counterflow, and opens binds and disperses glomus.

d) Stomach vacuity food stagnation and water-rheum can give rise to a glomus pattern characterized by a hard glomus below the heart, dry belching with food malodor, water qì under the rib-side, and intestinal rumbling and diarrhea. Fresh Ginger Heart-Draining Decoction (*shēng jiāng xiè xīn tāng*) is used to harmonize the stomach, dissipate rheum, and disperse glomus.

e) When inappropriate precipitation is used repeatedly and the stomach qì becomes severely vacuous, the appropriate formula is Licorice Heart-Draining Decoction (*gān cǎo xiè xīn tāng*), which supplements the center, harmonizes the stomach, and disperses glomus. In this pattern visiting qì ascends counterflow and gives rise to a hard glomus below the heart that is accompanied by local fullness. Other signs that may be observed include diarrhea and intestinal rumbling, dry retching, and heart vexation.

Although the five patterns above are the most common glomus patterns, other glomus patterns exist that are not treated with these five formulae. These patterns are discussed below:

a) Water amassment in the lower burner can give rise to a glomus pattern in which along with a glomus below the heart, other signs such as thirst, vexation and agitation, and inhibited urination are also present. This pattern is treated with Poria (Hoelen) Five Powder (*wǔ líng sǎn*) to transform qì, disinhibit water, and disperse glomus.
b) Inula and Hematite Decoction (*xuán fù dài zhě tāng*), which harmonizes the stomach, downbears counterflow, and flushes rheum, is used for glomus that occurs after the promotion of sweating, the use of precipitation, or the use of vomiting. In this pattern stomach qì is vacuous and turbid qì ascends counterflow. The main signs are hard glomus below the heart and belching.
c) In the Halloysite and Limonite Decoction (*chì shí zhī yǔ yú liáng tāng*) glomus pattern, a hard glomus below the heart is accompanied by incessant diarrhea. This pattern is glomus and efflux desertion; therefore, the main action of this formula is to secure and astringe the lower burner.

Line 151

脉浮而紧，而复下之，紧反入里，则作痞，按之自濡，但气痞耳。

Mài fú ér jǐn, ér fù xià zhī, jǐn fǎn rù lǐ, zé zuò pǐ, àn zhī zì rú, dàn qì pǐ ěr.

[When] the pulse is floating and tight, yet precipitation is used, the tightness instead enters the interior[1] and makes a glomus, which when pressed is soft. It is only a qì glomus.[2]

Text Notes

1. The tightness instead enters the interior, 紧反入里 *jǐn fǎn rù lǐ*: Here, "tightness," does not denote a pulse quality, but is used metonymically to refer to cold, the evil indicated by a tight pulse; hence the phrase is taken to mean that the cold evil falls inward following the inappropriate use of precipitation.
2. Qì glomus, 气痞 *qì pǐ*: A qì glomus is soft and full, but not painful. This type of glomus results from congestion of the qì dynamic.

Synopsis

The causes and distinguishing signs of glomus.

Commentary

A pulse that is floating and tight usually indicates greater yáng cold damage; therefore, it is appropriate to promote sweating. Zhāng Jī writes that here, precipitation has instead been used; he uses the word "yet" 复 *fù*, to mean that this is not the correct treatment. That is, the physician observes a pulse indicative of exterior disease, but uses a treatment that is appropriate only when an exterior pattern is absent.

The use of precipitation damages the qì of the spleen and stomach. A formless evil exploits this weakness and falls inward, binding below the heart. The term "formless evil" is used because in these cases of glomus no water or phlegm evil binds with the exterior evil, as in chest bind. Pain and hardness are absent, confirming that this is not chest bind. Instead, a soft glomus is present, the manifestation of a formless evil binding in the interior when precipitation has damaged the center burner qì and impaired the qì dynamic. Normal upbearing and downbearing cannot occur and the qì becomes congested in the center burner.

Glomus may occur in the absence of mistreatment in people who have vacuity of the spleen and stomach. In these people, glomus may occur spontaneously or following the contraction of an external evil.

4.12.1 Heat Glomus Patterns

4.12.1.1 Rhubarb and Coptis Heart-Draining Decoction Patterns

LINE 154

心下痞，按之濡，其脉关上浮者，大黄黄连泻心汤主之。

Xīn xià pǐ, àn zhī rú, qí mài guān shàng fú zhě, dà huáng huáng lián xiè xīn tāng zhǔ zhī.

When there is a glomus below the heart that is soft when pressure is applied, and the pulse is floating on the bar,* Rhubarb and Coptis Heart-Draining Decoction (*dà huáng huáng lián xiè xīn tāng*) governs.

TEXT NOTE

* The pulse is floating on the bar, 脉关上浮 *mài guān shàng fú*: The pulse is floating only in the bar position. Qián Huáng comments, "[In the expression] "the pulse is floating on the bar," "floating" means a yáng evil, and floating governs the upper [burner]. The bar [position] means the center burner. The inch [position] means the upper burner. Because the evil is in the center burner, [the pulse] is floating on the bar." This term is thought to have been created by Zhāng Jī.

FORMULA

Rhubarb and Coptis Heart-Draining Decoction (*dà huáng huáng lián xiè xīn tāng*)

∘ Drain heat and disperse glomus.

大黄二两　黄连一两

上二味以麻沸汤二升渍之须臾，绞去滓，分温再服。

Dà huáng èr liǎng　huáng lián yī liǎng

Shàng èr wèi yǐ má fèi tāng èr shēng zì zhī xū yú, jiǎo qù zǐ, fēn wēn zài fú.

rhubarb (大黄 *dà huáng*, Rhei Rhizoma) 2 liǎng
coptis (黄连 *huáng lián*, Coptidis Rhizoma) 1 liǎng

[For] the above two ingredients use two shēng of boiled water and steep for a moment. [Pour through a cloth and] wring [out the juice]* and remove the dregs. Divide [into two parts], and take warm twice a day.

Formula Note

* [Pour through a cloth and] wring [out the juice], 绞 *jiǎo*: After the ingredients are steeped, the decoction is poured through a cloth and the dregs are squeezed in the cloth to extract the juice.

Synopsis

The signs and treatment of heat glomus.

Commentary

According to Zhāng Jī's description, a glomus below the heart that is soft when pressed is a "qì glomus." This line specifically mentions that the bar pulse is floating. The bar pulse reflects the state of the center burner, and a pulse that is floating indicates exterior disease or heat. In view of the formula that is suggested, Rhubarb and Coptis Heart-Draining Decoction (*dà huáng huáng lián xiè xīn tāng*), one can infer that heat is present in the center burner. The process of glomus formation is that a formless heat evil binds below the heart, congesting the qì dynamic of the center burner.

Rhubarb and Coptis Heart-Draining Decoction (*dà huáng huáng lián xiè xīn tāng*) clears heat and disperses glomus. Bitter, cold rhubarb (*dà huáng*) drains heat, harmonizes the stomach, and opens binds. Coptis (*huáng lián*), also bitter and cold, clears fire from the heart and stomach. The preparation method is unique. The ingredients are only steeped, not boiled, and then they are pressed to remove the juice. This method is said to extract the light, buoyant qì without getting the heavy, turbid flavor. In this way the formula is made more moderate. Rhubarb and Coptis Heart-Draining Decoction (*dà huáng huáng lián xiè xīn tāng*), when prepared in this way, clears formless heat evil from the upper burner, but does not have the repletion-draining strength the ingredients would have if they were boiled normally.

According to both Lín Yì and the *Qiān Jīn Yì Fāng*, this formula should also contain scutellaria (*huáng qín*), which would strengthen the formula's ability to clear heat and disperse glomus. This assertion is based on the fact that the original Heart-Draining Decoction (*xiè xīn tāng*) contains rhubarb (*dà huáng*), coptis (*huáng lián*), and scutellaria (*huáng qín*). This point of view may be considered, but in our opinion, although the original Heart-Draining Decoction (*xiè xīn tāng*) contains scutellaria (*huáng qín*), Zhāng Jī writes "Rhubarb and Coptis Heart-Draining Decoction" rather than "Heart-Draining Decoction" to reflect a variation in the latter formula that does not contain scutellaria (*huáng qín*). Therefore, it may not, in fact, contain scutellaria (*huáng qín*).

LINE 164

(一) 伤寒大下后，复发汗，心下痞，恶寒者，表未解也。(二) 不可攻痞，当先解表，表解乃可攻痞。(三) 解表宜桂枝汤，攻痞宜大黄黄连泻心汤。

(1) *Shāng hán dà xià hòu, fù fā hàn, xīn xià pǐ, wù hán zhě, biǎo wèi jiě yě.* (2) *Bù kě gōng pǐ, dāng xiān jiě biǎo, biǎo jiě nǎi kě gōng pǐ.* (3) *Jiě biǎo yí guì zhī tāng, gōng pǐ yí dà huáng huáng lián xiè xīn tāng.*

(1) When in cold damage, after great precipitation has been used, sweating is then promoted, and [as a result there is] a glomus below the heart and aversion to cold, this means that the exterior has not yet been resolved. (2) One cannot attack the glomus, but should first resolve the exterior and [after] the exterior is resolved, then one can attack the glomus. (3) Cinnamon Twig Decoction (*guì zhī tāng*) is appropriate for resolving the exterior and Rhubarb and Coptis Heart-Draining Decoction (*dà huáng huáng lián xiè xīn tāng*) is appropriate for attacking the glomus.

SYNOPSIS

The signs and treatment of heat glomus occurring with an exterior pattern.

COMMENTARY

In greater yáng cold damage, the exterior should first be resolved before treating any interior pattern that may be present. To first precipitate and then promote sweating constitutes an inappropriate treatment, which may cause the exterior evil to fall inward and damage the qì of the center burner. When the exterior evil enters the interior and transforms to heat it binds below the heart, congesting the qì dynamic and forming a qì glomus. The presence of aversion to cold indicates that the exterior pattern is still unresolved, as Zhāng Jī explicitly states.

Glomus is an interior pattern which, as Zhāng Jī stresses, cannot be attacked when an exterior pattern remains unresolved. One must first resolve the exterior pattern and then treat the interior. Zhāng Jī suggests Cinnamon Twig Decoction (*guì zhī tāng*) to resolve the exterior on the grounds that sweating has already been promoted once and inappropriate precipitation has damaged the qì. Cinnamon Twig Decoction (*guì zhī tāng*) is a mild formula for resolving exterior patterns and harmonizing the construction and defense. Rhubarb and Coptis Heart-Draining Decoction (*dà huáng huáng lián xiè xīn tāng*) is the formula of choice for glomus that is the result of an exterior evil falling inward and transforming to heat.

4.12.1.2 Aconite Heart-Draining Decoction Patterns

LINE 155

心下痞，而复恶寒汗出者，附子泻心汤主之。

Xīn xià pǐ, ér fù wù hán hàn chū zhě, fù zǐ xiè xīn tāng zhǔ zhī.

When [there is] a glomus below the heart, yet also aversion to cold and sweating, Aconite Heart-Draining Decoction (*fù zǐ xiè xīn tāng*) governs.

FORMULA

Aconite Heart-Draining Decoction (*fù zǐ xiè xīn tāng*)

∘ Drain heat and disperse glomus; support yáng and secure the exterior.

大黄二两 黄连一两 黄芩一两 附子一枚（炮，去皮，破，别煮取汁）

右四味，切三味，以麻沸汤二升渍之，须臾，绞去滓，内附子汁，分温再服。

Dà huáng èr liǎng huáng lián yī liǎng huáng qín yī liǎng fù zǐ yī méi (pào, qù pí, pò, bié zhǔ qǔ zhī)

Yòu sì wèi, qiē sān wèi, yǐ má fèi tāng èr shēng zì zhī, xū yú, jiǎo qù zǐ, nà fù zǐ zhī, fēn wēn zài fú.

rhubarb (大黄 *dà huáng*, Rhei Rhizoma) 2 liǎng
coptis (黄连 *huáng lián*, Coptidis Rhizoma) 1 liǎng
scutellaria (黄芩 *huáng qín*, Scutellariae Radix) 1 liǎng
aconite (附子 *fù zǐ*, Aconiti Tuber Laterale) 1 piece (blast-fry, remove skin, break, boil separately to get the juice)

[For] the above four ingredients, cut the [first] three ingredients and use two shēng of boiled water to steep for a moment. [Pour through a cloth] and wring out [the juice]. Remove the dregs and add aconite (*fù zǐ*) juice. Divide [into two parts], and take warm twice a day.

SYNOPSIS

The signs and treatment of heat glomus occurring with an exterior yáng vacuity pattern.

COMMENTARY

In line 154, p. 230, Rhubarb and Coptis Heart-Draining Decoction (*dà huáng huáng lián xiè xīn tāng*) is used to attack a qì glomus. The previous line instructs physicians to resolve exterior conditions prior to attacking a glomus, which is an interior pattern. In this line the signs of glomus, aversion to cold, and sweating are present simultaneously. If aversion to cold alone is present as in the previous line, it indicates an unresolved exterior condition that must be addressed first. One would expect to see a pulse that is floating, a headache, or other exterior signs. Aversion to cold with sweating, however, in the absence of other exterior signs, means yáng vacuity. Although differing interpretations of the pathomechanism exist, the basic explanation of this pattern is vacuity of the exterior yáng, as Chéng Wú-Jǐ writes. Yóu Yí agrees that "[there is] insufficient yáng qì." In the *Yī Zōng Jīn Jiàn* the explanation is narrower, referring directly to the exterior yáng: "[this is] not an unresolved exterior [pattern]. [It is] vacuity of the exterior yáng." Qián Huáng further narrows this explanation: "the defensive yáng is not sound ... and sweat issues.... Vacuous yáng cannot control the external qì...and [there is] aversion to cold...."

Therefore, the treatment chosen is to drain heat and disperse the glomus while simultaneously supporting yáng and securing the exterior. The formula used is Aconite Heart-Draining Decoction (*fù zǐ xiè xīn tāng*). Rhubarb (*dà huáng*), coptis (*huáng lián*), and scutellaria (*huáng qín*) clear heat and disperse glomus. Acrid, hot aconite (*fù zǐ*) warms the channels, supports yáng, and secures the exterior. The preparation of this formula is slightly different from that of the preceding one. Rhubarb (*dà huáng*), scutellaria (*huáng qín*), and coptis (*huáng lián*) are prepared in the same way. Aconite (*fù zǐ*), however, is boiled separately and its juice is then added to the juice from the other three ingredients. In this way a mild preparation of the first three ingredients drains bound heat from below the heart, and the full strength of aconite (*fù zǐ*) supports yáng.

According to *Qiān Jīn Yì Fāng*, this formula is Rhubarb and Coptis Heart-Draining Decoction (*dà huáng huáng lián xiè xīn tāng*) plus aconite (*fù zǐ*). This classification supports the inclusion of scutellaria (*huáng qín*) in Rhubarb and Coptis Heart-Draining Decoction (*dà huáng huáng lián xiè xīn tāng*). See the commentary for line 154, p. 230, for further discussion of this issue.

4.12.2 Cold-Heat Complex Glomus Patterns

4.12.2.1 Pinellia Heart-Draining Decoction Patterns

LINE 149

(一) 伤寒五六日，呕而发热者，柴胡汤证具，而以他药下之，柴胡证仍在者，复与柴胡汤。(二) 此虽已下之，不为逆，必蒸蒸而振，却发热汗出而解。(三) 若心下满而硬痛者，此为结胸也，大陷胸汤主之。(四) 但满而不痛者，此为痞，柴胡不中与之，宜半夏泻心汤。

(1) *Shāng hán wǔ liù rì, ǒu ér fā rè zhě, chái hú tāng zhèng jù, ér yǐ tā yào xià zhī, chái hú zhèng réng zài zhě, fù yǔ chái hú tāng.* (2) *Cǐ suī yǐ xià zhī, bù wéi nì, bì zhēng zhēng ér zhèn, què fā rè hàn chū ér jiě.* (3) *Ruò xīn xià mǎn ér yìng tòng zhě, cǐ wéi jié xiōng yě, dà*

xiàn xiōng tāng zhǔ zhī. (4) *Dàn mǎn ér bù tòng zhě, cǐ wéi pǐ, chái hú bù zhōng yǔ zhī, yí bàn xià xiè xīn tāng.*

(1) When cold damage [has lasted for] five or six days, [and is marked by] retching and heat effusion, and [Minor] Bupleurum Decoction ([*xiǎo*] *chái hú tāng*) signs are present, [if] other medicinals [are used] to precipitate, [and the] [Minor] Bupleurum [Decoction] ([*xiǎo*] *chái hú* [*tāng*]) signs are still present, one can still give [Minor] Bupleurum Decoction ([*xiǎo*] *chái hú tāng*). (2) Although precipitation has already [been used], it is not an adverse [treatment] [and after the formula is given] there will be steaming and quivering,* then heat effusion and sweating [by which the disease] resolves. (3) If [there is] fullness, hardness, and pain below the heart, this indicates chest bind; [therefore,] Major Chest Bind Decoction (*dà xiàn xiōng tāng*) governs. (4) [If there is] fullness only, without pain, this indicates a glomus; [therefore,] one should not give [Minor] Bupleurum [Decoction] [and] Pinellia Heart-Draining Decoction (*bàn xià xiè xīn tāng*) is appropriate.

TEXT NOTE

* Steaming and quivering, 蒸蒸而振 *zhēng zhēng ér zhèn*: "Steaming" describes the force of the heat moving from the interior out to the exterior. "Quivering" means the shivering and trembling movement that is a physical expression of shiver sweating.

FORMULA

Pinellia Heart-Draining Decoction (*bàn xià xiè xīn tāng*)

◦ Harmonize the center, downbear counterflow, and disperse glomus.

半夏半升（洗） 黄芩 干姜 人参 甘草（炙）各三两 黄连一两 大枣十二枚（擘）

(一)右七味，以水一斗，煮取六升，去滓，再煎取三升，温服一升，日三服。(二)须大陷胸汤者，方用前第二法。

Bàn xià bàn shēng (*xǐ*) *huáng qín gān jiāng rén shēn gān cǎo* (*zhì*) *gè sān liǎng huáng lián yī liǎng dà zǎo shí èr méi* (*bò*)

(1) *Yòu qī wèi, yǐ shuǐ yī dǒu, zhǔ qǔ liù shēng, qù zǐ, zài jiān qǔ sān shēng, wēn fú yī shēng, rì sān fú.* (2) *Xū dà xiàn xiōng tāng zhě, fāng yòng qián dì èr fǎ.*

pinellia (半夏 *bàn xià*, Pinelliae Tuber) half shēng (washed)
scutellaria (黄芩 *huáng qín*, Scutellariae Radix) 3 liǎng
dried ginger (干姜 *gān jiāng*, Zingiberis Rhizoma Exsiccatum) 3 liǎng
ginseng (人参 *rén shēn*, Ginseng Radix) 3 liǎng
mix-fried licorice (甘草 *gān cǎo*, Glycyrrhizae Radix) 3 liǎng
coptis (黄连 *huáng lián*, Coptidis Rhizoma) 1 liǎng

jujube (大枣 *dà zǎo*, Ziziphi Fructus) 12 pieces (broken)

(1) [For] the above seven ingredients use one dǒu of water and boil to get six shēng. Remove the dregs and decoct again to get three shēng. Take one shēng warm three times a day. (2) If Major Chest Bind Decoction (*dà xiàn xiōng tāng*) is needed, the second previously mentioned method for the formula should be used.*

FORMULA NOTE

* The final sentence is not included in the *Zhù Jiě Shāng Hán Lùn* (注解伤寒论 "Annotated *Shāng Hán Lùn*").

SYNOPSIS

Possible treatments of a lesser yáng disease, after inappropriate use of precipitation, with Minor Bupleurum Decoction (*xiǎo chái hú tāng*), Major Chest Bind Decoction (*dà xiàn xiōng tāng*), and Pinellia Heart-Draining Decoction (*bàn xià xiè xīn tāng*).

COMMENTARY

When cold damage signs have persisted for five or six days and then one sees retching and heat effusion, it suggests that the evil has shifted into the lesser yáng. In that case, Minor Bupleurum Decoction (*xiǎo chái hú tāng*) is the appropriate treatment. (See line 96, p. 410.) In the first part of this line, Minor Bupleurum Decoction (*xiǎo chái hú tāng*) should be used, but precipitation is used instead.

After the use of precipitation three possible transmutations are described. In the first the lesser yáng disease is still present. The patient's right qì is still strong and although precipitation has been used erroneously, the damage was not great and the evil remains in the lesser yáng. Because no transmutation has occurred, one can still use Minor Bupleurum Decoction (*xiǎo chái hú tāng*) and this mistreatment is not considered an adverse treatment. Once Minor Bupleurum Decoction (*xiǎo chái hú tāng*) is given, the evil will be expelled from the lesser yáng. This expulsion is described by the phrase "steaming and quivering," in which the movement of the heat evil outward from the lesser yáng causes heat effusion and shiver sweating. Once the sweat issues, the disease will resolve.

In the second of the three possible transmutations, the patient is not strong and the use of precipitation causes the evil in the lesser yáng to fall inward, binding with water-rheum and causing chest bind. Pain, fullness, and hardness below the heart indicates chest bind, and Major Chest Bind Decoction (*dà xiàn xiōng tāng*) is the formula of choice.

In the third transmutation, the use of precipitation results in damage to the spleen and stomach. The evil in the lesser yáng exploits this weakness and attacks the center. When this occurs the evil binds in the interior and congests the qì dynamic in the center, causing abnormal upbearing and downbearing. Fullness below the heart without pain indicates a glomus. Minor Bupleurum Decoction (*xiǎo chái hú tāng*) should not be used because the main problem is not an evil in the lesser yáng, but congestion of the qì dynamic in the center burner due to the presence of a bound, formless evil. Pinellia Heart-Draining Decoction (*bàn xià xiè xīn tāng*) is used to harmonize the center, downbear counterflow, and disperse glomus. On the basis of the ingredients in the formula, this pattern is considered to be one of mixed heat and cold. A heat evil binds below the heart, causing a glomus.

Cold in the stomach and intestines is the result of damage from precipitation. This formula may be used for a pattern of mixed heat and cold, even without adverse treatment. It is suitable for the treatment of glomus below the heart accompanied by cold-type diarrhea, particularly when the tongue fur is thick and yellow.

Pinellia Heart-Draining Decoction (*bàn xià xiè xīn tāng*) is a modification of Minor Bupleurum Decoction (*xiǎo chái hú tāng*). It is Minor Bupleurum Decoction (*xiǎo chái hú tāng*) without bupleurum (*chái hú*) and fresh ginger (*shēng jiāng*), with the addition of coptis (*huáng lián*) and dried ginger (*gān jiāng*). Pinellia (*bàn xià*) is the sovereign ingredient. Acrid and warm, pinellia (*bàn xià*) downbears counterflow, checks retching, and dissipates glomus qì. Dried ginger (*gān jiāng*), also acrid and warm, warms the spleen and dissipates cold. Bitter and cold scutellaria (*huáng qín*) and coptis (*huáng lián*) clear heat. Ginseng (*rén shēn*), licorice (*gān cǎo*), and jujube (*dà zǎo*) supplement and boost the spleen and stomach. They help restore the qì dynamic of the center burner to normal. The combination of these ingredients illustrates some basic guidelines for choosing medicinals. Acrid flavors open, bitter flavors downbear, and sweet flavors regulate.

The directions for the preparation of this formula include the instruction to remove the dregs and cook the decoction again. This formula is an example of a harmonizing formula and it is cooked a second time to insure that the formula is moderate and harmonized. This method is suggested for all the bupleurum formulae and the three Heart-Draining Decoctions: Fresh Ginger Heart-Draining Decoction (*shēng jiāng xiè xīn tāng*), Pinellia Heart-Draining Decoction (*bàn xià xiè xīn tāng*), and Licorice Heart-Draining Decoction (*gān cǎo xiè xīn tāng*).

4.12.2.2 Fresh Ginger Heart-Draining Decoction Patterns

Line 157

伤寒汗出，解之后，胃中不和，心下痞硬，干噫食臭，胁下有水气，腹中雷鸣，下利者，生姜泻心汤主之。

Shāng hán hàn chū, jiě zhī hòu, wèi zhōng bù hé, xīn xià pǐ yìng, gān yì shí chòu, xié xià yǒu shuǐ qì, fù zhōng léi míng, xià lì zhě, shēng jiāng xiè xīn tāng zhǔ zhī.

When in cold damage after sweat has issued and brought resolution [of the exterior], the stomach is in disharmony, [there is] a hard glomus below the heart, dry belching with malodor of food,[1] water qì under the rib-side,[2] thunderous rumbling in the abdomen, and diarrhea, Fresh Ginger Heart-Draining Decoction (*shēng jiāng xiè xīn tāng*) governs.

Text Notes

1. Dry belching with malodor of food, 干噫食臭 *gān yī shí chòu*: Belching that does not produce any fluid or reflux, but has a putrid odor.
2. Water qì under the rib-side, 胁下有水气 *xié xià yǒu shuǐ qì*: Water-rheum inside the lower lateral part of the rib-cage.

FORMULA

Fresh Ginger Heart-Draining Decoction (*shēng jiāng xiè xīn tāng*)

∘ Harmonize the stomach and downbear counterflow; transform rheum and disperse glomus.

生姜四两（切） 甘草三两（炙） 人参三两 干姜一两 黄芩三两 半夏半升（洗） 黄连一两 大枣十二枚（擘）

右八味，以水一斗，煮取六升，去滓，再煎取三升，温服一升，日三服。

Shēng jiāng sì liǎng (qiē) gān cǎo sān liǎng (zhì) rén shēn sān liǎng gān jiāng yī liǎng huáng qín sān liǎng bàn xià bàn shēng (xǐ) huáng lián yī liǎng dà zǎo shí èr méi (bò)

Yòu bā wèi, yǐ shuǐ yī dǒu, zhǔ qǔ liù shēng, qù zǐ, zài jiān qǔ sān shēng, wēn fú yī shēng, rì sān fú.

fresh ginger (生姜 *shēng jiāng*, Zingiberis Rhizoma Recens) 4 liǎng (cut)
mix-fried licorice (甘草 *gān cǎo*, Glycyrrhizae Radix) 3 liǎng
ginseng (人参 *rén shēn*, Ginseng Radix) 3 liǎng
dried ginger (干姜 *gān jiāng*, Zingiberis Rhizoma Exsiccatum) 1 liǎng
scutellaria (黄芩 *huáng qín*, Scutellariae Radix) 3 liǎng
pinellia (半夏 *bàn xià*, Pinelliae Tuber) half shēng (washed)
coptis (黄连 *huáng lián*, Coptidis Rhizoma) 1 liǎng
jujube (大枣 *dà zǎo*, Ziziphi Fructus) 12 pieces (broken)

[For] the above eight ingredients use one dǒu of water and boil to get six shēng. Remove the dregs and decoct again to get three shēng. Take one shēng warm, three times a day.

SYNOPSIS

The signs and treatment of glomus that is the result of stomach vacuity, water-rheum, and non-transformation of food.

COMMENTARY

After sweating and the resolution of an exterior cold damage disease, the patient in this line has disharmony of the stomach. This disharmony may be the result of damage from the loss of fluids or it may be constitutional. In either case a weakness in the center is exploited by a residual evil which attacks the center and binds in the interior, causing congestion of the qì dynamic and the loss of normal upbearing and downbearing. This congestion manifests as a hard glomus below the heart.

Previously glomus has been described as being soft, not hard. Hardness means that the bound evil and the resultant congestion are more severe. Here, this sign is not described as being painful, with or without pressure; hence it is not chest bind.

Stomach function may become impaired as the result of a disease process or a constitutional weakness. In either case weakness of the stomach and qì congestion in the center burner results in congestion of the qì dynamic. Food cannot be properly digested and assimilated; consequently, belching with the odor of rotten food is observed. Because the qì dynamic is congested, turbidity, which should move downward, rises. The presence of water qì, or water-rheum, further impairs the function of the center and lower burners. This water-rheum may have been present prior to the onset of the disease or it may have resulted from abnormal accumulation of water, stemming from impaired spleen-stomach function. The clear and turbid qì move abnormally, causing diarrhea. Intestinal rumbling reflects disharmony in the center burner.

Fresh Ginger Heart-Draining Decoction (*shēng jiāng xiè xīn tāng*) is Pinellia Heart-Draining Decoction (*bàn xià xiè xīn tāng*) with the addition of fresh ginger (*shēng jiāng*) and a reduced amount of dried ginger (*gān jiāng*). The action of the formula is similar to that of Pinellia Heart-Draining Decoction (*bàn xià xiè xīn tāng*); it opens with acrid medicinals, downbears with bitter medicinals, and regulates with sweet medicinals. In this formula, however, fresh ginger (*shēng jiāng*) is the sovereign. Acrid and warm, it opens the stomach qì, repels foul turbidity, and dissipates water qì. The pairing of fresh ginger (*shēng jiāng*) and dried ginger (*gān jiāng*) is very important to the action of this formula. The qì of fresh ginger (*shēng jiāng*) is thin, so it diffuses and dissipates. Dried ginger (*gān jiāng*) has thick qì, so it promotes contraction. Thin and thick qì refer to mild and rich flavors, respectively. Fresh ginger (*shēng jiāng*) penetrates and does not confine; dried ginger (*gān jiāng*) confines and does not penetrate. Used together, contraction occurs within dissipation and confinement occurs within penetration. The pair is able to diffuse and dissipate water-rheum, while simultaneously warming and supplementing the center burner. Fresh ginger (*shēng jiāng*) and pinellia (*bàn xià*) downbear counterflow, transform rheum, and harmonize the stomach. The addition of coptis (*huáng lián*) and scutellaria (*huáng qín*) clears heat and disperses the glomus. Ginseng (*rén shēn*), jujube (*dà zǎo*), and licorice (*gān cǎo*) support the center and supplement vacuity.

4.12.2.3 Licorice Heart-Draining Decoction Patterns

Line 158

㈠伤寒中风，医反下之，其人下利日数十行，谷不化，腹中雷鸣，心下痞硬而满，干呕，心烦不得安。㈡医见心下痞，谓病不尽，复下之，其痞益甚，此非结热，但以胃中虚，客气上逆，故使硬也，甘草泻心汤主之。

(1) *Shāng hán zhòng fēng, yī fǎn xià zhī, qí rén xià lì rì shù shí xíng, gǔ bù huà, fù zhōng léi míng, xīn xià pǐ yìng ér mǎn, gān ǒu, xīn fán bù dé ān.* (2) *Yī jiàn xīn xià pǐ, wèi bìng bù jìn, fù xià zhī, qí pǐ yì shèn, cǐ fēi jié rè, dàn yǐ wèi zhōng xū, kè qì shàng nì, gù shǐ yìng yě, gān cǎo xiè xīn tāng zhǔ zhī.*

(1) [When] in cold damage [or] wind strike, the physician has used precipitation, the person [will have] diarrhea about ten times per day

[containing] food that has not been transformed, [with] thunderous rumbling in the abdomen, fullness and a hard glomus below the heart, dry retching, and vexation that cannot be quieted. (2) [When] the physician sees a glomus below the heart, suggesting the illness has not finished, and again uses precipitation, [yet as a result] the glomus increases in severity, [it is because] heat bind is absent; only stomach vacuity [is present] with counterflow ascent of visiting qì, causing hardness; [therefore,] Licorice Heart-Draining Decoction (*gān cǎo xiè xīn tāng*) governs.

FORMULA

Licorice Heart-Draining Decoction (*gān cǎo xiè xīn tāng*)

∘ Harmonize the stomach and supplement the center; disperse glomus and check diarrhea.

甘草四两（炙） 黄芩三两 干姜三两 半夏半升（洗） 大枣十二枚（擘） 黄连一两

右六味，以水一斗，煮取六升，去滓，再煎取三升，温服一升，日三服。

Gān cǎo sì liǎng (zhì) huáng qín sān liǎng gān jiāng sān liǎng bàn xià bàn shēng (xǐ) dà zǎo shí èr méi (bò) huáng lián yī liǎng

Yòu liù wèi, yǐ shuǐ yī dǒu, zhǔ qǔ liù shēng, qù zǐ, zài jiān qǔ sān shēng, wēn fú yī shēng, rì sān fú.

mix-fried licorice (甘草 *gān cǎo*, Glycyrrhizae Radix) 4 liǎng
scutellaria (黄芩 *huáng qín*, Scutellariae Radix) 3 liǎng
dried ginger (干姜 *gān jiāng*, Zingiberis Rhizoma Exsiccatum) 3 liǎng
pinellia (半夏 *bàn xià*, Pinelliae Tuber) half shēng (washed)
jujube (大枣 *dà zǎo*, Ziziphi Fructus) 12 pieces (broken)
coptis (黄连 *huáng lián*, Coptidis Rhizoma) 1 liǎng

[For] the above six ingredients use one dǒu of water and boil to get six shēng. Remove the dregs and decoct again to get three shēng. Take one shēng warm, three times a day.

SYNOPSIS

The signs and treatment of the pattern in which the inappropriate use of precipitation causes spleen and stomach vacuity, leading to severe glomus and diarrhea.

COMMENTARY

Both cold damage and wind strike are exterior conditions that are treated with exterior-resolving formulae. If precipitation is used it will damage the center qì and possibly result in the evil falling into the interior. Precipitation causes vacuity in the spleen, stomach, and intestines. The exterior evil exploits the vacuity and falls inward, resulting in a hard glomus below the heart. When an exterior evil falls inward it easily impairs the qì dynamic. When the qì dynamic is impaired normal upbearing and downbearing cannot occur, which can lead to a self-perpetuating cycle. For example, vacuity cold in the lower burner impairs the movement of qì. Because of this impairment, the spleen and stomach are unable to move and transform clear and turbid qì properly. This impairment causes diarrhea, exacerbating the spleen and stomach vacuity as clear essence qì is lost through the diarrhea. The increasing vacuity means less qì is available to move and the qì stagnation increases.

The use of precipitation results in an exterior evil falling inward and obstructing the qì dynamic. It also damages the qì of the center burner. The damage to center qì from the use of precipitation results in frequent diarrhea with non-transformed food and rumbling intestines. Here, precipitation causes severe diarrhea, perhaps indicating that originally the center burner was vacuous. Frequent diarrhea with non-transformed food, accompanied by intestinal rumbling, indicates extreme vacuity of spleen and stomach qì.

These signs are accompanied by dry retching and heart vexation, signs of upper burner heat; hence this pattern is a mixed pattern of heat and cold, with vacuity cold in the lower burner and heat in the upper burner. The retching and vexation further indicate impairment of the qì dynamic and the resultant loss of normal upbearing and downbearing.

If the physician misdiagnoses this pattern and uses precipitation again, it will exacerbate the vacuity in the center burner. This mistreatment will cause further irregularity in the qì dynamic and the glomus will become worse. This glomus is not the result of repletion heat bound in the interior, as in chest bind. As Zhāng Jī explains, when the spleen and stomach are vacuous and evil qì falls inward, upbearing and downbearing become abnormal, the qì dynamic is congested, and a hard glomus forms.

Licorice Heart-Draining Decoction (*gān cǎo xiè xīn tāng*) is Pinellia Heart-Draining Decoction (*bàn xià xiè xīn tāng*) with a larger dose of licorice (*gān cǎo*). Licorice (*gān cǎo*) enters the spleen and stomach, fortifying the center burner and securing center qì. A large dose of licorice (*gān cǎo*) boosts the center and moderates counterflow. If one accepts the point of view of both Lín Yì and the *Qiān Jīn Yì Fāng*, this formula should contain ginseng (*rén shēn*). The combination of jujube (*dà zǎo*) and ginseng (*rén shēn*) strengthens the formula's qì-boosting action. Pinellia (*bàn xià*) downbears counterflow and harmonizes the stomach, and disperses glomus and checks retching. Coptis (*huáng lián*) clears heat and resolves vexation. Dried ginger (*gān jiāng*) warms the center and dissipates cold.

4.12.3 Severe Patterns of Efflux Desertion, Glomus, and Diarrhea Affecting the Lower Burner (Halloysite and Limonite Decoction Patterns)

LINE 159

(一) 伤寒服汤药，下利不止，心下痞硬。(二) 服泻心汤已，复以他药下之，利不止。(三) 医以理中与之，利益甚。(四) 理中者，理中焦，此利在下焦，赤石脂禹余粮汤主之。(五) 复不止者，当利其小便。

(1) *Shāng hán fú tāng yào, xià lì bù zhǐ, xīn xià pǐ yìng.* (2) *Fú xiè xīn tāng yǐ, fù yǐ tā yào xià zhī, lì bù zhǐ.* (3) *Yī yǐ lǐ zhōng yǔ zhī, lì yì shèn.* (4) *Lǐ zhōng zhě, lǐ zhōng jiāo, cǐ lì zài xià jiāo, chì shí zhī yǔ yú liáng tāng zhǔ zhī.* (5) *Fù bù zhǐ zhě, dāng lì qí xiǎo biàn.*

(1) In cold damage, a decoction medicine* has been taken and [there is] incessant diarrhea and a hard glomus below the heart. (2) Heart-Draining Decoction (*xiè xīn tāng*) has already been taken, and then, because other medicinals [are used] to precipitate, [there is] incessant diarrhea. (3) The physician gives [a formula] to rectify the center and the diarrhea increases in severity. (4) Rectifying the center rectifies the center burner, [but] this diarrhea is in the lower burner, so Halloysite and Limonite Decoction (*chì shí zhī yǔ yú liáng tāng*) governs. (5) If [the diarrhea] persists, one should disinhibit the urine.

TEXT NOTE

* Decoction medicine, 汤药 *tāng yào*: A decocted formula for offensive precipitation. Yù Chāng writes, "Decoction medicine means medicinals to flush the stomach and intestines."

FORMULA

Halloysite and Limonite Decoction (*chì shí zhī yǔ yú liáng tāng*)

- Stem desertion and check diarrhea.

赤石脂一斤（碎） 太一禹余粮一斤（碎）

右二味，以水六升，煮取二升，去滓，分温三服。

Chì shí zhī yī jīn (suì) tài yī yǔ yú liáng yī jīn (suì)
Yòu èr wèi, yǐ shuǐ liù shēng, zhǔ qǔ èr shēng, qù zǐ, fēn wēn sān fú.

halloysite (赤石脂 *chì shí zhī*, Halloysitum Rubrum) 16 liǎng (broken)
limonite (太一余粮 *tài yī yú liáng*, Limonitum) 16 liǎng (broken)

[For] the above two ingredients use six shēng of water and boil to get three shēng. Remove the dregs, separate [into] three [doses] and take warm.

SYNOPSIS

The signs and treatment of the pattern in which inappropriate precipitation leads to a glomus and incessant diarrhea.

COMMENTARY

Since cold damage is an exterior pattern it should be treated with a formula to resolve the exterior. It is not clear what formula was given here, but it appears that it was a precipitating formula because the result is incessant diarrhea and a hard glomus below the heart. The treatment suggested in the text is one of the Heart-Draining Decoctions (*xiè xīn tāng*), probably Licorice Heart-Draining Decoction (*gān cǎo xiè xīn tāng*) or Fresh Ginger Heart-Draining Decoction (*shēng jiāng xiè xīn tāng*).

One of these formulae is given, but then precipitation is used again and the diarrhea does not cease. The original inappropriate treatment damaged the qì of the spleen and stomach and caused the formation of a glomus below the heart. A second mistreatment exacerbated the condition and the diarrhea continues.

The physician perceives the diarrhea to be an indication of cold in the center burner; therefore, Center-Rectifying Decoction (*lǐ zhōng tāng*) is chosen to warm the center burner. Nevertheless, after ingestion of the decoction the diarrhea becomes worse. Center-Rectifying Decoction (*lǐ zhōng tāng*) is appropriate for cases of diarrhea that are the result of spleen vacuity and cold. In more serious cases or in protracted illness, the original qì and the yáng qì of not only the spleen, but the kidney, may be damaged. Zhāng Jī explains that the diarrhea arises from the lower burner, not the center burner. Repeated mistreatment damages the original qì and the yáng qì of the spleen and kidney. The securing and containing functions of the spleen and kidney are impaired, producing a desertion pattern in the form of incessant diarrhea. This pattern must be treated with medicinals that astringe the lower burner.

Halloysite and Limonite Decoction (*chì shí zhī yǔ yú liáng tāng*) contains sweet, warm, and astringent halloysite (*chì shí zhī*), which astringes the intestines, stanches bleeding, and stems desertion. Sweet, neutral, astringent limonite (*yǔ yú liáng*) stanches bleeding and checks diarrhea, but also supplements the spleen, secures the stomach qì, and thickens the large intestine.

If a formula for checking diarrhea is used unsuccessfully, one should investigate urination. If urination is inhibited, it suggests that the clear and turbid are not being separated and that dampness is percolating into the large intestine. If one then disinhibits the urine, this treatment will restore proper separation of the turbid and clear, remove the dampness from the lower burner, and check the diarrhea.

4.12.4 Water Glomus Patterns (Poria Five Powder Patterns)

LINE 156

㈠ 本以下之，故心下痞，与泻心汤。 ㈡ 痞不解，其人渴而口燥烦，小便不利者，五苓散主之。

(1) *Běn yǐ xià zhī, gù xīn xià pǐ, yǔ xiè xīn tāng.* (2) *Pǐ bù jiě, qí rén kě ér kǒu zào fán, xiǎo biàn bù lì zhě, wǔ líng sǎn zhǔ zhī.* (3) *Yī fāng yún, rěn zhī yī rì nǎi yù.*

(1) When, because originally precipitation was used, [there is] therefore, a glomus below the heart, give Heart-Draining Decoction (*xiè xīn tāng*). (2) If the glomus does not resolve, and the person is thirsty, has a dry mouth, vexation, and inhibited urination, Poria (Hoelen) Five Powder (*wǔ líng sǎn*) governs. (3) According to another method, if [the patient] puts up with it for a day,* he/she will recover [without medication].

FORMULA NOTE

* Putting up with it for a day, 忍之一日 *rěn zhī yī rì*: This is taken to mean that the patient should put up with the thirst without drinking for one day. Note that Chéng Wú-Jǐ's *Zhù Jiě Shāng Hán Lùn* does not include this final sentence, and some modern commentators believe it should be removed.

SYNOPSIS

The signs and treatment of glomus below the heart in water amassment patterns.

COMMENTARY

When precipitation is used improperly it may result in the formation of a glomus, as it does in this line. Generally, one of the Heart-Draining Decoctions (*xiè xīn tāng*) is used, as it is here. The glomus should resolve, but it does not, suggesting that it is not a typical heat glomus. From the signs that occur after the ingestion of the original formula and the formula that is suggested, it is considered to be a water glomus.

Water glomus occurs when the qì transformation of the bladder is impaired. It may be the result of inappropriate precipitation, causing an exterior evil to shift from the greater yáng channel into the bladder, or it may be a constitutional problem. In either case inhibited urination, thirst, a dry mouth, and vexation are clear signs of the impairment of fluid movement in the body. Water collects in the lower burner and then attacks upward, resulting in congestion of the qì dynamic in the center burner. The typical treatment for glomus is not appropriate here, but instead, one must transform qì and move water.

A typical qì glomus causes signs that reflect congestion of the qì dynamic like retching counterflow and diarrhea. In comparison, in water glomus patterns signs of qì dynamic congestion are accompanied by signs of water amassment, such as inhibited urination and thirst.

Although some present-day commentators believe the last line should be removed, others believe that it has clinical significance. Because water amassment often results from excessive intake of water, the patient only has to put up with the thirst and desist from drinking for a day for the amassed water to be discharged from the body without need of any medication.

4.12.5 Phlegm Qì Glomus Patterns (Inula and Hematite Decoction Patterns)

LINE 161

伤寒发汗，若吐若下，解后，心下痞硬，噫气不除者，旋覆代赭汤主之。

Shāng hán fā hàn, ruò tù ruò xià, jiě hòu, xīn xià pǐ yìng, yì qì bù chú zhě, xuán fù dài zhě tāng zhǔ zhī.

When in cold damage, sweating is promoted or vomiting or precipitation [is used] and after resolution [of the exterior disease], [there is] a hard glomus below the heart and belching* that cannot be eliminated, Inula and Hematite Decoction (*xuán fù dài zhě tāng*) governs.

TEXT NOTE

* Belching, 噫气 *yì qì*: Expulsion of gas (qì) from the stomach that occurs after eating to satiation or eating too quickly, and in stomach diseases. It is one manifestation of counterflow ascent of stomach qì. The same as 嗳气 *ài qì*.

FORMULA

Inula and Hematite Decoction (*xuán fù dài zhě tāng*)

○ Harmonize the stomach and transform phlegm; subdue the liver and downbear counterflow.

旋覆花三两　人参二两　生姜五两　代赭一两　甘草三两（炙）　半夏半升（洗）　大枣十二枚（擘）

右七味，以水一斗，煮取六升，去滓，再煎取三升，温服一升，日三服。

Xuán fù huā sān liǎng rén shēn èr liǎng shēng jiāng wǔ liǎng dài zhě yī liǎng gān cǎo sān liǎng (zhì) bàn xià bàn shēng (xǐ) dà zǎo shí èr méi (bò)

Yòu qī wèi, yǐ shuǐ yī dǒu, zhǔ qǔ liù shēng, qù zǐ, zài jiān qǔ sān shēng, wēn fú yī shēng, rì sān fú.

inula flower (旋覆花 *xuán fù huā*, Inulae Flos) 3 liǎng
ginseng (人参 *rén shēn*, Ginseng Radix) 2 liǎng

fresh ginger (生姜 *shēng jiāng*, Zingiberis Rhizoma Recens) 5 liǎng
hematite (代赭石 *dài zhě shí*, Haematitum) 1 liǎng
mix-fried licorice (甘草 *gān cǎo*, Glycyrrhizae Radix) 3 liǎng
pinellia (半夏 *bàn xià*, Pinelliae Tuber) half shēng (washed)
jujube (大枣 *dà zǎo*, Ziziphi Fructus) 12 pieces (broken)

[For] the above seven ingredients use one dǒu of water. Boil to get six shēng, remove the dregs, and cook again to get three shēng. Take one shēng warm, three times a day.

SYNOPSIS

The signs and treatment of phlegm-qì glomus.

COMMENTARY

Here, following the resolution of a greater yáng cold damage pattern, a hard glomus below the heart and belching arise. The presence of these signs means that although the exterior pattern has resolved, the treatment method used was inappropriate. The use of vomiting or precipitation is clearly an inappropriate method, but the promotion of sweating is appropriate treatment for an exterior pattern. Here, sweating was promoted excessively or too strongly for the patient's constitution; hence although the principle was correct, its execution was not.

The inappropriate use of sweating, vomiting, or precipitation damages the qì of the spleen and stomach, impairing digestate decomposition. Movement and transformation become abnormal and phlegm-rheum is engendered. The signs in this pattern do not necessarily reflect phlegm-rheum, but when viewed in combination with the suggested formula, strongly suggest its presence. Phlegm-rheum, a result of the treatment or a reflection of the patient's original constitution, congests below the heart. It obstructs the qì dynamic and causes qì counterflow. The congestion below the heart manifests as a hard glomus and the belching provides evidence of the qì counterflow.

The phrase "which cannot be eliminated" may be interpreted in two ways. It may refer to the belching and mean that it is incessant and difficult to resolve. It may, however, also refer to the glomus. That is, after belching, the patient feels no relief from the discomfort below the heart.

The formula Inula and Hematite Decoction (*xuán fù dài zhě tāng*) harmonizes the stomach and transforms phlegm, as well as subdues the liver and downbears counterflow. Inula flower (*xuán fù huā*) is the sovereign agent. It disperses phlegm and downbears qì, and softens hardness and dissipates binds; it is an important agent for the resolution of phlegm glomus. Hematite (*dài zhě shí*) settles the liver and subdues counterflow. Thus, these two agents alone perform the main actions of the formula. Acrid, warm fresh ginger (*shēng jiāng*) and pinellia (*bàn xià*) harmonize the stomach, transform phlegm, and disperse glomus. Ginseng (*rén shēn*), mix-fried licorice (*gān cǎo*), and jujube (*dà zǎo*) supplement the spleen and stomach in order to fortify the vacuity present in the original condition. The combination of these agents disperses phlegm and harmonizes the qì of the center burner. In this way it allows for normal upbearing of the clear and downbearing of the turbid. When the clear and the turbid move normally, and the spleen and stomach are fortified, the disease will resolve.

Because this formula subdues the liver, counterflow ascent of the liver qì and the liver exploiting the vacuity of the spleen has been suggested as part of the pathomechanism. Wú Yí-Luò (吴仪洛) writes:

> Vacuity of earth is exploited by liver wood, and [stomach qì] ascends counterflow with the qì [of liver]. Thus the sovereign [agent] is ginseng (*rén shēn*), which supplements vacuity. The minister, bitter, cold hematite (*dài zhě shí*), is a heavy settler which enters the liver and guides ginseng (*rén shēn*) down to subdue and quiet the qì counterflow. Salty, warm inula flower (*xuán fù huā*) softens hardness, moves water, and precipitates qì.

This perspective may be compared with that offered by Chéng Wú-Jǐ, who makes no reference to the liver at all:

> Salty flavors can soften hardness. Salty inula flower (*xuán fù huā*) is used to soften the hard glomus. [When there is] vacuity, the qì floats [upward]. Heavy formulae can subdue. Heavy hematite (*dài zhě shí*) is used to subdue the vacuity counterflow. Acridity dissipates. Acrid fresh ginger (*shēng jiāng*) and pinellia (*bàn xià*) dissipate the vacuity glomus. Sweetness moderates. Sweet ginseng (*rén shēn*), mix-fried licorice (*gān cǎo*), and jujube (*dà zǎo*) supplement the stomach vacuity.

Both perspectives provide insight into the mechanism of the formula.

Inula and Hematite Decoction (*xuán fù dài zhě tāng*), which harmonizes the stomach, transforms phlegm, subdues the liver and downbears counterflow, may be compared with Minor Bupleurum Decoction (*xiǎo chái hú tāng*), which harmonizes and resolves the lesser yáng, since the ingredients are very similar. The former contains inula flower (*xuán fù huā*) and hematite (*dài zhě shí*), whereas the latter contains bupleurum (*chái hú*) and scutellaria (*huáng qín*). The remaining ingredients, ginseng (*rén shēn*), licorice (*gān cǎo*), jujube (*dà zǎo*), pinellia (*bàn xià*), and fresh ginger (*shēng jiāng*), are the same in both.

4.13 Upper Burner Heat and Lower Burner Cold Patterns: Coptis Decoction Patterns

Line 173

伤寒胸中有热，胃中有邪气，腹中痛，欲呕吐者，黄连汤主之。

Shāng hán xiōng zhōng yǒu rè, wèi zhōng yǒu xié qì, fù zhōng tòng, yù ǒu tù zhě, huáng lián tāng zhǔ zhī.

When in cold damage, [there is] heat in the chest, evil qì in the stomach, pain in the abdomen, and a desire to vomit, Coptis Decoction (*huáng lián tāng*) governs.

Formula

Coptis Decoction (*huáng lián tāng*)

○ Clear upper [burner heat] and warm lower [burner cold]; harmonize the center and downbear counterflow.

黄连三两 甘草三两（炙） 干姜三两 桂枝三两（去皮） 人参二两 半夏半升（洗） 大枣十二枚（擘）

(一) 右七味，以水一斗，煮取六升，去滓，温服，昼三、夜二。(二) 疑非仲景方。

Huáng lián sān liǎng gān cǎo sān liǎng (zhì) gān jiāng sān liǎng guì zhī sān liǎng (qù pí) rén shēn èr liǎng bàn xià bàn shēng (xǐ) dà zǎo shí èr méi (bò)

(1) *Yòu qī wèi, yǐ shuǐ yī dǒu, zhǔ qǔ liù shēng, qù zǐ, wēn fú, zhòu sān、yè èr.* (2) *Yí fēi zhòng jǐng fāng.*

coptis (黄连 *huáng lián*, Coptidis Rhizoma) 3 liǎng
mix-fried licorice (甘草 *gān cǎo*, Glycyrrhizae Radix) 3 liǎng
dried ginger (干姜 *gān jiāng*, Zingiberis Rhizoma Exsiccatum) 3 liǎng
cinnamon twig (桂枝 *guì zhī*, Cinnamomi Ramulus) 3 liǎng (remove bark)
ginseng (人参 *rén shēn*, Ginseng Radix) 2 liǎng
pinellia (半夏 *bàn xià*, Pinelliae Tuber) half shēng (washed)
jujube (大枣 *dà zǎo*, Ziziphi Fructus) 12 pieces (broken)

(1) [For] the above seven ingredients use one dǒu of water. Boil to get six shēng and remove the dregs. Take warm, three times [during] the day and twice at night. (2) It is doubted that this is [Zhāng] Zhòng Jǐng's formula.*

Formula Note

* It is doubted that this is [Zhāng] Zhòng Jǐng's formula, 疑非[张]仲景方 *yí fēi zhòng jǐng fāng*: This is an addition to the text by an unknown author.

Synopsis

The signs and treatment of abdominal pain with a desire to retch and vomit in a pattern of upper burner heat and lower burner cold.

Commentary

The reader is told that a heat evil is present in the chest, that is, above the diaphragm. An evil, not described as being hot or cold, is present in the stomach. The region of the stomach is considered to include the stomach, spleen, and intestines or, more generally, the abdomen. An analysis of the formula suggests that it treats cold in the abdomen. Thus, this line presents a case of heat in the upper body and cold in the lower body. It should be noted here that the area affected by this disease is larger than that treated with Pinellia Heart-Draining Decoction (*bàn xià xiè xīn tāng*), although the sign pattern is similar.

Because of the cold evil, the spleen and stomach are damaged. The cold congeals and the qì stagnates; hence the abdomen becomes painful. When the qì is stagnant, the stomach cannot downbear turbidity properly; hence the patient desires to vomit. Because a desire to vomit may also be the result of heat in the upper body, it may here be a sign of heat in the upper body, congestion of the qì dynamic, or a combination of both. In this pattern no evidence of either glomus or chest bind exists, although evils are present in the interior. The absence of these signs is another point differentiating this pattern from the one Pinellia Heart-Draining Decoction (*bàn xià xiè xīn tāng*) treats.

Treatment must aim to clear heat from the upper burner, warm the center burner, harmonize the stomach, and downbear counterflow. Coptis Decoction (*huáng lián tāng*) is Pinellia Heart-Draining Decoction (*bàn xià xiè xīn tāng*) without scutellaria (*huáng qín*) and with cinnamon twig (*guì zhī*). Bitter, cold coptis (*huáng lián*) clears heat in the upper body. Acrid, hot dried ginger (*gān jiāng*) warms the lower body. Acrid, warm cinnamon twig (*guì zhī*) dissipates cold and frees yáng. The emphasis of Coptis Decoction (*huáng lián tāng*) lies in using acrid agents to free the qì dynamic. In Pinellia Heart-Draining Decoction (*bàn xià xiè xīn tāng*) on the other hand, the emphasis is on the use of bitter agents to downbear the qì. Ginseng (*rén shēn*), licorice (*gān cǎo*), and jujube (*dà zǎo*) boost the qì and harmonize the center. In combination these medicinals restore normal upbearing and downbearing in the center burner. By downbearing counterflow, harmonizing the stomach, and checking retching, pinellia (*bàn xià*) strengthens one of the chief actions of the formula.

4.14 Adverse Treatment by Fire Patterns

Adverse treatment by fire patterns occurs as the result of inappropriate use of fire methods. Treatment by fire is an ancient practice that was particularly popular in the Hàn Dynasty. This treatment category includes warm needling, red-hot needling, moxibustion, fuming, and hot packs. Fire methods, used to promote sweating, dissipate cold, open impediment, and relieve pain, are appropriate for use with patients suffering from severe cold patterns.

Many of these treatments are not commonly used today, but the patterns discussed in this section still do appear in clinical practice. They typically involve yīn damage and stirring of blood or yáng hyperactivity and stirring of wind.

The signs in adverse treatment by fire patterns vary according to the treatment used, the original disease, and the patient's constitution. When fire evil attacks the interior, damaging the heart yáng, it may give rise to a pattern in which the heart spirit strays outward. This pattern is characterized by vexation and agitation, fright mania, and disquiet lying and sitting. When fire evil instead damages yīn and construction, it may stir the blood, giving rise to signs such as blood ejection and bloody stool. In certain patterns, the blood dissipates from the pulse and a yáng evil becomes depressed in the upper burner. The yáng evil cannot outthrust and this pattern is characterized by the absence of sweating below the lumbus, impediment, and aversion to cold in the soles of the feet.

LINE 110

㈠ 太阳病二日，反躁，凡熨其背而大汗出，大热入胃，胃中水竭，躁烦，必发谵语。㈡ 十余日，振栗，自下利者，此为欲解也。㈢ 故其汗从腰以下不得汗，欲小便不得，反呕，欲失溲，足下恶风，大便硬，小便当数而反不数及不多；大便已，头卓然而痛，其人足心必热， 谷气下流故也。

(1) *Tài yáng bìng èr rì, fǎn zào, fán yùn qí bèi, ér dà hàn chū, dà rè rù wèi, wèi zhōng shuǐ jié, zào fán, bì fā zhān yǔ.* (2) *Shí yú rì, zhèn lì, zì xià lì zhě, cǐ wéi yù jiě yě.* (3) *Gù qí hàn, cóng yāo yǐ xià bù dé hàn, yù xiǎo biàn bù dé, fǎn ǒu yù shī sōu, zú xià wù fēng, dà biàn yìng, xiǎo biàn dāng shuò ér fǎn bù shuò jí bù duō; dà biàn yǐ, tóu zhuó rán ér tòng, qí rén zú xīn bì rè, gǔ qì xià liú gù yě.*

(1) When greater yáng disease [has lasted] two days, but [there is] agitation whenever a hot pack[1] is used on the back, and [as a result there is] great sweating, [then] great heat enters the stomach, the stomach water[2] is exhausted, [there is] vexation and agitation, [and] there will be delirious speech. (2) If [after] more than ten days, [there is] shivering and spontaneous diarrhea, this means [that the disease] is about to resolve. (3) Consequently, sweating from the lumbus down cannot be obtained. [The person] desires but is unable to urinate, and instead retches. [The person is] verging on urinary incontinence and has aversion to wind in the soles of the feet and hard stool. Urination should be frequent, but instead it is infrequent and not copious. Defecation [occurs] and the head is suddenly painful. This patient will feel heat in the soles, because grain qì[3] flows downward.

TEXT NOTES

1. A hot pack, 熨 *yùn*: A cloth bag that contains medicinals warmed by stir-frying, and applied to the body to relieve pain, force sweating, or dissipate cold. The same as 热熨 *rè yùn*.
2. Stomach water, 胃中水 *wèi zhōng shuǐ*: The water in the stomach.
3. Grain qì, 谷气 *gǔ qì*: Indicates the clear yáng qì derived from food.

SYNOPSIS

Transmuted patterns and the mechanism of spontaneous recovery in greater yáng disease after the inappropriate use of a fire method.

COMMENTARY

Vexation is not generally seen in greater yáng disease. Its presence in the beginning of this line suggests that the evil heat qì has moved into the interior, as

Chéng Wú-Jǐ writes. At that point, using a fire method to force sweating is clearly inappropriate treatment. One should use acrid, cool medicinals to resolve the heat. When a heating method is used and great sweat issues, the fluids are damaged, the yīn of the stomach is exhausted, and what was originally only vexation becomes the more severe sign of agitation and vexation. The heat evil enters the stomach and because it is exuberant, it gives rise to delirious speech. A yáng brightness pattern in which the stomach domain is replete is already starting as the result of adverse treatment with heat.

If, after ten days, the disease has not become worse, it means that the patient's constitution was strong enough to withstand the evil and the heat evil is becoming debilitated. Once the evil is debilitated, the fluids begin to return to normal. Shivering and spontaneous diarrhea are, in that case, a sign of recovery and the elimination of the residual evil qì.

The third part of this line describes one other possible transmutation, following the use of an inappropriate treatment method. A modern student may wonder about the value of this section since modern physicians do not use these methods of treatment, but it is possible that one may see clinical signs that are similar to these, even if a hot pack is not used. Perhaps more significantly, the value of this section lies in the analysis of the pathomechanism. A group of signs are presented that provide insight into both normal and abnormal mechanisms of physiological function. The writing of Chéng Wú-Jǐ describes the significance of this section in the following words:

> If [there is] absence of sweating from lumbus down, then the fluids are unable to flow downward; consequently, [the patient] desires but is unable to urinate and the heat qì ascends counterflow and instead, [he/she] retches. [If this patient is] verging on urinary incontinence and has aversion to cold in the soles of the feet, the qì is unable to flow downward and [there is] vacuity. [If] the fluids are tending to percolate [out of the intestines], this makes the stool hard and should [make] urination frequent.... Here, because the fire heat has dried the interior, the fluids cannot flow downward; hence urination is not frequent and not copious. If the fire heat disperses, the fluids harmonize, then the bound stool will be moistened and will spontaneously evacuate. After the stool [passes], [there is] a sudden headache. At first, there was hard stool and the yáng qì could not flow downward. As the stool has passed, the yáng qì downbears and [there is] vacuity in the head; consequently, [there is] a sudden headache.... At first, when the yáng qì could not flow downward, there was aversion to cold in the soles of the feet. Now, the yáng qì is able to descend, so the soles [of the feet] are warm.

The use of inappropriate treatment damages both yīn and yáng. The signs, as described by Chéng Wú-Jǐ, represent vacuity of both yáng and yīn. Heat evils tend to attack upward, so sweat issues in the upper body. Because the fluids have been damaged, as has the yáng qì, neither is distributed properly and no sweat issues in the lower body. A desire to urinate exists, but because the fluids cannot flow downward, no urine is discharged. The inability to urinate reflects damage to the yáng qì and insufficient fluids. Damage to the yáng qì also results in an inability to control urination normally and a feeling of imminent incontinence. Often, hard stool indicates that the fluids are percolating out of the intestines and exiting the body through the urine, but this is not the case here because interior heat has caused dryness. Aversion to cold in the soles of the feet indicates that the yáng qì is unable to flow downward. When the stool becomes moistened and can move, the yáng qì spontaneously flows downward and a headache is the result of yáng vacuity in the head. This downward flow of qì also warms the soles of the feet.

Line 111

㈠ 太阳病中风，以火劫发汗，邪风被火热，血气流溢，失其常度，两阳相熏灼，其身发黄。㈡ 阳盛则欲衄，阴虚小便难。㈢ 阴阳皆虚竭，身体则枯燥，但头汗出，剂颈而还，腹满微喘，口干咽烂，或不大便，久则谵语，甚者至哕，手足躁扰，捻衣摸床，小便利者，其人可治。

(1) *Tài yáng bìng zhòng fēng, yǐ huǒ jié fā hān, xié fēng bèi huǒ rè, xuè qì liú yì, shī qí cháng dù, liǎng yáng xiāng xūn zhuó, qí shēn fā huáng.* (2) *Yáng shèng zé yù nǜ, yīn xū xiǎo biàn nán.* (3) *Yīn yáng jù xū jié, shēn tǐ zé kū zào, dàn tóu hàn chū, jì jǐng ér huán, fù mǎn wēi chuǎn, kǒu gān yān làn, huò bù dà biàn, jiǔ zé zhān yǔ, shèn zhě zhì yuē, shǒu zú zào rǎo, niǎn yī mó chuáng, xiǎo biàn lì zhě, qí rén kě zhì.*

(1) [When in] greater yáng wind strike disease, fire forcing[1] is used to promote sweating, the evil wind is exacerbated by fire-heat; [then] blood and qì flow and spill,[2] losing their normalcy.[3] (2) The two yáng[4] fume and scorch each other and [there is] generalized yellowing. (3) Yáng is exuberant, so [there is] about to be spontaneous external bleeding. Yīn is vacuous, so urination is difficult. (4) Yīn and yáng are both exhausted; [there is] generalized desiccation[5] and sweating only from the head that stops just at the neck, abdominal fullness, slight panting, dry mouth, putrefecation of the throat,[6] or inability to defecate. [If this] endures, there will be delirious speech, and when severe, hiccuping, agitation of the extremities, and picking at bedclothes.[7] When urination is uninhibited, the person can be treated.

Text Notes

1. Fire forcing, 火劫 *huǒ jié*: A fire method is used to force sweating. Fire methods include warm or hot needling, application of hot medicinals to the exterior of the body, and fuming.
2. Flow and spill, 流溢 *liú yì*: Abnormal movement of the blood, which may involve blood seeping out of the vessels.

3. Losing their normalcy, 失其常度 *shī qí cháng dù*: As above, a loss of normal movement of the qì and blood.
4. The two yáng, 两阳 *liǎng yáng*: Here, the use of the term "yáng" means wind and fire evils, not the yáng qì of the body.
5. Generalized desiccation, 身体枯燥 *shēn tǐ kū zào*: Emaciation, accompanied by dry, lusterless skin.
6. Putrefecation of the throat, 咽烂 *yān làn*: A condition in which the interior of the throat is red, swollen, and eroded. Also known as "damage in the throat," 咽中伤 *yān zhōng shāng*.
7. Picking at bedclothes, 捻衣摸床 *niǎn yī mō chuáng*: The patient unconsciously rubs and fingers the clothes and/or the bedclothes.

SYNOPSIS

Transmuted patterns and the prognosis for greater yáng wind strike patterns in which fire forcing is used to promote sweating.

COMMENTARY

In this line Zhāng Jī explains the mechanism of damage that occurs following inappropriate use of a fire method to force sweating. Wind and fire are both yáng evils. When fire is used to treat a yáng evil, yáng reinforces yáng and the strength of the evil is increased. This mistreatment engenders internal heat and damages both the qì and blood. The qì is stirred and the blood is harassed, which results in the loss of normal movement of both.

Fire forcing damages yīn and engenders internal heat. If fuming is then used, the heat will become exuberant and scorch the blood. When the blood is damaged in this way it becomes dry and part of it moves out of the vessels, resulting in generalized yellowing. Modern authors attribute the yellowing to a loss of normal function in the liver and gallbladder, which results in the abnormal movement of gall, but this explanation was unknown to Zhāng Jī and subsequent generations of doctors. See the Introduction for a further discussion of this issue.

Spontaneous external bleeding results from attack of exuberant yáng heat, since the heat forces the blood out of the vessels. Exuberant internal heat also damages yīn humor, resulting in yīn vacuity and difficult urination.

Inappropriate treatment with fire damages both yáng and yīn. When yīn and blood are exhausted, they cannot moisten the skin. When yáng and qì become exhausted, they cannot warm the body's exterior. Thus, in this condition, the skin is dry and lusterless.

As discussed previously, heat evils tend to attack upward. The heat causes sweating, but only from the head. The area of sweating is reduced because of the damage to the fluids caused by the heat evil. The heat evil flames in the upper part of the body, scorching the fluids and resulting in a dry mouth and inflamed throat. Dryness in the interior indicates that fluids cannot move normally, which also causes stagnation of the qì. When the qì is stagnant, the qì dynamic is congested, the abdomen becomes full, and the patient pants. Dryness and qì stagnation may also result in inability to pass the stool.

If the heat evil remains in the interior for a long time, it can affect the heart and lead to delirious speech and a more serious pattern. Hiccuping means that the stomach fluids have been seriously damaged and the stomach qì has lost regulation. Agitation of the extremities and picking at the bedclothes are indicative of exuberant heat desiccating the fluids and disrupting the ability of yīn to contain yáng. These signs suggest that the patient is stuporous and are very dangerous signs.

If, however, urination is inhibited, the patient may still be treated successfully. Although the heat evil is exuberant and yīn humor have been damaged, uninhibited urination indicates that there has not been total fluid collapse and that the bowels and viscera are still functioning; therefore, recovery is still possible. If urination is inhibited, it indicates fluid collapse and that the bowels and viscera are incapable of processing the fluids. In this pattern, successful treatment is less likely.

LINE 113

形作伤寒，其脉不弦紧而弱，弱者必渴，被火必谵语，弱者发热脉浮，解之当汗出愈。

Xíng zuò shāng hán, qí mài bù xián jǐn ér ruò, ruò zhě bì kě, bèi huǒ bì zhān yǔ, ruò zhě fā rè mài fú, jiě zhī dāng hàn chū yù.

[When] the form [of the illness] is that of cold damage[1] and the pulse is not stringlike [or] tight, and is weak, weakness [means] there will be thirst. [When] fire is used,[2] there will be delirious speech. When [in such cases the pulse] is weak, [if there is] heat effusion and the pulse is floating, sweating should [bring about] recovery.

TEXT NOTES

1. [When] the form [of the illness] is that of cold damage, 形作伤寒 *xíng zuò shāng hán*: An unspecified disease with signs that are similar to cold damage.
2. [When] fire is used, 被火 *bèi huǒ*: The patient is treated with a fire method.

SYNOPSIS

When warm disease damages yīn, the use of fire methods is contraindicated.

COMMENTARY

This disease is similar to cold damage, which suggests that heat effusion, headache, or other signs commonly seen in cold damage may be present, although differences also exist. The pulse in cold damage is generally floating and tight, whereas here the pulse is weak and floating. In the *Huáng Dì Nèi Jīng*, heat effusion with a pulse that is weak means internal heat. Accordingly, Zhāng Jī writes that in a disease like cold damage with signs such as heat effusion, when the pulse is weak, thirst arises from internal heat.

If a fire method is used to treat a patient with internal heat, the fire will boost the internal heat. Exuberant heat damages the fluids and affects the stomach, causing delirious speech.

The pulse is weak and floating and heat effusion is present, indicating that an evil is still present in the exterior. The disease will resolve if sweat issues.

LINE 114

太阳病，以火熏之，不得汗，其人必躁，到经不解，必清血，名为火邪。

Tài yáng bìng, yǐ huǒ xūn zhī, bù dé hàn, qí rén bì zào, dào jīng bù jiě, bì qīng xuè, míng wéi huǒ xié.

In greater yáng disease, because fire fuming is used and sweating is not obtained, the person will be agitated. [If the evil] reaches the [original] channel[1] and [the disease] does not resolve, there will be bloody stool.[2] [This pattern] is called fire evil.

TEXT NOTES

1. [If the evil] reaches the [original] channel, 到经 *dào jīng*: In six days, the evil is said to make a complete passage through the channels. On the seventh day it returns to the greater yáng channel.
2. Bloody stool, 清血 *qīng xuè*: 清 *qīng* is used as 圊 *qīng* and means toilet or using the toilet. Thus, this term means blood in the stool.

SYNOPSIS

An aggravated pattern in which fire evil descends and damages the yīn network vessels.

COMMENTARY

Greater yáng disease is treated by resolving the exterior. Here, fire fuming is used to force sweating, but it is unsuccessful. Because no sweat issues, the heat evil is trapped in the interior, unable to move outward and exacerbated by the fire treatment. Heat evil in the interior easily harasses the spirit and causes agitation.

If the evil makes a complete passage through the channel system and does not resolve, it means that the yáng evil is severe and that the heat has fallen deep into the interior. Heat deep in the interior cannot be eliminated through sweating. It scorches the yīn channels and harasses the blood, causing frenetic movement of the blood and ultimately the appearance of blood in the stool. Because this pattern occurs following adverse treatment with a heat method that causes exuberant heat in the interior, it is termed fire evil.

LINE 115

脉浮热甚，而反灸之，此为实，实以虚治，因火而动，必咽燥吐血。

Mài fú rè shèn, ér fǎn jiǔ zhī, cǐ wéi shí, shí yǐ xū zhì, yīn huǒ ér dòng, bì yān zào tù xuè.

[When] the pulse is floating and the heat is severe, but moxibustion [is used], this is repletion and [here] repletion is being treated as vacuity;

because [the blood] is stirred[1] by the fire, there will be dry throat and blood ejection.[2]

Text Notes

1. Stirred, 动 *dòng*: The blood moves in abnormal patterns.
2. Blood ejection, 吐血 *tù xuè*: The expulsion from the mouth of blood that comes from the stomach (vomiting of blood) or the lung and throat (coughing of blood).

Synopsis

Blood ejection and dry throat from counterflow ascent of fire evil, following the inappropriate use of moxibustion.

Commentary

A floating pulse and great heat generally indicate an exterior pattern in which the heat evil is exuberant. This is a repletion pattern, but it is treated as if it is a vacuity pattern and moxibustion is used. The physician may have thought that this was a case of extreme yáng debilitation, in which the pulse was floating and the heat was a result of the yáng qì floating to the surface of the body, prior to desertion.

The heat evil is further strengthened by the use of fire and it attacks the interior. Exuberant heat scorches the blood vessels and damages the yīn. Because the yīn is damaged, the throat becomes dry. The heat evil also causes stirring of the blood and frenetic movement of the blood outside the vessels. Blood from the stomach or from the lung and throat is ejected from the mouth.

Line 116

㈠ 微数之脉，慎不可灸。㈡ 因火为邪，则为烦逆，追虚逐实，血散脉中，火气虽微，内攻有力，焦骨伤筋，血难复也。㈢ 脉浮，宜以汗解。㈣ 用火灸之，邪无从出，因火而盛，病从腰以下，必重而痹，名火逆也。㈤ 欲自解者，必当先烦，烦乃有汗而解。㈥ 何以知之？脉浮，故知汗出解。

(1) Wēi shuò zhī mài, shèn bù kě jiǔ. (2) Yīn huǒ wéi xié, zé wéi fán nì, zhuī xū zhú shí, xuè sàn mài zhōng, huǒ qì suī wēi, nèi gōng yǒu lì, jiāo gǔ shāng jīn, xuè nán fù yě. (3) Mài fú, yí yǐ hàn jiě. (4) Yòng huǒ jiǔ zhī, xié wú cóng chū, yīn huǒ ér shèng, bìng cóng yāo yǐ xià, bì zhòng ér bì, míng huǒ nì yě. (5) Yù zì jiě zhě, bì dāng xiān fán, fán nǎi yǒu hàn ér jiě. (6) Hé yǐ zhī zhī? Mài fú, gù zhī hàn chū jiě.

(1) [When] the pulse is faint and rapid, [one must be] cautious and not use moxibustion. (2) Because fire is an evil, it will [cause] vexation

counterflow,[1] [as if] seeking vacuity and pursuing repletion,[2] and [it will] dissipate the blood from the pulse.[3] Although the fire qì is mild, it attacks the interior forcefully, parching the bones and damaging the sinews;[4] and [one knows] the blood is difficult to restore.[5] (3) When the pulse is floating, it is appropriate to resolve [the exterior] through sweating. (4) Using fire and moxibustion, the evil has no [place] from which to effuse and because of the fire, [it becomes] exuberant. From the lumbus down, there will be heaviness and impediment[6] and this is called adverse [treatment by] fire. (5) When [the disease] is about to resolve, there will first be vexation, then sweating and resolution. (6) How does one know this? The pulse is floating; hence one knows that sweating will resolve [the disease].

Text Notes

1. Vexation counterflow, 烦逆 *fán nì*: Depressed heat in the interior and counterflow ascent of fire qì.
2. [As if] seeking vacuity and pursuing repletion, 追虚逐实 *zhuī xū zhú shí*: The use of a fire method increases the vacuity and the repletion. Originally, yīn vacuity and heat repletion were present; hence the use of a fire method exacerbates yīn vacuity and fortifies heat repletion.
3. Dissipate the blood from the pulse, 血散脉中 *xuè sàn mài zhōng*: Blood vacuity is a component of yīn vacuity. Because the heat is severe, it damages the yīn and blood and causes an empty feeling in the pulse.
4. Parching the bones and damaging the sinews, 焦骨伤筋 *jiāo gǔ shāng jīn*: The heat disperses and scorches the yīn humors. The bones and sinews lose normal moistening and nourishment.
5. The blood is difficult to restore, 血难复也 *xuè nán fù yě*: Once an evil enters the blood, it becomes more difficult to treat. Furthermore, blood is a yīn substance and it is generally accepted that it is easier to boost yáng than to enrich yīn.
6. Heaviness and impediment 重而痹 *zhòng ér bì*: A feeling of heaviness in the lower limbs and difficulty in walking. Here, 痹 *bì*, often used to denote a category of diseases that are caused by wind, cold, and dampness invading the channels and that manifest in limb pain and joint pain (notably conditions classified as rheumatism or sciatica in modern medicine), is used descriptively to mean impeded physical movement.

Synopsis

Transmuted patterns following the inappropriate use of moxibustion in vacuity heat or unresolved exterior patterns.

Commentary

This line comprises three sections, each presenting a basic concept. The first is the first two sentences, from the beginning of the line to "the blood is difficult to restore." The second is the third and fourth sentences, ending at "adverse [treatment by] fire"; and the last is from there to the end of the line.

The first section presents the concept that in cases of vacuity heat, one cannot use heat methods. Moxibustion is the example given in the text, but in vacuity heat patterns, any heat method is inappropriate. The pulse is faint and rapid, indicating yīn vacuity with effulgent heat; therefore, one should enrich yīn and clear heat. Fire, although it can be used therapeutically, also represents an evil. If a fire method is used here, the fire will further damage yīn and assist the heat. The fire evil distresses the interior and contends with the vacuity heat, causing both the heat and the vacuity to become more severe. As heat generally has a tendency to rise in the body, this severe heat attacks upward and harasses the heart spirit, causing vexation, named "vexation counterflow."

When yīn is damaged, the blood becomes vacuous. The original vacuity is made worse by the use of an inappropriate method, damaging the blood to the point that it dissipates from the pulse and the pulse begins to move abnormally. Although the heat method used, perhaps moxibustion, is described as mild, its effect on a patient with yīn vacuity heat is still quite strong. By dispersing the fluids and scorching yīn, it causes the loss of normal moistening and nourishment. This dries out the bones and sinews and also is likely to affect the skin and flesh. At this point, because the damage to yīn and blood is severe, restoring it to normal is difficult.

When the pulse is floating, it is important to determine the presence or absence of an exterior condition. If an exterior condition is present, it is appropriate to resolve the exterior through the promotion of sweating, making the evil follow the sweat out of the body. Use of a fire method constitutes using a supplementing method to treat repletion and will deprive the evil of any path out of the body. The fire boosts the heat evil, causing exuberant heat. The heat rises up, forcing the qì and blood up with it. Heaviness and impediment in the lower body result from the lack of qì and blood. This pattern is called "adverse [treatment by] fire."

When the patient is about to recover, the pulse is floating and vexation and then sweating occur. A pulse that is floating indicates that right qì is rising up to dispel the evil from the exterior. When the right qì becomes hyperactive and contends with the evil, vexation may be observed. Following vexation, sweat issues and the disease resolves. One knows that vexation is a sign of imminent recovery because the pulse is floating. Vexation is not a sign of an internal disease process, but is a sign of right qì contending with the evil in the exterior.

4.15 Recovery Pattern Identification

Line 58

凡病，若发汗、若吐、若下、若亡血、亡津液，阴阳自和者，必自愈。

Fán bìng, ruò fā hàn、 ruò tù、 ruò xià、 ruò wáng xuè、 wáng jīn yè, yīn yáng zì hé zhě, bì zì yù.

In any illness, if sweating is promoted, [or] if vomiting [or] if precipitation [has been used], [and] if [as a result] the blood collapses* [or] liquid and humor collapse, when yīn and yáng spontaneously harmonize, [the person] will spontaneously recover.

Text Note

* Blood collapses, 亡血 *wáng xuè*: This term means blood vacuity, which can be the result of blood or fluid loss and does not necessarily mean a pattern of critical blood loss, as the modern usage of this term might suggest. See also line 347, p. 555, and line 87, p. 104, for other examples of this term.

Synopsis

In any disease, when yīn and yáng spontaneously harmonize, there can be spontaneous recovery.

Commentary

This line is a general commentary on the process of recovery from disease. The use of the term "all diseases" means that it is a discussion of any disease condition, not specifically cold damage or greater yáng disease. It does not matter what treatment was used, be it vomiting, precipitation, or the promotion of sweating, or what disharmonies exist, including fluid or blood collapse. In all these cases, yīn and yáng must harmonize before recovery can occur.

The goal of pattern identification and treatment determination is to provide treatment that allows yīn and yáng to return to a harmonious balance. The underlying principle of this concept and the reason the word "spontaneous," 自 *zì*, is used, is that the restoration of this balance is dependent on the ability of the body itself to return to harmony. In many situations, the restorative process occurs without the patient ingesting any medicine; when medicines are used, one must remember that they provide assistance to a natural process, rather than being entirely responsible for the cure.

Line 59

㈠ 大下之后，复发汗，小便不利者，亡津液故也。㈡ 勿治之，得小便利，必自愈。

(1) *Dà xià zhī hòu, fù fā hàn, xiǎo biàn bù lì zhě, wáng jīn yè gù yě.* (2) *Wù zhì zhī, dé xiǎo biàn lì, bì zì yù.*

(1) When after great precipitation, sweating is then promoted, and [as a result] urination is inhibited, [this] is because liquid and humor have collapsed. (2) Do not treat [this]; [once] the urine is disinhibited, [the person] will spontaneously recover.

Synopsis

A pattern of inhibited urination from liquid damage following inappropriate treatment.

COMMENTARY

If one patient is given both precipitation and sweating, it is normally in the order of first promoting sweating and then precipitation, although this general rule may be modified when the interior pattern is severe and the exterior pattern is mild. In this case, precipitation is used first and it fails to resolve the exterior condition and damages the fluids. Sweating is then promoted in an attempt to resolve a condition that has probably shifted into the interior, and the fluids are further damaged. Following these treatments, urination becomes inhibited, indicating that the mistreatment has caused fluid collapse.

Zhāng Jī advises us not to treat this patient and his admonition has been interpreted in two ways. Chéng Wú-Jǐ writes, "... one cannot disinhibit [the urine] with medicinals. Wait until the fluids are sufficient and the urine is uninhibited, then there will be spontaneous recovery." In this interpretation, one should provide no treatment and should wait for the natural processes of the body to restore the fluids. This interpretation reminds one of the previous line and the process of the restoration of harmony between yīn and yáng.

Kē Qín, however, offers a slightly different perspective: "[The admonition] not to treat is a contraindication of [treatment] to disinhibit the urine. It does not suggest that one should wait for spontaneous recovery. When a patient with fluid collapse is not [treated] to engender liquid, how can the urine be disinhibited? [If one] desires to disinhibit the urine, [one should] treat by boosting the fluids." According to this point of view, Zhāng Jī is cautioning against the use of medicinals to disinhibit the urine, not the use of all medicinals. If one engenders the fluids, it will assist the natural processes of the body, restore harmony, and bring about recovery.

In either case, once the urine is disinhibited, one knows that the fluids have been restored, either through the natural processes of the body or the assistance of medicinal therapy. Once the fluids are restored, the disease will resolve.

LINE 93

㈠ 太阳病，先下而不愈，因复发汗，以此表里俱虚，其人因致冒。㈡ 冒家汗出自愈。㈢ 所以然者，汗出表和故也。㈣ 里未和，然后复下之。

(1) *Tài yáng bìng, xiān xià ér bù yù, yīn fù fā hàn, yǐ cǐ biǎo lǐ jù xū, qí rén yīn zhì mào.* (2) *Mào jiā hàn chū zì yù.* (3) *Suǒ yǐ rán zhě, hàn chū biǎo hé gù yě.* (4) *Lǐ wèi hé, rán hòu fù xià zhī.*

(1) [When in] greater yáng disease, initial precipitation fails to bring about recovery [and] sweating is then promoted, and because of this [there is] dual interior-exterior vacuity, the person [will be] encumbered by veiling [dizziness].* (2) Veiling [dizziness] patients will recover spontaneously after sweating. (3) This is because sweating harmonizes the

exterior. (4) The interior is not yet harmonized, so afterwards one should precipitate.

TEXT NOTE

* Veiling [dizziness], 冒 *mào*: A feeling of cloudiness and dizziness in the head and eyes, as if something is obscuring them.

SYNOPSIS

The treatment of veiling dizziness that occurs in greater yáng disease after the promotion of sweating and use of precipitation.

COMMENTARY

In greater yáng disease, it is generally not appropriate to precipitate first. This treatment may damage right qì and result in the evil falling into the interior. Here precipitation is used, and because it is inappropriate treatment, the exterior pattern does not resolve. Sweating is then promoted in an attempt to resolve the exterior evil. The result of this mistreatment is that both the exterior and the interior become vacuous. When the right qì is vacuous, the evil lingers and clouds the clear yáng in the upper body, causing veiling dizziness.

Chéng Wú-Jǐ explains the sign of veiling as follows: "Veiling means depression. Precipitation results in interior vacuity and blood collapse. Sweating results in exterior vacuity and yáng collapse. The exterior and the interior are both vacuous, the cold [evil] qì is depressed, [the clear yáng qì cannot ascend] and as a result, the person [experiences] veiling."

The use of precipitation causes interior vacuity. The promotion of sweating causes exterior vacuity. In this situation, the evil obstructs the exterior and the yáng qì does not ascend properly. When the clear yáng does not ascend, the patient feels dizzy and unclear.

In this pattern, mistreatment causes vacuity of right qì, but this vacuity is not severe. If right qì naturally returns, it will be able to overcome the evil qì. At that point, sweating will occur and the disease will resolve. As Zhāng Jī explains in the text, this resolution occurs because the outward movement of sweat dispels evil qì and harmonizes the exterior. Because the patient was originally mistreated and has some mild vacuity, it is possible that no treatment should be given to assist in the process of resolving the exterior. Nonetheless, one could gently effuse the exterior, while simultaneously supporting right qì in order to expedite this process.

After the patient sweats, if the veiling dizziness resolves, but the interior is still in disharmony and the stool is blocked, one can again use a formula to precipitate the interior. This treatment will free the stool and harmonize the stomach.

This treatment process illustrates the importance of correct timing when treating simultaneous diseases of the interior and exterior. One must first identify the exterior pattern and the interior pattern, then decide which is most severe. At that point one can decide the order in which the two patterns should be treated. In general, it is important to resolve an exterior pattern prior to treating the interior pattern, as the example above illustrates.

Line 94

㈠ 太阳病未解，脉阴阳俱停，必先振栗汗出而解。㈡ 但阳脉微者，先汗出而解；但阴脉微者，下之而解。㈢ 若欲下之，宜调胃承气汤。

(1) *Tài yáng bìng wèi jiě, mài yīn yáng jù tíng, bì xiān zhèn lì hàn chū ér jiě.* (2) *Dàn yáng mài wēi zhě, xiān hàn chū ér jiě; dàn yīn mài wēi zhě, xià zhī ér jiě.* (3) *Ruò yù xià zhī, yí tiáo wèi chéng qì tāng.*

(1) In greater yáng disease that has not yet resolved, [if] the yīn yáng pulses both stop,[1] [the person] will first shiver, [then] sweat, and then [the disease] will resolve. (2) If only the yáng pulse [moves] slightly,[2] first sweat [will] issue and then [the disease] will resolve. If only the yīn pulse [moves] slightly, precipitate and then [the disease] will resolve. (3) If one desires to precipitate, Stomach-Regulating Qì-Coordinating Decoction (*tiáo wèi chéng qì tāng*) is appropriate.

Text Notes

1. The yīn yáng pulses both stop, 脉阴阳俱停 *mài yīn yáng jū tíng*: The inch and cubit pulses are both hidden and cannot be felt.
2. Pulse moves slightly, 脉微 *mài wēi*: Slight movement can be felt, in comparison to the beginning of the line, in which the pulse is hidden and cannot be felt. Because 微 *wēi* can be interpreted as "faint," Wāng Hǔ writes, "This is not the 'faint' of a pulse that is faint and weak."

Synopsis

The relationship between the pulse suddenly stopping and shiver sweating.

Commentary

When a greater yáng disease has not resolved, one would expect the pulse to be floating, but here it is hidden and cannot be felt. This pulse indicates that the qì and blood have been depressed by the evil and cannot outthrust. It is one manifestation of the struggle between right qì and evil qì. When right qì is able to counter evil qì, the patient shivers, indicating that evil qì is being forced out and is no longer depressed. Sweat will then issue and the disease will resolve. This pattern is known as shiver sweating.

In the second part of this line, the pulse manifestation is used to determine what course the disease will follow. Wāng Hǔ writes, "[When] the evil stagnates in the channel, the exterior qì cannot outthrust orderly; hence the yáng pulse [moves] slightly. [When] the evil stagnates in the bowel, the interior qì cannot flow freely; hence the yīn pulse [moves] slightly." If the yáng pulse moves slightly, it means that the exterior yáng has been blocked and depressed by the exterior evil. Once sweat issues, the disease will resolve. Modern commentators suggest that, although no treatment is offered in the text, it may be necessary to supplement yīn, yáng, qì, or blood of vacuous patients in order to assist the source of the sweat. If this type of treatment is not provided, the patient may be unable to sweat.

If the yīn pulse moves slightly, indicating that the evil is blocking the free flow of qì in the interior, one must attack the interior. When the evil is discharged, the qì will be able to flow freely. Stomach-Regulating Qì-Coordinating Decoction (*tiáo wèi chéng qì tāng*) is suggested because it is a moderate formula for precipitating the interior.

5 PATTERNS SIMILAR TO GREATER YÁNG DISEASE

The section below presents two patterns that are similar to greater yáng disease. These patterns must be carefully distinguished because the formulae used to treat them are harsh and easily damage the right qi. The first is a pattern of collected rheum in the chest and rib-side, and it is treated with Ten Jujubes Decoction (*shí zǎo tāng*), a harsh formula that expels water-rheum. The second is phlegm repletion in the chest and diaphragm, which is treated with Melon Stalk Powder (*guā dì sǎn*), a formula that causes the patient to vomit.

5.1 TEN JUJUBES DECOCTION PATTERNS

LINE 152

㈠ 太阳中风，下利，呕逆，表解者，乃可攻之。㈡ 其人漐漐汗出，发作有时，头痛，心下痞硬满，引胁下痛，干呕短气，汗出不恶寒者，此表解里未和也，十枣汤主之。

(1) *Tài yáng zhòng fēng, xià lì, ǒu nì, biǎo jiě zhě, nǎi kě gōng zhī.* (2) *Qí rén zhé zhé hàn chū, fā zuò yǒu shí, tóu tòng, xīn xià pǐ yìng mǎn, yǐn xié xià tòng, gān ǒu duǎn qì, hàn chū bù wù hán zhě, cǐ biǎo jiě lǐ wèi hé yě, shí zǎo tāng zhǔ zhī.*

(1) When, in greater yáng wind strike with diarrhea[1] and retching counterflow, the exterior has resolved, one can attack. (2) When the person has drizzly sweating[2] that occurs at [set] times, headache, hard glomus and fullness below the heart and pain extending under the rib-side, dry retching, shortness of breath, sweating, and absence of aversion to cold, this means [that] the exterior has resolved and the interior is not yet harmonized. Ten Jujubes Decoction (*shí zǎo tāng*) governs.

TEXT NOTES

1. Diarrhea, 下利 *xià lì*: Here the character 利 *lì*, which means disinhibit, uninhibited, or benefit, is used in the specific sense of uninhibited movement of stool, i.e., diarrhea. In this sense, 利 *lì* has to some extent been replaced by its homophone 痢 *lì*, diarrhea or dysentery.

2. Drizzly sweating, 桀桀汗出 *zhé zhé hàn chū*: Slight sweating. The character 桀 *zhé* was originally used in descriptions of small amounts of rain or small amounts of sweat.

FORMULA

Ten Jujubes Decoction (*shí zǎo tāng*)

∘ Attack and expel water-rheum.

芫花（熬） 甘遂 大戟

(一) 右三味，等分，各别捣为散。(二) 以水一升半，先煮大枣肥者十枚，取八合，去滓，内药末。(三) 强人服一钱匕，羸人服半钱，温服之，平旦服。(四) 若下少，病不除者，明日更服加半钱，得快下利后，糜粥自养。

Yuán huā (*áo*) *gān suì* *dà jǐ*

(1) *Yòu sān wèi, děng fēn, gè bié dǎo wéi sǎn.* (2) *Yǐ shuǐ yī shēng bàn, xiān zhǔ dà zǎo féi zhě shí méi, qǔ bā gě, qù zǐ, nà yào mò.* (3) *Qiáng rén fú yī qián bǐ, léi rén fú bàn qián, wēn fú zhī, píng dàn fú.* (4) *Ruò xià shǎo, bìng bù chú zhě, míng rì gèng fú jiā bàn qián, dé kuài xià lì hòu, mí zhōu zì yǎng.*

genkwa (芫花 *yuán huā*, Daphnes Genkwa Flos) (dry-fry)
kansui (甘遂 *gān suì*, Kansui Radix)
euphorbia/knoxia (大戟 *dà jǐ*, Euphorbiae seu Knoxiae Radix)
jujube (大枣 *dà zǎo*, Ziziphi Fructus) 10 pieces

(1) [For] the above three ingredients [use] equal parts. Pound separately and [make into] a powder. (2) Use one and a half shēng of water to first boil ten plump jujube (*dà zǎo*) to get eight gě. Remove the dregs and add the medicinal powder. (3) Strong people [can] take one and a half qián. Weak people [can] take a half qián. Take warm, at calm dawn.* (4) If diarrhea is scant and the disease is not eliminated, take again the next day and add a half qián [more]. As soon as diarrhea occurs, [the person should eat] rice gruel for nourishment.

FORMULA NOTES

* Calm dawn, 平旦 *pīng dàn*: Early in the morning. According to some sources, this is 5–7 A.M., and according to others it is 3–5 A.M.

SYNOPSIS

The signs and treatment of collected rheum in the chest and rib-side, and the differentiation between this pattern and greater yáng wind strike.

COMMENTARY

Greater yáng wind strike is an exterior condition characterized by signs such as aversion to cold, heat effusion, and headache. When in the course of wind strike disease one does not see these signs, but instead sees diarrhea and retching counterflow, this transmutation indicates that the exterior pattern has resolved and water-rheum has formed in the interior. Water-rheum accumulating in the lower burner causes diarrhea and when it ascends counterflow, attacking the stomach, it causes retching counterflow. After the exterior pattern has resolved one can attack the water-rheum in the interior. Zhāng Jī reinforces the idea that the exterior pattern has resolved by reminding the reader, in the second line, of the absence of aversion to cold.

This pattern is suspended rheum evil in the chest and rib-side. The presence of this evil congests the qì dynamic and results in a hard glomus with fullness and pain. One may ask if the presence of rheum evil directly causes the glomus or if the glomus is the result of congestion of the qì dynamic. Both answers are valid. A suspended rheum evil is thought to be able to cause a glomus directly and its presence also congests the qì dynamic, one of the causes of glomus.

Rheum evil disrupts the qì dynamic and covers the clear yáng, impairing its ascent and giving rise to headache. The stomach likes dryness and when the rheum seeps into the stomach, it causes disharmony and impairs downbearing; therefore, stomach qì ascends counterflow. The rheum follows this counterflow ascent and harasses the lungs, causing an inhibition of lung qì and shortness of breath.

The presence of headache, sweating, and retching counterflow may indicate a wind strike pattern, but the sweat only issues slightly and aversion to cold is absent. These points are the keys to the differentiation of this pattern.

This pattern of suspended water rheum in the chest and rib-side is a repletion pattern; therefore, one can attack and expel the water-rheum. Ten Jujubes Decoction (*shí zǎo tāng*) is a harsh formula for expelling water-rheum and must be used carefully. Genkwa (*yuán huā*), kansui (*gān suì*), and euphorbia/knoxia (*dà jǐ*) are cold, bitter, and toxic. They drastically precipitate and drain water, and are the sovereign medicinals in the formula. The nature of the formula is drastic and fierce, and when its use is appropriate, the effect is very rapid. Because these medicinals are toxic and attack evil, they can also damage the qì of the spleen and stomach, as well as right qì; consequently, jujube (*dà zǎo*) is included in the formula to supplement the spleen and support the right. Jujube (*dà zǎo*) also moderates and harmonizes toxic medicinals. The amount of jujube (*dà zǎo*) used is large when compared to the other ingredients, which is why the formula is named after jujube (*dà zǎo*).

The preparation and ingestion method is designed to moderate the harshness of the precipitating agents. Jujube (*dà zǎo*) is cooked to extract all of its supplementing action, but the other agents are made into powder and simply added to the decoction; they are not cooked at all. This method is similar to the one used for Rhubarb and Coptis Heart-Draining Decoction (*dà huáng huáng lián xiè xīn tāng*) and Aconite Heart-Draining Decoction (*fù zǐ xiè xīn tāng*) in that the qì of the harsh ingredients is extracted without the full flavor of those ingredients. One qián seven fēn of this formula may be used with strong patients and for weaker patients, only a half qián should be used. This formula should not be used at all for patients who are pregnant. The powdered ingredients can be irritating to the throat, so modern texts suggest putting the powder into capsules.

If after taking the formula the disease has not been eliminated and mild diarrhea is present, a slightly larger amount of the formula may be given the following day. The dosage should be regulated on the basis of the patient's constitution and the disease condition. The patient should eat rice gruel in order to nourish the spleen and stomach and consolidate the effect of the treatment.

5.2 Melon Stalk Powder Patterns

Line 166

病如桂枝证，头不痛，项不强，寸脉微浮，胸中痞硬，气上冲喉咽不得息者，此为胸有寒也，当吐之，宜瓜蒂散。

Bìng rú guì zhī zhèng, tóu bù tòng, xiàng bù jiàng, cùn mài wēi fú, xiōng zhōng pǐ yìng, qì shàng chōng hóu yān bù dé xī zhě, cǐ wéi xiōng yǒu hán yě, dāng tù zhī, yí guā dì sǎn.

When in an illness that resembles a Cinnamon Twig [Decoction] pattern, headache and stiff nape are absent, the inch pulse is slightly floating, [there is] hard glomus in the chest, and qì surges upward to the throat so [the person] cannot breathe, this indicates that [there is] cold in the chest and that vomiting should be used; [therefore,] Melon Stalk Powder (*guā dì sǎn*) is appropriate.

Formula

Melon Stalk Powder (*guā dì sǎn*)

◦ Eject phlegm repletion.

瓜蒂一分（熬黄） 赤小豆一分 (一) 右二味，各别捣筛，为散已，合治之，取一钱匕，以香豉一合，用热汤七合，煮作稀糜，去滓。(二) 取汁和散，温，顿服之。(三) 不吐者，少少加，得快吐乃止。诸亡血虚家，(四) 不可与瓜蒂散。

Guā dì yī fēn (áo huáng) chì xiǎo dòu yī fēn

(1) *Yòu èr wèi, gè bié dǎo shāi, wéi sǎn yǐ, hé zhì zhī, qǔ yī qián bǐ, yǐ xiāng chǐ yī gě, yòng rè tāng qī gě, zhǔ zuò xī mí, qù zǐ.* (2) *Qǔ zhī huò sǎn, wēn, dùn fú zhī.* (3) *Bù tù zhě, shǎo shǎo jiā, dé kuài tù nǎi zhǐ.* (4) *Zhū wáng xuè xū jiā, bù kě yǔ guā dì sǎn.*

melon stalk (瓜蒂 *guā dì*, Cucumeris Melonis Pedicellus) 1 fēn (dry-fry until yellow)
rice bean (赤小豆 *chì xiǎo dòu*, Phaseoli Calcarati Semen) 1 fēn

(1) [For] the above two ingredients pound and sieve separately. [Make into] a powder and combine to treat, using a qián-spoonful. Take one gě of fermented soybean (*xiāng chǐ*); use seven gě of hot water and boil to make a thin gruel. (2) Remove the dregs and combine the juice with the powder. Take warm as a single dose. (3) [If the person] does not vomit, add a little [more]. As soon as [the person] vomits, stop. (4) All blood collapse and vacuity patients cannot be given Melon Stalk Powder (*guā dì sǎn*).

Synopsis

The signs and treatment of phlegm repletion in the chest and diaphragm, and the differentiation between this pattern and greater yáng wind strike.

COMMENTARY

This pattern is described as being similar to wind strike, suggesting that heat effusion, aversion to cold, and sweating may be present. The absence of headache and neck stiffness and a pulse that is only slightly floating indicate that this pattern perhaps is slightly different from an exterior condition. Furthermore, the most important signs are hard glomus in the chest, qì surging up to the throat, and inability to breathe normally. Zhāng Jī tells us that cold is present in the chest. This information, when combined with an analysis of the formula, suggests the presence of phlegm-rheum congested in the area of the chest and diaphragm.

Phlegm-rheum repletion in the chest congests the qì dynamic and causes a hard glomus to form. Qì ascends counterflow followed by phlegm surging up into the throat and impairing normal breathing. The inch pulse reflects the status of the upper burner. Phlegm-rheum congests in the chest and the right qì contends with the evil; hence the inch pulse is floating. Because a repletion evil is present in the upper burner, vomiting treatment is used.

Melon Stalk Powder (*guā dì săn*) eliminates phlegm repletion in the upper burner by causing the patient to vomit. The sovereign ingredient, melon stalk (*guā dì*) is extremely bitter, and causes vomiting. Sour rice bean (*chì xiăo dòu*) increases the ability of the formula to cause vomiting.

6 CHAPTER APPENDIX

LINE 76A

发汗后，水药不得入口，为逆；若更发汗，必吐下不止。

Fā hàn hòu, shuĭ yào bù dé rù kŏu, wéi nì; ruò gèng fā hàn, bì tù xià bù zhĭ.

After sweating is promoted, water medicinals have not entered the mouth [and there is vomiting] because of [stomach qì] counterflow. If sweating is again promoted, there will be incessant vomiting and diarrhea.

SYNOPSIS

If vomiting occurs after the promotion of sweating, further promotion of sweating is contraindicated.

COMMENTARY

This line is the first part of line 76 and the rest of the line can be found under line 76B, p. 144.

If after the promotion of sweating, the patient is vomiting before a decoction even is swallowed, this means that the stomach qì is ascending counterflow. It is possible that the stomach yáng qì is constitutionally vacuous and accompanied by abiding rheum. The promotion of sweating causes the yáng qì to stray to the exterior, leaving the interior yáng even more vacuous and stirring the abiding rheum in the interior which then ascends counterflow. In this situation, although the exterior has not yet resolved, one cannot further promote sweating. If sweating is again promoted, it will exacerbate the previous mistake and further damage the qì of the spleen and stomach. This further damage will cause incessant vomiting and diarrhea.

This line can be compared with line 74, p. 198, in which the patient vomits after ingesting water. That is a pattern of water counterflow and it is treated with Poria (Hoelen) Five Powder (*wǔ líng sǎn*).

LINE 141A

㈠ 病在阳，应以汗解之，反以冷水潠之，若灌之，其热被劫不得去，弥更益烦，肉上粟起，意欲饮水，反不渴者，服文蛤散；若不差者，与五苓散。...

(1) *Bìng zài yáng, yīng yǐ hàn jiě zhī, fǎn yǐ lěng shuǐ sùn zhī, ruò guàn zhī, qí rè bèi jié bù qù, mí gèng yì fán, ròu shàng sù qǐ, yì yù yǐn shuǐ, fǎn bù kě zhě, fú wén gé sǎn.* (2) *Ruò bù chài zhě, yǔ wǔ líng sǎn....*

(1) When disease is in the yáng, [one] should [promote] sweating to resolve it, but here cold water is sprayed [on the patient].* If [cold water is] poured [over the patient], the heat will be plundered [but] it will not be eliminated and in addition [there will be] vexation, millet [papules] on the skin, a desire to drink water but absence of [actual] thirst [so] take Meretrix Clam Shell Powder (*wén gé sǎn*). (2) If [there is] no recovery, give Poria (Hoelen) Five Powder (*wǔ líng sǎn*)....

TEXT NOTES

* Cold water is sprayed [on the patient], 冷水潠 *lěng shuǐ sùn*: A treatment method in which cold water held in the mouth was sprayed on the patient in order to reduce heat in the body.

FORMULAE

Meretrix Clam Shell Powder (*wén gé sǎn*).

○

文蛤五两

㈠ 右一味，为散。㈡ 以沸汤和一方寸匕服，汤用五合。

Wén gé wǔ liǎng. (1) *Yòu yī wèi, wéi sǎn.* (2) *Yǐ fèi tāng huò yī fāng cùn bǐ fú, tāng yòng wǔ gě.*

meretrix clam shell (文蛤 *wén gé*, Meretricis Concha) 5 liǎng

(1) [For] the ingredient above, [crush it into] a powder. (2) Mix a square-inch-spoon [of the powder] into the boiled decoction. Use 5 gě of the decoction.

Poria (Hoelen) Five Powder (*wǔ líng sǎn*) See line 71, p. 195, for a discussion of this formula.

SYNOPSIS

The signs and treatment of cold depressed in the exterior.

COMMENTARY

This line is the first part of line 141 and the rest of the line can be found under line 141B, p. 223.

Disease of the yáng means that there is a greater yáng exterior pattern. The appropriate treatment is to promote sweating in order to eliminate the evil from the exterior. Here sweating is not promoted and cold water is instead sprayed on the patient. Not only does this not resolve the exterior, it also causes the evil to become depressed in the interstices. As a result, the heat effusion is not eliminated and defense yáng becomes increasingly blocked and depressed, causing vexation. Cold governs contraction and when cold water fetters the fleshy exterior it causes millet-papules to arise on the skin.

The patient has a desire to drink water in order to alleviate the vexation, but becasue there is no heat in the interior actual thirst is absent. This manifestation is one way to distinguish between vexation caused by depression of the exterior yáng and that caused by interior heat damaging fluid.

Meretrix Clam Shell Powder (*wén gé sǎn*) consists of only one ingredient, meretrix clam shell (*wén gé*), which is salty, cold and drying. It dissipates water-qì in order to resolve the exterior depression in this pattern. Once the yáng is unblocked, the vexation should be eliminated. However, if this formula does not have the desired effect, one can use Poria (Hoelen) Five Powder (*wǔ líng sǎn*), which warms yáng, transforms qì, disinhibits water, and harmonizes the exterior.

LINE 30

㈠ 问曰：证象阳旦，按法治之而增剧，厥逆，咽中干，两胫拘急而谵语。㈡ 师曰：言夜半手足当温，两脚当伸，后如师言。㈢ 何以知此？㈣ 答曰：寸口脉浮而大，浮为风，大为虚，风则生微热，虚则两胫挛，病形象桂枝，因加附子参其间，增桂令汗出，附子温经，亡阳故也。㈤ 厥逆，咽中干，烦躁，阳明内结，谵语烦乱，更饮甘草干姜汤。㈥ 夜半阳气还，两足当热，胫尚微拘急，重与芍药甘草汤，尔乃胫伸。㈦ 以承气汤微溏，则止其谵语，故知病可愈。

(1) *Wèn yuē: zhèng xiàng yáng dàn, àn fǎ zhì zhī ér zēng jù, jué nì, yān zhōng gān, liǎng jìng jū jí ér zhān yǔ.* (2) *Shī yuē: yán yè bàn shǒu zú dāng wēn, liǎng jiǎo dāng shēn, hòu rú shī yán.* (3) *Hé yǐ zhī cǐ?* (4) *Dá yuē: cùn kǒu mài fú ér dà, fú wéi fēng, dà wéi xū, fēng zé shēng wēi rè, xū zé liǎng jìng luán, bìng xíng xiàng guì zhī,*

yīn jiā fù zǐ cān qí jiān, zēng guì lìng hàn chū, fù zǐ wēn jīng, wáng yáng gù yě. (5) *Jué nì, yān zhōng gān, fán zào, yáng míng nèi jié, zhān yǔ fán luàn, gèng yǐn gān cǎo gān jiāng tāng.* (6) *Yè bàn yáng qì huán, liǎng zú dāng rè, jìng shàng wēi jū jí, zhòng yǔ sháo yào gān cǎo tāng, ěr nǎi jìng shēn.* (7) *Yǐ chéng qì tāng wēi táng, zé zhǐ qí zhān yǔ, gù zhī bìng kě yù.*

(1) Question: In a pattern similar to yáng dawn,[1] [if the physician] treats [the patient] according to [the appropriate] method,[2] but [the disease] becomes more acute, [then] there is reverse-flow, dryness in the throat, hypertonicity of the lower legs, and delirious speech. (2) The master[3] says: "In the middle of the night the extremities should be warm and the two legs should be able to extend." From here on, proceed as the master said. (3) How does one know this? (4) Answer: The inch pulse is floating and large; floating means wind and large means vacuity. The wind engenders mild heat, and [because of] vacuity, [there is] hypertonicity of the lower legs. The form of the illness is like a Cinnamon Twig [Decoction pattern], and because aconite (*fù zǐ*) is added, it increases [the ability of] cinnamon [twig] to cause sweat to issue, and aconite (*fù zǐ*) [also] warms the channels, so [there is] yáng collapse. (5) [When there is] reverse-flow, dryness in the throat, vexation and agitation, yáng brightness internal bind, delirious speech, and vexation and derangement, change to Licorice and Dried Ginger Decoction (*gān cǎo gān jiāng tāng*). (6) In the middle of the night, the yáng qì returns, so the legs should become warm, [but if] [there is] still slight hypertonicity of the lower legs, give a large [dose] of Peony and Licorice Decoction (*sháo yào gān cǎo tāng*), so that the lower legs will be able to extend. (7) Because Qì-Coordinating Decoctions (*chéng qì tāng*) [cause] slightly sloppy [stool] and then suppress the delirious speech, one knows [the person] can recover from the disease.

TEXT NOTES

1. In a pattern similar to yáng dawn, 证象阳旦 *zhèng xiàng yáng dàn*: Yáng dawn pattern, 阳旦证 *yáng dàn zhèng*, is another name for the Cinnamon Twig Decoction (*guì zhī tāng*) pattern. Nevertheless, on the basis of information contained in *Lèi Zhèng Huó Rén Shū* (类证活人书 "The Life-Saving Book in Systematized Patterns"), some commentators believe that 阳旦汤 *yáng dàn tāng* is Cinnamon Twig Decoction (*guì zhī tāng*) plus scutellaria (*huáng qín*).
2. [if the physician] treats [the patient] according to [the appropriate] method, 按法治 *àn fǎ zhì*: Cinnamon Twig Decoction (*guì zhī tāng*) should be given according to the previous instructions for its ingestion.

3. The master, 师 *shī*: It is not known to whom "the master" refers.

SYNOPSIS

Using a question and answer format, this line discusses the pathomechanism of a pattern similar to yáng dawn.

COMMENTARY

In this line, we are told that the patient exhibits signs that appear similar to a Cinnamon Twig Decoction (*guì zhī tāng*) pattern. We may refer back to line 29, p. 187, and see such signs as a pulse that is floating and spontaneous sweating, but also observed are heart vexation, hypertonicity in the limbs, and frequent urination, which are uncharacteristic of exterior vacuity patterns. Cinnamon Twig Decoction (*guì zhī tāng*) is used to treat the patient, but instead of recovery, we observe counterflow cold in the extremities, dry throat, hypertonicity of the lower legs, and delirious speech.

As the line continues, it becomes more difficult to understand. We are told that aconite (*fù zǐ*) warms the channels and as a result, the yáng collapses. This sequence of events does not seem logical. Furthermore, the author combines yáng brightness internal bind signs of delirious speech, vexation, and derangement, with reverse flow, dry throat, and vexation and agitation, leaving the reader with the impression that in this pattern, yáng vacuity and exuberant heat appear simultaneously.

This line is placed in the appendix because of the difficulties in determining its clinical significance, and because "master" may refer to Zhāng Jī, in which case the reference would have been added to the original text.

LINE 75

㈠ 未持脉时，病人手叉自冒心，师因教试令咳，而不咳者，此必两耳聋无闻也，所以然者，以重发汗虚故如此。㈡ 发汗后，饮水多必喘，以水灌之亦喘。

(1) *Wèi chí mài shí, bìng rén shǒu chā zì mào xīn, shī yīn jiāo shì lìng ké, ér bù ké zhě, cǐ bì liǎng ěr lóng wú wén yě, suǒ yǐ rán zhě, yǐ chóng fā hàn xū gù rú cǐ.* (2) *Fā hàn hòu, yǐn shuǐ duō bì chuǎn, yǐ shuǐ guàn zhī yì chuǎn.*

(1) [The master has] not yet felt the pulse and the person has their hands crossed over their heart. The master, because [of seeing this], instructs the person to try to cough; and [if the person] does not cough, this must be [because] the two ears are deaf and do not hear. Why [this] is so is because of the repeated promotion of sweating, which [caused] vacuity. (2) When, following the promotion of sweating, [the person] drinks copious amounts of water, there will be panting; [and if] water is poured [onto the body]* [there will] also be panting.

TEXT NOTE

* Water is poured [onto the body], 以水灌 *yǐ shuǐ guàn*: The patient takes a bath or shower.

SYNOPSIS

a) A diagnostic method for combining the looking examination with inquiry.

b) Issues to which one should attend during the convalescent period after sweating and a transmuted pattern that can occur if inappropriate actions are taken.

COMMENTARY

This line is best understood when divided into two sections: the first, comprising the first two sentences; and the second, comprising the final sentence. When the patient covers his/her heart, a pattern of heart vacuity and palpitations is likely. The physician instructs the patient to cough, perhaps to investigate whether the action of coughing will produce pain in the chest region. The patient does not respond and it appears that the patient's hearing is impaired. Deafness may be differentiated into vacuity and repletion patterns. When combined with the sign of covering the heart, it appears that this pattern belongs to vacuity. This conclusion is reinforced by the statement in the text that the promotion of sweating has caused vacuity. The reader is reminded that excessive promotion of sweating can damage the essence qì of the heart and kidney. Although no treatment is indicated in the text, one might consider using Cinnamon Twig and Licorice Decoction (*guì zhī gān cǎo tāng*) with the addition of ingredients such as ginseng (*rén shēn*) and aconite (*fù zǐ*), which warm the kidney yáng.

In the second section of the line, following the promotion of sweating the patient drinks a large amount of water. When sweating is promoted excessively, the fluids are discharged through the exterior and the patient feels thirsty. If, however, a large amount of water is ingested, it may collect in the interior leading to a pattern of water amassment. In this pattern, the collected water-rheum counterflow ascends and attacks the lungs, causing panting. Following the promotion of sweating, the fleshy exterior is vacuous and the patient should be cautioned against bathing too soon after the treatment. According to the authors of *Gāo Děng Cóng Shū*, if the patient showers or bathes, water-cold qì can easily enter the body through skin and body hair, to which the lung is connected. The evil, entering through the skin, then blocks the lung qì and causes panting. These two panting patterns occur because the patient is not sufficiently prudent following an illness. This line reinforces the idea that a physician must not only diagnose and treat effectively, but also counsel the patient with regard to prudent behavior.

Line 105

㈠ 伤寒十三日，过经谵语者，以有热也，当以汤下之。㈡ 若小便利者，大便当硬，而反下利，脉调和者，知医以丸药下之，非其治也。㈢ 若自下利者，脉当微厥，今反和者，此为内实也，调胃承气汤主之。

(1) *Shāng hán shí sān rì, guò jīng zhān yǔ zhě, yǐ yǒu rè yě, dāng yǐ tāng xià zhī.* (2) *Ruò xiǎo biàn lì zhě, dà biàn dāng yìng, ér fǎn xià lì, mài tiáo hé zhě, zhī yī yǐ wán yào xià zhī, fēi qí zhì yě.* (3) *Ruò zì xià lì zhě, mài dāng wēi jué, jīn fǎn hé zhě, cǐ wéi nèi shí yě, tiáo wèi chéng qì tāng zhǔ zhī.*

(1) When, in cold damage [that has lasted for] thirteen days, [there is] channel passage[1] and delirious speech, [it is] because of heat, and one should precipitate with a decoction. (2) If urination is uninhibited, the stool should be hard; but [if] instead [there is] diarrhea and the pulse is in harmony,[2] one knows the physician[3] precipitated with a pill medicine and this is not the [correct] treatment. (3) If [there is] spontaneous diarrhea, the pulse should be faint and [there should be] reversal [cold],[4] but now [there is] harmony,[5] which means internal repletion; [therefore,] Stomach-Regulating Qì-Coordinating Decoction (*tiáo wèi chéng qì tāng*)[6] governs.

Text Notes

1. Channel passage, 过经 *guò jīng*: The movement of evils from one channel to another during the course of cold damage disease. The original disease pattern ceases and a new pattern begins.
2. The pulse is in harmony, 脉调和 *mài tiáo hé*: Two interpretations have been offered for this term. The first is that the pulse is in harmony; that is normal. The problem with this interpretation is that if the pulse were normal, disease would be absent. The second and likelier interpretation is that the pulse is in harmony with the current pattern, in this case a yáng brightness disease. Wāng Hǔ writes, "Now the pulse is instead harmonious. 'Instead harmonious' means that this pulse is not contrary to the yáng brightness bowel pattern. If the pulse were truly harmonious, disease would be absent."
3. The physician, 医 *yī*: A physician other than Zhāng Jī himself. This is one of a number of instances where Zhāng Jī is referring to the mistreatment of a patient by another physician. In his preface to the text he is critical of contemporary physicians and their poor skills.
4. The pulse should be faint and [there should be] reversal [cold], 脉当微厥 *mài dāng wēi jué*: This term may also be interpreted as meaning that the pulse should be faint and reverting. The authors of *Gāo Děng Cóng Shū* do not

accept this interpretation on the grounds that it would be difficult to imagine what a "reverting pulse" is.

5. Harmony, 和 *hé*: Harmony means that the pulse is not faint and there is no reversal, as one would expect, but instead the patient appears normal.
6. Stomach-Regulating Qì-Coordinating Decoction (*tiáo wèi chéng qì tāng*): A complete discussion of this formula can be found with line 248, p. 327.

SYNOPSIS

The signs and treatment of diarrhea that is the result of the inappropriate use of a pill medicine for offensive precipitation in yáng brightness bowel repletion pattern.

COMMENTARY

When a cold damage disease persists for more than ten days and then delirious speech is observed, it is likely that the evil has shifted from the greater yáng into the yáng brightness. Heat in the yáng brightness causes dry stool, which is the root of delirious speech. When this pattern is observed, it is appropriate to precipitate, probably using one of the Qì-Coordinating Decoctions (*chéng qì tāng*) in order to flush dryness-repletion, discharge heat, and harmonize the stomach.

In yáng brightness heat repletion internal bind patterns, dryness-heat can distress the fluids, so that they percolate into the bladder and cannot enter the intestines; consequently, urination is uninhibited and the stool is hard and bound. In the pattern presented above, instead of hard bound stool the patient experiences diarrhea. Nonetheless, the pulse conforms with a heat repletion internal bind pattern, in that it is likely to be sunken, replete, and large, and no signs of vacuity exist. Because of this sign pattern, one can deduce that the patient was treated inappropriately with a pill medicine. Inappropriate precipitation cannot resolve the dryness-repletion and instead causes diarrhea.

Inappropriate precipitation damages the spleen and stomach and may lead to vacuity cold diarrhea. The pattern of vacuity cold diarrhea should be differentiated from the pattern described in this line. If the diarrhea is accompanied by a pulse that is faint and reversal cold of the extremities, the pattern is one of vacuity cold. In this pattern, however, the occurrence of diarrhea is marked by the word "instead" in order to emphasize that it is unexpected and different from diarrhea that occurs in the absence of erroneous treatment. Furthermore, the pulse is described as being "in harmony," suggesting that it is replete, not faint as would be seen in a vacuity cold pattern.

This pattern is described as "internal repletion" and therefore precipitation is used to drain repletion. Nonetheless, the patient has already undergone harsh precipitation that has damaged the stomach qì, so further harsh precipitation is inappropriate. Stomach-Regulating Qì-Coordinating Decoction (*tiáo wèi chéng qì tāng*) is suggested because it will address the internal repletion and harmonize the stomach qì.

Line 108

伤寒腹满谵语，寸口脉浮而紧，此肝乘脾也，名曰纵，刺期门。

Shāng hán fù mǎn zhān yǔ, cùn kǒu mài fú ér jǐn, cǐ gān chéng pí yě, míng yuē zòng, cì qī mén.

When in cold damage, [there is] abdominal fullness, delirious speech, and the inch opening[1] is floating and tight, this means the liver is exploiting the spleen and it is called restraint.[2] One should needle Cycle Gate (*qī mén,* LR-14).

Text Notes

1. Inch opening, 寸口 *cùn kǒu*: The wrist pulse or specifically the inch position.
2. Restraint, 纵 *zòng*: A five-phase relationship in which one viscus restrains another viscus following the restraining sequence. An example of this is wood restraining earth. This is the normal restraining sequence, 相克 *xiāng kè*.

   Rebellion, 横 *héng*, stands in opposition to restraint and expresses the situation in which one viscus restrains another viscus, but instead of following the restraining cycle, the action is counter to the cycle. An example of this is wood restraining metal. In the normal restraining sequence metal restrains wood. This pattern is counter to the normal sequence, 相侮 *xiāng wǔ*.

Synopsis

The signs and treatment of the liver exploiting the spleen.

Commentary

This line describes a pattern of the liver exploiting the spleen. However, the signs are suggestive of yáng míng disease, while the pulse is reminiscent of cold damage.

The appearance of abdominal fullness and delirious speech during the course of an external contraction is normally understood to indicate yáng brightness. Here, however, the pulse is not sunken, replete, and large, as one would expect in a yáng brightness disease, but instead is floating and tight. Furthermore, because tidal heat effusion and abdominal pain are absent, one knows that this is probably not a yáng brightness pattern. The attribution of the signs described in this line to the liver exploiting the spleen reflect lines from the *Huáng Dì Nèi Jīng* which read, "The liver governs speech... When the liver qì is exuberant, speech is profuse... The spleen governs the abdomen...." When liver qì is exuberant, speech may become delirious and the abdomen may become full, indicating that the spleen has been restrained by the liver qì. In the present line, the term "restraint" (纵 *zòng*) is used to describe this pathomechanism.

A pulse that is floating and tight is a further indication that this is not yáng brightness disease. Nonetheless, how such a pulse would reflect the liver exploiting the spleen is not immediately apparent, since it is normally considered to be characteristic of cold damage. The rationale is supplied by *Biàn Mài Fǎ* (辨脉法 "Identifying Pulses") which states, "A pulse that is floating and tight is called stringlike." Moreover, the text of the present line specifically states that the pulse is floating and tight at the "inch opening." If this term is taken to mean the inch position, then the pulse would be tight and floating, which is characteristic of cold damage.

In the present line, the needling treatment suggested would appear to throw more light on the precise nature of the condition. Two different patterns may arise when the liver exploits the spleen. One is a pattern of repletion, in which exuberant liver qì rebels against a healthy spleen. The other is a pattern of vacuity, in which the spleen is vacuous and the liver exploits the weakness. The vacuity pattern must be treated by fortifying the spleen, whereas the repletion pattern is treated by draining the liver. Needling Cycle Gate (*qī mén,* LR-14) courses and drains repletion of the liver qì; hence one knows that this is a repletion pattern.

LINE 109

伤寒发热，啬啬恶寒，大渴欲饮水，其腹必满，自汗出，小便利，其病欲解，此肝乘肺也，名曰横，刺期门。

Shāng hán fā rè, sè sè wù hán, dà kě yù yǐn shuǐ, qí fù bì mǎn, zì hàn chū, xiǎo biàn lì, qí bìng yù jiě, cǐ gān chéng fèi yě, míng yuē héng, cì qī mén.

In cold damage with heat effusion, huddled aversion to cold, and great thirst with desire to drink water, there will be abdominal fullness. Spontaneous sweating and uninhibited urination indicate the disease is about to resolve. This is because the liver is exploiting the lung and is called rebellion.* One should needle Cycle Gate (*qī mén,* LR-14).

TEXT NOTE

* Rebellion, 横 *héng*: The opposite of the restraining sequence. Normally, metal (lung) restrains wood (liver), but here the opposite occurs, which is called "rebellion."

SYNOPSIS

The signs and treatment of the liver exploiting the lung.

COMMENTARY

In cold damage disease patterns, the simultaneous appearance of a) heat effusion and aversion to cold which suggest greater yáng disease and b) great thirst and abdominal fullness, which suggest yáng brightness disease, is a strong indication of greater yáng and yáng brightness combination disease. Nonetheless, in this pattern, combination disease is absent and the pattern is described as "the liver exploiting the lung."

When the liver qì is exuberant it can rebel against the lung, particularly if the lung is weak. The lung governs the skin and [body] hair and when exuberant liver qì exploits the lung, the opening and closing of the interstices is impaired and the exterior becomes blocked, giving rise to heat effusion and aversion to cold. The lung governs regulation of the waterways and when its functions are impaired, fluids are not properly distributed to the bladder, causing inhibited urination. When wood fire torments metal and the lung is scorched, the patient feels thirst and desires to drink. Water collects in the interior and is not transformed. This amassment causes stagnation of the qì dynamic and abdominal fullness. Although the text does not explicitly state that urination is inhibited or that sweating is absent, the presence of both signs is implied by the phrase "spontaneous sweating and uninhibited urination indicates the disease is about to resolve." Furthermore, the most important aspect of this pattern is impairment of lung function; therefore, the appearance of spontaneous sweating and uninhibited urination indicates that normal lung function is returning. This pattern may resolve spontaneously, although resolution is not certain. Because the root of this pattern lies in exuberant liver qì, the liver is treated in order to benefit the lung. Cycle Gate (*qī mén,* LR-14) is drained and when the liver qì is not exuberant, lung function will return to normal.

Line 119

太阳伤寒者，加温针，必惊也。

Tài yáng shāng hán zhě, jiā wēn zhēn, bì jīng yě.

When in greater yáng cold damage, a warm needle is used, there will be fright.

Synopsis

A transmuted pattern that occurs when a warming needle is used in a cold damage pattern, which is inappropriate.

Commentary

Greater yáng cold damage is characterized by heat effusion, aversion to cold, absence of sweating, generalized pain, and a pulse that is floating and tight. It is appropriate to promote sweating with acrid, warm Ephedra Decoction (*má huáng tāng*), which expels cold evils. If warm needling is used, not only will the exterior disease fail to resolve, but the construction-blood will be damaged and the heart qì will be dissipated and chaotic, leading to fright and disquietude.

Another explanation of this line is that fright is a direct reaction to the needling, not a reaction to changes in the body brought about by the needling. The idea is that warm needling is a strong exterior stimulus that can elicit fright in certain patients.

Chén Niàn-Zǔ writes that warm needling may not always be inappropriate: "In greater yáng cold damage, if [the evil] is in the channels, [one] should needle. If [it] is in the exterior [or] the flesh, then the promotion of sweating is appropriate [and] resolving the flesh is appropriate; needling is not appropriate. If [one] adds a warm needle and damages the channels then the spirit qì of the channel vessels floats outward; consequently, [there] will be fright."

Line 121

太阳病吐之，但太阳病当恶寒，今反不恶寒，不欲近衣，此为吐之内烦也。

Tài yáng bìng tù zhī, dàn tài yáng bìng dāng wù hán, jīn fǎn bù wù hán, bù yù jìn yī, cǐ wéi tù zhī nèi fán yě.

[In] greater yáng disease, vomiting [has been used], but[1] [since in] greater yáng disease there should be aversion to cold, and now [there is] no aversion to cold and the person has no desire to put on [additional] clothes, this means [the use of] vomiting [caused] internal vexation.[2]

Text Notes

1. But 但 *dàn*: Originally, this character was most commonly used to mean "only," and this is its most common usage in the *Shāng Hán Lùn*. Here, however, it is used in the sense of "but" which developed in the Hàn Dynasty.
2. Internal vexation 内烦 *nèi fán*: Several different interpretations are offered for this term.
   a) The authors of *Gāo Děng Cóng Shū* describe this sign as vexation and oppression in the heart. "Internal" refers to the heart and "vexation" refers to vexation and oppression.
   b) The authors of *Shāng Hán Lùn Yì Shì* write that when right qì is damaged, vexation may be engendered in the interior. This type of vexation is different from that which is the result of external evil and so it is called "internal vexation."
   c) The authors of *Shāng Hán Lùn Yán Jiū Dà Cí Diǎn* describe internal vexation as vexation and oppression in the chest which is the result of internal heat. They refer to the following commentary from Yóu Yí: "This is a transmuted pattern [following] the erroneous [use of] vomiting. The absence of aversion to cold and no desire to wear [more] clothes indicates that although obvious exterior heat is absent, the heat is in the interior; consequently, [the pattern] is called internal vexation. In internal vexation, vomiting causes fluid collapse, dryness in the stomach, and internal heat vexation."

Synopsis

The signs of vexation heat in the stomach that occur when vomiting is used in greater yáng disease, which is inappropriate.

Commentary

In greater yáng exterior patterns the evil is in the fleshy exterior, and sweating should be promoted to expel the evil. Although vomiting treatment can effuse and dissipate evils and may resolve the exterior evil, the use of this method easily damages the stomach fluids. Stomach dryness engenders heat and internal heat engenders vexation; consequently, the patient feels vexation and oppression in the heart. The absence of aversion to cold, as well as no desire for additional clothing, reinforces the idea that the evil has left the exterior and entered the yáng brightness.

When vomiting treatment is used in greater yáng exterior patterns, the transmutations may vary depending on the original constitution of the patient and on what medicinals were given. In this pattern, fluid damage and a transformation to dryness leads to dryness-heat in the stomach and internal vexation. If, however, the treatment damages yáng and gives rise to vacuity cold in the stomach, signs such as vomiting in the evening of food eaten in the morning may be observed.

With regard to the treatment for this pattern, although none is included in the text, we may look to other similar lines for information. In line 71, p. 195, Stomach-Regulating Qì-Coordinating Decoction (*tiáo wèi chéng qì tāng*) is used for a pattern with heat and no aversion to cold to harmonize the stomach. The same formula is used in line 212, p. 338, to resolve heart vexation. For a pattern with constipation and abdominal fullness and distention, this formula may be used to discharge heat and harmonize the stomach. If, in addition to the signs described above, heat effusion and aversion to heat are also observed, further diagnosis is necessary and a different formula may be required.

LINE 123

㈠ 太阳病，过经十余日，心下温温欲吐，而胸中痛，大便反溏，腹微满，郁郁微烦，先此时自极吐下者，与调胃承气汤。㈡ 若不尔者，不可与。㈢ 但欲呕，胸中痛，微溏者，此非柴胡汤证，以呕，故知极吐下也。

(1) *Tài yáng bìng, guò jīng shí yú rì, xīn xià yùn yùn yù tù, ér xiōng zhōng tòng, dà biàn fǎn táng, fù wēi mǎn, yù yù wēi fǎn, xiān cǐ shí zì jí tù xià zhě, yǔ tiáo wèi chéng qì tāng.* (2) *Ruò bù ěr zhě, bù kě yǔ.* (3) *Dàn yù ǒu, xiōng zhōng tòng, wēi táng zhě, cǐ fēi chái hú tāng zhèng, yǐ ǒu, gù zhī jí tù xià yě.*

(1) When in greater yáng disease, ten or more days after channel passage [there is] seething below the heart with a desire to vomit[1] and chest pain, but sloppy stool, slight abdominal fullness, depression [and] mild vexation;[2] [and if] before this time, extreme vomiting and precipitation [were used], give Stomach-Regulating Qì-Coordinating Decoction (*tiáo wèi chéng qì tāng*). (2) If it is not like this [pattern], one cannot give [this formula]. (3) A desire only to retch with chest pain and slightly sloppy [stool] is not a [Minor] Bupleurum Decoction ([*xiǎo*] *chái hú tāng*) pattern. Because of the retching, one knows extreme vomiting and precipitation [were used].

TEXT NOTES

1. Seething below the heart with a desire to vomit, 心下温温欲吐 *xīn xià yùn yùn yù tù*: Vexation and oppression felt below the heart accompanied by nausea

and a desire but inability to vomit. See line 324, p. 477, for an occurrence of a similar sign.

2. Depression [and] mild vexation, 郁郁微烦 *yù yù wēi fán*: Inhibition of normal emotional activity, expressing itself in the form of oppression, frustration, and irascibility, accompanied by heart vexation. See line 103, p. 431, for another occurrence of this sign.

SYNOPSIS

a) The signs and treatment of transmuted patterns that occur when vomiting and precipitation are used in greater yáng disease, which is inappropriate.

b) Distinguishing between these patterns and the Minor Bupleurum Decoction (*xiǎo chái hú tāng*) pattern.

COMMENTARY

In greater yáng disease, when the exterior disease has been resolved for more than a week and the patient exhibits signs such as vexation and oppression below the heart, nausea, and depression, one may notice the similarity with a lesser yáng disease. Nonetheless, abdominal fullness and sloppy stool are generally not characteristic of lesser yáng disease; therefore, one should conclude that this is not a lesser yáng pattern. Abdominal distention and heart vexation can appear in yáng brightness patterns, but sloppy stool is unlikely in those patterns; therefore, a yáng brightness pattern is unlikely. This patient was treated with both vomiting and precipitating medicinals which damaged the fluids, causing stomach dryness that transformed to heat. The heat evil became depressed in the interior. This pattern is a transmuted pattern that is the result of erroneous treatment. A desire to vomit and sloppy stool are a continuing manifestation of the medicinals used to cause vomiting and precipitation. Pain in the chest is the result of qì counterflow following vomiting. In this case one must remove stomach dryness-heat, but a harsh formula would not be appropriate since the patient has already been through several mistreatments. Stomach-Regulating Qì-Coordinating Decoction (*tiáo wèi chéng qì tāng*) is appropriate to discharge heat, moisten dryness, and harmonize the stomach.

In the second line of the text we are told that if the pattern does not present in this particular way, one should not precipitate. This line applies to a situation in which inappropriate treatment has led to a negative transmutation. If these same signs arise spontaneously, a different treatment should be used. For example, in the absence of precipitating treatment the combination of sloppy stool and abdominal fullness can indicate a greater yīn disease in which the spleen and stomach yáng is damaged by cold evil. If no medicinals have been used to cause vomiting and the patient exhibits sign such as seething below the heart and desire to vomit, it may indicate a greater yáng evil has shifted into the lesser yáng. In either of these patterns, Stomach-Regulating Qì-Coordinating Decoction (*tiáo wèi chéng qì tāng*) is not appropriate.

The final section of this line emphasizes that the nausea that is present in this pattern is the result of inappropriate vomiting and precipitation, it does not represent a lesser yáng disease that can be treated with [Minor] Bupleurum Decoction ([*xiǎo*] *chái hú tāng*).

It should be noted that several commentators interpret the second and third sentences of this line differently than the commentary above. Kē Qín agrees that the second line, "if it is not like this [pattern], one cannot give [this formula]," refers to whether or not the patient has received treatment with medicinals to cause vomiting and precipitation. However, he interprets the word 温 *yùn*, as meaning "warm," and this choice is not accepted by most other commentators.

Line 139

(一) 太阳病，二三日，不能卧，但欲起，心下必结，脉微弱者，此本有寒分也。(二) 反下之，若利止，必作结胸，未止者，四日复下之，此作协热利也。

(1) *Tài yáng bìng, èr sān rì, bù néng wò, dàn yù qǐ, xīn xià bì jié, mài wēi ruò zhě, cǐ běn yǒu hán fèn yě.* (2) *Fǎn xià zhī, ruò lì zhǐ, bì zuò jié xiōng, wèi zhǐ zhě, sì rì fù xià zhī, cǐ zuò xié rè lì yě.*

(1) When greater yáng disease [has lasted] two or three days, [and the person] is unable to sleep, and desires only to get up, [then] there will be a bind below the heart and a pulse that is faint and weak, which means that originally [there were] cold elements.* (2) But if precipitation is used, and the [resulting] diarrhea is checked, there will be chest bind; [if the diarrhea] is unchecked and, after four days, precipitation is used again, this will cause complex diarrhea.

Text Note

* Cold elements, 寒分 *hán fèn*: Different interpretations have been offered for this term. Kē Qín explains it as cold rheum. Chéng Wú-Jǐ explains it simply as cold evil. In the *Qiān Jīn Yì Fāng*, *Mài Jīng*, and *Jīn Guì Yù Hán Jīng*, the character 分 *fēn* is eliminated, and in the *Wài Tái Mì Yào* (外台秘要 "Essential Secrets from Outside the Metropolis") the term "cold," 寒分 *hán fēn*, is replaced with "enduring cold," 久寒 *jiǔ hán*.

Synopsis

In people who normally have phlegm-rheum, and who contract greater yáng disease, the use of precipitation is inappropriate and can lead to the transmuted patterns of chest bind or complex heat diarrhea.

Commentary

This line describes the consequences of mistreating a greater yáng exterior pattern with precipitation. After a short period of time ("two or three days"), the greater yáng exterior pattern is still present. At the same time, the patient cannot lie or sleep quietly, prefers to sit up, and has a bind below the heart. These signs are suggestive of an exterior evil falling into the interior and entering the yáng brightness, but in that case the pulse would be surging, large, slippery, and replete. Here, instead, the pulse is faint and weak, suggesting that this is not a pattern of yáng brightness repletion heat, but one of cold. This patient has cold-rheum amassment in the area below the heart, which congests the yáng qì in the chest, giving rise to bind. Cold-rheum also congests the movement of the qì in the vessels; consequently, the pulse is faint and weak.

This pattern is simultaneous exterior cold and interior rheum so it should be treated by resolving the exterior and transforming cold-rheum. If bind below the heart from the presence of cold-rheum is taken as an indication of repletion heat and offensive precipitation is used, the evil will fall inward, giving rise to diarrhea. If the diarrhea ceases, evil will bind with cold-rheum in the interior and form chest bind. No explanation is provided for the mechanism by which the diarrhea ceases. If the diarrhea persists and precipitation is used again in an attempt to resolve the original bind, this further mistreatment will damage the spleen and stomach. Diarrhea from internal vacuity and an unresolved exterior evil will exist together, in a pattern described as complex diarrhea.

LINE 140

太阳病，下之，其脉促，不结胸者，此为欲解也；脉浮者，必结胸；脉紧者，必咽痛；脉弦者，必两胁拘急；脉细数者，头痛未止；脉沉紧者，必欲呕；脉沉滑者，协热利；脉浮滑者，必下血。

Tài yáng bìng, xià zhī, qí mài cù, bù jié xiōng zhě, cǐ wéi yù jiě yě; mài fú zhě, bì jié xiōng; mài jǐn zhě, bì yān tòng; mài xián zhě, bì liǎng xié jū jí; mài xì shuò zhě, tóu tòng wèi zhǐ; mài chén jǐn zhě, bì yù ǒu; mài chén huá zhě, xié rè lì; mài fú huá zhě, bì xià xuè.

When in greater yáng disease, precipitation is used and the pulse is skipping, this is not chest bind, and it means [the disease] is about to resolve. If the pulse is floating, there will be chest bind. If the pulse is tight, there will be sore throat. If the pulse is stringlike, there will be hypertonicity of both rib-sides. If the pulse is fine and rapid, there will be an unrelieved headache. If the pulse is sunken and tight, there will be desire to retch. If the pulse is sunken and slippery, there will be complex diarrhea. If the pulse is floating and slippery, there will be blood descent.

SYNOPSIS

After the inappropriate use of precipitation in greater yáng disease, the pulse can be used to infer the different kinds of transmutations.

COMMENTARY

This line is a discussion of the significance of different pulse qualities in a greater yáng pattern following the inappropriate use of precipitation. In general, Zhāng Jī stresses the correlating signs and pulses,. and, as he states in his own preface, he was critical of the practice already prevalent in his own time of taking the pulse and ignoring the signs. This line places an emphasis on the pulse considered to be inconsistent with the rest of the text, and for this reason is thought by some to be the work of Wáng Shū-Hé, who is not only known to have laid great emphasis on the pulse, but also suspected of having altered the original text when compiling the *Shāng Hán Lùn* from the sections relating to externally contracted disease contained in the now lost *Shāng Hán Zá Bìng Lùn*.

In greater yáng disease the promotion of sweating is generally the most appropriate treatment and it will expel the evil. If precipitation is used instead, many different transmutations are possible. This line outlines a group of these transmutations, on the basis of the associated pulse.

If the pulse is skipping, evil qì will not bind in the chest and the disease will resolve. In the *Shāng Hán Lùn* "skipping" refers to a pulse that is urgent, but this is not the same pulse as is denoted by the term "skipping pulse," in which the pulse is rapid and interrupted. It is considered a yáng pulse that indicates the movement of qì upward and outward. It is through this dynamic that the evil is expelled outward and the disease resolves.

If the pulse is floating, it indicates that the exterior evil is still exuberant and has not been debilitated by the precipitating treatment. Because precipitation causes interior vacuity, the exterior evil exploits the interior weakness, falls into the upper burner, and becomes bound with phlegm-water evil, causing chest bind.

If the pulse is tight, it indicates that exterior cold evil has entered the interior. Following precipitation, cold evil directly enters the lesser yīn. Yīn cold distresses the lower burner, vacuous from the precipitating treatment. It follows the channel, surging upward and causing sore throat.

A pulse that is stringlike suggests that following precipitation, the evil has shifted into the lesser yáng. The course of the lesser yáng channel moves through the rib-sides and consequently, the patient feels hypertonicity in these areas.

Following precipitation, a pulse that is fine indicates vacuity and a pulse that is rapid indicates heat. Yáng becomes vacuous and agitated and it runs upward to the head, causing pain.

Inappropriate precipitation can damage the yáng qì, causing yáng vacuity. Vacuous yáng is unable to move the pulse normally and it becomes sunken. When the pulse is tight, it may indicate cold-rheum collecting in the interior. Vacuous yáng is unable to expel the cold-rheum and so it ascends counterflow, causing a desire to retch.

In the case of a pulse that is sunken and slippery because this pattern is characterized by complex diarrhea, the sunken quality is not thought to indicate yáng vacuity, as above, but rather an interior pattern. A pulse that is slippery indicates internal repletion; here, evil heat follows the force of erroneous precipitation and distresses the lower burner, causing food to stray downward and diarrhea to appear.

After precipitation, if the pulse is still floating and is also slippery it indicates that the exterior evil has not been eliminated, but has instead fallen into the interior. This heat evil harasses the blood and causes bloody stool.

Line 142

(一) 太阳与少阳并病，头项强痛，或眩冒，时如结胸，心下痞硬者，当刺大椎第一间、肺俞、肝俞，慎不可发汗，发汗则谵语，脉弦。(二) 五日谵语不止，当刺期门。

(1) *Tài yáng yǔ shào yáng bìng bìng, tóu xiàng jiàng tòng, huò xuàn mào, shí rú jié xiōng, xīn xià pǐ yìng zhě, dāng cì dà zhuī dì yì jiān、fèi shū、gān shū, shèn bù kě fā hàn, fā hàn zé zhān yǔ, mài xián.* (2) *Wǔ rì zhān yǔ bù zhǐ, dāng cì qī mén.*

(1) When in greater yáng and lesser yáng dragover disease, [there is] stiffness and pain of the head and nape, or veiling dizziness, and it is sometimes like chest bind with a hard glomus below the heart, one should needle Great Hammer (*dà zhuī,* GV-14), Lung Transport (*fèi shū,* BL-13), and Liver Transport (*gān shū,* BL-18). Be cautious and do not promote sweating [because if] sweating is promoted [it will] cause delirious speech and a pulse that is stringlike. (2) [If after] five days the delirious speech does not stop, one should needle Cycle Gate (*qī mén,* LR-14).

Synopsis

In greater yáng and lesser yáng dragover disease, one should use acupuncture and not promote sweating.

Commentary

When a greater yáng disease has not ceased and signs of a lesser yáng disease appear, the resultant pattern is called a greater yáng and lesser yáng combination disease. Stiffness and pain of the head and nape is a sign of the greater yáng channel contracting an exterior evil. Veiling dizziness means that gallbladder fire has followed the lesser yáng channel and assaulted the clear orifices. A periodic sign similar to chest bind is not true chest bind, but reflects an inhibition of lesser yáng channel qì. A hard glomus is present in the area below the heart. When the qì congestion is severe, the area becomes painful and the pattern appears to be chest bind. Nonetheless, the fullness and pain of chest bind is not periodic, but persistent; therefore, one may conclude that this sign does not constitute chest bind.

One way of approaching this line is to consider theory loosely characterized by the idea that diseases of the organs are best treated with a decoction, while diseases of the channels can be treated with acupuncture. Although this theory is not universally accepted, it is one way to explain the use of acupuncture here. The main signs of this pattern involve the greater yáng and lesser yáng channels. Great Hammer (*dà zhuī,* GV-14) is an intersection point for the three yáng channels. It has a strong action to dispel wind. Lung Transport (*fèi shū,* BL-13) rectifies the qì and dissipates evil qì. These two points resolve the greater yáng exterior evil. Liver Transport (*gān shū,* BL-18), the liver transport point, drains gallbladder fire and harmonizes the lesser yáng.

If acupuncture is not used here and instead a decoction is given to promote sweating, the fluids will be damaged. This damage allows lesser yáng fire to become intense. Intense wood fire rebels against earth, heat exploits the stomach, and the stomach qì becomes disharmonious. This process leads to delirious speech. The pulse is stringlike, a quality associated with lesser yáng patterns. If the delirious speech continues unabated, one can needle Cycle Gate (*qī mén,* LR-14) to drain wood fire. Once the fire is cleared, the delirious speech will cease.

Line 150

太阳少阳并病，而反下之，成结胸，心下硬，下利不止，水浆不下，其人心烦。

Tài yáng shào yáng bìng bìng, ér fǎn xià zhī, chéng jié xiōng, xīn xià yìng, xià lì bù zhǐ, shuǐ jiāng bù xià, qí rén xīn fán.

When in greater yáng and lesser yáng dragover disease, instead precipitation is used, [it will] cause chest bind, hardness below the heart, incessant diarrhea, [inability to get] fluids down, and heart vexation.

Synopsis

The critical signs of chest bind that may occur in greater yáng and lesser yáng dragover disease following the inappropriate use of precipitation.

Commentary

Greater yáng disease and lesser yáng disease are appropriately treated through the promotion of sweating and harmonizing treatment, respectively. Neither of these patterns nor the combination of the two is appropriately treated through precipitation. Appropriate treatment consists in harmonizing the lesser yáng and resolving the exterior using a formula such as Bupleurum and Cinnamon Twig Decoction (*chái hú guì zhī tāng*) or using acupuncture points such as Lung Transport (*fèi shū,* BL-13), Great Hammer (*dà zhuī,* GV-14), and Heart Transport (*xīn shū,* BL-15). The use of precipitation causes the evil in the greater yáng and lesser yáng channels to fall inward. In this case, this evil heat combines with phlegm evil in the interior and forms chest bind; consequently, the patient feels pain and hardness below the heart. Because of the presence of a repletion evil in the chest, the patient is unable to swallow fluids normally. Furthermore, the presence of a yáng evil in the interior causes heart vexation. At the same time, the use of precipitation also damages the qì of the center burner, causing vacuity cold of the spleen and stomach. The center qì falls and incessant diarrhea occurs. This pattern is repletion in the upper burner and vacuity in the lower burner.

The formation of chest bind in this pattern is similar to heat repletion chest bind, as described in line 131, p. 212. "[When] the disease springs from yáng, yet precipitation is used, the heat enters [the interior] and causes chest bind."

Both patterns are the result of erroneous precipitation in a greater yáng disease; but in this pattern, in addition to the repletion pattern in the upper burner, a vacuity pattern is also present, whereas the pattern in line 131 is a pure repletion pattern.

The treatment of this pattern presents a difficult problem. The presence of a repletion evil in the chest suggests that attacking is appropriate, but incessant diarrhea indicates vacuity of the right qì and the need for supplementation. To attack the repletion would be to damage further the right qì and to supplement the vacuity would be to boost the repletion. No treatment is suggested in the text, but one may consider first supplementing the center vacuity and then addressing the repletion. The rationale for this approach is that incessant diarrhea is an indication of severe damage to right qì. Right qì is already straying and about to expire; therefore, it must be supplemented before the repletion evil can be attacked.

LINE 153

(一) 太阳病，医发汗，遂发热恶寒。(二) 因复下之，心下痞，表里俱虚，阴阳气并竭，无阳则阴独。(三) 复加烧针，因胸烦。(四) 面色青黄，肤瞤者，难治；今色微黄，手足温者，易愈。

(1) *Tài yáng bìng, yī fā hàn, suì fā rè wù hán.* (2) *Yīn fù xià zhī, xīn xià pǐ, biǎo lǐ jù xū, yīn yáng qì bìng jié, wú yáng zé yīn dú.* (3) *Fù jiā shāo zhēn, yīn xiōng fán.* (4) *Miàn sè qīng huáng, fū rùn zhě, nán zhì; jīn sè wēi huáng, shǒu zú wēn zhě, yì yù.*

(1) In greater yáng disease, the physician promotes sweating and then [there is] heat effusion and aversion to cold. (2) Because precipitation is then used, [there is] a glomus below the heart, dual interior-exterior vacuity, exhaustion of yīn, yáng, and qì, and no yáng only yīn.* (3) A hot needle is then added, so [there is] chest vexation. (4) If the complexion is green-blue and yellow and [there is] twitching of the flesh, this is difficult to treat. Now, the complexion is slight yellow and the extremities are warm so [the patient will] easily recover.

TEXT NOTE

* No yáng only yīn 无阳则阴独 *wú yáng zé yīn dú*: No exterior signs (yáng), only interior signs (yīn). After sweating and precipitation, evil qì falls into the interior. Chéng Wú-Jǐ writes, "'No yáng' means that the exterior pattern ceases. 'Only yīn' means a glomus [is present] in the interior."

SYNOPSIS

The transmuted patterns and determination of prognosis following the use of sweating, precipitation, and hot needles.

COMMENTARY

In greater yáng disease the promotion of sweating is an appropriate treatment;

but after sweat issues, if heat effusion and aversion to cold are still observed, as they are here, it suggests that the treatment was ineffective and the exterior evil is still present. Generally, it is appropriate to promote sweating again, mildly, but in this case the physician instead uses precipitation. Precipitation is inappropriate in greater yáng disease and damages the qì of the spleen and stomach. The evil qì exploits the weakness in the interior and falls inward, impairing upbearing and downbearing. The qì dynamic becomes congested and a glomus forms below the heart. The promotion of sweating damages the exterior, and precipitation damages the interior; therefore, both become vacuous, "dual interior-exterior vacuity." After the evil falls inward, the exterior pattern ceases and only signs of an interior pattern are present. This situation is described in the text as "no yáng only yīn," since the exterior is yáng and the interior is yīn.

The glomus in this pattern is the result of an evil that falls inward following the inappropriate use of precipitation in a greater yáng disease. It is a mixed pattern of heat, from the repletion evil, and cold, from the vacuity of the spleen and stomach. It would be appropriate to use a formula such as Pinellia Heart-Draining Decoction (*bàn xià xiè xīn tāng*) to harmonize the stomach, disperse glomus, fortify the spleen, and boost qì. Nonetheless, the physician in this line instead uses hot needling to force further sweating. Fire evil attacks the interior and causes vexation in the chest. This mistreatment exacerbates and further complicates the original pattern.

Because of the mistreatment not only has the evil not been resolved but the exterior and interior are both vacuous. At this point, if the complexion is blue-green and yellow, the liver qì is exploiting the spleen. When wood restrains earth, yáng becomes vacuous and cannot warm the fleshy exterior; consequently, twitching is observed. The appearance of this sign indicates that the qì of the bowels and viscera has been greatly damaged and the prognosis is poor. If the complexion is slightly yellow and the extremities are warm, it indicates that the qì of the spleen and stomach is still able to outthrust to the extremities. The stomach qì is still present and the source of transformation has not expired. The patient still has the strength to counter the evil and can recover.

Line 160

伤寒吐下后，发汗，虚烦，脉甚微，八九日心下痞硬，胁下痛，气上冲咽喉，眩冒，经脉动惕者，久而成痿。

Shāng hán tù xià hòu, fā hàn, xū fán, mài shèn wēi, bā jiǔ rì xīn xià pǐ yìng, xié xià tòng, qì shàng chōng yān hóu, xuàn mào, jīng mài dòng tì zhě, jiǔ ér chéng wěi.

When in cold damage, vomiting and precipitation [are used] and then sweating is promoted, [there is] vacuity vexation, and the pulse is severely faint. After eight or nine days, [there is] a hard glomus below the heart, pain under the rib-side, qì surging upward to the throat, veiling dizziness, and jerking of the channel vessels.[1] [If] this endures, it will become wilting.[2]

TEXT NOTES

1. Jerking of the channel vessels, 经脉动惕 *jīng mài dòng tì*: Spasmodic movement of the flesh and sinews of the body.
2. Wilting, 痿 *wěi*: Weakness and limpness of the sinews that in severe cases prevents the lifting of the arms and legs. The condition is mainly found to affect the legs, preventing the patient from walking.

SYNOPSIS

In cold damage, the inappropriate use of vomiting, precipitation, and sweating can lead to water-rheum stirring in the interior and if this endures and is not treated, it can lead to wilting.

COMMENTARY

In this line, vomiting and precipitation are used to treat a greater yáng disease and the disease does not resolve. As a result, sweating is then promoted. The combination of these mistreatments damages right qì and liquid. The evil harasses the vacuous interior and causes heart vexation. Because the yáng qì is insufficient, the pulse becomes faint. After eight or nine days, right qì has not recovered and yáng vacuity is severe. Vacuous yáng is unable to control water and water qì ascends counterflow, causing a hard glomus to form below the heart and pain in the rib-sides. Water qì congests in the center burner and impairs stomach downbearing. Stomach qì ascends counterflow and causes a sensation of qì surging upward into the throat. Furthermore, when the clear yáng cannot ascend normally, the patient feels veiling dizziness. Not only is the yáng qì vacuous, but the fluids have also been damaged. The sinews and vessels are not nourished and moistened because the fluids are insufficient; they are also not warmed because the yáng qì is vacuous. As a result, jerking of the channels occurs and if this sign is not addressed properly, it can progress into the more severe sign of wilting.

A comparison between this line with line 67, p. 171, shows that although the signs and pathomechanisms are similar, yáng vacuity in this line is more severe. In both lines, a greater yáng disease is treated inappropriately, resulting in an exterior evil falling inward. In line 67, the signs are counterflow fullness below the heart, qì surging upward to the chest, dizziness, and a pulse that is sunken and tight. In the line preceding, the pulse is faint and the patient also feels pain under the rib-side. Following the promotion of sweating, generalized quivering and trembling is observed in line 67, whereas in the preceding line, sweating gives rise to jerking and then wilting. These differences illustrate that yáng vacuity in this line is more severe than in line 67.

Although no treatment is suggested in this line, on the basis of the information gleaned from line 67 one can surmise that a formula such as Poria (Hoelen), Cinnamon Twig, Ovate Atractylodes, and Licorice Decoction (*fú líng guì zhī bái zhú gān cǎo tāng*) would be used to warm the yáng and control water. It is possible that aconite (*fù zǐ*) would possibly be added.

It should be noted that although most commentators agree on the general meaning of this line, two different interpretations are offered for the pathomechanism. Chéng Wú-Jǐ represents one school of thought, which is that erroneous treatment damages both the qì and fluids and rheum evil is also present. The authors of the *Yī Zōng Jīn Jiàn* represent the other interpretation, in which vacuity of yīn, yáng, qì, and blood exists in this patient, without a rheum evil. Nonetheless, the first explanation seems more plausible since it is able to explain the entire line, without suggesting that errors exist in the original text, which the second explanation requires. Furthermore, if one considers the comparison with line 67 and the formula that is used, the suggestion of rheum evil seems quite plausible.

Line 171

太阳少阳并病，心下硬，颈项强而眩者，当刺大椎、肺俞、肝俞，慎勿下之。

Tài yáng shào yáng bìng bìng, xīn xià yìng, jǐng xiàng jiàng ér xuàn zhě, dāng cì dà zhuī、fèi shū、gān shū, shèn wù xià zhī.

When in greater yáng and lesser yáng dragover disease, [there is] hardness below the heart, stiffness of the neck and nape, and dizziness, one should needle Great Hammer (*dà zhuī,* GV-14), Lung Transport (*fèi shū,* BL-13), and Liver Transport (*gān shū,* BL-18), and should be careful not to use precipitation.

Synopsis

In greater yáng and lesser yáng dragover disease, it is appropriate to use acupuncture and one cannot use offensive precipitation.

Commentary

In greater yáng and lesser yáng dragover disease, stiffness of the neck and nape indicates that the greater yáng evil has not resolved, and hardness below the heart and dizziness indicate that the lesser yáng has contracted the evil. These signs can all be seen as a reflection of inhibited movement of channel qì; therefore, the use of acupuncture is recommended in this line. Great Hammer (*dà zhuī,* GV-14) and Lung Transport (*fèi shū,* BL-13) resolve the greater yáng evil, and Liver Transport (*gān shū,* BL-18) resolves the lesser yáng evil. When a hard glomus is observed below the heart following the inappropriate use of precipitation, a formula such as Pinellia Heart-Draining Decoction (*bàn xià xiè xīn tāng*) may be used and one should not precipitate further. Here a hard glomus occurs in dragover disease of the greater and lesser yáng. The channel qì is inhibited and depressed in the interior; hence acupuncture is used and one is cautioned against the use of precipitation. If a hard glomus appears in lesser yáng and yáng brightness dragover disease, one may use Major Bupleurum Decoction (*dà chái hú tāng*) to harmonize the lesser yáng and attack interior repletion.

If one considers this line and line 142, p. 284, together, it is clear that in greater yáng and lesser yáng dragover disease neither the promotion of sweating nor the use of precipitation is appropriate treatment. This line cautions against the use of precipitation but does not record the outcome of using precipitation. Line 150, p. 285, however, does record the following signs and symptoms as the result of this mistreatment: "chest bind, hardness below the heart, incessant diarrhea, [inability to get] fluids down, and heart vexation."

LINE 174

㈠ 伤寒八九日，风湿相搏，身体疼烦，不能自转侧，不呕不渴，脉浮虚而濇者，桂枝附子汤主之。㈡ 若其人大便硬，小便自利者，去桂加白术汤主之。

(1) *Shāng hán bā jiǔ rì, fēng shī xiāng bó, shēn tǐ téng fán, bù néng zì zhuǎn cè, bù ǒu bù kě, mài fú xū ér sè zhě, guì zhī fù zǐ tāng zhǔ zhī.* (2) *Ruò qí rén dà biàn yìng, xiǎo biàn zì lì zhě, qù guì jiā bái zhú tāng zhǔ zhī.*

(1) When cold damage [has lasted] eight or nine days, [and] wind and dampness contend with each other,[1] [there is] generalized vexing pain,[2] inability to turn sides,[3] absence of retching, absence of thirst, and a pulse that is floating, vacuous, and rough; Cinnamon Twig and Aconite Decoction (*guì zhī fù zǐ tāng*) governs. (2) If the person has hard stool and the urine is spontaneously uninhibited, Minus Cinnamon Plus Ovate Atractylodes Decoction (*qù guì jiā bái zhú tāng*) governs.

TEXT NOTES

1. Wind and dampness contend with each other, 风湿相搏 *fēng shī xiāng bó*: Wind and dampness are understood to exacerbate each other and cause each other to persist. When these two evils are in contention, they remain in the flesh and inhibit the movement of qì and blood.
2. Generalized vexing pain, 身体疼烦 *shēn tǐ téng fán*: Severe pain felt throughout the body. Here, 烦 *fán* is an indication of severity, not vexation in the sense of vexation and agitation, 烦躁 *fán zào*. Yamada Seichin (山田正珍) writes, "'Vexing pain' means pain that is severe."
3. Inability to turn sides, 不能转侧 *bù néng zhuǎn cé*: Difficulty turning from side to side or rolling over.

FORMULAE

Cinnamon Twig and Aconite Decoction (*guì zhī fù zǐ tāng*)

- Warm the channels and assist yáng; dispel wind and eliminate dampness.

桂枝四两（去皮） 附子三枚（炮，去皮，破） 生姜三两（切） 大枣十二枚（擘） 甘草二两（炙）

右五味，以水六升，煮取二升，去滓，分温三服。

guì zhī sì liǎng (qù pí) fù zǐ sān méi (pào, qù pí, pò) shēng jiāng sān liǎng (qiē) dà zǎo shí èr méi (bò) gān cǎo èr liǎng (zhì)

Yòu wǔ wèi, yǐ shuǐ liù shēng, zhǔ qǔ èr shēng, qù zǐ, fēn wēn sān fú.

cinnamon twig (桂枝 *guì zhī*, Cinnamomi Ramulus) 4 liǎng (remove bark)
aconite (附子 *fù zǐ*, Aconiti Tuber Laterale) 3 pieces (blast-fry, remove skin, crush)

fresh ginger (生姜 *shēng jiāng*, Zingiberis Rhizoma Recens) 3 liǎng (cut)
jujube (大枣 *dà zǎo*, Ziziphi Fructus) 12 pieces (broken)
mix-fried licorice (甘草 *gān cǎo*, Glycyrrhizae Radix) 2 liǎng

[For] the above five ingredients use six shēng of water. Boil to get two shēng, and remove the dregs. Separate into three [doses] and take warm.

Minus Cinnamon Plus Ovate Atractylodes Decoction (*qù guì jiā bái zhú tāng*)

附子三枚（炮，去皮，破） 白术四两 生姜三两（切） 甘草二两（炙） 大枣十二枚（擘）

㈠ 右五味，以水六升，煮取二升，去滓，分温三服。㈡ 初一服，其人身如痹，半日许复服之，三服都尽，其人如冒状，勿怪，此以附子、术并走皮内，逐水气未得除，故使之耳，法当加桂四两。㈢ 此本一方二法：以大便硬、小便自利，去桂也；以大便不硬、小便不利，当加桂。㈣ 附子三枚，恐多也。㈤ 虚弱家及产妇，宜减服之。

Fù zǐ sān méi (pào, qù pí, pò) bái zhú sì liǎng shēng jiāng sān liǎng (qiē) gān cǎo èr liǎng (zhì) dà zǎo shí èr méi (bò)

(1) *Yòu wǔ wèi, yǐ shuǐ liù shēng, zhǔ qǔ èr shēng, qù zǐ, fēn wēn sān fú.* (2) *Chū yī fú, qí rén shēn rú bì, bàn rì xǔ fù fú zhī, sān fú dōu jìn, qí rén rú mào zhuàng, wù guài, cǐ yǐ fù zǐ、zhú bìng zǒu pí nèi, zhú shuǐ qì wèi dé chú, gù shǐ zhī ěr, fǎ dāng jiā guì sì liǎng.* (3) *Cǐ běn yī fāng èr fǎ: yǐ dà biàn yìng、xiǎo biàn zì lì, qù guì yě; yǐ dà biàn bù yìng、xiǎo biàn bù lì, dāng jiā guì.* (4) *Fù zǐ sān méi, kǒng duō yě.* (5) *Xū ruò jiā jí chǎn fù, yí jiǎn fú zhī.*

aconite (附子 *fù zǐ*, Aconiti Tuber Laterale) 3 pieces (blast-fry, remove skin and break)
ovate atractylodes (白术 *bái zhú*, Atractylodis Ovatae Rhizoma) 4 liǎng
fresh ginger (生姜 *shēng jiāng*, Zingiberis Rhizoma Recens) 3 liǎng (cut)
mix-fried licorice (*gān cǎo*) 2 liǎng
jujube (大枣 *dà zǎo*, Ziziphi Fructus) 12 pieces (broken)

(1) [For] the above five ingredients, use six shēng of water and boil to get two shēng. Remove the dregs, separate into three [doses] and take warm. (2) [If after] the first [dose], the person [has a condition] like generalized impediment, take again in about half a day. In three doses, [the formula] is finished and [if the person has a condition] like veiling, this is not strange, [but] is because the aconite (*fù zǐ*) and ovate atractylodes (*bái zhú*) have penetrated the interior of the skin to expel the water qì, [which] has not yet been eliminated, so [there is this pattern]. As a rule, one should add 4 liǎng of cinnamon [twig] (*guì* [*zhī*]). (3) This is one formula with two methods. When the stool is hard and the urine is spontaneously uninhibited, remove cinnamon [twig] (*guì* [*zhī*]). When the stool is not hard and the urine is inhibited, add cinnamon [twig] (*guì* [*zhī*]). (4) [In some cases] three pieces of aconite (*fù zǐ*) may be feared too much. (5) For weak patients and women who have just given birth, it is appropriate to take less.

SYNOPSIS

The signs and treatment of wind-cold-damp evil impediment in the fleshy exterior.

COMMENTARY

In this line, wind, damp, and cold contend and give rise to generalized pain, an inability to turn sides, and a pulse that is floating, vacuous, and rough. This is a pattern of impediment, a description of which can be found in the *Sù Wèn*, "Three miscellaneous qì—wind, cold, damp—combine [into] impediment." As a result of wind-cold-damp in the fleshy exterior, construction and defense become disharmonious, and movement of qì and blood is inhibited, giving rise to generalized pain and inability to turn sides.

Although in cold damage patterns generalized pain is present, here the pain is severe and the patient cannot turn freely, a sign not generally seen in cold damage patterns. Furthermore, in Ephedra Decoction (*má huáng tāng*) patterns, the pulse is generally floating and tight, indicating that wind-cold has fettered the exterior and right qì is replete. Here, the pulse is floating, vacuous, and rough, indicating that the exterior yáng is insufficient and that the wind-damp contention has caused congestion in the channels and vessels. Retching and thirst are indicative of lesser yáng and yáng brightness disease, respectively, and the absence of these signs corroborate the absence of these patterns.

Cinnamon Twig and Aconite Decoction (*guì zhī fù zǐ tāng*) is suggested to warm the channels, reinforce yáng, dispel wind, and overcome dampness. Cinnamon twig (*guì zhī*) frees yáng and dispels wind. Aconite (*fù zǐ*) warms the channels and relieves pain. These two ingredients reinforce yáng in order to warm the channels and dissipate wind, cold, and dampness from the channels. Fresh ginger (*shēng jiāng*) is acrid and penetrates outward. It assists the other ingredients in warming and dissipating. Licorice (*gān cǎo*) and jujube (*dà zǎo*) combine with fresh ginger (*shēng jiāng*) to transform yáng with acridity and sweetness and harmonize construction and defense.

If the stool is hard and urination is uninhibited, it suggests that the fluids are percolating. Therefore, cinnamon twig (*guì zhī*), which transforms qì and disinhibits water, is removed from the formula and ovate atractylodes (*bái zhú*), which fortifies the spleen, dries dampness, and distributes liquid, is added.

One final note: Cinnamon Twig and Aconite Decoction (*guì zhī fù zǐ tāng*) and Cinnamon Twig Decoction Minus Peony Plus Aconite (*guì zhī qù sháo yào jiā fù zǐ tāng*) are identical except that the quantities of each ingredient differ. As a consequence, the two formulae are used differently and these differences are significant. The former is used for wind, cold, and dampness causing impediment, with signs such as vexing pain and an inability to turn to the side. Large doses of cinnamon twig (*guì zhī*) and aconite (*fù zǐ*) are used because the emphasis is on warming the channels and expelling cold and damp in order to relieve pain. Peony (*sháo yào*) is not used, because it is cool, sour, and constraining and may cause congealing in the channels. The latter formula is used in greater yáng exterior vacuity patterns with chest fullness, aversion to cold, and a pulse that is faint. Smaller doses of cinnamon twig (*guì zhī*) and aconite (*fù zǐ*) are used to warm the channels and restore yáng, in order to treat the milder signs of aversion to cold and a pulse that is faint. Here, peony (*sháo yào*) is not used for fear that it would further congest the chest yáng.

LINE 175

风湿相搏，骨节疼烦，掣痛不得屈伸，近之则痛剧，汗出短气，小便不利，恶风不欲去衣，或身微肿者，甘草附子汤主之。

Fēng shī xiāng bó, gǔ jié téng fán, chè tòng bù dé qū shēn, jìn zhī zé tòng jù, hàn chū duǎn qì, xiǎo biàn bù lì, wù fēng bù yù qù yī, huò shēn wēi zhǒng zhě, gān cǎo fù zǐ tāng zhǔ zhī.

When wind and dampness contend with each other, [and there is] vexing pain in the joints,* pulling pain, and an inability to bend and stretch, pain that is exacerbated when [anyone even comes] near, sweating, shortness of breath, inhibited urination, aversion to wind with no desire to remove the clothes, or mild generalized swelling, Licorice and Aconite Decoction (*gān cǎo fù zǐ tāng*) governs.

TEXT NOTE

* Vexing pain in the joints, 骨节疼烦 *gǔ jié téng fán*: Severe joint pain.

FORMULA

Licorice and Aconite Decoction (*gān cǎo fù zǐ tāng*)

∘ Warm yáng and dissipate cold; dispel dampness and relieve pain.

甘草二两（炙） 附子二枚（炮，去皮，破） 白术二两 桂枝四两（去皮）

㈠ 右四味，以水六升，煮取三升，去滓，温服一升，日三服。㈡ 初服得微汗则解。㈢ 能食汗止复烦者，将服五合，恐一升多者，宜服六七合为始。

Gān cǎo èr liǎng (zhì) fù zǐ èr méi (pào, qù pí, pò) bái zhú èr liǎng guì zhī sì liǎng (qù pí)

(1) *Yòu sì wèi, yǐ shuǐ liù shēng, zhǔ qǔ sān shēng, qù zǐ, wēn fú yī shēng, rì sān fú.* (2) *Chū fú dé wēi hàn zé jiě.* (3) *Néng shí hàn zhǐ fù fán zhě, jiāng fú wǔ gě, kǒng yī shēng duō zhě, yí fú liù qī gě wéi shǐ.*

licorice (甘草 *gān cǎo*, Glycyrrhizae Radix) 2 liǎng
aconite (附子 *fù zǐ*, Aconiti Tuber Laterale) 2 pieces (blast-fry, remove skin, break)
ovate atractylodes (白术 *bái zhú*, Atractylodis Ovatae Rhizoma) 2 liǎng
cinnamon twig (桂枝 *guì zhī*, Cinnamomi Ramulus) 4 liǎng (remove bark)

(1) [For] the above four ingredients, use six shēng of water and boil to get three shēng. Remove the dregs and take one shēng warm, three times a day. (2) In the beginning, [after] taking [a dose] there should be slight sweating and resolution. (3) [If the person] can eat, the sweating stops, and vexation returns, give five gě. [If there is] fear that one shēng is too much, it is appropriate to take six or seven gě to start with.

SYNOPSIS

The signs and treatment of wind-cold-damp evil impediment in the joints.

COMMENTARY

In this pattern wind and dampness contend and become bound in the joints, resulting in severe joint pain. The pain is so severe that it is exacerbated when one even tries to approach the patient. In the previous line retching and thirst are absent, suggesting that the interior is in harmony. Here, sweat issues and the patient feels aversion to wind and does not desire to remove any clothes. These signs suggest that the defensive yáng is vacuous and insecure. Furthermore, when damp evil congests the interior, qì transformation and diffusion are impaired. In the upper burner the breath, becomes short, and in the lower burner, urination becomes inhibited. Generalized swelling may be observed as a further indication of damp congestion.

Licorice and Aconite Decoction (*gān cǎo fù zǐ tāng*) is used to warm yáng and dissipate cold, and to dispel dampness and relieve pain. When wind and dampness contend in the interior, cold is often engendered, and thus the formula contains ingredients to address the cold evil. Aconite (*fù zǐ*) warms the channels and dissipates cold. Ovate atractylodes (*bái zhú*) fortifies the spleen and dries dampness. Cinnamon twig (*guì zhī*) warms and frees yáng. These ingredients warm the exterior yáng in order to secure the defensive yáng, dispel wind-damp, and warm the channels. When the wind, damp, and cold are dispelled, the pain will cease. Once the defensive yáng is secure, aversion to wind and sweating will cease. These ingredients also transform and move the qì to address the issues of inhibited urination, shortness of breath, and generalized swelling. Licorice (*gān cǎo*) harmonizes the ingredients and supplements the center burner in order to support right qì.

This pattern is more severe than the one treated with Cinnamon Twig and Aconite Decoction (*guì zhī fù zǐ tāng*), but a smaller dosage of aconite (*fù zǐ*) is used in Licorice and Aconite Decoction (*gān cǎo fù zǐ tāng*). The reason is that in the previous pattern wind-damp evil collects in the flesh, but here it pours into the joints—a location that is considered to be deeper. Wind-damp in the joints is difficult to eliminate quickly, and if too large a dosage of medicinals is employed, the wind will be eliminated but the dampness will remain. Furthermore, licorice (*gān cǎo*) moderates the harsh nature of aconite (*fù zǐ*) and ovate atractylodes (*bái zhú*) so that their actions slowly come into play, eliminating both wind and dampness. Thus, the importance of licorice (*gān cǎo*) in this formula should not be underestimated.

Three formulae are used to treat wind-cold-damp. Cinnamon Twig and Aconite Decoction (*guì zhī fù zǐ tāng*) is suggested for patterns in which wind-damp invades the fleshy exterior and exterior wind is prevalent. Cinnamon Twig Decoction Minus Cinnamon Twig Plus Poria (Hoelen) and Ovate Atractylodes (*guì zhī qù guì jiā fú líng bái zhú tāng*) is used when wind-damp invades the fleshy exterior and interior dampness is prevalent. Licorice and Aconite Decoction (*gān cǎo fù zǐ tāng*) is used when wind-damp invades the joints and both evils are equally prevalent.

Chapter Two

Yáng Brightness Disease

Pulses and Signs; Treatment

辨阳明病脉证并治

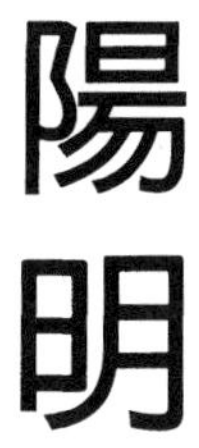

1 OVERVIEW

Yáng brightness disease is the stage of externally contracted disease in which yáng qì is hyperactive and evil qì is exuberant. The pathomechanism of yáng brightness disease is explained by the term "stomach domain is replete" (胃家实 *wèi jiā shí*). "Stomach domain" refers to the stomach and intestines, and "replete" refers to an evil transforming to heat and entering the interior, and food accumulation and stagnation. In general, when an exterior evil enters the yáng brightness, it transforms to dryness and heat, resulting in a pattern of interior heat repletion.

Yáng brightness disease can originate in the greater yáng channel, in the lesser yáng channel, or directly in the yáng brightness channel. Yáng brightness disease can also originate in the yīn channels, although these transmutations are less frequently encountered. Enduring depressed greater yīn cold-damp can transform into heat and give rise to a yáng brightness pattern. A lesser yīn evil can also transform to heat and damage the fluids, giving rise to a yáng brightness pattern. In rare cases, if stomach yáng is vacuous, yáng brightness patterns of stomach cold with qì counterflow can be observed. Also, an evil can fall inward and enter the three yīn channels, giving rise to a pattern of vacuity cold. The yáng brightness is the final yáng channel through which an evil passes prior to entering the three yīn channels; therefore, it is said that "yáng brightness is the outer shelter of the three yīn" (阳明为三阴之外蔽 *yáng míng wéi sān yīn zhī wài bì*).

Yáng brightness disease may be divided into heat patterns and repletion patterns. Heat patterns, also referred to as yáng brightness channel patterns, involve formless dryness-heat and are characterized by great generalized heat effusion, great sweating, great thirst, and a pulse that is surging and large or slippery and rapid (the four greats). Aversion to heat and heart vexation are also commonly observed in yáng brightness channel patterns. Repletion patterns, also referred to as yáng brightness bowel patterns, involve formed heat bind and are characterized by afternoon tidal heat effusion, sweat streaming from the limbs, abdominal distention, fullness and pain, inability to defecate or heat bind with circumfluence, and a pulse that is sunken, slow, and forceful, or slippery and rapid.

Yáng brightness disease generally involves the qì aspect, but yáng brightness heat can enter the blood aspect. In yáng brightness blood amassment patterns heat contends with enduring static blood and gives rise to signs such as forgetfulness and hard, black stool that is easy to expel.

In yáng brightness disease we can also see wind strike or cold strike patterns in which a wind or cold evil strikes yáng brightness directly. Both these patterns differ from the basic yáng brightness patterns by the absence of heat and dryness signs. These two patterns are differentiated primarily on the basis of whether or not the patient is able to eat. In wind strike, the patient is able to eat, indicating that stomach yáng is still exuberant and a replete evil is absent from the bowel. In cold strike, the patient is unable to eat because stomach yáng is insufficient, as a result of damage from cold evil.

1.1 SIGNS

Aversion to heat 恶热 *wù rè*: Aversion to heat occurs instead of aversion to cold because the exterior evil has entered the interior and transformed into heat, giving rise to heat both in the exterior and the interior. Aversion to cold may be seen in the early stages of yáng brightness disease, but it should quickly give way to aversion to heat and must be clearly differentiated from that which occurs in greater yáng disease.

Heat effusion 发热 *fā rè*: In yáng brightness disease heat patterns, heat effusion is strong and results from interior heat steaming outward. It is much stronger than the feather-warm heat effusion of greater yáng. In yáng brightness repletion patterns, heat binds in the interior and the outward effusion of heat is not strong, but instead manifests as afternoon tidal heat effusion.

Spontaneous sweating 自汗出 *zì hàn chū*: In yáng brightness disease, sweating is copious and streams outward, in contrast to sweating that occurs in greater yáng wind strike, which is scant and issues slowly. In heat patterns, the sweat is said to be copious over the whole body, whereas in repletion patterns, it is said to stream from the limbs. Nonetheless, in yáng brightness patterns, sweating may be absent or only observed on a small part of the body. If sweating is absent, it generally suggests that yīn liquid is vacuous; if sweating is present only on a small part of the body (i.e., the head), it may be the result of dampness and heat depressed in the interior—as occurs in yellowing patterns.

Thirst with desire to drink water 渴欲饮水 *kě yù yǐn shuǐ*: Thirst occurs in both heat and repletion patterns because intense interior heat damages the stomach liquid and humor. For this reason, thirst is an important indication that an evil has shifted into the yáng brightness. In these patterns the patient has a dry mouth and tongue, and drinks copious amounts of water. Although thirst may also be observed in greater yáng water amassment patterns, the patient does not drink copious amounts of water, and may vomit water. Furthermore, the tongue and mouth are not dry in water amassment patterns.

Abdominal fullness, distention, and pain 腹胀、满、痛 *fù zhàng, mǎn, tòng*: These signs are observed primarily in yáng brightness repletion patterns as a manifestation of formed dryness bind. Because a replete evil is bound in the interior, these signs are usually severe and persistent. Furthermore, this is abdominal pain that refuses pressure. These signs can be clearly distinguished from vacuity cold abdominal fullness, which occurs in greater yīn patterns and which is mild and intermittent.

Inability to defecate 不大便 *bù dà biàn*: Inability to defecate refers to absence of defecation, difficult defecation, and hard stool, all of which are a manifestation of dryness repletion in yáng brightness repletion patterns. Nonetheless, inability to defecate should not be viewed as an unequivocal indicator of yáng brightness disease because it can occur in the absence of replete interior heat, and is sometimes seen in exterior patterns. Furthermore, diarrhea can also be observed in repletion patterns. Referred to as "heat bind with circumfluence," it occurs when loose stool passes out around hard stool that partially obstructs the intestines. Inability to defecate is also seen in straitened spleen patterns in which stomach heat fetters and constrains the spleen, such that the spleen is unable to move fluids. The fluids percolate into the bladder and the stool becomes hard. In this pattern, inability to defecate does not generally cause abdominal fullness or pain.

Delirious speech 谵语 *zhān yǔ*: Delirious speech may occur in either heat or repletion patterns as the result of replete heat ascending to the upper body. The speech is incoherent and the voice is heavy and forceful. Furthermore, the spirit may be clouded so that the person seems to be seeing apparitions. These are signs of repletion. If there is repetitious speech, the voice is faint and forceless, and the spirit-mind seems clear but then does not, this is not called "delirious speech," but is called "muttering," and is considered to be a vacuity pattern.

Yellowing 发黄 *fā huáng*: Yáng brightness disease includes jaundice patterns, which in the *Shāng Hán Lùn* are called "yellowing." Yellowing is divided into two basic types: yáng yellowing and yīn yellowing. Yáng yellowing occurs when heat and dampness combine in the interior giving rise to signs such as generalized yellowing (in which the yellow is a bright color), inhibited urination, generalized heat, dry mouth, heart vexation, glomus, possible blocked stool, red tongue with a yellow fur, and a pulse that is soggy and rapid. Yīn yellowing occurs when cold and dampness combine in the interior giving rise to signs such as generalized yellowing in which the yellow color is dark and dull, aversion to cold and desire for warmth, no heat effusion, sloppy stool, pale tongue with white fur, and a pulse that is sunken and slow.

1.2 TREATMENT

Heat patterns (yáng brightness channel patterns) should be treated with a formula such as White Tiger Decoction (*bái hǔ tāng*) to clear and resolve yáng brightness heat. Repletion patterns (yáng brightness bowel patterns) should be treated with one of the Qì-Coordinating Decoctions (*chéng qì tāng*).

In the straitened spleen pattern, Hemp Seed Pill (*má zǐ rén wán*) is used to precipitate with moistness.

Yáng yellowing patterns are treated with Capillaris Decoction (*yīn chén hāo tāng*) or Gardenia and Phellodendron Decoction (*zhī zǐ bǎi pí tāng*) to clear heat, eliminate dampness, and abate yellowness. In yáng yellowing patterns with exterior signs, Ephedra, Forsythia, and Rice Bean Decoction (*má huáng lián qiáo chì xiǎo dòu tāng*) may be used. Although the text suggests no formulae to treat yīn yellowing, this pattern is treated by warming the center, dissipating cold, and drying dampness.

Yáng brightness blood amassment patterns in which heat enters the blood aspect and contends with static blood is treated with Dead-On Decoction (*dǐ dàng tāng*) to break stasis and expel blood.

1.3 Schematic Overview

Basic Yáng Brightness Disease Patterns

- **Heat patterns**
  - Exuberant dryness heat (Channel repletion): with great heat, great sweating, great thirst and desire to drink, great vexation, and a pulse that is surging and large: White Tiger Decoction (*bái hǔ tāng*)
  - Other heat patterns
    * Heart vexation and anguish: Gardenia and Fermented Soybean Decoction (*zhī zǐ chǐ tāng*)
    * Damage to qì and yīn with dry mouth, great thirst and desire to drink, and vexation: White Tiger Decoction Plus Ginseng (*bái hǔ jiā rén shēn tāng*)
    * Unresolved heat, yīn damage, and collected water with a pulse that is floating, heat effusion, thirst with desire to drink, and inhibited urination: Polyporus Decoction (*zhū líng tāng*)
- **Bowel repletion patterns**
  - Treated by precipitation
    * Mild dryness repletion with hard stool or inability to defecate, steaming heat effusion, sweating, heart vexation, and dry yellow tongue fur: Stomach-Regulating Qì-Coordinating Decoction (*tiáo wèi chéng qì tāng*)
    * Heat bind repletion with hard stool or inability to defecate, abdominal distention and fullness, tidal heat effusion and delirious speech: Minor Qì-Coordinating Decoction (*xiǎo chéng qì tāng*)
    * Severe bowel repletion with inability to defecate or heat bind with circumfluence, abdominal fullness, hardness and pain, tidal heat effusion, and delirious speech: Major Qì-Coordinating Decoction (*dà chéng qì tāng*)
  - Treated by moistening and enema
    * Straitened spleen with difficult defecation, mild abdominal fullness, copious urination: Hemp Seed Pill (*má zǐ rén wán*)

  - Enema: Honey Brew Formula (*mì jiān fāng*), Cucumber Gourd Root Formula (*tǔ guā gēn fāng*), Pig's Bile Formula (*zhū dǎn zhī fāng*)

Transmuted Patterns

- **Damp-heat yellowing patterns**
  - Generalized yellowing, yellow inhibited urination, absence of sweating, thirst, and abdominal fullness: Capillaris Decoction (*yīn chén hāo tāng*)
  - Yellowing, heat effusion, heart vexation and anguish, and thirst: Gardenia and Phellodendron Decoction (*zhī zǐ bǎi pí tāng*)
  - Yellowing, inhibited urination, heat effusion and aversion to cold, absence of sweating, and generalized itching: Ephedra, Forsythia, and Rice Bean Decoction (*má huáng lián qiáo chì xiǎo dòu tāng*)
- **Blood heat patterns** with the possibility of spontaneous external bleeding, dry mouth, heat effusion, delirious speech, black stool that is easy to pass, or pus and blood in the stool: Dead-On Decoction (*dǐ dàng tāng*).
- **Vacuity cold** with retching, inability to eat, and hiccup: Evodia Decoction (*wú zhū yú tāng*)

2 ESSENTIAL FEATURES OF YÁNG BRIGHTNESS DISEASE

This section of the yáng brightness chapter presents the essential features of this disease: its causes, pathomechanisms, and signs.

Line 180

阳明之为病，胃家实是也。

Yáng míng zhī wéi bìng, wèi jiā shí shì yě.

In disease of yáng brightness, the stomach domain is replete.

Synopsis

The essential feature of yáng brightness heat repletion patterns.

Commentary

The essential feature of yáng brightness heat repletion patterns is that the "stomach domain is replete." We should first of all explain the meaning of "stomach domain." This term is interpreted as the stomach and the large intestine because in the channel and network vessels both of these belong to yáng brightness. However, the term can also be taken to mean the stomach, the large intestine, and the small intestine. This interpretation rests on the statement contained in the *Líng Shū* (灵枢 "The Magic Pivot") that "the large and small intestine both belong to the stomach." The stomach is connected to the small intestine and large intestine below, and all three bowels are engaged in the conveyance and transformation of food.

In the phrase "the stomach domain is replete," the word "replete" is most clearly explained by Yú Wú-Yán, who states: "The word 'replete' in 'the stomach domain is replete' has two meanings. One is repletion from food accumulation and stagnation. The other is repletion from exterior heat passing into the interior." Both these meanings are included in the notion of "repletion of evil qì," which derives from the statement contained in the *Sù Wèn* which reads: "When evil qì is exuberant, there is repletion; when essential qì is despoliated, there is vacuity."

Since yáng brightness governs dryness, when an evil enters the yáng brightness it tends to transform into dryness. As it transforms into dryness the interior heat becomes exuberant and damages the fluids. Yáng brightness disease can take either of two forms: a channel pattern or a bowel pattern. If the patient is not suffering from abiding waste and stagnation in the stomach and intestines when yáng brightness disease develops, this exuberant heat follows the channels, so that it affects both the inner and outer body, giving rise to great heat, great thirst, great sweating, and a pulse that is large and surging—a pattern known as a yáng brightness channel pattern. If, by contrast, exuberant dryness-heat contends with abiding stagnation in the stomach and intestines, it may cause the stool to become bound and dry, blocking the intestines. Bound stool blocking the intestines may cause tidal heat effusion, absence of defecation, and abdominal fullness, hardness, and pain; in severe cases it may cause delirious speech. This pattern is known as a yáng brightness repletion pattern. Both these conditions are manifestations of "evil qì repletion"; hence "the stomach domain is replete" constitutes the essential feature of yáng brightness disease.

The essential features of all the channel diseases other than yáng brightness are expressed in terms of signs and pulses. Only that of yáng brightness disease is expressed in terms of a pathomechanism. This pathomechanism does not explain all the variants of yáng brightness disease since there are also conditions of cold, dampness, and/or vacuity.

2.1 CAUSES AND PATHOMECHANISMS

LINE 179

(一) 问曰：病有太阳阳明，有正阳阳明，有少阳阳明，何谓也？(二) 答曰：太阳阳明者，脾约是也；正阳阳明者，胃家实是也；少阳阳明者，发汗利小便已，胃中燥烦实，大便难是也。

(1) *Wèn yuē: bìng yǒu tài yáng yáng míng, yǒu zhèng yáng yáng míng, yǒu shào yáng yáng míng, hé wèi yě?* (2) *Dá yuē: tài yáng yáng míng zhě, pí yuē shì yě; zhèng yáng yáng míng zhě, wèi jiā shí shì yě; shào yáng yáng míng zhě, fā hàn lì xiǎo biàn yǐ, wèi zhōng zào fán shí, dà biàn nán shì yě.*

(1) Question: [Yáng brightness] disease includes greater yáng yáng brightness,[1] right yáng yáng brightness,[2] and lesser yáng yáng brightness.[3] What does this mean? (2) Answer: In greater yáng yáng brightness, the spleen is straitened.[4] In right yáng yáng brightness, the stomach domain is replete. In lesser yáng yáng brightness, when sweating is promoted and urine is disinhibited, [there is] dry vexing repletion in the stomach[5] and difficult defecation.

Text Notes

1. Greater yáng yáng brightness, 太阳阳明 *tài yáng yáng míng*: The evil passes from the greater yáng channel into the yáng brightness channel.
2. Right yáng yáng brightness, 正阳阳明 *zhèng yáng yáng míng*: The evil invades directly into the yáng brightness channel.
3. Lesser yáng yáng brightness, 少阳阳明 *shào yáng yáng míng*: The evil passes from the lesser yáng channel into the yáng brightness channel as a result of inappropriate treatment.
4. The spleen is straitened, 脾约 *pí yuē*: Stomach heat binds the spleen, disturbing the spleen's functions of movement and transformation. This disturbance causes dryness in the intestines and constipation.
5. Dry vexing repletion in the stomach, 胃中燥烦实 *wèi zhōng zào fán shí*: A repletion evil in the stomach engendering exuberant dryness and heat that causes vexation.

Synopsis

The causes and origins of yáng brightness disease.

Commentary

Yáng brightness disease is characterized by dryness-heat repletion. It has many causes. This line proposes three causes on the basis of the laws governing the development of disease in the triple yáng and the processes of passage from one to the other.

The first possibility is that an exterior evil in the greater yáng shifts into the yáng brightness. This shift may occur as a result of mistreatment or in the absence of timely treatment. In either case an exterior evil enters the interior and transforms to heat. The stomach becomes hot and the intestines become dry. The fluids are damaged and the spleen's function of movement and transformation is restrained, giving rise to bound stool without hardness, fullness, and pain in the abdomen. This is called "straitened spleen."

In the second situation an exterior evil directly invades the yáng brightness. This happens in patients with hyperactive stomach yáng. When the evil enters the yáng brightness, it transforms into dryness, further damages liquid, and further transforms into heat. If the patient happens to have accumulation and stagnation in the stomach and intestines, the dryness-heat will exacerbate the congestion so that the stool will become blocked.

Zhāng Jī includes the term "the stomach domain is replete" in this line to emphasize that exuberant dryness-heat in the stomach and intestines is a major characteristic of yáng brightness disease. In all three of these patterns, the stomach domain is replete.

The third situation is that an evil from the lesser yáng shifts into the yáng brightness. Appropriate treatment for lesser yáng disease is harmonization. In this case, however, sweating is promoted and urination is disinhibited. This mistreatment damages the fluids and the evil easily transforms to heat and dryness. The heat and dryness enter the yáng brightness and disturbs the movement of the stool, which becomes difficult to expel.

Modern commentators tend to agree that the present line is misleading because it suggests that yáng brightness disease varies in form depending on the provenance of the evil. This line is notably contradicted by line 181, p. 304, which states that yáng brightness disease coming from greater yáng may take the form of no change of clothes, internal repletion, or difficult defecation, depending on the severity. It is therefore now believed that irrespective of where the evil comes from, the three different forms mentioned may arise.

LINE 181

(一) 问曰：何缘得阳明病？(二) 答曰：太阳病，若发汗，若下，若利小便，此亡津液，胃中干燥，因转属阳明。(三) 不更衣，内实，大便难者，此名阳明也。

(1) *Wèn yuē: hé yuán dé yáng míng bìng?* (2) *Dá yuē: tài yáng bìng, ruò fā hàn, ruò xià, ruò lì xiǎo biàn, cǐ wáng jīn yè, wèi zhōng gān zào, yīn zhuǎn shǔ yáng míng.* (3) *Bù gēng yī, nèi shí, dà biàn nán zhě, cǐ míng yáng míng yě.*

(1) Question: Why does one gets yáng brightness disease? (2) Answer: In greater yáng disease, if sweating is promoted, if precipitation [is used,] or if urination is disinhibited, this [causes] liquid and humor collapse and dryness in the stomach; hence [there is a] shift to the yáng brightness. (3) No change of clothes,* internal repletion, and difficult defecation; these [signs] are called yáng brightness.

TEXT NOTE

* No change of clothes, 不更衣 *bù gēng yī*: Formerly it was customary to change one's clothes after defecation, and so the expression "changing one's clothes" was a euphemism for defecation.

SYNOPSIS

When greater yáng disease is treated inappropriately, it can shift into yáng brightness disease.

COMMENTARY

When in greater yáng disease an inappropriate treatment is used, it can cause the evil to move into the yáng brightness. The mistreatments described in this line are the (excessive) promotion of sweating, precipitation, and disinhibiting the urine.

The promotion of sweating is normally an appropriate treatment for greater yáng exterior patterns. Appropriate promotion of sweating should give rise to a generalized mild sweating. If the sweating is excessive or incomplete, it can induce the evil to enter the interior. Incomplete sweating is discussed in the following line. Copious sweating can damage the fluids and the qì, so that if the evil passes into the interior it easily transforms into dryness, causing the disease to shift into yáng brightness. Inappropriate precipitation or disinhibition of urine instead of sweating can likewise damage the fluids and encourage the disease to shift into yáng brightness. Furthermore, as stated in the commentary on the first line of yáng brightness disease, preexisting stagnation of the stomach and intestines is another major disposing factor for development of yáng brightness repletion pattern. When the evil enters the interior and transforms into dryness it contends with the waste in the intestines, causing the bowel qì to become bound and blocked.

The three signs in the second part of this line may be seen as a single description of a yáng brightness disease or as separate signs. Chéng Wú-Jǐ (成无己) writes: "When people in ancient times went to the toilet, they would change their clothes. Not changing clothes meant failure to defecate. Not changing clothes means that the stomach contents cannot be discharged; hence [there is] internal repletion. [When] there are no fluids in the stomach, and, in addition, there is heat amassment, defecation is difficult and this is yáng brightness internal repletion." In his explanation, all three terms describe the same condition. The authors of *Yī Zōng Jīn Jiàn* write that these signs refer back to the preceding line: "Stomach repletion disease can be divided into three forms: not changing clothes, which is greater yáng yáng brightness straitened spleen; internal repletion, which is right yáng yáng brightness repletion in the stomach domain; and difficult stool, which is lesser yáng yáng brightness difficult stool. These three signs can all be treated by precipitation, but differ in severity. Straitened spleen is milder than difficult defecation; difficult defecation is milder than repletion in the stomach domain." Thus, these signs are considered three different conditions or as a single condition.

LINE 185

㈠ 本太阳初得病时，发其汗，汗先出不彻，因转属阳明也。㈡ 伤寒发热无汗，呕不能食，而反汗出濈濈然者，是转属阳明也。

(1) *Běn tài yáng chū dé bìng shí, fā qí hàn, hàn xiān chū bù chè, yīn zhuǎn shǔ yáng míng yě.* (2) *Shāng hán fā rè wú hán, ǒu bù néng shí, ér fǎn hàn chū jí jí rán zhě, shì zhuǎn shǔ yáng míng yě.*

(1) Originally, at the beginning of greater yáng disease, sweating is promoted, [but it] is incomplete, which causes a shift to yáng brightness. (2) When in cold damage, [there is] heat effusion, sweating is absent,

[and there is] retching and inability to eat, and [sweating occurs] but it is a streaming sweat,* this means a shift to yáng brightness.

TEXT NOTE

* Streaming sweat, 汗出濈濈然 *hàn chū jí jí rán*: A continuous flow of sweat. The word 濈 *jí* comes from 戢 *jí*, which means "to collect" or "to gather." This phrase would appear to describe how the sweat gathers into rivulets or streams. According to traditional commentators, yáng brightness disease is usually characterized by profuse sweating. "Streaming sweat" is normally taken to imply profusion, although in the following line, the phrase 濈然微汗出 *jí rán wéi hàn chū* means "mild streaming sweat." For this reason, "streaming sweat" is generally assumed to emphasize continuity rather than profusion. Nevertheless, mild continuous sweating implies the discharge of a large amount of sweat over time.

SYNOPSIS

Greater yáng disease with incomplete promotion of sweating or cold damage with exuberant evil heat can shift into yáng brightness disease.

COMMENTARY

The two sentences of this line present different situations in which greater yáng disease shifts to the yáng brightness. The first arises after sweating has been promoted, while in the second, no inappropriate treatment has been given.

The first condition arises after the promotion of sweating. The promotion of sweating is the appropriate treatment in greater yáng diseases, but here it leads to a pathological transmutation. Sweating is promoted, but it is incomplete; that is, the sweating started and then stopped, or was of excessively short duration, or the sweating was too mild and failed to occur over the entire body. Thus the evil has not been expelled, and owing to hyperactivity of stomach yáng, it has entered the interior, transformed to heat, and settled in the yáng brightness. This is therefore a transmutation that is ascribed to constitutional factors.

The second part of the line presents another situation in which greater yáng evil shifts into the yáng brightness. Here there is no mention of any treatment. We assume, therefore, that there has been no promotion of sweating and no inappropriate treatment. In the shift into yáng brightness, the original heat effusion and absence of sweating of greater yáng cold damage gives way to a "streaming sweat" characteristic of yáng brightness. We infer from this development that the aversion to cold of greater yáng has given way to heat effusion, sweating, and aversion to heat rather than cold. The line seems to suggest that the original greater yáng condition was also marked by retching and inability to eat. Given the subsequent shift into yáng brightness, retching and inability to eat is usually taken to reflect hyperactivity of stomach yáng, which is a predisposing factor for yáng brightness disease. Hyperactivity of stomach yáng easily leads to impairment of the harmony and downbearing of the stomach, in which counterflow ascent of stomach qì gives rise to retching and impairment of the stomach's governing of intake causes inability to eat.

Whether inappropriate treatment, or exuberant interior heat, causes the evil to enter the yáng brightness, the result is streaming sweat. This type of continuous sweating leads to a great loss of sweat, which is the external sign of yáng brightness disease. It reflects dryness-heat in the stomach and intestines, steaming the fluids and forcing them towards the exterior. However, this type of sweating not only fails to resolve the evil, it also damages liquid. The only method of treatment is to clear and drain yáng brightness dryness-heat. When the evil is eliminated, the sweating will stop and the fluids will be safeguarded.

This line and the preceding one present three situations in which a greater yáng evil may shift into the yáng brightness. In the first, sweating is promoted excessively and the fluids are damaged. In the second, sweating is promoted incompletely and the evil heat enters the interior. In the third, without promotion of sweating or inappropriate treatment, hyperactive interior heat encourages an exterior evil to enter the interior spontaneously.

Line 188

伤寒转系阳明者，其人濈然微汗出也。

Shāng hán zhuǎn xì yáng míng zhě, qí rén jí rán wēi hàn chū yě.

When [the evil] in cold damage* shifts to yáng brightness, the person will have slight streaming sweat.

Text Note

* Cold damage, 伤寒 *shāng hán*: In this context the term is used in its broader sense of externally contracted heat disease, not in the narrower sense of greater yáng cold damage, since any evil entering yáng brightness, not only disease passing from the greater yáng to yáng brightness, will give rise to streaming sweat.

Synopsis

The signs appearing when cold damage shifts into the yáng brightness.

Commentary

Yáng brightness governs the flesh and diseases affecting the fluids. When exterior evil enters yáng brightness, dryness-heat steams the fluids and forces them out through the interstices of the flesh. Consequently, sweating is a major feature of yáng brightness. "Slight streaming sweat" in this line describes a mild, continuous flow of sweat. This sign is insufficient to determine that the disease is in yáng brightness; the presence of heat effusion with no aversion to cold, but rather aversion to heat, is required as corroboration. Further, in formless yáng brightness dryness-heat, there is usually also great thirst and a large surging pulse; in yáng brightness dryness-heat contending with formed accumulation and stagnation, there is usually also abdominal fullness, hardness, and pain; inability to evacuate; and tidal heat effusion and delirious speech. The most important references to sweating in yáng brightness disease are to be found in the following lines: line 182, p. 308; line 219, p. 318; line 213, p. 331; line 230, p. 422; and line 253, p. 343.

In certain conditions, yáng brightness disease does not manifest in sweating. Absence of sweating occurs when, owing to insufficiency of fluids, sweat cannot be produced, despite exuberant heat. Absence of sweating, or sweating from the head only, is observed when yáng brightness heat binds with internal dampness evil, obstructing the qì dynamic, causing absence of sweating or sweating from the head only, and inhibited urination. In such cases yellowing is more likely to occur.

2.2 Pulses and Signs

Line 182

(一) 问曰：阳明病外证云何？ (二) 答曰：身热，汗自出，不恶寒，反恶热也。

(1) *Wèn yuē: yáng míng bìng wài zhèng yún hé?* (2) *Dá yuē: shēn rè, hàn zì chū, bù wù hán, fǎn wù rè yě.*

(1) Question: What are the outward signs of yáng brightness disease? (2) Answer: [There is] generalized heat [effusion], spontaneous sweating and no aversion to cold, but aversion to heat.

Synopsis

The exterior signs of yáng brightness disease.

Commentary

Yáng brightness disease is caused by evil heat entering the interior, and is characterized by dryness-heat repletion. Dryness-heat in the interior is not directly accessible to the senses. Its presence is deduced from outward signs that are detected through the four examinations.

Heat is formless. When it originates in the stomach and steams the flesh, both the inner body and the outer body are hot. Hence the outward sign is generalized heat. Generalized heat may be seen in diseases of all of the six channels, so one must differentiate carefully. When it occurs in greater yáng disease, it is accompanied by aversion to cold, a pulse that is floating, headache, and sweating or no sweating, depending on whether it is exterior repletion or vacuity. In lesser yáng disease, generalized heat alternates with aversion to cold. Heat effusion does not normally appear in disease of the triple yīn because generally the sign patterns do not include heat. If it does occur, it indicates more complex patterns, which will be discussed later.

Heat effusion in yáng brightness disease differs from that of any other channel disease in that the heat is more exuberant, is (with minor exceptions) always accompanied by—but not abated by—sweating, and is associated with aversion to heat rather than to cold. The heat effusion is accompanied by sweating because the dryness-heat causes the yáng brightness bowel's copious qì and blood to steam. The heat effusion is associated with no aversion to cold because the exterior pattern has already ceased and the disease evil has completely entered the yáng brightness. Because yáng brightness is marked by exuberant interior heat, there is also aversion to heat rather than aversion to cold. This marks a clear difference between yáng brightness and greater yáng.

The present line makes no mention of tidal heat [effusion] and delirious speech, which are also outward signs of yáng brightness disease. However, these signs are only observed in severe or critical conditions. If one waits for the appearance of these signs to identify yáng brightness disease, one will have missed an early opportunity for successful treatment.

Line 183

㈠问曰：病有得之一日，不发热而恶寒者，何也？㈡答曰：虽得之一日，恶寒将自罢，即自汗出而恶热也。

(1) *Wèn yuē: bìng yǒu dé zhī yī rì, bù fā rè ér wù hán zhě, hé yě?* (2) *Dá yuē: suī dé zhī yī rì, wù hán jiāng zì bà, jí zì hán chū ér wù rè yě.*

(1) Question: What of disease [that has lasted for] a day, [when] heat effusion is absent [and there is] aversion to cold? (2) Answer: Although [there has been disease for] only a day, the aversion to cold will spontaneously cease and then there will be spontaneous sweating and aversion to heat.

Synopsis

Signs presenting when the yáng brightness contracts external evil right at the onset of illness.

Commentary

In the present line, yáng brightness has just contracted external evil, but the evil has not yet transformed into heat. This line describes an illness that is in the early stages, probably the first couple of days, not necessarily the first day. The disease is still in the process of development, and so the classical signs of yáng brightness have not yet developed. Hence there is aversion to cold without heat effusion.

We can analyze the differences between the aversion to cold described in the present line and that of other patterns from three angles. As regards the manifestation of disease, aversion to cold here is not accompanied by heat effusion. Nevertheless, since yáng brightness is essentially dryness-heat, the aversion to cold is mild and may be accompanied by signs such as vexation and agitation or red tongue. Hence this is not the aversion to cold of greater yáng, which is accompanied by heat effusion. As regards the course of the disease, the appearance of aversion to cold at onset of yáng brightness disease is temporary and will swiftly disappear without being treated. This is different from the aversion to cold appearing in other patterns. As regards pathomechanism, although disease entering yáng brightness is marked by dryness-heat which normally manifests as heat effusion with aversion to heat, nevertheless, aversion to cold can arise when an external evil, having just entered, has not yet given rise to exuberant dryness-heat, and blocks the yáng qì, preventing it from reaching outward.

Yáng brightness disease develops very swiftly, giving rise to heat effusion with aversion to heat rather than to cold, and with profuse sweating. Although the classical yáng brightness signs have not fully developed, the phrase "the aversion to cold will cease," hints that they are about to appear. When one recognizes that the aversion to cold is different from that seen in greater yáng disease, one will be able to anticipate the change to the yáng brightness and treat the patient correctly.

LINE 184

(一) 问曰：恶寒何故自罢？(二) 答曰：阳明居中，主土也，万物所归，无所复传，始虽恶寒，二日自止，此为阳明病也。

(1) *Wèn yuē: Wù hán hé gù zì bà?* (2) *Dá yuē: yáng míng jū zhōng, zhǔ tǔ yě, wàn wù suǒ guī, wú suǒ fù chuán, shǐ suī wù hán, èr rì zì zhǐ, cǐ wéi yáng míng bìng yě.*

(1) Question: Why does aversion to cold cease spontaneously? (2) Answer: Yáng brightness resides in the center and governs earth. All things converge [here and] nothing passes further. Although at the beginning [there is] aversion to cold, in two days [it will] spontaneously cease, indicating yáng brightness disease.

SYNOPSIS

Continuing from the preceding line, an explanation of why aversion to cold spontaneously ceases.

COMMENTARY

The foot yáng brightness stomach is dry earth. The hand yáng brightness large intestine is dry metal. The qì of these two channels is the same; consequently, the yáng brightness governs dryness. Since the greater yīn and the yáng brightness stand in interior-exterior relationship, stomach dry earth receives enriching and moistening from the damp earth of the spleen, and large intestine dry metal is cleared and harmonized by the clear metal of the lung. Under normal circumstances, yáng brightness and greater yīn balance each other, so that the dryness of yáng brightness is not apparent. It becomes apparent only when this balance is upset. If yáng brightness dryness becomes excessive, then greater yīn dampness is insufficient, giving rise to a yáng brightness dryness-heat repletion pattern. If yáng brightness dryness becomes insufficient, then greater yīn dampness is excessive, giving rise to a yáng brightness cold pattern or shifting to the greater yīn. The present line discusses excessive yáng brightness dryness with insufficient greater yīn dampness. Yáng brightness is characterized by dryness transformation, and however long or short the course of the disease so far, aversion to cold is bound to cease spontaneously, as explained in the preceding line. The practitioner needs to be aware that aversion to cold can appear in yáng brightness disease, although only at its onset.

Aversion to cold can appear in disease of any of the six channels. However, there are certain distinguishing features. In greater yáng disease, aversion to cold appears and recedes as the disease begins and ends. If greater yáng disease persists and timely treatment is not given, aversion to cold can continue for eight or nine days. When aversion to cold appears in lesser yáng disease, it is generally as part of alternating aversion to cold and heat effusion. In disease of the three yīn, aversion to cold appears without heat effusion and will persist unless treatment to warm the center and return yáng is given.

The present line explains the spontaneous cessation of aversion to cold in yáng brightness disease in terms of the doctrine of the five phases. In the natural world, earth engenders and fosters all things. All things grow, develop, become debilitated, and die, after which they return to the earth. In the body, the spleen and stomach are center earth, because they are located in the center burner and because food and drink taken in are transformed into essence and distributed through the body, nourishing the body and engendering life activity. The phrase "All things converge [here and] nothing passes further" is explained as meaning that any evil—exterior or interior, cold or heat—can, under certain conditions, converge in the yáng brightness, just as all things return to earth. Yáng brightness governs dryness transformation; all evils can transform into dryness. After an evil has transformed into dryness and formed repletion, the bowel qì is blocked, and the condition can only be treated by clearing and precipitation. "Nothing passes further" is understood to allude to this situation, rather than meaning that the evil in yáng brightness cannot pass to another channel. Indeed, yáng brightness disease can shift into the yīn channels, such as when yáng brightness disease marked by exuberant heat stirring the blood manifests in nosebleed. If, in this condition, the clearing and precipitating treatment is excessive, it can cause the evil to pass into the triple yīn.

Line 186

伤寒三日，阳明脉大。

Shāng hán sān rì, yáng míng mài dà.

In cold damage[1] [that has lasted] three days,[2] the yáng brightness pulse is large.

Text Notes

1. Cold damage, 伤寒 *shāng hán*: Here, cold damage should be understood in the broad sense of externally contracted disease, since it is not only in greater yáng cold damage that one may find a pulse that is large following the shift to the yáng brightness.
2. Three days, 三日 *sān rì*: A short period of time has passed, not necessarily exactly three days.

Synopsis

The primary pulse for yáng brightness disease.

Commentary

Yáng brightness has copious qì and blood, and insofar as it is equated with the stomach, it is the sea of grain and water. For these reasons, yáng brigbtness disease is characterized by a pulse that is large. Because the yáng brightness governs dryness, when an evil enters, it easily transforms into dryness-heat and spreads throughout the body. It steams and distresses the qì and blood, forcing movement and causing the pulse to become large.

A pulse that is large is not the only pulse seen in yáng brightness. In yáng brightness disease, formless dryness-heat rampant in the interior and exterior can cause the pulse to be surging, large, slippery, and rapid. Nevertheless, when heat-dryness forms repletion and causes stoppage of bowel qì, the pulse becomes sunken, replete, and in some cases slow.

A large pulse is also seen in disease other than yáng brightness. For example, line 25, p. 125, describes an exterior pattern arising in greater yáng disease in which the pulse is surging and large. Again, line 30, p. 269, states, "The inch pulse is floating and large; floating means wind and large means vacuity." Here "large" as a sign of vacuity clearly refers to a pulse that is large and forceless. In the present line, however, "the yáng brightness pulse is large" refers to a pulse that is large and forceful. We may infer from these examples that according to Zhāng Jī's usage, "large" refers to breadth of the pulse only, and has no connotations of strength.

3 BASIC YÁNG BRIGHTNESS DISEASE PATTERNS

3.1 HEAT PATTERNS

3.1.1 Gardenia and Fermented Soybean Decoction Patterns

The following two lines describe the Gardenia and Fermented Soybean Decoction (*zhī zǐ chǐ tāng*) pattern occurring in yáng brightness disease. This pattern may also occur in greater yáng disease, but the initial course of the disease is different. In greater yáng disease, it is mostly the result of exterior evil shifting into the interior and becoming depressed in the region of the chest and diaphragm after inappropriate treatment. In yáng brightness disease, this pattern occurs as a result of residual heat following precipitation. In both cases, this pattern is characterized by heart vexation and anguish as the main sign, and is attributable to the pathomechanism of formless evil heat harassing the upper burner. For this reason, the treatment is the same in both cases.

LINE 221

㈠阳明病，脉浮而紧，咽燥口苦，腹满而喘，发热汗出，不恶寒，反恶热，身重。㈡若发汗则躁，心愦愦，反谵语；若加温针，必怵惕，烦躁不得眠；若下之，则胃中空虚，客气动膈，心中懊侬，舌上胎者，栀子豉汤主之。

Yáng míng bìng, mài fú ér jǐn, yān zào kǒu kǔ, fù mǎn ér chuǎn, fā rè hàn chū, bù wù hán, fǎn wù rè, shēn zhòng, ruò fā hàn zé zào, xīn kuì kuì, fǎn zhān yǔ; ruò jiā wēn zhēn, bì chù tì, fán zào bù dé mián; ruò xià zhī, zé wèi zhōng kōng xū, kè qì dòng gé, xīn zhōng ào nóng, shé shàng tāi zhě, zhī zǐ chǐ tāng zhǔ zhī.

When in yáng brightness disease, the pulse is floating and tight, the throat is dry and [there is] a bitter taste in the mouth, abdominal fullness, panting, heat effusion, sweating, absence of aversion to cold, and instead, aversion to heat [is present] and [there is] generalized heaviness, if sweating is promoted, there will be agitation, restiveness of the heart[1] but[2] delirious speech. If one adds a warm needle, there will be apprehensiveness and vexation and agitation with inability to sleep. If one precipitates, there will be empty vacuity in the stomach, visiting qì stirring the diaphragm, anguish in the heart, and if fur [arises] on the tongue, Gardenia and Fermented Soybean Decoction (*zhī zǐ chǐ tāng*) governs.

Text Note

1. Restiveness of the heart, 心愦愦 *xīn kuì kuì*: A feeling of disorder, vexation, and unrest centered in the heart.
2. But 反 *fǎn*: This occurrence of 反 *fǎn* is considered by many commentators to be a mistake because the appearance of delirious speech seems reasonable given that a yáng brightness disease is mistakenly treated with an acrid, warm, exterior-resolving formula, which exacerbates the heat, disturbing the heart and resulting in delirious speech. Its presence might however be justified, if it suggests that the mistaken use of this formula not only exacerbates the heat, but also damages heart liquid, resulting in a complex pattern of heat repletion and yīn vacuity. In patterns of vacuity, muttering, not delirious speech, is often observed; therefore, we can understand the phrase as, "but instead of muttering, there is delirious speech."

Synopsis

a) Transmuted patterns that may occur following inappropriate treatment of yáng brightness heat patterns.

b) The signs and treatment of heat remaining in the chest and diaphragm following precipitation in yáng brightness heat patterns.

Commentary

As stated in the commentary on the preceding line, a pulse that is large is the main pulse of yáng brightness disease. The present line describes yáng brightness disease with a pulse that is floating and tight. The pulse here is a mutation. A pulse that is tight generally indicates cold or pain; it may also occur in abiding food or phlegm-rheum. The reason why a pulse that is tight occurs in these cases is because of fierce contention between right qì and evil qì. The condition described in the present line is one of repletion of evil and repletion of right, arising when exuberant yáng brightness dryness-heat contends with right qì. The tension between evil and right results in a pulse that is tight. When the pulse is floating, one usually considers the possibility of an exterior pattern. In yáng brightness disease, however, a pulse that is floating indicates dryness-heat rampant in both the interior and exterior. In both cases, when light pressure is applied, the pulse is superabundant; for this reason the pulse is described as floating. However, when heavy pressure is applied, there is a difference. In exterior patterns, the pulse is less forceful, but it is not empty when heavy pressure is applied. This pulse is due to right qì thrusting toward the exterior to expel the evil. In yáng brightness disease, by contrast, it is still forceful under pressure, reflecting exuberant interior heat. Furthermore, of course, these patterns can be differentiated on the basis of the other signs present, such as heat effusion, aversion to cold, and headache, in the case of greater yáng disease, or aversion to heat, thirst, and streaming sweat, in the case of yáng brightness disease.

Dry throat and bitter taste in the mouth reflect steaming dryness-heat impairing stomach harmony and downbearing and causing turbid heat qì to surge upward. These two signs also appear in the description of the essential features of lesser yáng disease (see line 263, p. 407). However, it is not difficult to distinguish the two conditions since the accompanying signs are different in each case. For example, in lesser yáng disease, fullness in the chest and under the rib-side and a pulse that is stringlike and fine are also present. Here, the fullness is in the abdomen, and the pulse is floating and tight.

Abdominal fullness and panting arise when internally exuberant dryness-heat causes congestion of qì dynamic and counterflow ascent of lung qì. Abdominal fullness and panting occur in both formless yáng brightness dryness-heat and repletion patterns, which are readily distinguished by other presenting signs.

Heat effusion, sweating, and aversion to heat instead of cold are attributable to dryness-heat in the interior steaming the fluids and forcing them out to the exterior. These are the outward indicators of yáng brightness disease. Yáng brightness heat patterns usually include vexation and agitation. However, the present line speaks of generalized heaviness. This arises when interior heat damages original qì, causing congestion in the channel vessels.

This line discussed several inappropriate mistreatments, including two that exacerbate the heat. The signs enumerated in the first part of the line are all attributable to internal dryness-heat. In this situation, "treating heat with heat" (以热治热 *yǐ rè zhì rè*) constitutes "replenishing repletion" (实实 *shí shí*). If heat effusion and a pulse that is floating and tight are misinterpreted as an exterior pattern, and sweating is inappropriately applied, it will exacerbate the condition. Warm, acrid exterior-resolving medicinals will exacerbate the heat, and the promotion of sweating will further damage the fluids. As a result, the even more exuberant evil heat will harass the heart spirit, causing agitation and restiveness, and in severe cases delirious speech. Again, the presence of generalized heaviness and a pulse that is floating and tight, if taken to indicate internal cold-damp, might prompt the use of warm needling. However, such treatment would be inappropriate because it would boost the interior heat, which would harass the heart spirit and cause apprehension, vexation and agitation, and sleeplessness as well.

Precipitation is appropriate for treating yáng brightness repletion patterns. It is not suitable for a condition caused by formless dryness-heat in the interior such as is described in the present line. Precipitation in this case will damage the stomach and intestines; it will not promote but even hinder the elimination of evil heat, which will then harass the [region of the] chest and diaphragm. This is described as "visiting qì stirring the diaphragm," which gives rise to anguish in the heart, as well as a white, yellow, or mixed yellow and white tongue fur.

Gardenia and Fermented Soybean Decoction (*zhī zǐ chǐ tāng*) is used to clear and diffuse depressed heat in the chest and diaphragm. (See line 76B, p. 144, for a discussion of this formula.) In the present line, the depressed heat in the chest and diaphragm is due to the inappropriate use of precipitation in yáng brightness formless heat. In the greater yáng section, the same formula was used to treat depressed heat in the chest and diaphragm resulting from the inappropriate treatment (vomiting or precipitation). These two cases differ as to the location of the evil prior to inappropriate treatment (exterior in greater yáng and interior in yáng brightness). However, in both cases, inappropriate treatment causes heat to become depressed in the chest and diaphragm region, giving rise to anguish in the heart, even though the accompanying signs are slightly different.

Line 228

阳明病，下之，其外有热，手足温，不结胸，心中懊憹，饥不能食，但头汗出者，栀子豉汤主之。

Yáng míng bìng, xià zhī, qí wài yǒu rè, shǒu zú wēn, bù jié xiōng, xīn zhōng ào nóng, jī bù néng shí, dàn tóu hàn chū zhě, zhī zǐ chǐ tāng zhǔ zhī.

When in yáng brightness disease, precipitation is used and [there is] heat in the exterior,* warm extremities, no chest bind, anguish in the heart, hunger with inability to eat, and sweating only from the head, Gardenia and Fermented Soybean Decoction (*zhī zǐ chǐ tāng*) governs.

Text Note

* Heat in the exterior, 其外有热 *qí wài yǒu rè*: Generalized heat expressed to the outside of the body.

Synopsis

The signs and treatment of yáng brightness disease when, following precipitation, residual heat that has not been eliminated, harasses the chest and diaphragm.

Commentary

The present line describes another Gardenia and Fermented Soybean Decoction (*zhī zǐ chǐ tāng*) pattern arising after precipitation in yáng brightness disease. Here, yáng brightness dryness repletion with bowel qì stoppage is appropriately treated by attacking with coldness and bitterness, but although the dryness bind has been freed, the treatment is not completely successful, since residual heat remains. In such a situation, precipitation cannot be used again, and the correct treatment is to clear and diffuse the residual heat to provide a final adjustment.

Heat in the exterior with warm extremities after precipitation is the outward manifestation of residual heat. It suggests that the heat was even more severe prior to precipitation.

The absence of chest bind is a key pattern-identification point in the present line. It reflects formless evil heat harassing the region of the chest and diaphragm, rather than heat repletion chest bind resulting from heat and water-rheum binding together in the chest. Here there is no pain in the diaphragm that refuses pressure, or hard fullness below the heart; rather, there is only anguish in the heart with no pain or only slight pain, but no hardness and fullness. Hence both conditions are caused by heat in the chest and diaphragm, but should not be confused.

The anguish in the heart is due to evil heat harassing the inner body. Hunger with inability to eat is explained as meaning a sensation "similar to hunger but not hunger," which is often called "clamoring stomach" (嘈杂 *cáo zá*). This is caused by heat harassing the stomach duct disturbing normal digestion. Finally, when yáng brightness heat is pronounced, there is great sweating or sweat streaming from the hands and feet. However, in this case, heat has been reduced by precipitation and is only strong enough to manifest in warmth in the extremities. The residual heat rises upwards; it is incapable of producing a generalized sweat and merely causes sweating from the head.

3.1.2 White Tiger Decoction Patterns

The White Tiger Decoction (*bái hǔ tāng*) pattern is one of exuberant yáng brightness dryness-heat. The characteristic signs are great heat, great thirst, great sweating, and a pulse that is surging and large. The pulse may also be floating and slippery. The primary signs presented for this pattern are abdominal fullness and generalized heaviness, difficulty turning sides, insensitivity of the mouth, grimy complexion, delirious speech, and enuresis.

Frequent aversion to wind, great thirst, dry tongue, and increased desire to drink water, heart vexation, and slight aversion to cold in the back are all considered signs of fluid damage, in which case White Tiger Decoction Plus Ginseng (*bái hǔ jiā rén shēn tāng*) is suggested.

These formulae should generally not be used if the exterior pattern has not yet resolved.

LINE 176

伤寒，脉浮滑，此表有热，里有寒，白虎汤主之。

Shāng hán, mài fú huá, cǐ biǎo yǒu rè, lǐ yǒu hán, bái hǔ tāng zhǔ zhī.

When in cold damage the pulse is floating and slippery, this [means there is] heat in the exterior and cold in the interior.* White Tiger Decoction (*bái hǔ tāng*) governs.

TEXT NOTE

* Cold in the interior, 里有寒 *lǐ yǒu hán*: Lín Yì (林亿) et al., the editors of the Sòng version, believe that this is an error and that the text should read "heat in the interior," 里有热 *lǐ yǒu rè*. They state, "[When there is] heat bound in the interior, and [there is] heat in both the interior and exterior, White

Tiger Decoction (*bái hǔ tāng*) governs...." This interpretation is generally accepted.

FORMULA

White Tiger Decoction (*bái hǔ tāng*)

∘ Clear heat with cold and acridity.

知母六两　石膏一斤（碎）　甘草二两（炙）　粳米六合

右四味，以水一斗，煮米熟，汤成去滓，温服一升，日三服。

Zhī mǔ liù liǎng　shí gāo yī jīn (suì)　gān cǎo èr liǎng (zhì)　gēng mǐ liù gě

Yòu sì wèi, yǐ shuǐ yī dǒu, zhǔ mǐ shú, tāng chéng qù zǐ, wēn fú yī shēng, rì sān fú.

anemarrhena (知母 *zhī mǔ*, Anemarrhenae Rhizoma) 6 liǎng
gypsum (石膏 *shí gāo*, Gypsum) 1 jīn (crushed)
mix-fried licorice (甘草 *gān cǎo*, Glycyrrhizae Radix) 2 liǎng
rice (粳米 *gēng mǐ*, Oryzae Semen) 6 gě

[For] the above four ingredients use one dǒu of water. Boil until the rice is cooked. When the decoction is ready,* remove the dregs and take one shēng warm, three times a day.

FORMULA NOTE

* When the decoction is ready, 汤成 *tāng chéng*: Since the instructions state that one shēng should be taken warm, three times a day, the phrase "when the decoction is ready" is taken to mean "when the decoction has been reduced to three shēng."

SYNOPSIS

The pulse, signs, and treatment of yáng brightness disease with heat in both the exterior and interior.

COMMENTARY

The present line begins with the phrase "cold damage," which is here meant in its broader sense of any externally contracted heat disease. The line describes the signs and treatment of a condition resulting from externally contracted disease evil that passes from the exterior into the interior and enters yáng brightness.

The line discusses a pathomechanism on the basis of the pulse alone, without consideration of signs. Here we can infer from the formula that the signs will be those of formless exuberant dryness-heat mentioned in line 26, p. 156; line 168, p. 323; and line 182, p. 308.

The pulse is described as floating and slippery. Here, floating does not signify evil in the exterior; rather it is the outward manifestation of exuberant internal heat, and accompanying signs ought to include heat effusion, spontaneous sweating, and aversion to heat rather than to cold. Hence the text attributes the floating quality of the pulse to "heat in the exterior." However, this is not to be misinterpreted as greater yáng exterior heat. "Slippery" is the direct manifestation of exuberant internal heat. This is because exuberant internal heat stirs qì and blood, so that the pulse comes and goes smoothly (往来流利 *wǎng lái liú lì*), like "pearls rolling in a dish" (如盘走珠 *rú pán zǒu zhū*), and accompanying signs should include great vexation and thirst with intake of fluid, and a dry yellow tongue fur. On the basis of the descriptions of pulses in yáng brightness disease given in line 186, p. 311, and line 221, p. 312, we can assume that in the present line the pulse is forceful when heavy pressure is applied.

White Tiger Decoction (*bái hǔ tāng*) is used to treat formless internal dryness-heat spreading through the whole body so that there is heat in both the interior and exterior. Gypsum (*shí gāo*) is acrid, sweet, and very cold, and clears heat. Anemarrhena (*zhī mǔ*) is bitter, cold, and moistening; it discharges fire and enriches dryness. Together, these two ingredients clear exuberant yáng brightness heat and safeguard stomach liquid. Mix-fried licorice (*gān cǎo*) and rice (*gēng mǐ*) together boost the qì and harmonize the center, since when qì is sufficient, the fluids will be engendered. Furthermore, these two ingredients help avoid damage to the stomach from the use of cold medicinals.

Line 219

(一) 三阳合病，腹满身重，难以转侧，口不仁面垢，谵语遗尿，发汗则谵语，下之则额上生汗，手足厥冷。(二) 若自汗出者，白虎汤主之。

(1) *Sān yáng hé bìng, fù mǎn shēn zhòng, nán yǐ zhuǎn cè, kǒu bù rén miàn gòu, zhān yǔ yí niào, (fā hàn zé zhān yǔ, xià zhī zé é shàng shēng hàn, shǒu zú jué lěng).* (2) *Ruò zì hàn chū zhě, bái hǔ tāng zhǔ zhī.*

(1) In combination disease of the three yáng,[1] [there is] abdominal fullness, generalized heaviness, difficulty turning sides, insensitivity of the mouth,[2] grimy face,[3] delirious speech and enuresis. ([If] sweating is promoted, there will be delirious speech[4] and [if] precipitation is used, sweat will arise on the forehead and [there will be] reversal cold of the extremities.) (2) If sweat spontaneously issues, White Tiger Decoction (*bái hǔ tāng*) governs.

Text Notes

1. Combination disease of the three yáng, 三阳合病 *sān yáng hé bìng*: Simultaneous appearance of the signs of greater yáng, lesser yáng, and yáng brightness disease.
2. Insensitivity of the mouth, 口不仁 *kǒu bù rén*: Inhibition of normal speech and a loss of normal taste.
3. Grimy face, 面垢 *miàn gòu*: The face appears as if concealed by a layer of oily dirt.

4. [If] sweating is promoted, there will be delirious speech, 发汗则谵语 *fā hán zé zhān yǔ*: The *Jīn Guì Yù Hán Jīng* version reads 发汗则谵语甚 *fā hàn zé zhān yǔ shèn*, "[if] sweating is promoted, delirious speech will be [more] pronounced." This would make more sense in the context, since delirious speech is said to be present prior to promotion of sweating.

SYNOPSIS

The signs, treatment, and contraindications for combination disease of the three yáng with the emphasis strongly on yáng brightness.

COMMENTARY

The latter part of this line takes the form of grammatical inversion. The last sentence, "If sweat spontaneously issues, White Tiger Decoction (*bái hǔ tāng*) governs," should logically follow after "enuresis."

This line starts off with "simultaneous disease of the three yáng," but the signs enumerated can all be explained in terms of yáng brightness disease, and the treatment suggested is a formula specifically addressing yáng brightness disease. One explanation put forward for this discrepancy is that although this illness may have begun as simultaneous disease of the three yáng, at this point the emphasis has already shifted to yáng brightness. Because yáng brightness dryness-heat is congested in the interior, stomach qì cannot descend and the qì stagnates in the abdomen, causing abdominal fullness. However, the abdominal fullness is milder than the abdominal fullness with absence of defecation observed in yáng brightness bowel repletion. Exuberant yáng brightness heat damages liquid and consumes qì, causing generalized heaviness and difficulty turning sides. Damage to liquid also causes the mouth and tongue to be parched and dry, which leads to a loss of normal taste sensation and an inhibition of normal speech. Both the foot yáng brightness and the hand yáng brightness channel are distributed over the face. Consequently yáng brightness evil heat congested in the interior steams turbid qì of the stomach and intestines, and causes it rise to the face, giving the face a grimy or dirty appearance. Exuberant stomach heat rising to harass the spirit-light causes delirious speech. In clouded spirit with delirious speech due to exuberant heat, the bladder loses restraint, resulting in urinary incontinence. The above-mentioned signs are attributed to exuberant yáng brightness heat in the inner body. Whether or not White Tiger Decoction (*bái hǔ tāng*) is used depends on whether or not there is sweating. If sweat spontaneously issues, it means that although the fluids have been damaged, they have not been completely exhausted. White Tiger Decoction (*bái hǔ tāng*) clears internal heat and safeguards liquid. If there is no sweating, this is because of severe damage to fluids, which may give rise to a yáng brightness repletion pattern. White Tiger Decoction (*bái hǔ tāng*) treats formless dryness-heat, and is inadequate to treat severe damage to fluids. The appropriate treatment will depend on the signs and pulse.

If heat effusion and generalized heaviness are misinterpreted as an exterior pattern and sweating is promoted with warm acrid agents, this treatment will exacerbate the internal heat and the resultant loss of sweat will exacerbate the damage to liquid caused by the stomach heat. Consequently, the delirious speech will become more pronounced.

If the abdominal fullness is misinterpreted as constituting yáng brightness bowel repletion, and precipitation is given, this treatment will lead to exhaustion of yīn humor in the lower body. Yáng will then have nothing to depend on and will stray to the upper body. As a result, sweat will issue only from the forehead. When yáng strays to the head from the rest of the body, it cannot warm the limbs, hence the reversal cold of the extremities.

3.1.3 White Tiger Decoction Plus Ginseng Patterns

LINE 170

伤寒，脉浮，发热无汗，其表不解，不可与白虎汤；渴欲饮水，无表证者，白虎加人参汤主之。

Shāng hán, mài fú, fā rè wú hàn, qí biǎo bù jiě, bù kě yǔ bái hǔ tāng; kě yù yǐn shuǐ, wú biǎo zhèng zhě, bái hǔ jiā rén shēn tāng zhǔ zhī.

When in cold damage, the pulse is floating, [and there is] heat effusion [and] sweating is absent, the exterior has not resolved; one cannot give White Tiger Decoction (*bái hǔ tāng*); if [there is] thirst with a desire for fluids and no exterior signs, White Tiger Decoction Plus Ginseng (*bái hǔ jiā rén shēn tāng*) governs.

SYNOPSIS

a) Before an exterior pattern has resolved, White Tiger Decoction (*bái hǔ tāng*) is contraindicated.

b) The signs and treatment of yáng brightness disease with exuberant heat and liquid damage.

COMMENTARY

As in line 176, p. 316, the phrase "cold damage" in the present line refers to externally contracted heat disease in general. The first half of the present line discusses a greater yáng exterior pattern (cold damage in the narrow sense), as we can tell from the signs and pulse. The latter half describes the signs and treatment of an externally contracted disease evil entering yáng brightness, transforming into heat, and damaging liquid.

Since a pulse that is floating and slippery can appear in a White Tiger Decoction (*bái hǔ tāng*) pattern (see line 176, p. 316), and a pulse that is floating and tight can appear in exuberant yáng brightness heat (see line 221, p. 312), a pulse that is floating is not necessarily an indication of a greater yáng exterior pattern. A pulse that is floating may (as in line 1, p. 41), reflect right qì hastening toward the exterior to resist an externally contracted disease evil, or (as in line 176, p. 316), it may be the outward manifestation of exuberant internal heat. Identification is made on the basis of accompanying signs.

In the first part of the present line, a pulse that is floating with heat effusion and absence of sweating is explained as being a greater yáng cold damage pattern.

Since the phrase "the exterior has not resolved" means that the exterior evil has not yet been eliminated, we may expect aversion to cold to be present. When a pulse that is floating occurs in yáng brightness dryness-heat, it will be accompanied by heat effusion, aversion to heat rather than to cold, and spontaneous sweating. Before a greater yáng exterior pattern has resolved, the method of treatment is promoting sweating to resolve the exterior, as with Ephedra Decoction (*má huáng tāng*). Even if yáng brightness interior heat appears simultaneously, the treatment is dual resolution of the exterior and interior as with Major Green-Blue Dragon Decoction (*dà qīng lóng tāng*). Zhāng Jī emphasizes that when "the exterior has not resolved, one cannot give White Tiger Decoction (*bái hǔ tāng*)" because cold and cool medicinals will not only fail to eliminate the external evil, but will also damage center yáng and cause the external evil to fall inward, giving rise to transmuted patterns.

In the latter part of the present line, the absence of exterior signs means that the exterior has resolved, and that the disease evil has completely entered the interior. The presence of thirst with a desire to drink means that the disease evil has transformed into yáng brightness dryness-heat and has damaged liquid and consumed qì. In view of this, we assume that the pulse is still floating or surging and large, but since liquid and qì have been damaged, it is likely to be relatively forceless when heavy pressure is applied. The absence of sweating in the first half of the line should now have given way to spontaneous sweating, and although heat effusion persists, aversion to cold should have given way to aversion to heat. These are the outward manifestations of yáng brightness dryness-heat. White Tiger Decoction Plus Ginseng (*bái hǔ jiā rén shēn tāng*) is suggested because it clears heat and engenders liquid, boosts qì, and nourishes yīn.

Line 169

伤寒无大热，口燥渴，心烦，背微恶寒者，白虎加人参汤主之。

Shāng hán wú dà rè, kǒu zào kě, xīn fán, bèi wēi wù hán zhě, bái hǔ jiā rén shēn tāng zhǔ zhī.

When in cold damage great heat [effusion] is absent[1] [and there is] a dry mouth, thirst, heart vexation, and slight aversion to cold in the back,[2] White Tiger Decoction Plus Ginseng (*bái hǔ jiā rén shēn tāng*) governs.

Text Notes

1. Great heat [effusion] is absent, 无大热 *wú dà rè*: No great heat in the exterior.
2. Slight aversion to cold in the back, 背微恶寒 *bèi wēi wù hán*: A mild fear of cold felt in the back of the body. Different interpretations of the pathomechanism of this, sign are discussed below.

Synopsis

The signs and treatment of yáng brightness disease in which the interior heat is very exuberant and damages both liquid and qì.

Commentary

The phrase "great heat is absent" appears in several places in the descriptions of triple yáng disease. In the present line, as in several other lines (line 63, p. 154, and line 136, p. 218), it refers to great heat present in the interior but absent from the exterior, although the precise location of the heat in the interior is different. In one place (line 61, p. 181), it refers to false heat arising when vacuous yáng floats to the exterior.

Exuberant interior heat damages the fluids causing dry mouth and thirst. Furthermore, heat in the yáng brightness easily ascends and harasses the heart, causing heart vexation. In such cases there is usually "generalized heat" (line 182, p. 308). In the present line, however, profuse sweating due to exuberant yáng brightness dryness-heat has damaged liquid and qì—on the one hand causing the interstices of the flesh to loosen, and on the other causing yáng qì to become depressed in the interior—so that the body cannot resist wind and cold. As a result, not only has the original heat effusion abated ("great heat is absent"), but there is even slight aversion to cold in the back. Although the outward signs of the yáng brightness dryness-heat have abated, the internal heat is still pronounced. Here, slight aversion to cold in the back should not be misinterpreted as constituting an exterior pattern or interior cold pattern. Because there is interior heat, the aversion to cold in the back is only "slight," and, in addition, there is dry mouth and heart vexation. Although the pulse is not described in the present line, it should support this conclusion. As to treatment, White Tiger Decoction (*bái hŭ tāng*) is still recommended because of exuberant interior heat. Nevertheless, ginseng (*rén shēn*) is added to boost qì and engender liquid, addressing the looseness of the interstices of the flesh.

"Slight aversion to cold in the back" must be clearly distinguished from the aversion to cold occurring at the onset of disease. Line 183, p. 309, describes a condition in which externally contracted evil enters the yáng brightness directly. There is aversion to cold at the onset of disease, but as yáng brightness dryness-heat develops, it quickly ceases. The situation described in the present line differs in that the "slight aversion to cold in the back" appears not at onset, but after great heat and greater sweating, and that owing to damage to liquid and qì it will not cease spontaneously. "Slight aversion to cold in the back" must also be distinguished from the aversion to cold occurring in greater yáng disease and the aversion to cold of triple yīn disease. Aversion to cold in greater yáng disease is generalized over the whole body and is associated with heat effusion, headache, generalized pain, and a pulse that is floating. It appears with onset of greater yáng disease and disappears with its cessation. Aversion to cold in diseases of the three yīn channels is likewise generalized; it is associated with curled lying posture, cold limbs, and a pulse that is sunken and faint. In greater yáng and triple yīn disease, the aversion to cold is pronounced, never "slight," and never limited to the back; it is never accompanied by thirst with heart vexation, which is strictly a manifestation of exuberant internal yáng brightness heat.

LINE 168

伤寒若吐若下后，七八日不解，热结在里，表里俱热，时时恶风，大渴，舌上干燥而烦，欲饮水数升者，白虎加人参汤主之。

Shāng hán ruò tù ruò xià hòu, qī bā rì bù jiě, rè jié zài lǐ, biǎo lǐ jù rè, shí shí wù fēng, dà kě, shé shàng gān zào ér fán, yù yǐn shuǐ shuò shēng zhě, bái hǔ jiā rén shēn tāng zhǔ zhī.

When in cold damage, if vomiting [is used], or if precipitation [is used] and after seven or eight days [there is] no resolution, the heat is bound in the interior, with heat in both the exterior and interior, frequent aversion to wind,* great thirst, dry tongue, vexation, and a desire to drink several shēng of water, [then] White Tiger Decoction Plus Ginseng (*bái hǔ jiā rén shēn tāng*) governs.

TEXT NOTE

* Frequent aversion to wind, 时时恶风 *shí shí wù fēng*: Recurrent sensation of cold on exposure to wind or drafts.

SYNOPSIS

The signs and treatment of cold damage when, after the use of vomiting and precipitation, there is heat bound in the interior, and exuberant heat damages liquid.

COMMENTARY

If greater yáng cold damage is mistreated with vomiting or precipitating treatment, the disease will not resolve through the exterior. Instead, the damage to liquid caused by the mistreatment may cause the evil to fall into the interior and transform into yáng brightness dryness-heat, causing further damage to liquid. This is described in the present line, and bound heat in the interior gives rise to symptoms in the interior and exterior. On the one hand, great thirst, dry tongue, vexation, and desire to drink large amounts of water indicate yáng brightness interior heat; on the other, generalized heat (with aversion to heat rather than to cold) and spontaneous sweating are the outward signs of yáng brightness heat. This is what is meant by "heat in both the exterior and interior."

Frequent aversion to wind is not the aversion to wind of greater yáng cold damage. Rather it arises for the same reasons as "aversion to cold in the back" in the preceding line, i.e., exuberant interior heat steaming the fluids, causing profuse sweating, which loosens interstices of the flesh and damages both qì and yīn.

The major difference between the two lines is the presence or absence of great heat in the exterior. This difference, however, is not of major importance, since the underlying pathomechanism is the same.

Exuberant dryness-heat in the interior damages the fluids and the qì; hence White Tiger Decoction Plus Ginseng (*bái hǔ jiā rén shēn tāng*) is used to clear yáng brightness interior heat, boost the qì, and engender liquid.

Line 222

若渴欲饮水，口干舌燥者，白虎加人参汤主之。
Ruò kě yù yǐn shuǐ, kǒu gān shé zào zhě, bái hǔ jiā rén shēn tāng zhǔ zhī.

If [there is] thirst with desire to drink water, dry mouth, and dry tongue, [then] White Tiger Decoction Plus Ginseng (*bái hǔ jiā rén shēn tāng*) governs.

Synopsis

Continuing from line 221, p. 312, a description of the signs and treatment of yáng brightness disease in which exuberant heat damages liquid.

Commentary

This line is regarded as a further discussion of the situation presented in line 221, p. 312. When formless dryness-heat in the yáng brightness is mistreated through the use of precipitation or sweating, the heat may remain in the chest and diaphragm, harassing the heart. This pattern is treated with Gardenia and Fermented Soybean Decoction (*zhī zǐ chǐ tāng*). If the evil does not resolve and the fluid damage becomes more severe, thirst with desire to drink and a dry mouth and tongue may arise. In this case, White Tiger Decoction Plus Ginseng (*bái hǔ jiā rén shēn tāng*) is used to clear interior heat and engender liquid.

3.1.4 Polyporus Decoction Patterns

In a yáng brightness disease, following inappropriate precipitation, yīn may be damaged and residual heat may remain in the presence of collected water. Polyporus Decoction (*zhū líng tāng*) may then be used to clear heat, disinhibit water, and foster yīn. Nonetheless, following copious sweating and fluid damage, with signs such as thirst and inhibited urination, one must identify patterns carefully to determine if this formula is appropriate.

Line 223

若脉浮发热，渴欲饮水，小便不利者，猪苓汤主之。
Ruò mài fú fā rè, kě yù yǐn shuǐ, xiǎo biàn bù lì zhě, zhū líng tāng zhǔ zhī.

If the pulse is floating and [there is] heat effusion, thirst with a desire to drink water, and inhibited urination, [then] Polyporus Decoction (*zhū líng tāng*) governs.

Formula

Polyporus Decoction (*zhū líng tāng*)

- Clear heat and disinhibit water; foster yīn and moisten dryness.

猪苓（去皮） 茯苓 泽泻 阿胶 滑石（碎）各一两

右五味，以水四升，先煮四味取二升，去滓，内阿胶烊消，温服七合，日三服。

Zhū líng (qù pí) fú líng zé xiè ē jiāo huá shí (suì) gè yī liǎng

Yòu wǔ wèi, yǐ shuǐ sì shēng, xiān zhǔ sì wèi qǔ èr shēng, qù zǐ, nà ē jiāo yáng xiāo, wēn fú qī gě, rì sān fú.

polyporus (猪苓 *zhū líng*, Polyporus) (remove skin)
poria (茯苓 *fú líng*, Poria)
alisma (泽泻 *zé xiè*, Alismatis Rhizoma)
ass hide glue (阿胶 *ē jiāo*, Asini Corii Gelatinum)
talcum (滑石 *huá shí*, Talcum) (crushed)
each ingredient 1 liǎng

[For] the above five ingredients use four shēng of water. First boil the four ingredients [not including ass hide glue (*ē jiāo*)] to get two shēng. Remove the dregs and blend in the ass hide glue (*ē jiāo*). Take seven gě warm three times a day.

Synopsis

Continuing from line 221, p. 312, an explanation of the signs and treatment of yáng brightness disease with liquid damage and bound water and heat.

Commentary

This line presents a scenario that may occur following the inappropriate treatment of yáng brightness disease. Line 221, p. 312, line 222, p. 324, and line 223, p. 324, present three possibilities; in this line, a fourth is presented. After the mistreatment, the interior heat evil is not eliminated and severely damages the fluids. However, a water evil is also present as the result of another disease process or the patient's constitution. Water and heat become bound in the interior and the qì cannot transform fluids. Thirst with a desire to drink indicates that the fluids have been damaged by exuberant interior heat and that the internal bind has obstructed normal qì transformation, so the fluids are not being transformed properly. Inhibited urination indicates that water amassment in the lower burner has obstructed the normal movement of fluids. Heat effusion and a pulse that is floating are exterior expressions of exuberant yáng brightness heat.

Polyporus Decoction (*zhū líng tāng*) clears heat, disinhibits the urine, and moistens dryness. Polyporus (*zhū líng*), poria (*fú líng*), and alisma (*zé xiè*) percolate dampness and disinhibit the urine. Talcum (*huá shí*) disinhibits binds in the six bowels, and because it is cold in nature, it not only disinhibits bound water but it also clears heat. Salty and cold, ass hide glue (*ē jiāo*) fosters yīn and clears heat. It is particularly appropriate in patterns where damage to yīn humor occurs with collected water and heat. Polyporus Decoction (*zhū líng tāng*) clears heat without causing dryness and disinhibits water without damaging yīn.

This line is similar to line 71, p. 195, in which the pulse is floating, and inhibited urination, slight heat, and dissipation thirst are observed. Although the signs are similar, the pathomechanisms are completely different. That pattern arises from a greater yáng exterior evil that shifts into the bladder, impairing the qì transformation, whereas this pattern arises when a yáng brightness interior heat evil binds with collected water. In the preceding pattern, Poria (Hoelen) Five Powder (*wǔ líng sǎn*) is used because it contains not only ingredients to disinhibit the urine, but also contains cinnamon twig (*guì zhī*), which warms the yáng and restores the qì dynamic. In this case, Polyporus Decoction (*zhū líng tāng*) is given because it does not include cinnamon twig (*guì zhī*), but instead contains talcum (*huá shí*) and ass hide glue (*ē jiāo*), which clear heat and moisten dryness. Polyporus Decoction (*zhū líng tāng*) is used when the heat is considered to be deeper in the body; hence the tongue color may be deep red or even purple, whereas in line 71, it will probably be light red.

Line 224

阳明病，汗出多而渴者，不可与猪苓汤，以汗多胃中燥，猪苓汤复利其小便故也。

Yáng míng bìng, hàn chū duō ér kě zhě, bù kě yǔ zhū líng tāng, yí hàn duō wèi zhōng zào, zhū líng tāng fù lì qí xiǎo biàn gǔ yě.

When in yáng brightness disease, [there is] copious sweating and thirst, one cannot give Polyporus Decoction (*zhū líng tāng*) because with copious sweat the stomach is dry and Polyporus Decoction (*zhū líng tāng*) disinhibits the urine.

Synopsis

Contraindications for the use of Polyporus Decoction (*zhū líng tāng*).

Commentary

In yáng brightness disease, exuberant interior heat steams the fluids and forces them out to the exterior, resulting in copious sweating and fluid damage. Fluid damage may give rise to thirst and inhibited urination. Although inhibited urination is not explicitly described in the text, its presence is likely because Zhāng Jī is discussing Polyporus Decoction (*zhū líng tāng*), which is generally used when urination is inhibited. An important differentiation that should be made here is that fluid damage may cause thirst and inhibited urination, but water amassment bound with internal heat may also cause these signs. In the first situation, one is cautioned against using Polyporus Decoction (*zhū líng tāng*), while in the second situation, Polyporus Decoction (*zhū líng tāng*) is the formula of choice. In this case copious sweating causes stomach dryness. When internal dryness is the pattern, one must not disinhibit the urine. Although Polyporus Decoction (*zhū líng tāng*) clears heat and nourishes the yīn, one of its primary actions is to disinhibit the urine; hence it should not be used. If, as in the preceding line, sweat has not issued, yet the patient is thirsty and has inhibited urination, then one may consider using Polyporus Decoction (*zhū líng tāng*).

3.2 Repletion Patterns

3.2.1 Qì-Coordinating Decoction Patterns

It is helpful first to understand the name of the "Qì-Coordinating Decoction." The stomach is the sea of grain and water; it decomposes food and passes it on to the small intestine, which separates the clear and the turbid. The turbid part passes on down to the large intestine, where it is formed into stool ready for expulsion from the body. According to the *Líng Shū*, when food enters the stomach, "the stomach fills and the intestines are vacuous," and when food passes downward, "the intestines fill and the stomach is vacuous." In this way, "vacuity gives way to fullness, and fullness to vacuity." The name of this formula alludes to its ability to promote the continuity of this movement. The Chinese 承 *chéng* means to "continue," "carry on," or "inherit." Coordinating the qì means promoting the harmonious action of the stomach and intestines.

The Stomach-Regulating Qì-Coordinating Decoction (*tiáo wèi chéng qì tāng*) pattern is a mild pattern of yáng brightness bowel repletion. The primary pathomechanism in this pattern is that dryness-heat binds in the interior and the bowel qì is blocked. The main signs are mild glomus and fullness, and steaming heat effusion may also be observed. The formula drains heat and moistens dryness, and harmonizes the stomach. Medicinals to rectify the qì and disperse glomus are not included in this formula because the signs are not severe.

In Minor Qì-Coordinating Decoction (*xiǎo chéng qì tāng*) pattern, dryness-heat also binds in the interior, blocking the bowel qì. Glomus and fullness are the main signs, but they are more severe than in the pattern described above and may be accompanied by hard stool. This formula drains heat and frees the stool, and disperses glomus and fullness. The formula contains ingredients to rectify the qì and disperse glomus, but does not contain hardness-softening mirabilite (*máng xiāo*) because severe hardness is absent in these patterns.

The Major Qì-Coordinating Decoction (*dà chéng qì tāng*) pattern is the most severe of these three. Glomus, fullness, dryness, and repletion are all present. The commonly observed signs are tidal heat effusion, delirious speech, bound stool or heat bind with circumfluence, abdominal fullness, hardness and pain, streaming sweat, a dry yellow tongue, and a pulse that is sunken and replete or slow and forceful. This formula offensively precipitates heat repletion and flushes dryness bind. It is the harshest of these three formulae and must be used cautiously. This pattern is sometimes observed in fatal conditions.

3.2.1.1 Stomach-Regulating Qì-Coordinating Decoction Patterns

LINE 248

太阳病三日，发汗不解，蒸蒸发热者，属胃也，调胃承气汤主之。

Tài yáng bìng sān rì, fā hàn bù jiě, zhēng zhēng fā rè zhě, shǔ wèi yě, tiáo wèi chéng qì tāng zhǔ zhī.

When greater yáng disease [has lasted for] three days, and sweating is promoted [but there is] no resolution [of the disease] and [there is] steaming heat effusion,* this belongs to the stomach, and Stomach-Regulating Qì-Coordinating Decoction (*tiáo wèi chéng qì tāng*) governs.

Text Note

* Steaming heat effusion, 蒸蒸发热 *zhēng zhēng fā rè*: A feeling of strong heat, as if it is moving from the interior of the body to the exterior, like steam rising from boiling water.

Formula

Stomach-Regulating Qì-Coordinating Decoction (*tiáo wèi chéng qì tāng*)

∘ Drain heat and harmonize the stomach; moisten dryness and soften hardness.

大黄四两（去皮，清酒洗） 甘草二两（炙） 芒消半升

右三味，切，以水三升，煮二物至一升，去滓，内芒消，更上火一二沸，温顿服之以调胃气。

Dà huáng sì liǎng (qù pí, qīng jiǔ xǐ) gān cǎo èr liǎng (zhì) máng xiāo bàn shēng

Yòu sān wèi, qiē, yǐ shuǐ sān shēng, zhǔ èr wù zhì yī shēng, qù zǐ, nà máng xiāo, gèng shàng wēi huǒ yī èr fèi, wēn dùn fú zhī, yǐ tiáo wèi qì.

rhubarb (大黄 *dà huáng*, Rhei Rhizoma) 4 liǎng (washed with clear wine*)
mix-fried licorice (甘草 *gān cǎo*, Glycyrrhizae Radix) 2 liǎng
mirabilite (芒硝 *máng xiāo*, Mirabilitum) half shēng

[For] the above three ingredients, cut [them] and use three shēng of water. Boil [the first] two ingredients down to one shēng and remove the dregs. Add the mirabilite (*máng xiāo*). Place [the decoction] again on a mild flame and boil once or twice. Take warm as a single dose, to regulate the stomach qì.

Formula Note

* Washed in clear wine, 清酒洗 *qīng jiǔ xǐ*: Rhubarb (*dà huáng*) may be prepared with wine in one of two ways:

a) It may be placed in wine, allowed to steep briefly, and then stir-fried until the color changes slightly.

b) It may be sprayed with wine, steamed briefly, and then dried.

The goal of processing rhubarb (*dà huáng*) with liquor is to give it ascending properties. Raw, its main direction of action is downward. In diseases with signs in the center or upper burners, the liquor-treated agent is more suitable.

Synopsis

The signs and treatment of greater yáng disease that shifts to yáng brightness stomach repletion following the promotion of sweating.

COMMENTARY

The appropriate treatment for greater yáng disease is the promotion of sweating. After three days, when sweating has been promoted and the disease has not resolved, one should consider that the evil may have fallen into the interior. Steaming heat effusion is a sign of exuberant internal heat. Exuberant heat steams in the interior, resulting in a feeling of heat moving from the interior to the exterior. This sign may be accompanied by streaming sweat, a sign of interior heat steaming the fluids, or aversion to heat. This pattern belongs to the yáng brightness, or as in the text, "belongs to the stomach."

Stomach-Regulating Qì-Coordinating Decoction (*tiáo wèi chéng qì tāng*) is used to treat yáng brightness bowel repletion in cases where dryness repletion is primary. These patterns are characterized by abdominal fullness, absence of defecation, and a dry tongue with yellow fur. In severe cases the patient may be vexed and speak deliriously. In this case, abdominal fullness and blocked stool are not yet observed, so Stomach-Regulating Qì-Coordinating Decoction (*tiáo wèi chéng qì tāng*) is used to clear heat and harmonize the stomach, and the attacking and bind-breaking ability of Major Qì-Coordinating Decoction (*dà chéng qì tāng*) is not considered necessary. The identification of this pattern, on the basis of the text alone, would be very difficult; therefore, this line is another example of the formula being used to work back to the pattern.

In this line, blocked bowel qì and yáng brightness heat are thought to be present. White Tiger Decoction (*bái hǔ tāng*) would clear the heat, but not address the bowel repletion. Major Qì-Coordinating Decoction (*dà chéng qì tāng*) would also not be appropriate because great repletion and great fullness are absent. The ability of Minor Qì-Coordinating Decoction (*xiǎo chéng qì tāng*) to regulate the qì and eliminate fullness is not considered necessary because clear distention and fullness are also absent. Stomach-Regulating Qì-Coordinating Decoction (*tiáo wèi chéng qì tāng*) is used for mild repletion, fullness, and dryness. It drains dryness-heat, supports and normalizes the stomach qì, and safeguards the fluids. Bitter, cold rhubarb (*dà huáng*) drains heat and eliminates repletion. It pushes out the old to make room for the new. In patterns for which this formula is used, abdominal signs are generally present. Rhubarb (*dà huáng*) is treated with liquor so that its actions will ascend into the abdomen, as well as descend into the bowels. Salty, cold mirabilite (*máng xiāo*) drains heat, moistens dryness, and softens hardness. The two together clear heat, open the bowel, attack hardness, and break binds. These actions are moderated by the addition of mix-fried licorice (*gān cǎo*). Mix-fried licorice (*gān cǎo*) supplements the center and protects the stomach qì and fluids from being damaged by the cold, bitter ingredients.

The method of taking the formula should be noted. In line 29, p. 187, taking a small amount of Stomach-Regulating Qì-Coordinating Decoction (*tiáo wèi chéng qì tāng*) is suggested for disharmony of the stomach qì and delirious speech. That is a pattern of stomach heat in which bowel repletion is absent. A small amount of the formula is taken to clear stomach heat, illustrating moderate use of a moderate formula. In this line, the dryness-heat is more severe and the bowel qì is blocked. Although great repletion and fullness are absent, if only a small amount of a mild formula is taken, it may be difficult to resolve the disease. In order to avoid this problem, the formula is prepared and taken as a single dose; this is an example of using a larger dose of a mild formula in an severe pattern.

LINE 249

伤寒吐后，腹胀满者，与调胃承气汤。

Shāng hán tù hòu, fù zhàng mǎn zhě, yǔ tiáo wèi chéng qì tāng.

When in cold damage, [if] after vomiting [is used], [there is] abdominal distention and fullness, give Stomach-Regulating Qì-Coordinating Decoction (*tiáo wèi chéng qì tāng*).

SYNOPSIS

The signs and treatment of yáng brightness dryness repletion with abdominal fullness.

COMMENTARY

The use of vomiting treatment for cold damage is inappropriate treatment. When vomiting is used, an evil in the center or upper burner may be expelled, but an evil in the lower burner will remain. This evil, due to the patient's constitution or to environmental factors, may transform to dryness-heat and bind in the bowel, causing blocked bowel qì. This pattern may be precipitated, but since the only sign is abdominal distention and fullness, and all of the Qì-Coordinating Decoction (*chéng qì tāng*) patterns contain this sign, how should one choose? The choice is made by the process of elimination, on the basis of the severity of the signs. In this line, signs of great repletion or great fullness are absent, as are delirious speech and tidal heat effusion. It is unlikely that the strength of Major Qì-Coordinating Decoction (*dà chéng qì tāng*) is required. The abdominal fullness and distention is not described as painful or where the patient refuses pressure, so Minor Qì-Coordinating Decoction (*xiǎo chéng qì tāng*) is not considered to be necessary. Zhāng Jī suggests using Stomach-Regulating Qì-Coordinating Decoction (*tiáo wèi chéng qì tāng*) to precipitate mildly and clear heat.

In previous cases, following the inappropriate use of vomiting, the qì of the center burner was damaged. When the center burner qì is damaged, the spleen and stomach are vacuous and movement and transformation is impaired. This results in stagnation of the qì dynamic and fullness and distention in the abdomen. In cases of center burner vacuity with fullness and distention, one should warm the center and fortify the spleen, and move the qì and disperse fullness. Although it does mildly supplement the qì of the center burner, this is not the main action of Stomach-Regulating Qì-Coordinating Decoction (*tiáo wèi chéng qì tāng*), which suggests that the abdominal fullness in this line is different from that observed in cases of vacuity. When fullness and distention are the result of center burner vacuity, the signs are generally periodic, not constant, and the discomfort decreases with warmth and pressure and may not be painful. In this line, it is likely that the abdominal fullness and distention is persistent, aggravated by heat and pressure, and accompanied by other signs of yáng brightness interior heat repletion, such as thirst, vexation, and heat effusion.

Line 207

阳明病，不吐不下，心烦者，可与调胃承气汤。

Yáng míng bìng, bù tù bù xià, xīn fán zhě, kě yǔ tiáo wèi chéng qì tāng.

When in yáng brightness disease, neither vomiting nor precipitation [was used] and [there is] heart vexation, one can give Stomach-Regulating Qì-Coordinating Decoction (*tiáo wèi chéng qì tāng*).

Synopsis

The signs and treatment of yáng brightness repletion with depressed heat and heart vexation.

Commentary

In yáng brightness disease, repletion dryness-heat is present in the interior. It rises up and harasses the heart, causing spirit disorders such as vexation. It should also be noted that the stomach channel divergence passes into the heart and heat may follow the channel and enter the heart through this pathway.

Because Stomach-Regulating Qì-Coordinating Decoction (*tiáo wèi chéng qì tāng*) is suggested, one would expect that the heart vexation in this pattern is accompanied by absence of defecation, fullness and distention in the abdomen that is aggravated by pressure, steaming heat effusion, and sweating. These accompanying signs help one differentiate between the heart vexation in this pattern, which may be termed "repletion vexation," and the heart vexation seen in Gardenia and Fermented Soybean Decoction (*zhī zǐ chǐ tāng*) patterns which is termed "vacuity vexation." In vacuity vexation patterns, precipitation or vomiting has already been used and the substantial repletion evil has been eliminated. Residual heat harasses the region of the chest and diaphragm, leading to heart vexation, but painful abdominal distention and blocked stool are absent. One other type of vexation that should be considered is that which occurs when the use of precipitation or vomiting damages the qì of the spleen and stomach, leading to interior qì vacuity. This vacuity may also lead to vexation, but in these cases, other signs of qì vacuity should be observed, and if abdominal fullness and distention is present, it should be soft and alleviated by pressure.

3.2.1.2 Minor Qì-Coordinating Decoction Patterns

Line 213

㈠阳明病，其人多汗，以津液外出，胃中燥，大便必硬，硬则谵语，小承气汤主之。㈡若一服谵语止者，更莫复服。

(1) *Yáng míng bìng, qí rén duō hàn, yǐ jīn yè wài chū, wèi zhōng zào, dà biàn bì yìng, yìng zé zhān yǔ, xiǎo chéng qì tāng zhǔ zhī.* (2) *Ruò yī fú zhān yǔ zhǐ zhě, gèng mò fù fú.*

(1) [When] in yáng brightness disease, the person is sweating copiously, because liquid and humor are issuing outwards, the stomach becomes dry and the stool will be hard. With hard [stool], delirious speech will follow, and Minor Qì-Coordinating Decoction (*xiǎo chéng qì tāng*) governs. (2) If after one dose the delirious speech stops, no more should be taken.

FORMULA

Minor Qì-Coordinating Decoction (*xiǎo chéng qì tāng*)

◦ Drain heat and free the stool; disperse stagnation and eliminate fullness.

大黄四两（酒洗） 厚朴二两（炙，去皮） 枳实三枚（大者，炙）

㈠ 右三味，以水四升，煮取一升二合，去滓，分温二服。㈡ 初服汤当更衣，不尔者尽饮之，若更衣者，勿服之。

Dà huáng sì liǎng (jiǔ xǐ) hòu pò èr liǎng (zhì, qù pí) zhǐ shí sān méi (dà zhě, zhì)

(1) *Yòu sān wèi, yǐ shuǐ sì shēng, zhǔ qǔ yī shēng èr gě, qù zǐ, fēn wēn èr fú.* (2) *Chū fú tāng dāng gēng yī, bù ěr zhě jìn yǐn zhī, ruò gēng yī zhě, wù fú zhī.*

rhubarb (大黄 *dà huáng*, Rhei Rhizoma) 4 liǎng (washed with wine)
magnolia bark (厚朴 *hòu pò*, Magnoliae Cortex) 2 liǎng (remove bark and mix-fry)
unripe bitter orange (枳实 *zhǐ shí*, Aurantii Fructus Immaturus) 3 pieces ([choose] large [pieces]* and mix-fry)

(1) [For] the above three ingredients use four shēng of water. Boil to get one shēng and two gě. Remove the dregs and divide into two doses, and take warm. (2) [After] the first dose there should be a [bowel movement]; if not, finish the decoction. If [there is] a change of clothes [(a bowel movement)], do not take any more.

FORMULA NOTE

* Unripe bitter orange (*zhǐ shí*): "Pieces" here means whole pieces of the fruit. The large fruit is considered to have a weaker ability to move qì.

SYNOPSIS

The signs and treatment of hard stool and delirious speech that are the result of liquid damage from copious sweating in yáng brightness disease.

COMMENTARY

Yáng brightness bowel repletion with dryness bind generally occurs through one of two primary pathomechanisms. The first is that damage to the fluids results in dryness bind, and the second is that exuberant heat results in dryness bind. These patterns are similar, but slight differences exist in the signs and treatment.

Fluid damage and dryness bind generally occur after copious sweating or when the urine is disinhibited. The stomach and intestines become dry and the scant fluids cannot oppose the dryness-heat. Abiding waste in the bowels becomes dry and bound, blocking the intestines and obstructing the qì. When the stool is bound and the qì is blocked, abdominal fullness may be observed, although not the severe fullness and glomus seen in Major Qì-Coordinating Decoction (*dà chéng qì tāng*) patterns. Turbid qì follows the heat upward and harasses the heart, causing delirious speech. This pattern is treated with Minor Qì-Coordinating Decoction (*xiǎo chéng qì tāng*) because great repletion and great fullness are absent, but the signs are too severe to be treated with Stomach-Regulating Qì-Coordinating Decoction (*tiáo wèi chéng qì tāng*).

While Major Qì-Coordinating Decoction (*dà chéng qì tāng*) is used for patterns with glomus, fullness, dryness, and repletion, Minor Qì-Coordinating Decoction (*xiǎo chéng qì tāng*) is used for patterns with dry stool, glomus, and fullness, where the dryness-heat is less severe. Minor Qì-Coordinating Decoction (*xiǎo chéng qì tāng*) does not include mirabilite (*máng xiāo*) because in this pattern the dry heat is less severe and its ability to clear heat and moisten dryness is not necessary. Rhubarb (*dà huáng*) is sufficient to clear heat and precipitate. If the two were used together, precipitation would be too strong for this patient. Because the qì dynamic is congested and stagnant, and because Minor Qì-Coordinating Decoction (*xiǎo chéng qì tāng*) is suggested, the presence of at least mild abdominal distention and fullness is assumed. Magnolia bark (*hòu pò*) is used to move the qì and eliminate fullness. Cold, slightly bitter unripe bitter orange (*zhǐ shí*) rectifies the qì and disperses glomus. Because in this pattern the fullness and glomus are probably mild, the dosages of these two ingredients, particularly unripe bitter orange (*zhǐ shí*), are small in comparison to Major Qì-Coordinating Decoction (*dà chéng qì tāng*).

If after taking Minor Qì-Coordinating Decoction (*xiǎo chéng qì tāng*) the delirious speech stops, then one knows that the bowel qì is free and the dryness bind has resolved. Therefore, one should not take the formula again, since it may damage the qì of the stomach and spleen, potentially leading to further adverse diseases.

The second pattern mentioned above involves dryness that is the result of exuberant internal heat. This pattern is characterized by severe fluid damage, dryness, repletion, glomus, and fullness. Major Qì-Coordinating Decoction (*dà chéng qì tāng*) is used and will be discussed beginning with line 220, p. 336.

LINE 214

㈠阳明病，谵语，发潮热，脉滑而疾者，小承气汤主之。㈡因与承气汤一升，腹中转气者，更服一升，若不转气者，勿更与之，明日又不大便，脉反微濇者，里虚也，为难治，不可更与承气汤也。

(1) *Yáng míng bìng, zhān yǔ, fā cháo rè, mài huá ér jí zhě, xiǎo chéng qì tāng zhǔ zhī.* (2) *Yīn yǔ chéng qì tāng yī shēng, fù zhōng zhuǎn qì zhě, gèng fú yī shēng, ruò bù zhuǎn qì zhě, wù gèng yǔ zhī, míng rì yòu bù dà biàn, mài fǎn wēi sè zhě, lǐ xū yě, wéi nán zhì, bù kě gèng yǔ chéng qì tāng yě.*

(1) When in yáng brightness disease [there is] delirious speech, tidal heat effusion, and a pulse that is slippery and racing, Minor Qì-Coordinating Decoction (*xiǎo chéng qì tāng*) governs. (2) When, as a result of using one shēng of [Minor] Qì-Coordinating Decoction ((*xiǎo*) *chéng qì tāng*) [there is] shifting of qì* in the abdomen, again take one shēng; if [there is] no shifting of qì, do not give it again. The next day, [if there is] again inability to defecate, but the pulse is faint and rough, this indicates internal vacuity. [This] is difficult to treat and one cannot again give [Minor] Qì-Coordinating Decoction ((*xiǎo*) *chéng qì tāng*).

TEXT NOTE

* Shifting of qì, 转气 *zhuǎn qì*: A feeling of stirring in the intestines accompanied by frequent flatulence.

SYNOPSIS

The treatment and contraindications for the mild pattern of yáng brightness organ repletion.

COMMENTARY

In yáng brightness disease with delirious speech and tidal heat effusion, one knows that the stool is already bound, the bowel is replete, and the heat is severe. One may consider whether to use Minor Qì-Coordinating Decoction (*xiǎo chéng qì tāng*) or Major Qì-Coordinating Decoction (*dà chéng qì tāng*), seeing that the condition is severe. If the pulse is sunken, replete, and forceful, Major Qì-Coordinating Decoction (*dà chéng qì tāng*) should be used to drain repletion heat and break hardness. Here, although there are signs of exuberant interior heat (such as delirious speech and tidal heat effusion), the pulse is slippery and racing, which means that the heat, although exuberant, has not completely entered the bowel and the hardness bind is not severe. Minor Qì-Coordinating Decoction (*xiǎo chéng qì tāng*) is used to clear heat and open the bowel, and move the qì and disperse stagnation. As soon as the bowel opens, the dry heat will disperse and the delirious speech and tidal heat effusion will resolve.

In the second part of this line, Zhāng Jī explains a method of using Minor Qì-Coordinating Decoction (*xiǎo chéng qì tāng*) in which one observes the changes following ingestion and then decides if further ingestion is appropriate. The key sign is shifting of qì, which reflects the effect of the medicinals on the bowel. Once the heat is cleared and the qì moves, turbid qì in the stomach and intestines is stirred and descends. Shifting qì indicates that although the bowels are not yet open, the qì is moving and the dry stool can be expelled. If shifting qì is observed, the decoction may be taken again to continue this process. If, however, shifting qì is absent, it means that the stool is not moving and one must reassess the situation.

If, in the near future (not necessarily the next day), the stool again becomes bound, but the pulse is faint and rough, a new problem exists. The absence of stool indicates a repletion evil congesting the stomach and intestines, but the pulse has changed. A pulse that is weak indicates qì vacuity and a pulse that is rough indicates scant blood. Here, vacuity exists within repletion, and Minor Qì-Coordinating Decoction (*xiǎo chéng qì tāng*) cannot be used. In cases of vacuity one should not precipitate and in cases of repletion one should not supplement; therefore, Zhāng Jī writes that this disease is "difficult to treat." The authors of *Gāo Děng Cóng Shū* suggest that in this case one may consider using a formula like Yellow Dragon Decoction (*huáng lóng tāng*), which contains the following ingredients:

rhubarb (大黄 *dà huáng*, Rhei Rhizoma) 12g
mirabilite (芒硝 *máng xiāo*, Mirabilitum) 9g
unripe bitter orange (枳实 *zhǐ shí*, Aurantii Fructus Immaturus) 9g
magnolia bark (厚朴 *hòu pò*, Magnoliae Cortex) 12g
licorice (甘草 *gān cǎo*, Glycyrrhizae Radix) 3g
ginseng (人参 *rén shēn*, Ginseng Radix) 6g
tangkuei (当归 *dāng guī*, Angelicae Sinensis Radix) 9g

This formula clears heat and frees the stool, and supplements qì and blood, simultaneously treating both repletion and vacuity.

LINE 250

太阳病，若吐、若下、若发汗后，微烦，小便数，大便因硬者，与小承气汤和之愈。

Tài yáng bìng, ruò tù, ruò xià, ruò fā hàn hòu, wēi fán, xiǎo biàn shuò, dà biàn yīn yìng zhě, yǔ xiǎo chéng qì tāng hé zhī yù.

When in greater yáng disease, if after vomiting, precipitation, or the promotion of sweating, [there is] mild vexation, frequent urination, and as a result, hard stool, give Minor Qì-Coordinating Decoction (*xiǎo chéng qì tāng*) to harmonize and bring about recovery.

SYNOPSIS

The signs and treatment of heat repletion bind from liquid damage caused by inappropriate treatment of greater yáng disease.

COMMENTARY

The three treatment methods in the line above represent mistreatments. In greater yáng disease the use of vomiting and precipitation is clearly inappropriate and if sweating is promoted improperly, it, too, is inappropriate. Mistreatment of an exterior disease may result in the evil falling inward. In this case it enters the yáng brightness and transforms to heat and dryness. The heat causes vexation and frequent urination, further damaging the fluids (which may have already been damaged from the mistreatment), and the stool becomes hard. Minor Qì-Coordinating Decoction (*xiǎo chéng qì tāng*) is used to clear heat and free the stool. Once the stool is free and the yáng brightness bowel is open, the other signs will resolve because harmony has been restored. Major Qì-Coordinating Decoction (*dà chéng qì tāng*) is not used in this case because tidal heat effusion and delirious speech are absent and the vexation is described as mild. Although the fluids have been damaged, the dryness-heat does not appear to be severe; therefore Minor Qì-Coordinating Decoction (*xiǎo chéng qì tāng*) is sufficient.

Delirious speech and tidal heat effusion cannot be seen as unequivocal signs in the differentiation of Major Qì-Coordinating Decoction (*dà chéng qì tāng*) and Minor Qì-Coordinating Decoction (*xiǎo chéng qì tāng*) patterns. One must consider the entire pattern and the pathomechanism. In line 213, p. 331, hard stool and delirious speech are treated with Minor Qì-Coordinating Decoction (*xiǎo chéng qì tāng*) because these signs are the result of copious sweating damaging the fluids and causing dryness bind. The harsh precipitation used to treat exuberant internal heat with dryness bind is not necessary. In line 214, p. 333, delirious speech and tidal heat effusion are present, yet Minor Qì-Coordinating Decoction (*xiǎo chéng qì tāng*) is given. In that case the pulse is slippery and racing, indicating that the repletion bind in the bowel is not yet severe; therefore Major Qì-Coordinating Decoction (*dà chéng qì tāng*) is not yet necessary. Finally, in line 207, p. 331, heart vexation, similar to the mild vexation in the line above, is observed, yet Stomach-Regulating Qì-Coordinating Decoction (*tiáo wèi chéng qì tāng*) is used. In that case, clear signs of qì stagnation are absent and only signs of dryness-heat repletion are present; therefore Stomach-Regulating Qì-Coordinating Decoction (*tiáo wèi chéng qì tāng*) is used.

3.2.1.3 Major Qì-Coordinating Decoction Patterns

LINE 220

二阳并病，太阳证罢，但发潮热，手足漐漐汗出，大便难而谵语者，下之则愈，宜大承气汤。

Èr yáng bìng bìng, tài yáng zhèng bà, dàn fā cháo rè, shǒu zú zhé zhé hàn chū, dà biàn nán ér zhān yǔ zhě, xià zhī zé yù, yí dà chéng qì tāng.

When in dragover disease of the two yáng, the greater yáng disease has ceased and [there is] only tidal heat effusion, sweat streaming from the extremities, difficult defecation and delirious speech, precipitation will bring about recovery and [therefore,] Major Qì-Coordinating Decoction (*dà chéng qì tāng*) is appropriate.

FORMULA

Major Qì-Coordinating Decoction (*dà chéng qì tāng*)

◦ Offensively precipitate heat repletion; flush dryness bind.

大黄四两（酒洗） 厚朴半斤（炙，去皮） 枳实五枚（炙） 芒消三合

㈠ 右四味，以水一斗，先煮二物，取五升，去滓，内大黄，更煮取二升，去滓，内芒消，更上微火一两沸，分温再服。㈡ 得下，余勿服。

Dà huáng sì liǎng (jiǔ xǐ) hòu pò bàn jīn (zhì, qù pí) zhǐ shí wǔ méi (zhì) máng xiāo sān gě

(1) *Yòu sì wèi, yǐ shuǐ yī dǒu, xiān zhǔ èr wù, qǔ wǔ shēng, qù zǐ, nà dà huáng, gèng zhǔ qǔ èr shēng, qù zǐ, nà máng xiāo, gèng shàng wēi huǒ yī èr fèi, fēn wēn zài fú.* (2) *Dé xià, yú wù fú.*

rhubarb (大黄 *dà huáng*, Rhei Rhizoma) 4 liǎng (washed with wine)
processed magnolia bark (厚朴 *hòu pò*, Magnoliae Cortex) half jīn (remove bark)
processed unripe bitter orange (枳实 *zhǐ shí*, Aurantii Fructus Immaturus) 5 pieces
mirabilite (芒硝 *máng xiāo*, Mirabilitum) 3 gě

(1) [For] the above four ingredients use one dǒu of water. First boil [the first] two ingredients to get five shēng. Remove the dregs and add rhubarb (*dà huáng*); boil again to get two shēng. Remove the dregs, add mirabilite (*máng xiāo*). Place again on a mild flame and boil once or twice. Divide [into two parts], and take warm twice a day. (2) One precipitation has occurred, do not take any more.

SYNOPSIS

The signs and treatment of dragover disease of the two yáng that shifts into yáng brightness organ repletion.

COMMENTARY

In dragover disease one disease pattern leads into an another. Originally, a greater yáng disease pattern was observed and then yáng brightness disease signs began to appear. At this point, the greater yáng signs have already ceased and only yáng brightness signs are present.

Tidal heat effusion is the type of heat effusion generally seen in yáng brightness patterns. Nevertheless, as is clear from line 214, p. 333, tidal heat effusion, in the absence of other signs of yáng brightness repletion, is not sufficient to warrant the use of Major Qì-Coordinating Decoction (*dà chéng qì tāng*). Here, tidal heat effusion occurs with streaming sweat, difficult stool, and delirious speech. Tidal heat effusion is heat effusion with a set periodicity which, when associated with yáng brightness patterns, is generally said to occur in the late afternoon and early evening, roughly between the hours of 3 P.M.and 7 P.M.—the hours when the qì of the yáng brightness is effulgent.

Exuberant yáng brightness heat can steam the fluids and force them to the exterior, causing sweating. Yáng brightness governs the four limbs; therefore, streaming sweat issues only from the extremities when exuberant heat has damaged the fluids. Fluid depletion is also reflected in difficult defecation, which means that the stool is dry, hard, and difficult to expel. Exuberant heat in the stomach easily ascends and invades the heart—a process that has been explained in several previous lines. Here, delirious speech is the result of exuberant heat harassing the heart spirit.

This pattern of yáng brightness bowel repletion is treated by precipitation, using Major Qì-Coordinating Decoction (*dà chéng qì tāng*) to precipitate offensively and drain dryness-heat. Bitter, cold rhubarb (*dà huáng*) clears heat and removes repletion, flushing the stomach and intestines. When dryness bind and hardness are both present it is difficult to move the stagnation downward, so mirabilite (*máng xiāo*) is added to soften hardness and moisten dryness. Bound stool results in blockage of the intestines and congestion of the qì dynamic, which may cause glomus and fullness. Without including medicinals to move the qì, the qì congestion may block the action of the precipitants; therefore, magnolia bark (*hòu pò*) and unripe bitter orange (*zhǐ shí*) are added to move the qì and break binds. Zhāng Jī advises that once the stool moves, the formula should not be ingested again because excessive use of precipitation damages the qì.

Once again, we should examine the differences between the three Qì-Coordinating Decoctions (*chéng qì tāng*) formulae for clarity. Stomach-Regulating Qì-Coordinating Decoction (*tiáo wèi chéng qì tāng*) does not include unripe bitter orange (*zhǐ shí*) and magnolia bark (*hòu pò*) because qì stagnation is not evident in those patterns, but a large dose of mirabilite (*máng xiāo*) is used to increase the formula's ability to drain heat and moisten dryness. Minor Qì-Coordinating Decoction (*xiǎo chéng qì tāng*) does not contain mirabilite (*máng xiāo*) because in those patterns the dryness-heat is secondary, but unripe bitter orange (*zhǐ shí*) and magnolia bark (*hòu pò*), which rectify the qì, are used in small doses because the signs of qì stagnation are relatively mild. Major Qì-Coordinating Decoction (*dà chéng qì tāng*) treats patterns of severe repletion, dryness, fullness, and hardness.

LINE 212

㈠ 伤寒，若吐若下后，不解，不大便五六日，上至十余日，日晡所发潮热，不恶寒，独语如见鬼状，若剧者，发则不识人，循衣摸床，惕而不安，微喘直视，脉弦者生，濇者死；微者，但发热谵语者，大承气汤主之。㈡ 若一服利，则止后服。

(1) *Shāng hán, ruò tù ruò xià hòu, bù jiě, bù dà biàn wǔ liù rì, shàng zhì shí yú rì, rì bū suǒ fā cháo rè, bù wù hán, dú yǔ rú jiàn guǐ zhuàng, ruò jù zhě, fā zé bù shì rén, xún yī mō chuáng, tì ér bù ān, wēi chuǎn zhí shì, mài xián zhě shēng, sè zhě sǐ; wēi zhě, dàn fā rè zhān yǔ zhě, dà chéng qì tāng zhǔ zhī.* (2) *Ruò yī fú lì, zé zhǐ hòu fú.*

(1) In cold damage, if after vomiting or precipitation [there is] no resolution, inability to defecate for five or six days—even up to ten days or more—late afternoon tidal heat effusion, no aversion to cold, and soliloquy as if [the person is] seeing ghosts,* [then the following applies:] if serious, [when the disease] emerges, [the person] will not recognize people, will pick at the bedclothes, [feel] fear and disquiet, pant slightly, and stare forward. If the pulse is stringlike [the person will] live, and if the pulse is rough [the person will] die. When in mild [cases], [there is] only heat effusion and delirious speech, Major Qì-Coordinating Decoc-

tion (*dà chéng qì tāng*) governs. (2) If one dose disinhibits [the stool], then stop taking it afterwards.

TEXT NOTE

* Soliloquy as if [the person is] seeing ghosts. 独语如见鬼 *dú yǔ rú jiàn guǐ*: The patient talks to himself/herself and the spirit is clouded.

SYNOPSIS

Pattern identification, treatment, and prognosis for the severe yáng brightness bowel repletion pattern.

COMMENTARY

In cold damage patterns the use of vomiting or precipitation is inappropriate. If one of these methods is used many different transmutations may occur. In this line a transmutation to a yáng brightness disease is presented. It is a pattern of bowel repletion with absence of defecation for five, six, or even more than ten days. The bowel qì is clearly congested and abdominal fullness and glomus are also likely. Tidal heat effusion in the late afternoon is typical of yáng brightness patterns because that is the time the yáng brightness qì is effulgent. Furthermore, the absence of aversion to cold means that this is no longer an exterior pattern and suggests that exuberant dry heat is bound in the interior; consequently aversion to heat may be observed. When exuberant heat in the interior disturbs the heart spirit, it may result in delirious speech. Soliloquy as if seeing ghosts represents one type of delirious speech, which is seen in cases of more severe internal heat bind repletion.

In an extremely severe pattern, exuberant heat damages the fluids and harasses the spirit to the point that the patient becomes stuporous and no longer recognizes those around him/her. In this state of altered consciousness, the unconscious movements of picking at the bedclothes may be seen. This spirit disturbance is further reflected in the fear and disquiet of the patient. The patient easily becomes agitated and frightened and is difficult to calm. Heat from the stomach ascends and flames in the lungs, resulting in dryness. Lung downbearing and diffusing become abnormal and mild panting results. When exuberant heat in the interior scorches the fluids, the loss of normal moistening and nourishment impairs movement in the sinews and channels. The eyes cannot move normally, and stare straight ahead in a fixed position.

The pulse is used in this line to make a prognosis. A pulse that is stringlike indicates that the patient's constitution is strong and/or the fluids have not been totally exhausted and the qì is still vital. This patient may be treated successfully. If the pulse is rough, it indicates vacuity of right qì and desiccated fluids from extreme heat repletion in the interior. Here, the treatment will be very difficult and the prognosis is not good.

The final section of this line suggests the use of Major Qì-Coordinating Decoction (*dà chéng qì tāng*) if the disease is not severe, referring to the beginning of the line. The original condition, characterized by absence of defecation, heat effusion, delirious speech, and aversion to heat, should be treated with Major Qì-Coordinating Decoction (*dà chéng qì tāng*). If the disease becomes more severe, as in the second part of the line, no treatment is suggested. It is likely that Major Qì-Coordinating Decoction (*dà chéng qì tāng*) would be given again because this formula is already an extremely harsh attacking formula and its strength cannot be increased. This pattern is severe and will be difficult to resolve.

Line 241

(一) 大下后，六七日不大便，烦不解，腹满痛者，此有燥屎也。(二) 所以然者，本有宿食故也，宜大承气汤。

(1) *Dà xià hòu, liù qī rì bù dà biàn, fán bù jiě, fù mǎn tòng zhě, cǐ yǒu zào shǐ yě.* (2) *Suǒ yǐ rán zhě, běn yǒu sù shí gù yě, yí dà chéng qì tāng.*

(1) When after great precipitation [there is] inability to defecate for six or seven days, unresolved vexation, and abdominal fullness and pain, this [means] there is dry stool.[1] (2) Why [this] is so is because the root is abiding food,[2] for which Major Qì-Coordinating Decoction (*dà chéng qì tāng*) is appropriate.

Text Notes

1. Dry stool, 燥屎 *zào shǐ*: Dry and hard stool that is the result of abiding food in the intestines desiccated by internal heat.
2. Abiding food, 宿食 *sù shí*: Food and drink accumulating in the intestines.

Synopsis

The signs and treatment of dry stool that binds again following the use of precipitation.

Commentary

Yáng brightness repletion should be treated with precipitation. Following precipitation, if the patient has a bowel movement, abdominal pain and fullness are absent, and the appetite improves, then one knows the disease has been cured. In this case, after precipitation the stool remains bound; vexation, abdominal fullness and pain appear. After the initial precipitation, the patient may have evacuated stool, but now the stool is bound again. This pattern is described by Zhāng Jī as "dry stool," indicating that the intestinal matter is still being dried by internal heat. Bound stool with abdominal pain and distention indicate the presence of yáng brightness bowel repletion. The heat evil in the stomach rises up and harasses the heart, causing vexation. The vexation was present originally; therefore, following precipitation, when it is still present, it is called "unresolved vexation."

Zhāng Jī explains that the root of this disorder lies in abiding food, which impairs the qì dynamic of the stomach and intestines. Following the initial precipitation, the stool may have moved, but the interior heat is not completely eliminated. The fluids have not yet returned to normal, nor has the qì dynamic been restored; hence the stool easily becomes dry and bound again. Major Qì-Coordinating Decoction (*dà chéng qì tāng*) may be used again to expel the dry stool. This second treatment should eliminate any remaining heat and allow the fluids and the qì dynamic to return to normal.

Several different scenarios are possible following precipitation. In the first, the bowel qì is free, but residual heat remains, causing vexation and anguish. The absence of both bound stool and abdominal pain suggests that Gardenia and Fermented Soybean Decoction (*zhī zǐ chǐ tāng*), be used to clear residual heat and resolve the vexation. If, after precipitation, bound stool, vexation, delirious speech, and steaming heat effusion are observed, Stomach-Regulating Qì-Coordinating Decoction (*tiáo wèi chéng qì tāng*) is used. Minor Qì-Coordinating Decoction (*xiǎo chéng qì tāng*) treats bound stool, abdominal fullness, and heart vexation following precipitation. In short, following precipitation in yáng brightness bowel repletion, the patient may recover, may need additional precipitation, or may need a formula to clear residual heat.

LINE 242

病人小便不利，大便乍难乍易，时有微热，喘冒不能卧者，有燥屎也，宜大承气汤。

Bìng rén xiǎo biàn bù lì, dà biàn zhà nán zhà yì, shí yǒu wēi rè, chuǎn mào bù néng wò zhě, yǒu zào shǐ yě, yí dà chéng qì tāng.

When the person has inhibited urination, intermittently difficult and easy stool, periodic mild heat, panting and veiling,[1] and is unable to sleep,[2] [this means that] there is dry stool, and [therefore,] Major Qì-Coordinating Decoction (*dà chéng qì tāng*) is appropriate.

TEXT NOTES

1. Panting and veiling, 喘冒 *chuǎn mào*: The simultaneous appearance of hasty, rapid, labored breathing and clouded head and dizzy vision.
2. Inability to sleep, 不能卧 *bù néng wò*: Insomnia that is the result of a spirit disturbance caused by exuberant heat in the interior rising and harassing the heart spirit. According to the *Shāng Hán Lùn Yán Jiū Dà Cí Diǎn*, this term may mean insomnia or an inability to lie down.

SYNOPSIS

The signs and treatment of stool that is sometimes difficult, sometimes easy, in yáng brightness organ repletion internal bind.

COMMENTARY

In yáng brightness repletion, frequent urination and hard stool are often present due to the interior heat, but in the pattern described in the present line, urination is inhibited. Dryness-heat in the interior binds with waste, resulting in dry stool that is sometimes difficult to expel. The interior heat, however, also steams the fluids and a portion of the fluids are forced into the intestines. This portion of the fluids moistens the stool and so stool may occasionally pass easily. When dryness-heat forces the fluids into the intestines, the fluids cannot pass out through the urine, so urination is inhibited.

Periodic mild heat is a pattern of internal heat evil deep inside the body, in which evil qì only occasionally outthrusts to the exterior. Panting and veiling reflects heat from the stomach rising upward, which distresses the lungs and causes hasty, labored breathing. This rising heat harasses the head (causing dizziness and mental confusion) and the heart spirit (causing an inability to sleep). Furthermore, when the stomach is disharmonious, the patient is unable to sleep normally. "[When] the stomach is disharmonious, sleep is not quiet," 胃不和，卧者不安 *wèi bù hé, wò zhě bù ān.*

Here, dry stool, and sometimes easy, sometimes difficult stool, together with the suggestion of Major Qì-Coordinating Decoction (*dà chéng qì tāng*), indicate a pattern of yáng brightness bowel repletion with dry stool. In addition to the signs above, one should see abdominal fullness and pain, heat effusion, and other signs of a true repletion pattern before using this type of harsh precipitating formula.

LINE 252

伤寒六七日，目中不了了，睛不和，无表里证，大便难，身微热者，此为实也，急下之，宜大承气汤。

Shāng hán liù qī rì, mù zhōng bù liǎo liǎo, jīng bù hé, wú biǎo lǐ zhèng, dà biàn nán, shēn wēi rè zhě, cǐ wéi shí yě, jí xià zhī, yí dà chéng qì tāng.

When in cold damage [that has lasted for] six or seven days, [there is] unclear vision, disharmony of the eyes,[1] neither an exterior nor an interior pattern,[2] difficult defecation, and mild generalized heat, this indicates repletion, [so] precipitation is urgent and [therefore,] Major Qì-Coordinating Decoction (*dà chéng qì tāng*) is appropriate.

TEXT NOTES

1. Disharmony of the eyes, 睛不和 *jīng bù hé*: The eyes appear dull and cannot turn and move flexibly.
2. Neither an exterior nor an interior pattern, 无表里证 *wú biǎo lǐ zhèng*: No clear signs of either an exterior pattern (such as heat effusion or aversion to cold) or an interior pattern (such as abdominal fullness or tidal heat effusion).

SYNOPSIS

In cold damage, when there is unclear vision and disharmony of the eyes, one should urgently precipitate to preserve yīn.

COMMENTARY

In cold damage, if exterior signs are absent after six or seven days, one must consider that the disease has shifted into the interior. Here, this supposition is supported by the appearance of difficult defecation and generalized heat, which have both been discussed previously and may indicate yáng brightness bowel repletion. Zhāng Jī describes this as a repletion pattern and suggests urgent precipitation with Major Qì-Coordinating Decoction (*dà chéng qì tāng*). Precipitation is urgently required because of the appearance of unclear vision and disharmony of the eyes.

Unclear vision and disharmony of the eyes indicate that the interior heat has scorched the fluids to a more severe extent. In the *Líng Shū* it is written, "The essence of the five viscera and six bowels all pours upward to the eyes." Qián Huáng writes, "Heat evil scorches the interior, the fluids are desiccated, and then the essence-spirit cannot pour upward to the eyes. Thus, [there is] unclear vision and disharmony of the eyes." When the fluids are severely desiccated, the essence is also affected. Not only the stomach fluids, but also the kidney essence is damaged by the interior heat. As Yè Guì (叶桂, style 天士 Tiān-Shì) writes, "[When] heat evil does not dry the stomach liquid, it will consume the kidney humor." The eyes lose normal moistening and nourishment; consequently they are disharmonious and lack clarity. When the fluids and essence are damaged to this degree, the brain, which is the sea of essence and marrow, may also be affected. Urgent precipitation is appropriate to discharge heat and avoid complete fluid desiccation. This treatment, a method of eliminating repletion heat by freeing the stool with cold-natured draining precipitants, is referred to as "raking the firewood from beneath the cauldron," 釜底抽薪 *fǔ dǐ chōu xīn*.

LINE 253

阳明病，发热汗多者，急下之，宜大承气汤。

Yáng míng bìng, fā rè hàn duō zhě, jí xià zhī, yí dà chéng qì tāng.

When in yáng brightness disease [there is] heat effusion and copious sweating, precipitation is urgently [required and therefore,] Major Qì-Coordinating Decoction (*dà chéng qì tāng*) is appropriate.

SYNOPSIS

In yáng brightness disease with heat effusion and copious sweating, one should urgently precipitate to preserve yīn.

COMMENTARY

In yáng brightness disease, when Zhāng Jī suggests urgent precipitation, one may assume the presence of bowel repletion bind with absence of defecation and painful abdominal fullness and distention. In this situation, what is the significance of heat effusion and copious sweating? Yáng brightness diseases are generally characterized by tidal heat effusion and streaming sweat from the extremities. Here, the heat effusion is not tidal, but continuous, indicating that the interior and exterior heat is very strong. It steams the fluids and forces them to the exterior, causing copious sweating over the whole body. With strong interior heat and rapid loss of sweat, the fluids are damaged quickly, which may lead to fluid desiccation and the appearance of more critical signs. Although no critical signs are observed yet urgent precipitation is suggested in order to avoid the desiccation of the fluids and the transmutation to a critical condition.

Line 254

发汗不解，腹满痛者，急下之，宜大承气汤。

Fā hàn bù jiě, fù mǎn tòng zhě, jí xià zhī, yí dà chéng qì tāng.

When sweating is promoted, [but brings] no resolution, [and there is] abdominal fullness and pain, precipitation is urgent, and [therefore,] Major Qì-Coordinating Decoction (*dà chéng qì tāng*) is appropriate.

Synopsis

After the promotion of sweating has not brought resolution and there is yáng brightness organ repletion, it is appropriate to precipitate urgently to preserve yīn.

Commentary

Sweating is generally promoted in greater yáng disease. If the promotion of sweating does not resolve the disease, but instead results in abdominal fullness and pain, it means that the evil has already entered the interior and transformed to dryness-heat repletion. The bowel qì is congested, the stool is bound, and abdominal pain and fullness are present. This transmutation may have occurred due to the inappropriate promotion of sweating, excessive promotion of sweating, or the constitution of the patient.

Zhāng Jī suggests the use of urgent precipitation because of the speed with which this transmutation occurred. In previous lines, he refers to the passage of several days or even six or seven days, before suggesting the use of Major Qì-Coordinating Decoction (*dà chéng qì tāng*). This situation is urgent because immediately following the sweating, signs of yáng brightness bowel repletion appeared, suggesting that the heat and dryness is severe, the fluids have already been damaged, and the bowel qì is already blocked. If urgent precipitation is not used, a transmutation to a more serious pattern may occur.

Line 255

腹满不减，减不足言，当下之，宜大承气汤。

Fù mǎn bù jiǎn, jiǎn bù zú yán, dāng xià zhī, yí dà chéng qì tāng.

When abdominal fullness does not decrease, [or] decreases insufficiently to speak of, one should precipitate, and [in such cases] Major Qì-Coordinating Decoction (*dà chéng qì tāng*) is appropriate.

Synopsis

The signs and treatment of an abdominal fullness pattern for which precipitation is appropriate.

Commentary

Abdominal fullness has many causes. On the basis of the formula used here, the abdominal fullness in this line may be attributed to yáng brightness bowel repletion and is considered a reference to the preceding line. Internal dryness-heat repletion congests the qì dynamic; consequently, abdominal fullness is likely accompanied by bound stool, tidal heat effusion, and other signs of yáng brightness bowel repletion.

The abdominal fullness present in this line, although occasionally diminishing somewhat in severity, generally persists with very little change. Zhāng Jī calls attention to this point in order to differentiate this type of abdominal fullness from vacuity cold abdominal fullness. In vacuity cold abdominal fullness, the fullness periodically decreases. Vacuity cold abdominal fullness also responds well to warmth and pressure, factors that would exacerbate the dryness-heat repletion abdominal fullness presented in this line. Therefore, precipitation using Major Qì-Coordinating Decoction (*dà chéng qì tāng*) is appropriate.

LINE 256

㈠阳明少阳合病，必下利，其脉不负者，为顺也。㈡负者，失也，互相克贼，名为负也，脉滑而数者，有宿食也。㈢当下之，宜大承气汤。

(1) *Yáng míng shào yáng hé bìng, bì xià lì, qí mài bù fù zhě, wéi shùn yě.* (2) *Fù zhě, shī yě, hù xiāng kè zéi, míng wéi fù yě, mài huá ér shuò zhě, yǒu sù shí yě.* (3) *Dāng xià zhī, yí dà chéng qì tāng.*

(1) In yáng brightness and lesser yáng combination disease, there will be diarrhea and when the pulse is not contrary, it means [that the disease] is [in] favorable [sequence].* (2) When the [pulse] is contrary, [it means] deviation [from the normal sequence]* and mutual restraining and robbing, so it is called contrary. When the pulse is slippery and fast [it means there is] abiding food. (3) One should precipitate and [therefore,] Major Qì-Coordinating Decoction (*dà chéng qì tāng*) is appropriate.

TEXT NOTE

* When the pulse is not contrary, it means [that the disease] is [in] favorable [sequence], 其脉不负者，为顺也 *qí mài bù fù zhě, wéi shùn yě*; When the [pulse] is contrary, [it means] deviation [from the normal sequence], 负者，失也 *fù zhě, shī yě*: The pulse is used to determine if the disease is progressing according to the five-phase engendering sequence or counter to it. The appearance of a pulse that is in the five-phase sequence is a positive sign, and the appearance of a pulse that is counter to this sequence is considered a negative sign.

SYNOPSIS

The pulse, signs, and treatment of lesser yáng and yáng brightness combination disease when precipitation is appropriate.

Commentary

Yáng brightness belongs to earth and lesser yáng belongs to wood. The spleen and stomach belong to earth, and the liver and gallbladder belong to wood. In the normal five-phase sequence, wood restrains earth. In yáng brightness and lesser yáng combination disease, fire from the lesser yáng and dryness from the yáng brightness produce dryness-heat bind in the center, and force the fluids to hasten downward, causing a loss of normal conveyance and diarrhea. In this case the diarrhea is likely malodorous, sticky, and accompanied by a heat sensation in the anus.

In yáng brightness and lesser yáng combination disease, if the pulse is a yáng brightness pulse (such as slippery and rapid) it is not contrary and means that the wood evil has not restrained and damaged earth. The center qì is still effulgent and this situation is said to be in sequence. If, however, the pulse is stringlike, it is contrary, reflecting the influence of the lesser yáng and indicating that the yáng brightness is weak and is being restrained and harmed by the lesser yáng. This condition is described as deviating from the normal sequence.

When the pulse is slippery and rapid, it means that the yáng brightness qì is still effulgent and that abiding food has blocked the stomach and intestines. Heat-type diarrhea is likely accompanied by abdominal fullness and pain, and a thick yellow tongue fur, indicating a yáng brightness bowel repletion pattern that can be treated with Major Qì-Coordinating Decoction (*dà chéng qì tāng*).

In line 172, p. 159, Scutellaria Decoction (*huáng qín tāng*) is used to treat diarrhea that occurs in greater yáng and lesser yáng combination disease. In that case, an exterior evil shifts into the lesser yáng and distresses the stomach and intestines. Because abiding food is absent, a bitter, cold formula is used to clear heat and check the diarrhea. In line 32, p. 111, diarrhea in greater yáng and yáng brightness combination disease is treated with Pueraria Decoction (*gé gēn tāng*). In that case, clear signs of an exterior pattern exist, and interior heat and abiding food are absent. Pueraria Decoction (*gé gēn tāng*) is used to resolve the exterior, upbear the fluids, and check the diarrhea. These patterns all have diarrhea as a key sign, but the pathomechanisms and treatments are very different and must be clearly differentiated.

Line 239

病人不大便五六日，绕脐痛，烦躁，发作有时者，此有燥屎，故使不大便也。

Bìng rén bù dà biàn wǔ liù rì, rào qí tòng, fán zào, fā zuò yǒu shí zhě, cǐ yǒu zào shǐ, gù shǐ bù dà biàn yě.

When the patient has not defecated for five or six days, and has pain around the umbilicus and vexation and agitation that occur periodically,* this means [that there is] dry stool causing [the person] not to defecate.

TEXT NOTE

* That occur periodically, 发作有时 *fā zuò yǒu shí*: This periodicity refers to both the pain and the vexation.

SYNOPSIS

The signs of dry stool interior bind in yáng brightness organ repletion.

COMMENTARY

When a patient does not defecate for about one week, one cannot assume that it is a case of yáng brightness bowel repletion, but must investigate the other signs. The area around the umbilicus belongs to the intestines. Pain around the umbilicus, when defecation is absent, indicates intestinal blockage and stagnant bowel qì. Zhāng Jī explains that this is the result of dry stool. Dry, bound stool is generally caused by internal dryness-heat. When heat dries the bowels and the bowel qì cannot move, heat and turbid qì rises, harassing the heart and causing vexation and agitation. Because the turbid qì cannot pass out of the bowels normally, pain is felt in the umbilical region.

The periodicity of these signs is similar to tidal heat effusion. As Qián Huáng writes, "[These signs, which] occur periodically, [belong to the] same category as late-afternoon tidal heat effusion." Pain and vexation are the result of the movement of exuberant interior dryness-heat and turbid qì that cannot be expelled because the stool is blocked. During the yáng brightness period the qì is effulgent, and these signs are exacerbated. When the yáng brightness period passes and the qì subsides, the pain and vexation decrease.

Although no treatment is offered in this line, it is likely that precipitation would be used, as in line 238, p. 350, "If [there is] dry stool, Major Qì-Coordinating Decoction (*dà chéng qì tāng*) is appropriate."

In the text, many different sign patterns and criteria are used to identify the presence or absence of dry stool. Dry stool may be indicated by: a) absence of defecation for five or six days, pain in the umbilical region and vexation; b) tidal heat effusion, delirious speech, and sweat streaming from the extremities; c) persistent abdominal fullness; d) unclear vision and disharmony of the eyes; e) inhibited urination, intermittent easy and difficult stool, periodic mild heat, and panting and veiling; or f) shifting of qì following the ingestion of a small amount of Minor Qì-Coordinating Decoction (*xiǎo chéng qì tāng*).

LINE 215

㈠阳明病，谵语，有潮热，反不能食者，胃中必有燥屎五六枚也。㈡若能食者，但硬耳，宜大承气汤下之。

(1) *Yáng míng bìng, zhān yǔ, yǒu cháo rè, fǎn bù néng shí zhě, wèi zhōng bì yǒu zào shǐ wǔ liù méi yě.* (2) *Ruò néng shí zhě, dàn yìng ěr, yí dà chéng qì tāng xià zhī.*

(1) When in yáng brightness disease, [there is] delirious speech and tidal heat effusion, but inability to eat, [this means that] there must be five

or six pieces of dry stool in the stomach.[1] (2) (If [the person] is able to eat, [there is] only hard [stool].) Major Qì-Coordinating Decoction (*dà chéng qì tāng*) is appropriate for precipitation.[2]

TEXT NOTES

1. Dry stool in the stomach, 胃中燥屎 *wèi zhōng zào shǐ*: Dry stool in the intestines. The character 胃 *wèi* in this text is often thought to include the stomach and intestines. Here, because of the reference to stool, it is simply read as "intestines." Xú Dà Chūn (徐大椿, style 灵胎 Líng-Tāi) writes, "The stomach does not contain dry stool. This says 'stomach', but means the yáng brightness, which is the name for the stomach and intestines." In line 157, p. 237, however, the term 胃中 *wèi zhōng* refers only to the stomach.
2. Major Qì-Coordinating Decoction (*dà chéng qì tāng*) is appropriate for precipitation, 宜大承气汤下之 *yí dà chéng qì tāng xià zhī*: This line is regarded as another example of grammatical inversion. Although it appears at the end of the line, it actually refers to the pattern described in the first part of the line.

SYNOPSIS

The signs and treatment of the severe pattern of hard bound stool in yáng brightness organ repletion.

COMMENTARY

In yáng brightness bowel repletion, dryness-heat repletion blocks the bowel qì and causes an upward movement of heat and turbidity. Heat and turbidity harasses the heart spirit and causes delirious speech. Tidal heat effusion is the outward manifestation of the exuberant interior heat. Its periodicity is related to the periodicity of the qì of yáng brightness.

The appearance of delirious speech and tidal heat effusion indicates the presence of dry, bound stool in the intestines. Bowel repletion and dry stool may appear with different degrees of severity. In these two lines, the ability to eat is used to differentiate mild and severe patterns and to decide if precipitation is appropriate. In cases of bowel repletion and internal heat, the patient is usually still able to eat, and rapid hungering may be observed as a result of heat in the stomach. If the patient is unable to eat, it indicates, as Zhāng Jī explains, "dry stool in the stomach." Dry stool obstructs the movement of bowel qì and impairs stomach and intestinal function; hence not only is the stool bound, but the patient cannot eat either. Here, Major Qì-Coordinating Decoction (*dà chéng qì tāng*) is appropriate to expel the dry stool. When the stool is expelled, the qì dynamic will return to normal and the patient will be able to eat normally.

Delirious speech and tidal heat effusion in a patient who is able to eat suggests that although the stool is hard, it is not dry and bound. Precipitation with Major Qì-Coordinating Decoction (*dà chéng qì tāng*) is not necessary, although precipitation with a milder formula, such as Minor Qì-Coordinating Decoction (*xiǎo chéng qì tāng*) may be appropriate.

It is important to note here that the ability or inability to eat, although an important sign used in the differentiation of these patterns, should not be seen as an unequivocal indication of any one condition. In line 190, p. 382, inability to eat indicates cold strike, and ability to eat indicates wind strike. In line 194, p. 366, inability to eat indicates vacuity cold in the stomach. These lines are reminders that any individual sign must be interpreted in the context of the other signs and should not be viewed in isolation.

Line 217

㈠ 汗出谵语者，以有燥屎在胃中，此为风也，须下者，过经乃可下之。㈡ 下之若早，语言必乱，以表虚里实故也。㈢ 下之愈，宜大承气汤。

(1) *Hàn chū zhān yǔ zhě, yǐ yǒu zào shǐ zài wèi zhōng, cǐ wéi fēng yě, xū xià zhě, guò jīng nǎi kě xià zhī.* (2) *Xià zhī ruò zǎo, yǔ yán bì luàn, yǐ biǎo xū lǐ shí gù yě.* (3) *Xià zhī yù, yí dà chéng qì tāng.*

(1) When [there is] sweating and delirious speech because of dry stool in the stomach, this indicates wind. One must precipitate, [and since] [there has] been channel passage, one can precipitate. (2) Precipitation, if [used too] early, will [result in] deranged speech, this being because of exterior vacuity and interior repletion. (3) Precipitation [will bring about] recovery and [therefore,] Major Qì-Coordinating Decoction (*dà chéng qì tāng*) is appropriate.

Synopsis

The differentiation of exterior vacuity and interior repletion patterns and for which pattern precipitation should be used.

Commentary

The sweating mentioned in the first part of this line indicates exterior vacuity, which Zhāng Jī refers to as "wind" and which we may interpret as an unresolved greater yáng exterior vacuity pattern. In order to decide that sweating means greater yáng exterior vacuity, it is likely that one would also have to see aversion to cold, a pulse that is floating and/or other corroborating signs. Likewise, delirious speech indicates yáng brightness bowel repletion. Zhāng Jī explains that delirious speech is the result of dry stool in the stomach and intestines. It is likely that along with delirious speech, one would also observe bound stool, abdominal fullness, and/or other corroborating signs of yáng brightness bowel repletion. Zhāng Jī writes that one "must precipitate," but one must also be cautious about precipitating when an exterior pattern still exists. Once channel passage has occurred and the pattern is purely a yáng brightness pattern, one can safely precipitate.

If precipitation is used too early, before the exterior evil has been resolved, it will result in a negative transmutation. Generally, exterior-interior diseases are treated by first resolving the exterior condition and then treating the interior, unless the interior condition is urgent. In this case, precipitation prior to the resolution of the exterior evil results in an exacerbation of the delirious speech, which is described as deranged speech. This transmutation is the result of the exterior evil falling inward and boosting the heat that was present in the interior.

Exterior vacuity and interior repletion may be interpreted in two ways, both of which provide useful perspectives. Qián Huáng views this term as a description of the state of the patient following treatment, and he writes, "The evil in the exterior all falls into the interior; hence the exterior is empty; [there is] no evil. The evil is all in the interior; hence it is said that the exterior is vacuous and the interior is replete." According to this interpretation, vacuity and repletion refer to the presence or absence of evil qì. Following erroneous precipitation, all evil qì falls into the interior. Another perspective is provided by the authors of *Gāo Děng Cóng Shū* who write that "exterior vacuity and interior repletion" refers to the pattern of greater yáng exterior vacuity and yáng brightness interior repletion, prior to treatment. This pattern is considered simultaneous exterior-interior disease and should be treated by first resolving the exterior and then attacking the interior. Inappropriate precipitation causes the evil to fall inward and the speech to become deranged.

Line 238

阳明病，下之，心中懊侬而烦，胃中有燥屎者，可攻，腹微满，初头硬，后必溏，不可攻之，若有燥屎者，宜大承气汤。

Yáng míng bìng, xià zhī, xīn zhōng ào nóng ér fán, wèi zhōng yǒu zào shǐ zhě, kě gōng, fù wēi mǎn, chū tóu yìng, hòu bì táng, bù kě gōng zhī, ruò yǒu zào shǐ zhě, yí dà chéng qì tāng.

When in yáng brightness disease, precipitation is used and [there is] anguish and vexation in the heart and dry stool in the stomach, one can attack. [If there is] mild abdominal fullness, and [stool that is] hard at the beginning and then sloppy, one cannot attack. If [there is] dry stool, Major Qì-Coordinating Decoction (*dà chéng qì tāng*) is appropriate.

Synopsis

The differentiation of whether or not attacking is appropriate in a yáng brightness disease after precipitation has been used.

Commentary

Following the use of precipitation in yáng brightness disease, any of three outcomes are possible. The first is that it was the correct treatment and the disease resolves. The second is that it was the correct treatment, but the evil has not been totally eliminated and one must precipitate again. The last is that it was an inappropriate treatment or was used excessively and a negative transmutation occurs.

In this line, two transmutations that occur following the use of precipitation in yáng brightness disease are presented. The first is characterized by anguish in the heart, vexation, and dry stool in the stomach and intestines. Dry stool in the intestines blocks the movement of bowel qì; consequently dryness-heat cannot flow downward and heat and turbidity rise up, harassing the heart and causing anguish and vexation. The initial precipitation did not completely eliminate the evil repletion in the bowel, although it was the correct treatment, and further precipitation is required. It is likely that in addition to anguish and vexation, signs such as bound stool, abdominal pain and fullness, and pain around the umbilicus would be observed.

In the second transmutation, the abdomen is mildly painful. This sign is not the severe type of abdominal pain generally seen in yáng brightness bowel repletion. Furthermore, the stool is not dry and bound. It is hard at first and then sloppy. Therefore, this is no longer yáng brightness bowel repletion and precipitation should not be used.

Finally, Zhāng Jī writes that Major Qì-Coordinating Decoction (*dà chéng qì tāng*) should be used in cases of dry stool. This suggestion refers back to the beginning of the line, so we know that further precipitation is appropriate for the treatment of the first transmutation.

In line 228, p. 315, anguish in the heart following the use of precipitation is treated with Gardenia and Fermented Soybean Decoction (*zhī zǐ chǐ tāng*). In that case, substantial heat is absent from the interior and only residual heat remains in the chest. Dry stool and bowel repletion are absent; therefore precipitation is not appropriate. These two lines may be compared to illustrate the differentiation of post-precipitation transmutations.

3.2.2 Moistening and Enema Patterns

LINE 247

趺阳脉浮而濇，浮则胃气强，濇则小便数，浮濇相搏，大便则硬，其脾为约，麻子仁丸主之。

Fū yáng mài fú ér sè, fú zé wèi qì qiáng, sè zé xiǎo biàn shuò, fú sè xiāng bó, dà biàn zé yìng, qí pí wéi yuē, má zǐ rén wán zhǔ zhī.

[When] the instep yáng pulse[1] is floating and rough, floating [means] strong qì in the stomach,[2] and rough [means] urination is frequent. The floating and rough [qualities of the pulse] indicate contention and the stool is hard, [which means] the spleen is straitened; [therefore,] Hemp Seed Pill (*má zǐ rén wán*) governs.

TEXT NOTES

1. Instep yáng pulse, 趺阳脉 *fū yáng mài*: The pulse felt on the upper surface of the foot, approximately at the point Surging Yáng (*chōng yáng*, ST-42). This point is on the yáng brightness stomach channel and was used by Zhāng Jī to investigate the strength of the stomach qì and transmutations affecting the spleen and stomach.

2. Strong qì in the stomach, 胃气强 *wèi qì qiáng*: Strong evil qì in the stomach, not strength of the normal stomach qì.

FORMULA

Hemp Seed Pill (*má zǐ rén wán*)

◦ Moisten the intestines and enrich dryness; moderately free the stool.

麻子仁二升 芍药半斤 枳实半斤（炙） 大黄一斤（去皮） 厚朴一尺（炙，去皮） 杏仁一升（去皮尖，熬，别作脂）

㈠ 右六味，蜜和丸，如梧桐子大，饮服十丸，日三服。㈡ 渐加，以知为度。

Má zǐ rén èr shēng sháo yào bàn jīn zhǐ shí bàn jīn (zhì) dà huáng yī jīn (qù pí) hòu pò yī chǐ (zhì, qù pí) xìng rén yī shēng (qù pí jiān, áo, bié zuò zhī)

(1) *Yòu liù wèi, mì huò wán, rú wú tóng zǐ dà, yǐn fú shí wán, rì sān fú.* (2) *Jiàn jiā, yǐ zhī wéi dù.*

hemp seed (麻子仁 *má zǐ rén*, Cannabis Semen) 2 shēng

peony (芍药 *sháo yào*, Paeoniae Radix) half jīn

processed unripe bitter orange (枳实 *zhǐ shí*, Aurantii Fructus Immaturus) half jīn

rhubarb (大黄 *dà huáng*, Rhei Rhizoma) 1 jīn (remove bark)

magnolia bark (厚朴 *hòu pò*, Magnoliae Cortex) 1 chǐ[1](mix-fry, remove bark)

apricot kernel (杏仁 *xìng rén*, Armeniacae Semen) 1 shēng (remove skin and tips, dry-fry, grind into a fat-like [mixture])

(1) [For] the above six ingredients [grind first and then] mix with honey to form pills the size of firmiana seeds.[2] Take ten pills with water, three times a day. (2) Gradually increase [the dose] until [the patient] feels [the stool is freed].

FORMULA NOTES

1. One chǐ, 一尺 *yī chǐ*: A unit of measure from the Hàn Dynasty equal to approximately 23 centimeters or 9 inches.
2. Firmiana seed 梧桐子 *wú tóng zǐ*: These seeds are 6-8 mm in diameter, about the size of a pea. They are commonly taken as standard for pill size.

SYNOPSIS

The pulse, signs and treatment of straitened spleen.

COMMENTARY

When the pulse is taken at the instep, this gives particular information about the state of the stomach and the spleen. In this line, the pulse at the instep is both floating and rough. Zhāng Jī writes that the floating characteristic indicates strong qì in the stomach and the rough characteristic indicates that urination is frequent.

In this case, strong stomach qì refers to a strong evil present in the stomach, not strength of right qì, and is a negative sign. On the basis of the other signs and the formula used, one knows that this is dryness-heat evil.

In order to understand the significance of the floating and rough qualities of the pulse, one must understand fluid movement in the body. The stomach receives fluids, but these fluids are moved by the spleen, as it irrigates the four sides of the body. If the spleen moves and transforms properly, the stomach will not be dry. In the present case, dryness-heat is present in the stomach and the spleen cannot counter this evil; consequently, its functions are disturbed, with the result that the fluids do not move correctly. This pattern is referred to as "straitened spleen" because the spleen is controlled or constrained by the evil in the stomach. Because the spleen cannot perform its functions correctly and fluid movement is disturbed, excess water seeps into the bladder and insufficient water moves into the intestines. Internal heat forces the water out of the bladder; hence urination is frequent. The stool becomes hard because the water is insufficient to moisten the intestines. Too much water is in the bladder and not enough is in the intestines. Frequent urination and hard stool reflect the fact that the spleen has been straitened by the dry heat present in the stomach. Thus Zhāng Jī writes that the rough and floating qualities of the pulse are in contention. The floating quality represents the evil in the stomach and the rough quality represents the straitened spleen. The stomach evil contends with the spleen and spleen cannot perform its normal functions

This line presents a situation similar to line 244, p. 401, with "[the person]] will not change clothes for ten days, [but] will have discomfort." Although the stool is bound, abdominal pain and distention are absent or mild. Urination is copious or normal. No noticeable changes are observed in the intake of food and drink.

The pattern of straitened spleen belongs to yáng brightness, but should be differentiated from patterns for which one of the Qì-Coordinating Decoctions (*chéng qì tāng*) is used. In those patterns, dryness-heat repletion in the stomach damages the fluids in the center burner, resulting in aversion to heat, delirious speech, tidal heat effusion, and abdominal distention and pain. The pathomechanism is explained through the yáng brightness. In straitened spleen patterns, by contrast, dry heat in the stomach causes the spleen to lose its normal ability to move and transform fluids. The pathomechanism is explained through the function of the spleen and its relationship to the stomach.

Hemp Seed Pill (*má zǐ rén wán*) is used to moisten and free the stool. It is Minor Qì-Coordinating Decoction (*xiǎo chéng qì tāng*) with the addition of hemp seed (*má rén*), apricot kernel (*xìng rén*), and peony (*sháo yào*). Rhubarb (*dà huáng*), magnolia bark (*hòu pò*), and unripe bitter orange (*zhǐ shí*), which is Minor Qì-Coordinating Decoction (*xiǎo chéng qì tāng*), drain heat, eliminate repletion, and move the stool and abduct stagnation. When the stomach heat is reduced, the spleen will not be influenced by the dryness-heat and will begin to move the fluids properly again. Hemp seed (*má rén*), the sovereign, is added to moisten the intestines, enrich dryness, and disinhibit the stool. Apricot kernel (*xìng rén*) also moistens the intestines, as well as the lungs. Its action of depurative downbearing allows the qì to move down and helps the movement of qì in both the upper and lower burners. Peony (*sháo yào*) harmonizes the blood and relaxes tension. These ingredients are used together to resolve intestinal dryness and fluid desiccation.

LINE 233

(一) 阳明病，自汗出，若发汗，小便自利者，此为津液内竭，虽硬不可攻之，当须自欲大便，宜蜜煎导而通之。(二) 若土瓜根及大猪胆汁，皆可为导。

(1) *Yáng míng bìng, zì hàn chū, ruò fā hàn, xiǎo biàn zì lì zhě, cǐ wéi jīn yè nèi jié, suī yìng bù kě gōng zhī, dāng xū zì yù dà biàn, yí mì jiān dǎo ér tōng zhī.* (2) *Ruò tǔ guā gēn jí dà zhū dǎn zhī, jiē kě wéi dǎo.*

(1) In yáng brightness disease with spontaneous sweating, if sweating is promoted and urination is spontaneously uninhibited, this means liquid and humor are exhausted. Although [there is] hard [stool], one cannot attack, [but] should wait [until the person spontaneously] desires to defecate* and then it is appropriate abduct [stool] to free [the intestine] with [a] thickened honey [enema]. (2) If cucumber gourd root (*tǔ guā gēn*) and gall from a large pig [are available], both can be [used as] an enema.

TEXT NOTE

* Should wait until the person spontaneously desires to defecate, 当须自欲大便 *dāng xū zì yù dà biàn*: The physician should wait until the patient has the desire to defecate. That is the most appropriate time for the use of an enema. Because dry stool blocks the bowel, the patient has the desire, but not the ability to defecate. Here, 须 *xū* is translated as "wait," not as "must."

FORMULA

Honey Brew Formula (*mì jiān fāng*)

○ Clear heat and moisten dryness; abduct downward and free the stool.

食蜜七合

(一) 右一味，于铜器内，微火煎，当须凝如饴状，搅之勿令焦著。(二) 欲可丸，并手捻作挺，令头锐，大如指，长二寸许，当热时急作，冷则硬。(三) 以内谷道中，以手急抱，欲大便时乃去之。(四) 疑非仲景意，已试甚良。

Shí mì qī gě

(1) *Yòu yī wèi, yú tóng qì nèi, wēi huǒ jiān, dāng xū níng rú yí zhuàng, jiǎo zhī wù lìng jiāo zháo.* (2) *Yù kě wán, bìng shǒu niǎn zuò tǐng, lìng tóu ruì, dà rú zhǐ, cháng èr cùn xǔ, dāng rè shí jí zuò, lěng zé yìng.* (3) *Yǐ nà gǔ dào zhōng, yǐ shǒu jí bào, yù dà biàn shí nǎi qù zhī.* (4) *Yí fēi zhòng jǐng yì, yǐ shì shèn liáng.*

eating honey (食蜜 *shí mì*, Mel) 7 gě

(1) Place the above ingredient in a copper pot. Cook it with a mild flame. It must congeal to a form like malt sugar; stir to prevent it from burning and sticking [to the pot]. (2) [Wait until the consistency is correct] to form a pill, then roll it [into] a finger-like shape, leaving a sharp head, so that it is the size of a finger and about two cùn long. It is urgent to use it while hot, as it will harden when cold. (3) Insert into the grain tract[1] and hold [the buttocks closed] with the hand, releasing [the buttocks] when [the person] is about to defecate. (4) It is doubted that this is [Zhāng] Zhòng Jǐng's formula,[2] [but] it proves to be very effective.

FORMULA NOTES

1. Grain tract, 谷道 *gǔ dào*: A term used to indicate the anus and intestines.
2. It is doubted that this is [Zhāng] Zhòng Jǐng's formula, 疑非[张]仲景方 *yí fēi zhòng jǐng fāng*: This is an addition to the text by an unknown author.

Cucumber Gourd Root Formula (*tǔ guā gēn fāng*)

This formula has been lost. There is a great deal of disagreement among modern commentators with regard to its ingredients and usage.

Pig's Bile Formula (*zhū dǎn zhī fāng*)

又大猪胆一枚，泻汁，和少许法醋，以灌谷道内，如一食顷，当大便出宿食恶物，甚效。

Yòu dà zhū dǎn yī méi, xiè zhī, huò shǎo xǔ fǎ cù, yǐ guàn gǔ dào nèi, rú yī shí qǐng, dāng dà biàn chū sù shí wù wù, shèn xiào.

[Take] the gallbladder from one large pig and drain the juice. Mix with a small amount of cooking vinegar and pour into the grain tract, [leaving in for] about the time it takes to eat a meal. The stool should issue forth with the abiding food and bad substances. It is very effective.

SYNOPSIS

When there is hard stool from liquid damage and the patient desires to defecate but cannot, it is appropriate to use an enema.

COMMENTARY

In the original yáng brightness disease presented in this line, spontaneous sweat issues. If sweating is then promoted, it will damage the fluids and is not appropriate treatment. If, due to the patient's constitution or the disease progression, urination then becomes disinhibited, it will exhaust the fluids, leading to dry hard stool. The presence of dry hard stool, however, does not necessarily mean that one can precipitate. Here, Zhāng Jī cautions that, in fact, although the stool is hard, one cannot precipitate because the problem is fluid exhaustion, not exuberant interior dryness-heat. The stomach domain is probably not replete in the patient in this line. Mistreatment, not the patient's original constitution, has resulted in fluid damage and bound stool.

In this case the patient has the desire to defecate, but because dry stool blocks the bowel, is unable to defecate. An enema is used to enrich and moisten the stool, allowing it to flow out easily. After the stool is expelled, one should observe the patient and see if further treatment is necessary. The desire but inability to defecate means that the stool is near the end of the intestinal tract. Precipitation is unlikely to reach this area and will only damage the qì of the center burner; therefore Zhāng Jī cautions against attacking.

This pattern should also be differentiated from that in which Hemp Seed Pill (*má zǐ rén wán*) would be used. In that pattern, the stool is bound, but the patient feels no desire to defecate, which means that the spleen is unable to distribute the fluids properly. In this line, although the stool is bound, the patient desires to defecate, indicating that the stool is already in a position to be expelled, but because of fluid damage, it cannot.

Bee's honey (*fēng mì*) is sweet, balanced, and non-toxic. It enriches yīn and moistens dryness. Used locally, it is effective for the treatment of intestinal dryness with dry stool and blood-yīn debilitation dry stool. Bitter and cold, pig's bile (*zhū dǎn zhī*) clears heat, and when mixed with vinegar, it ejects and drains. It is appropriate for blocked stool from fluid damage, particularly when signs of heat are present. The ingredients for Cucumber Gourd Root Formula (*tǔ guā gēn fāng*) are unknown, except for cucumber gourd root (*tǔ guā gēn*), which is bitter, cold, and non-toxic. This root is juicy and is pounded to extract this juice, which can then be used as an enema to free the stool.

3.2.3 Precipitation Pattern Identification

The following four lines discuss the identification of yáng brightness disease that is suitable for precipitation. Further, the range of uses for Minor Qì-Coordinating Decoction (*xiǎo chéng qì tāng*) and Major Qì-Coordinating Decoction (*dà chéng qì tāng*) is discussed. This discussion focuses on the descriptions of the signs, evaluation of the severity of dryness-heat and bowel repletion, and the state of the fluids. All these issues must be considered prior to precipitation. Precipitation is generally not used if exterior signs are still present. None of the signs mentioned previously (such as tidal heat effusion) can be seen as an unequivocal indication that precipitation is necessary but when seen in relation to other signs, they are all important indicators that precipitation may be appropriate.

LINE 208

㈠ 阳明病，脉迟，虽汗出不恶寒者，其身必重，短气，腹满而喘，有潮热者，此外欲解，可攻里也。㈡ 手足濈然汗出者，此大便已硬也，大承气汤主之；若汗多，微发热恶寒者，外未解也，其热不潮，未可与承气汤；若腹大满不通者，可与小承气汤，微和胃气，勿令至大泄下。

(1) *Yáng míng bìng, mài chí, suī hàn chū bù wù hán zhě, qí shēn bì zhòng, duǎn qì, fù mǎn ér chuǎn, yǒu cháo rè zhě, cǐ wài yù jiě, kě gōng lǐ yě.* (2) *Shǒu zú jí rán hàn chū zhě, cǐ dà biàn yǐ yìng yě, dà chéng qì tāng zhǔ zhī; ruò hàn duō, wēi fā rè wù hán zhě, wài wèi*

jiě yě, qí rè bù cháo, wèi kě yǔ chéng qì tāng; ruò fù dà mǎn bù tōng zhě, kě yǔ xiǎo chéng qì tāng, wēi hé wèi qì, wù lìng zhì dà xiè xià.

(1) When in yáng brightness disease the pulse is slow, even though [there is] sweating, and aversion to cold is absent, there will be generalized heaviness, shortness of breath, abdominal fullness, panting, and tidal heat effusion, which means the exterior is about to resolve and one can attack the interior. (2) Sweat streaming from the extremities indicates the stool is already hard and [therefore,] Major Qì-Coordinating Decoction (*dà chéng qì tāng*) governs. If [there is] copious sweating, mild heat effusion and aversion to cold, the exterior has not yet resolved, [and given that] this heat [effusion] is not tidal, one cannot give Qì-Coordinating Decoctions (*chéng qì tāng*). If [there is] great abdominal fullness and [the stool is] blocked, one can give Minor Qì-Coordinating Decoction (*xiǎo chéng qì tāng*) to harmonize the stomach qì mildly, [but] must not cause great discharge and precipitation.

Synopsis

The differentiation of whether or not attacking is appropriate in a yáng brightness disease and the distinction between the patterns of Major Qì-Coordinating Decoction (*dà chéng qì tāng*) and Minor Qì-Coordinating Decoction (*xiǎo chéng qì tāng*).

Commentary

This line is best understood in three sections (as numbered in the text). In the first section, a yáng brightness pattern is present, but the pulse is slow. In yáng brightness channel patterns, the pulse is typically surging and large. In yáng brightness bowel repletion, the pulse is usually sunken and strong. One may consider that a slow quality indicates exuberant cold, but Major Qì-Coordinating Decoction (*dà chéng qì tāng*) is used to treat this pattern, so one must assume that it is not a cold pattern. Exuberant dryness-heat dries the stool and causes blockage of the bowel qì. When the bowel qì becomes blocked, the qì and blood may be affected by this congestion, and in some cases this congestion may cause a pulse that is slow. Sweat issues, but aversion to cold is absent, suggesting that the greater yáng exterior pattern has already ceased and the evil has entered the interior. Generalized heaviness is a result of the same process that makes the pulse slow. Internal heat repletion causes congestion and stagnation of the qì dynamic, resulting in a feeling of heaviness throughout the body. Congestion and stagnation of the qì also causes abdominal fullness, since normal upbearing and downbearing of the qì is disturbed. Here, the qì cannot move down and out through the bowel, but qì movement in the upper burner is also affected. Impaired movement of qì, in combination with internal heat repletion that rises up and attacks the lung, results in shortness of breath and panting. Tidal heat effusion is characteristic of yáng brightness bowel repletion and its presence reinforces the conclusion that this is yáng brightness disease. Zhāng Jī explains that the exterior pattern is about to resolve and one can precipitate the interior without concern about an exterior evil falling inward.

The stomach governs the extremities and yáng brightness heat repletion steams the fluids and forces a sweat streaming from the extremities. When this occurs, the fluids are forced out to the extremities by exuberant interior heat; consequently, the stool becomes hard. Exuberant interior dryness-heat with dry, hard stool is treated through precipitation with Qì-Coordinating Decoctions (*chéng qì tāng*).

In the second section of the line, although sweat issues, heat effusion and aversion to cold is also present, indicating that the exterior pattern has not yet resolved. Here, the heat effusion is not the tidal heat effusion of yáng brightness patterns because the exterior pattern is unresolved; therefore, one cannot use precipitation and none of the Qì-Coordinating Decoctions (*chéng qì tāng*) formulae are appropriate. If precipitation is used, this treatment may cause the exterior evil to fall inward

In the final section of the line, only abdominal fullness and blocked stool are observed and signs of exuberant interior heat (such as tidal heat effusion or streaming sweat from the extremities) and exterior disease are absent. Precipitation may be used to eliminate the fullness and unblock the intestines. In this case it is not appropriate to use a strong precipitating formula, such as Major Qì-Coordinating Decoction (*dà chéng qì tāng*) because indications of exuberant interior dryness-heat repletion are absent. Minor Qì-Coordinating Decoction (*xiǎo chéng qì tāng*) is sufficient to harmonize the stomach qì and allow the bowels to move freely.

LINE 209

㈠ 阳明病，潮热，大便微硬者，可与大承气汤，不硬者，不可与之。㈡ 若不大便六七日，恐有燥屎，欲知之法，少与小承气汤，汤入腹中，转失气者，此有燥屎也，乃可攻之；若不转失气者，此但初头硬，后必溏，不可攻之，攻之必胀满不能食也。㈢ 欲饮水者，与水则哕。㈣ 其后发热者，必大便复硬而少也，以小承气汤和之。㈤ 不转失气者，慎不可攻也。

(1) *Yáng míng bìng, cháo rè, dà biàn wēi yìng zhě, kě yǔ dà chéng qì tāng, bù yìng zhě, bù kě yǔ zhī.* (2) *Ruò bù dà biàn liù qī rì, kǒng yǒu zào shǐ, yù zhī zhī fǎ, shǎo yǔ xiǎo chéng qì tāng, tāng rù fù zhōng, zhuǎn shī qì zhě, cǐ yǒu zào shǐ yě, nǎi kě gōng zhī; ruò bù zhuǎn shī qì zhě, cǐ dàn chū tóu yìng, hòu bì táng, bù kě gōng zhī, gōng zhī bì zhàng mǎn bù néng shí yě.* (3) *Yù yǐn shuǐ zhě, yǔ shuǐ zé yuē.* (4) *Qí hòu fā rè zhě, bì dà biàn fù yìng ér shǎo yě, yǐ xiǎo chéng qì tāng hé zhī.* (5) *Bù zhuǎn shī qì zhě, shèn bù kě gōng yě.*

(1) When in yáng brightness disease, [there is] tidal heat effusion and slightly[1] hard stool, one can give Major Qì-Coordinating Decoction (*dà chéng qì tāng*), [but if there is] no hardness, one cannot give [this

formula]. (2) If [the patient] has not been able to defecate for six or seven days and one fears [there is] dry stool, the way to find out is to give a small amount of Minor Qì-Coordinating Decoction (*xiǎo chéng qì tāng*). When the decoction enters the abdomen, passing of [fecal] qì[2] indicates dry stool and one can attack; [but if there is] no passing of [fecal] qì, only hard first, then sloppy stool, one cannot attack, for if one attacks there will be abdominal fullness and inability to eat. (3) [There is] a desire to drink water and when water is given, [there is] immediate hiccupping. (4) After this, [there is] heat effusion and the stool will again be hard and scant, so use Minor Qì-Coordinating Decoction (*xiǎo chéng qì tāng*) to harmonize. (5) If [there is] no passing of [fecal] qì, one [should be] cautious and cannot attack.

TEXT NOTES

1. Slightly, 微 *wēi*: According to *Gāo Děng Cóng Shū*, this is an error in the text. This word should not appear, for if the stool were only slightly hard, Major Qì-Coordinating Decoction (*dà chéng qì tāng*) would not be given.
2. Passing of fecal qì, 转失气 *zhuǎn shī qì*: A feeling of stirring in the intestines, accompanied by frequent flatulence. This term is the same as "shifting of qì," 转气 *zhuǎn qì*.

   The character 失气 *shī*, "passing of qì," appears in many versions as 矢气 *shǐ qì*, in which 矢 *shǐ*, "arrow," stands euphemistically for its homophone 屎 , feces.

SYNOPSIS

A differentiation of the methods used with Major Qì-Coordinating Decoction (*dà chéng qì tāng*) and Minor Qì-Coordinating Decoction (*xiǎo chéng qì tāng*).

COMMENTARY

This line is best understood by dividing it into four sections. The first is from the beginning to "one cannot give [this formula]." The second is from "if [the patient] has not been able to defecate" to "one can attack." The third is from "[but if there is] no passing of [fecal] qì" to "immediate hiccupping." The fourth is from "After this, [there is] heat effusion" to the end.

The first section presents a case of yáng brightness disease with tidal heat effusion and hard stool. This pattern is yáng brightness bowel repletion with exuberant interior dryness-heat and it is treated with Major Qì-Coordinating Decoction (*dà chéng qì tāng*). If the stool is not hard, then this is not a case of bowel repletion with exuberant dryness-heat, and precipitation should not be used.

In the second section, the patient does not defecate for about a week, but no other clear signs of bowel repletion are present. If one is not positive that dry stool is blocking the bowels, a small dose of Minor Qì-Coordinating Decoction (*xiǎo chéng qì tāng*) may be given as a diagnostic indicator. If after ingesting the formula the patient feels stirring in the intestines and passes gas, it confirms that dry stool is blocking the bowels. In this case, one can use Major Qì-Coordinating Decoction (*dà chéng qì tāng*) to precipitate and unblock the intestines.

If, however, following the ingestion of Minor Qì-Coordinating Decoction (*xiǎo chéng qì tāng*) shifting of qì is absent, as in the third section, then precipitation must not be used. In this case, dry stool is absent, and the stool is hard at the beginning and then sloppy at the end. This type of stool may indicate heat without repletion, damp-heat, or even vacuity cold in the stomach, and must be further differentiated; precipitation should not be used. If precipitation is used, it will damage the qì of the spleen and the stomach, impair the qì dynamic in the center burner, and disturb normal upbearing and downbearing, causing abdominal fullness and inability to eat. When the qì of the stomach and spleen is damaged, the fluids are not properly transformed and thirst arises. When water is taken in, it ascends counterflow and causes hiccup.

In the final section, following precipitation, heat effuses and the stool again becomes hard and scant, indicating that although the use of precipitation was correct, the fluids were damaged and residual heat is present. The stool is not moving freely, but it is not completely obstructed. In this case, Major Qì-Coordinating Decoction (*dà chéng qì tāng*) is no longer necessary. Minor Qì-Coordinating Decoction (*xiǎo chéng qì tāng*) is sufficient to move the stool and harmonize the stomach.

The final caution regarding the use of precipitation emphasizes that if a small dose of Minor Qì-Coordinating Decoction (*xiǎo chéng qì tāng*) is given and there is no subsequent passing of fecal qì, precipitation must not be used.

LINE 251

㈠得病二三日，脉弱，无太阳、柴胡证，烦躁，心下硬，至四五日，虽能食，以小承气汤少少与，微和之，令小安，至六日，与承气汤一升。㈡若不大便六七日，小便少者，虽不受食，但初头硬，后必溏，未定成硬，攻之必溏。㈢须小便利，屎定硬，乃可攻之，宜大承气汤。

(1) *Dé bìng èr sān rì, mài ruò, wú tài yáng、chái hú zhèng, fán zào, xīn xià yìng, zhì sì wǔ rì, suī néng shí, yǐ xiǎo chéng qì tāng shǎo shǎo yǔ, wēi hé zhī, lìng xiǎo ān, zhì liù rì, yǔ chéng qì tāng yī shēng.* (2) *Ruò bù dà biàn liù qī rì, xiǎo biàn shǎo zhě, suī bù shòu shí, dàn chū tóu yìng, hòu bì táng, wèi dìng chéng yìng, gōng zhī bì táng.* (3) *Xū xiǎo biàn lì, shǐ dìng yìng, nǎi kě gōng zhī, yí dà chéng qì tāng.*

(1) [When] in an illness [that the person has] had for two or three days, the pulse is weak, [there is] neither a greater yáng [nor] a [Minor] Bupleurum [Decoction] ((*xiǎo*) *chái hú* (*tāng*)) pattern, and [there is] vexation and agitation, and hardness below the heart, [then] at four or

five days, although [the person] is able to eat, one can give a very small amount of Minor Qì-Coordinating Decoction (*xiǎo chéng qì tāng*) to harmonize and quiet. At six days, give one shēng of [Minor] Qì-Coordinating Decoction ([*xiǎo*] *chéng qì tāng*). (2) If [there is] inability to defecate for six or seven days and scant urination, although [the person] will not accept food and [there is] only stool that is hard at the beginning and then sloppy, [it is] not yet formed and hard, and [if] one attacks, there will be sloppy [stool]. (3) There must be uninhibited urination and hard formed stool, then one can attack and [therefore,] Major Qì-Coordinating Decoction (*dà chéng qì tāng*) is appropriate.

SYNOPSIS

A differentiation of the methods used with Major Qì-Coordinating Decoction (*dà chéng qì tāng*) and Minor Qì-Coordinating Decoction (*xiǎo chéng qì tāng*).

COMMENTARY

This line is best understood if divided into three sections (as numbered in the text). In the first section, the disease has lasted for two or three days and although this is a short period of time, signs of either a greater yáng exterior pattern or a lesser yáng Minor Bupleurum Decoction (*xiǎo chái hú tāng*) pattern are absent. The presence of vexation and agitation, and hardness below the heart, in light of the use of a Qì-Coordinating Decoction (*chéng qì tāng*), suggests a yáng brightness internal repletion pattern. One can assume that the stool is bound and a Qì-Coordinating Decoction (*chéng qì tāng*) is used in order to free the stool, but the pulse is weak, a quality not typically seen in interior repletion patterns. This pulse may be interpreted in two ways. Wāng Hǔ writes that the weak quality reinforces the idea that an exterior evil is absent; hence the pulse is not floating or tight. Kē Qín raises another issue, questioning if this "is evidence of no yáng" and a yīn pattern. In the three yīn patterns, however, the patient is generally unable to eat, whereas in this case, the patient is able to eat. It is unlikely that a yīn pattern is present in this case. Yù Chāng further emphasizes the importance of the patient's ability to eat, by referring to line 215, p. 347: "... inability to eat, [this means that] there must be five or six pieces of dry stool in the stomach." This patient is able to eat; therefore, dry stool is not present in the stomach and intestines. In this case, only mild precipitation is appropriate, and a very small amount of Minor Qì-Coordinating Decoction (*xiǎo chéng qì tāng*) is given to harmonize the stomach. If after six days, vexation and hardness below the heart persist, the internal heat has not been eliminated and it is likely that the stool will be bound. In that case, one can give a full shēng of Minor Qì-Coordinating Decoction (*xiǎo chéng qì tāng*).

If the stool is absent for six or seven days and vexation, agitation, and hardness below the heart are present, it suggests dry stool bound in the intestines and one may consider using Major Qì-Coordinating Decoction (*dà chéng qì tāng*) to precipitate. Nonetheless, inability to eat suggests that the stomach qì is not effulgent. Scanty urination accompanied by stool that is hard at the beginning and then sloppy suggests that the fluids are not being distributed properly. When the qì of the stomach and spleen is weak or obstructed, the clear and the turbid are not separated properly. Fluids do not move down into the bladder to be expelled, and consequently urination is scanty. Fluids are entering the intestines; therefore, the stool is not dry and bound, but is hard at the beginning, then sloppy. This is not dry, bound stool; therefore precipitation should not be used. If precipitation is used, sloppy stool will be exacerbated because the qì of the spleen and stomach will be further damaged.

If, however, urination becomes uninhibited, it means that the fluids are moving normally and are sufficient. In this case if the stool is absent for six or seven days, it indicates dry, bound stool in the intestines, and other signs (such as abdominal pain and distention, and a thick tongue fur) would likely be present. Precipitation with Major Qì-Coordinating Decoction (*dà chéng qì tāng*) is appropriate to unblock the intestines.

LINE 203

㈠ 阳明病，本自汗出，医更重发汗，病已差，尚微烦不了了者，此必大便硬故也。㈡ 以亡津液，胃中干燥，故令大便硬。㈢ 当问其小便，日几行。㈣ 若本小便日三四行，今日再行，故知大便不久出，今为小便数少，以津液当还入胃中，故知不久必大便也。

(1) *Yáng míng bìng, běn zì hàn chū, yī gèng chóng fā hàn, bìng yǐ chài, shàng wēi fán bù liǎo liǎo zhě, cǐ bì dà biàn yìng gù yě.* (2) *Yǐ wáng jīn yè, wèi zhōng gān zào, gù lìng dà biàn yìng.* (3) *Dāng wèn qí xiǎo biàn, rì jǐ xíng.* (4) *Ruò běn xiǎo biàn rì sān sì xíng, jīn rì zài xíng, gù zhī dà biàn bù jiǔ chū, jīn wéi xiǎo biàn shuò shǎo, yǐ jīn yè dāng huán rù wèi zhōng, gù zhī bù jiǔ bì dà biàn yě.*

(1) When in yáng brightness disease, there was originally spontaneous sweating and the physician again promoted sweating, and [the exterior] disease is already cured, [yet there is] still mild vexation that has not been clearly [resolved], this is because the stool is hard. (2) Due to liquid and humor collapse, the stomach is dry and this makes the stool hard. (3) One should ask how many times a day [the patient] urinates. (4) If originally there was urination three or four times a day and now [there is urination] twice a day* one knows the stool will issue soon. Now, the urine is frequent and scant because the fluids are entering the stomach; therefore, one knows defecation will occur soon.

TEXT NOTE

* Now, [there is] urination twice a day, 今日再行 *jīn rì zài xíng*: The character, 行 *xíng*, is used to mean the act of urinating. 日行 *rì xíng* would be once a day, so 日再行 *rì zài xíng* means twice a day.

Synopsis

On the basis of whether urination is copious or scanty, one can determine the degree of hardness of the stool.

Commentary

In yáng brightness disease, spontaneous sweating may occur due to exuberant internal heat. Although the promotion of sweating is appropriate in exterior patterns, it is not generally used in yáng brightness patterns, particularly when sweat has already issued. The use of this method further depletes fluids that have been damaged through the loss of sweat. At this point, exterior signs are absent; only mild vexation is observed. That the vexation is mild means that the internal dryness-heat is not severe. The indication that this sign is not clearly resolved, although the exterior disease has resolved, suggests internal damage that delays recovery.

Zhāng Jī explains that the stool is hard because the fluids have been depleted and the stomach is dry. It is possible that the stool is bound and one should use precipitation to resolve this pattern; Zhāng Jī writes that the urine may be used as an indication of the progress of the disease. If the patient normally urinates three or four times a day, but now only urinates twice, it means that the fluids are being redistributed within the body. When the urine is more scant than normal, one may consider that fluid is entering the stomach and intestines, instead of being expelled from the body. This fluid moistens the dryness in the stomach and intestines and allows the stool to be expelled. Thus, in this case one should not use precipitation.

In this line Zhāng Jī uses a comparison of the amount of urine to make a decision about the state of the fluids in the body. Nonetheless, one must consider the whole disease course when looking at any sign. In other lines, similar signs are given slightly different significance. In line 233, p. 354, uninhibited urination is taken as a sign of fluid debilitation and hard stool. Line 247, p. 351, discusses straitened spleen, and in that case frequent urination is related to hard stool. Hard stool and frequent urination are also related in line 250, p. 335. Frequent and/or uninhibited urination may indicate that the fluids are percolating out of the body, leaving the stomach and intestines dry, and the stool hard. In the line above, fluid collapse and hard stool are related to a decrease in the frequency and amount of the urine. Yáng brightness patterns with bound stool can be divided into two basic types. One is dryness-heat internal bind and the other is fluid depletion. In the first, heat should be drained through precipitation with cold, bitter medicinals; in the second, dryness should be moistened. Moistening may occur through the use of a decoction, an enema, or spontaneously, as above.

3.2.4 Contraindications for Precipitation

Line 204

伤寒呕多，虽有阳明证，不可攻之。

Shāng hán ǒu duō, suī yǒu yáng míng zhèng, bù kě gōng zhī.

In cold damage with frequent retching, although there are yáng brightness signs, one cannot attack.

SYNOPSIS

When in cold damage there is increased retching, the direction of the disease dynamic is upward and one cannot attack downward.

COMMENTARY

In the broad category of externally contracted diseases indicated by cold damage, patterns may arise in which an exterior evil shifts to the yáng brightness, resulting in signs such as bound stool, abdominal pain and distention, and tidal heat effusion. Generally, it is appropriate to attack with a precipitating formula in these cases. If the internal heat evil is not bound in the intestines and instead it ascends and insults the stomach, it may cause retching and vomiting. In this case the evil is not in the intestines, but in the region of the stomach and the diaphragm. When an evil insults the stomach and causes counterflow, one cannot use precipitation. If precipitation is used, it may damage the right qì and result in the evil falling deeper into the interior from the region of the stomach and the diaphragm.

Because lesser yáng disease may also be characterized by retching, one should differentiate carefully. In lesser yáng patterns (half interior-half exterior patterns), the pivot mechanism is involved. When heat enters the lesser yáng, the pivot mechanism becomes inhibited, gallbladder fire flames upward and invades the stomach, and retching counterflow occurs. This type of retching is often accompanied by alternating aversion to cold and heat effusion, and fullness in the chest and under the rib-side, and other signs of lesser yáng disease.

LINE 205

阳明病，心下硬满者，不可攻之，攻之利遂不止者死，利止者愈。

Yáng míng bìng, xīn xià yìng mǎn zhě, bù kě gōng zhī, gōng zhī lì suì bù zhǐ zhě sǐ, lì zhǐ zhě yù.

When in yáng brightness disease, [there is] hard fullness below the heart, [one] cannot attack, [for] attacking [will cause] incessant diarrhea, and [the person] will die; [but] if the diarrhea stops, [the person will] recover.

SYNOPSIS

When in cold damage there is excessive retching, the disease dynamic is upward; [therefore,] one cannot use offensive precipitation.

COMMENTARY

In yáng brightness disease with hardness and fullness in the abdomen, precipitation is generally suggested. In this case the hardness and fullness is not in the abdomen, but below the heart. This sign pattern suggests the absence of a substantial evil bound in the intestines and the presence of formless evil heat congesting the qì dynamic. Precipitation should not be used because it is ineffective for treating formless evils and it will damage right qì and the qì of the stomach and spleen, resulting in incessant diarrhea. If the damage to the qì is severe and the diarrhea cannot be checked, the right qì will desert and the patient will die. If the diarrhea can be checked, the patient may still recover.

Hard fullness below the heart appears to be similar to the main sign of chest bind. Generally in chest bind, heat and water bind in the area of the chest and diaphragm so that the area below the heart becomes hard, full, and painful to the degree that the patient refuses to allow palpation. This area of fullness and hardness may extend all the way down into the lesser abdomen. The appropriate treatment for chest bind is to drain heat and expel water. In the line above, Zhāng Jī states that in this case one cannot attack, indicating that the area of hardness and fullness is probably not painful and does not extend down into the lesser abdomen.

LINE 206

阳明病，面合色赤，不可攻之，必发热，色黄者，小便不利也。

Yáng míng bìng, miàn hé sè chì, bù kě gōng zhī, bì fā rè, sè huáng zhě, xiǎo biàn bù lì yě.

When in yáng brightness disease, [there is] redness of the whole face, one cannot attack, [otherwise] there will be heat effusion and yellowing. [In such cases,] the urine is inhibited.

SYNOPSIS

In yáng brightness disease when the whole face is red, precipitation is contraindicated. The line presents a transmuted pattern that may occur if precipitation is used inappropriately.

COMMENTARY

The yáng brightness channel spreads over the face. When exuberant heat in the yáng brightness channel becomes depressed and cannot diffuse and outthrust, it steams upward and causes a red complexion. In this case exuberant heat is depressed in the channel, not bound in the bowel; therefore, one should not attack with precipitation, but should diffuse and clear heat.

The use of precipitation causes heat effusion and yellowing through the following mechanism. Heat in the channel is not eliminated by attacking with precipitation and the spleen and stomach are damaged, resulting in impaired fluid movement and dampness. Heat and dampness combine and steam in the interior, producing heat effusion and yellowing. A yellow color is produced because yellow is the color associated with earth. This pattern is considered a case of yáng yellowing because the yellowing is accompanied by heat effusion. Inhibited urination is corroborating evidence that fluid movement is impaired and the fluids, instead of being expelled, remain in the interior.

Line 189

阳明中风，口苦咽干，腹满微喘，发热恶寒，脉浮而紧，若下之，则腹满，小便难也。

Yáng míng zhòng fēng, kǒu kǔ yān gān, fù mǎn wēi chuǎn, fā rè wù hán, mài fú ér jǐn, ruò xià zhī, zé fù mǎn, xiǎo biàn nán yě.

In yáng brightness wind strike with bitter taste in the mouth, dry throat, abdominal fullness, slight panting, heat effusion, aversion to cold, and a pulse that is floating and tight, if precipitation is used there will be abdominal fullness and difficult urination.

Synopsis

In yáng brightness disease when the exterior evil has not yet resolved and the interior is not yet replete, precipitation is contraindicated.

Commentary

Although this line begins with the words, "yáng brightness wind strike," it is a pattern of combination disease of the three yáng. Heat effusion and aversion to cold with a pulse that is floating and tight indicates a greater yáng exterior pattern. Abdominal fullness and panting belong to yáng brightness disease. Lesser yáng disease can be seen in the signs of bitter taste in the mouth and dry throat.

In yáng brightness disease, when abdominal fullness and panting are accompanied by tidal heat effusion, delirious speech, or other signs of bowel repletion, one may consider precipitation. In this case accompanying signs are absent and clear evidence of an unresolved exterior pattern exists. Therefore, even in the absence of lesser yáng signs, precipitation would not be the correct treatment. Because lesser yáng signs are observed, this pattern should be treated by harmonizing the lesser yáng, resolving the exterior, and clearing heat.

If precipitation is used, it will damage the center burner qì, impair the qì dynamic, and exacerbate the abdominal fullness. This disruption of the qì mechanism may impair fluid transformation and/or the fluids may be damaged by precipitation, resulting in difficult urination.

Line 194

㈠ 阳明病，不能食，攻其热必哕，所以然者，胃中虚冷故也。㈡ 以其人本虚，攻其热必哕。

(1) *Yáng míng bìng, bù néng shí, gōng qí rè bì yuē, suǒ yǐ rán zhě, wèi zhōng xū lěng gù yě.* (2) *Yǐ qí rén běn xū, gōng qí rè bì yuē.*

(1) When in yáng brightness disease, [there is] inability to eat, attacking the heat will result in hiccup. Why [this is] so is because [there is]

vacuity cold in the stomach. (2) Because the person was originally vacuous, there will be hiccup when the heat is attacked.

SYNOPSIS

When there is vacuity cold in the stomach, precipitation is contraindicated; this line presents a transmuted pattern that may occur if precipitation is used inappropriately.

COMMENTARY

In yáng brightness disease the patient may or may not be able to eat, and this sign is not an unequivocal indicator of any particular pattern. When stomach heat disperses food, or the bowel is replete and the stomach qì effulgent, the patient is usually able to eat. When dry stool binds in the intestines blocking the bowel qì, or vacuity cold is present in the stomach, the patient is usually unable to eat normally.

This line presents a case of vacuity cold in the stomach with inability to eat. The physician thought that this was a case of dry stool with internal heat and attacked the heat. If this treatment were correct, the heat bind would resolve and the patient would then be able to eat normally. Following the use of precipitation, however, there is hiccup. Zhāng Jī explains that this transmutation indicates vacuity cold in the stomach. Because originally the stomach qì was vacuous, the use of an attacking method further damages the qì; when the stomach qì is damaged, the qì ascends counterflow, resulting in hiccup.

In yáng brightness disease with inability to eat, one can differentiate the pattern on the basis of the accompanying signs. If accompanied by abdominal fullness, absence of defecation, tidal heat effusion, and delirious speech, it is clear that the inability to eat is a result of bowel repletion with dry stool and precipitation may be used. If, however, other signs of bowel repletion are absent, one must be cautious before using an attacking method.

4 YÁNG BRIGHTNESS DISEASE AND TRANSMUTED PATTERNS

4.1 YELLOWING PATTERNS

LINE 199

阳明病，无汗，小便不利，心中懊侬者，身必发黄。

Yáng míng bìng, wú hàn, xiǎo biàn bù lì, xīn zhōng ào nóng zhě, shēn bì fā huáng.

When in yáng brightness disease, sweating is absent, [and there is] inhibited urination and anguish in the heart, there will be generalized yellowing.*

Text Note

* Yellowing, 发黄 *fā huáng*: See line 125, p. 207, for an explanation, and see the Overview of the present chapter for further discussion of this sign. In the lines that follow, "yáng yellow," 阳黄 *yáng huáng*, means a pattern of bound damp-heat causing yellowing, while "yīn yellow," 阴黄 *yīn huáng*, means a pattern of bound cold-damp causing it.

Synopsis

The pattern of yellowing that occurs in yáng brightness disease from the steaming action of depressed damp-heat.

Commentary

Generally, in yáng brightness disease, exuberant dryness-heat in the interior steams the fluids and forces them to the exterior, resulting in copious sweating and frequent urination. In this case sweating is absent and urination is inhibited, indicating that the normal pathomechanism has been altered and that heat is congested and stagnant. Zhāng Jī tells us that in this situation generalized yellowing will occur. From this information one can deduce that not only is heat congested in the interior, but dampness also. Damp evil lodged in the center impairs qì transformation, causes stagnation of the qì dynamic, and disturbs fluid movement. Turbid fluids cannot move downward to the bladder, so urination is inhibited. Furthermore, since qì and fluid movement is abnormal, no sweat issues. The heat cannot move out of the body through the sweat or through the urine, and so it becomes depressed in the interior. The presence of anguish in the heart suggests that the heat, because it cannot pass out of the body, instead rises up and disturbs the heart spirit.

When heat is depressed in the interior, it can combine with dampness and cause generalized yellowing. This pathomechanism is explained in two ways. Commentators such as Zhāng Zhì-Cōng, Yóu Yí, and Qián Huáng refer to the effect of damp-heat on the spleen. Because yellow is the color associated with the spleen, damp-heat in the interior (without an external pathway through the urine or sweat) impairs the functions of the spleen and produces generalized yellowing. This pathomechanism reflects an understanding of yellowing or jaundice as being related to the spleen and stomach. This understanding persisted until the Qīng Dynasty, when Kē Qín and Yè Guì proposed the idea that yellowing was related to the liver and gallbladder. On the basis of that conceptualization, one may also understand generalized yellowing as being the result of damp-heat in the interior steaming the liver and gallbladder, and forcing gall out to the exterior of the body, although this was probably not the way Zhāng Jī understood this pathomechanism. (Please see the Introduction for a more complete discussion of this issue.) Zhāng Jī places this pattern in the category of yáng brightness disease, which belongs to the spleen and stomach, not the liver and gallbladder.

LINE 200

阳明病，被火，额上微汗出，而小便不利者，必发黄。

Yáng míng bìng, bèi huǒ, é shàng wēi hàn chū, ér xiǎo biàn bù lì zhě, bì fā huáng.

When a yáng brightness disease [is treated] with fire and [there is] slight sweating from the forehead and inhibited urination, there will be yellowing.

SYNOPSIS

Yellowing that is the result of the inappropriate use of fire treatment in yáng brightness disease.

COMMENTARY

Yáng brightness disease is characterized by internal dryness-heat repletion; appropriate treatments include clearing heat and precipitation. In this case, a fire method is used to treat the patient. This line presents an example of treating repletion with repletion. The use of fire assists, and does not eliminate, the dryness-heat evil. The fluids are damaged by severe heat. If copious sweat issues or urination is frequent, one knows that the fluids have not been exhausted and the heat can follow the sweat or urine out of the body. In this case, however, the fluid damage is already severe and as the internal heat forces the remaining fluids upward, only mild sweat issues from the head. The fluids are insufficient; hence urination is inhibited. The combination of dampness and heat in the interior when sweating is absent or insufficient and when urination is inhibited may produce yellowing.

LINE 236

阳明病，发热汗出者，此为热越，不能发黄也；但头汗出，身无汗，剂颈而还，小便不利，渴引水浆者，此为瘀热在里，身必发黄，茵陈蒿汤主之。

Yáng míng bìng, fā rè hàn chū zhě, cǐ wéi rè yuè, bù néng fā huáng yě; dàn tóu hàn chū, shēn wú hàn, jì jǐng ér huán, xiǎo biàn bù lì, kě yǐn shuǐ jiāng zhě, cǐ wéi yū rè zài lǐ, shēn bì fā huáng, yīn chén hāo tāng zhǔ zhī.

When in yáng brightness disease, [there is] heat effusion and sweating, this means that the heat is straying,* and unable [to cause] yellowing. Sweating only from the head, not from the body, [and] stopping at the neck, [as well as] inhibited urination and thirst with intake of fluids, indicates stasis heat in the interior; [hence] there will be generalized yellowing and [therefore,] Capillaris Decoction (*yīn chén hāo tāng*) governs.

Text Note

* Straying heat, 热越 *rè yuè*: The heat is able to effuse and is moving outward.

Formula

Capillaris Decoction (*yīn chén hāo tāng*)

∘ Clear heat, disinhibit dampness, and abate yellowing.

茵陈蒿六两　栀子十四枚（擘）　大黄二两（去皮）

(一) 右三味，以水一斗二升，先煮茵陈，减六升，右二味，煮取三升，去滓，分三服。(二) 小便当利，尿如皂荚汁状，色正赤。(三) 一宿腹减，黄从小便去也。

Yīn chén hāo liù liǎng zhī zǐ shí sì méi (bò) dà huáng èr liǎng (qù pí)

(1) *Yòu sān wèi, yǐ shuǐ yī dǒu èr shēng, xiān zhǔ yīn chén, jiǎn liù shēng, yòu èr wèi, zhǔ qǔ sān shēng, qù zǐ, fēn sān fú.* (2) *Xiǎo biàn dāng lì, niào rú zào jiá zhī zhuàng, sè zhèng chì.* (3) *Yī xiǔ fù jiǎn, huáng cóng xiǎo biàn qù yě.*

capillaris (茵陈蒿 *yīn chén hāo*, Artemisiae Capillaris Herba) 6 liǎng

gardenia (栀子 *zhī zǐ*, Gardeniae Fructus) 14 pieces (broken)

rhubarb (大黄 *dà huáng*, Rhei Rhizoma) 2 liǎng (remove skin)

(1) [For] the above three ingredients use one dǒu two shēng of water. First boil capillaris (*yīn chén hāo*) to reduce [the decoction by] six shēng. Add [the other] two ingredients and boil to get 3 shēng. Remove the dregs, separate into three doses, and take. (2) The urine should be disinhibited and like the juice of the gleditsia fruit (*zào jiá*), a pure red color. (3) [After] one night, the abdominal [signs] will be relieved* and the yellow will come out with the urine.

Text Note

* [After] one night, the abdominal [signs] will be relieved, 一宿腹减 *yī sù fù jiǎn*: This line has been explained in two ways according to the authors of *Gāo Děng Cóng Shū*. The first is that its inclusion suggests that in the original pattern, the stasis heat is severe, and abdominal fullness, although not mentioned in the text, is present, along with bound stool. The second is that after the patient takes the decoction, the stool will be freed and the stasis heat will be eliminated.

Synopsis

The signs and treatment of yellowing from static heat in the interior in yáng brightness disease.

Commentary

This line is Zhāng Jī's explanation of the pathomechanism of yellowing. In yáng brightness patterns with internal dryness-heat repletion, repletion heat causes heat effusion and sweating, and although this does not resolve the disease, it allows the heat to pass to the outside. When the heat can pass out of the body through effusion of heat or sweating, the process is described as "straying." When this occurs, the heat cannot combine with dampness and cause yellowing.

If, however, sweating only occurs on the head, and urination is inhibited, the heat cannot skip to the exterior and remains in the interior. The heat in the interior disturbs and congests the qì dynamic and the movement of fluids. When the fluids cannot move, they become stagnant. Sweat only issues from the head, not from the body, and urination is inhibited. The heat and dampness become bound in the interior and this binding is described here as "stasis heat." The heat cannot skip to the exterior; consequently the patient yellows.

Capillaris Decoction (*yīn chén hāo tāng*) is a primary formula for clearing heat, disinhibiting dampness, and abating yellow. Capillaris (*yīn chén*) treats yellowing by clearing heat and disinhibiting dampness. Modern writers list the stomach, spleen, liver, and gallbladder as its entering channels, perhaps reflecting the associations between jaundice and the liver and gallbladder. Nonetheless, a quote from the *Běn Cǎo Zhèng Yì* provides another insight: "The flavor of capillaris (*yīn chén*) is bland and it disinhibits water. It is a special agent for treating damp-heat in the two domains of the stomach and spleen." This categorization is probably closer to the one with which Zhāng Jī was familiar. Bitter and cold, gardenia (*zhī zǐ*) clears heat and disinhibits dampness in all three burners. It also has an action to open and regulate the waterways. Rhubarb (*dà huáng*), also bitter and cold, drains and precipitates. It is able to drain the stasis heat from the interior.

LINE 260

伤寒七八日，身黄如橘子色，小便不利，腹微满者，茵陈蒿汤主之。

Shāng hán qī bā rì, shēn huáng rú jú zǐ sè, xiǎo biàn bù lì, fù wēi mǎn zhě, yīn chén hāo tāng zhǔ zhī.

When in cold damage [that has lasted for] seven or eight days, [there is] generalized yellowing the color of a tangerine, inhibited urination, and mild abdominal fullness, Capillaris Decoction (*yīn chén hāo tāng*) governs.

SYNOPSIS

A further description of the signs and treatment of damp-heat yellowing.

COMMENTARY

This line can be seen as additional commentary on the preceding line. The preceding line, line 236, p. 369, provides an explanation of the pathomechanism of yellowing, while this line provides a more detailed description of the signs.

Although this line begins with the words "cold damage," it appears to present a case of yáng yellowing that belongs to the yáng brightness. An exterior evil from a cold damage condition may have entered the interior. Urination is inhibited and the heat and dampness become bound in the interior. Generalized yellowing occurs because the heat does not effuse, sweat does not issue, and urination is inhibited. This color, described as the color of a tangerine, is the color of yáng yellowing. Heat and dampness bound in the interior stagnate and disturb qì dynamic, producing abdominal fullness. Capillaris Decoction (*yīn chén hāo tāng*) is used to clear heat, disinhibit dampness, and abate yellowing.

LINE 261

伤寒身黄，发热，栀子蘖皮汤主之。

Shāng hán shēn huáng, fā rè, zhī zǐ bǎi pí tāng zhǔ zhī.

In cold damage with generalized yellowing and heat effusion, Gardenia and Phellodendron Decoction (*zhī zǐ bǎi pí tāng*) governs.

FORMULA

Gardenia and Phellodendron Decoction (*zhī zǐ bǎi pí tāng*)

∘ Clear and discharge damp-heat in order to abate yellowing.

肥栀子十五个（擘） 甘草一两（炙） 黄蘖二两。

右三味，以水四升，煮取一升半，去滓，分温再服。

Féi zhī zǐ shí wǔ ge (bò) gān cǎo yī liǎng (zhì) huáng bǎi èr liǎng.

Yòu sān wèi, yǐ shuǐ sì shēng, zhǔ qǔ yī shēng bàn, qù zǐ, fēn wēn zài fú.

fat gardenia (肥栀子 *zhī zǐ*, Gardeniae Fructus) 15 pieces (broken)
mix-fried licorice (甘草 *gān cǎo*, Glycyrrhizae Radix) 1 liǎng
phellodendron (黄蘖 *huáng bǎi*, Phellodendri Cortex) 2 liǎng

[For] the above three ingredients use four shēng of water. Boil to get one and a half shēng and remove the dregs. Divide [into two parts], and take warm twice a day.

SYNOPSIS

The signs and treatment of cold damage with yellowing and heat effusion.

COMMENTARY

As in the preceding line, generalized yellowing occurs in a cold damage pattern, indicating that dampness and heat are bound in the interior. Because yellowing occurs, it is likely that sweating is absent and urination is inhibited. In this pattern, heat effusion allows some of the heat from the interior to pass out of the body. Abdominal fullness or other signs of a severe interior pattern are absent, so Capillaris Decoction (*yīn chén hāo tāng*) is not used, but Gardenia and Phellodendron Decoction (*zhī zǐ bǎi pí tāng*) is suggested instead. The use of this formula, which clears heat and eliminates vexation, suggests that vexation, agitation, and/or anguish in the heart may be seen in this pattern. Because signs of an exterior pattern are absent, Ephedra, Forsythia, and Rice Bean Decoction (*má huáng lián qiáo chì xiǎo dòu tāng*), which is used to treat a similar pattern in the next line, is not used.

Gardenia (*zhī zǐ*) resolves anguish and vexation in the heart and depressed heat bind. It discharges fire from all three burners and opens and regulates the waterways; hence it is commonly used in damp-heat patterns with yellowing. Bitter and cold, phellodendron (*huáng bǎi*) clears heat, dries dampness, and abates yellow.

Licorice (*gān cǎo*), which harmonizes the center burner, moderates the effect of the bitter, cold agents so that they do not damage the spleen and stomach. When the heat is cleared and the dampness is eliminated, the functions of the spleen and stomach will return to normal and the yellowing will resolve.

LINE 262

伤寒瘀热在里，身必黄，麻黄连轺赤小豆汤主之。
Shāng hán yū rè zài lǐ, shēn bì huáng, má huáng lián qiáo chì xiǎo dòu tāng zhǔ zhī.

In cold damage with stasis heat in the interior, there will be generalized yellowing; Ephedra, Forsythia, and Rice Bean Decoction (*má huáng lián qiáo chì xiǎo dòu tāng*) governs.

FORMULA
Ephedra, Forsythia, and Rice Bean Decoction (*má huáng lián qiáo chì xiǎo dòu tāng*)

∘ Resolve the exterior and dissipate the evil; clear heat and eliminate dampness in order to abate yellow.

麻黄二两（去节） 连轺二两（连翘根是） 杏仁四十个（去皮尖） 赤小豆一升 大枣十二枚（擘）生梓白皮（切）一升 生姜二两（切） 甘草二两（炙）。

右八味，以潦水一斗，先煮麻黄再沸，去上沫，内诸药，煮取三升，去滓，分温三服，半日服尽。

Má huáng èr liǎng (qù jié) lián qiáo èr liǎng (lián qiáo gēn shì) xìng rén sì shí ge (qù pí jiān) chì xiǎo dòu yī shēng dà zǎo shí èr méi (bò) shēng zǐ bái pí (qiē) yī shēng shēng jiāng èr liǎng (qiē) gān cǎo èr liǎng (zhì)

Yòu bā wèi, yǐ liáo shuǐ yī dǒu, xiān zhǔ má huáng zài fèi, qù shàng mò, nà zhū yào, zhǔ qǔ sān shēng, qù zǐ, fēn wēn sān fú, bàn rì fú jìn.

ephedra (麻黄 *má huáng*, Ephedrae Herba) 2 liǎng (remove nodes)
forsythia (连翘 *lián qiáo*, Forsythiae Fructus) 2 liǎng (forsythia root (连翘根 *lián qiáo gēn*, Forsythiae Radix))*
apricot kernel (杏仁 *xìng rén*, Armeniacae Semen) 40 pieces (remove skin and tips)
rice bean (赤小豆 *chì xiǎo dòu*, Phaseoli Calcarati Semen) 1 shēng
jujube (大枣 *dà zǎo*, Ziziphi Fructus) 12 pieces (broken)
raw catalpa bark (梓白皮 *zǐ bái pí*, Catalpae Cortex) 1 shēng (cut)
fresh ginger (生姜 *shēng jiāng*, Zingiberis Rhizoma Recens) 2 liǎng (cut)
mix-fried licorice (甘草 *gān cǎo*, Glycyrrhizae Radix) 2 liǎng

[For] the above eight ingredients use one dǒu of rain water. First boil ephedra (*má huáng*), then boil again and remove the foam [collecting] on top. Add all [the other] medicinals and boil to get three shēng. Remove the dregs, divide into three [parts], and take warm. Finish [the decoction] in half a day.

FORMULA NOTE

* forsythia root (连翘根 *lián qiáo gēn*, Forsythiae Radix): Although this parenthetical appears to indicate forsythia root, in modern practice the fruit of the plant is used.

SYNOPSIS

The signs and treatment of yáng yellowing with an exterior pattern.

COMMENTARY

As in preceding lines, generalized yellowing occurs in a cold damage pattern. Zhāng Jī reminds us of the pathomechanism involved when he writes "stasis heat in the interior." Nonetheless, in this line he does not use Capillaris Decoction (*yīn chén hāo tāng*) or Gardenia and Phellodendron Decoction (*zhī zǐ bǎi pí tāng*), and instead suggests Ephedra, Forsythia, and Rice Bean Decoction (*má huáng lián qiáo chì xiǎo dòu tāng*). From this formula one can conclude that signs of an exterior pattern (such as aversion to cold and heat effusion) are present and sweating is absent. This pattern is a combination of an unresolved exterior pattern and stasis heat in the interior.

Ephedra (*má huáng*) and fresh ginger (*shēng jiāng*) are acrid and warm agents that promote sweating, and diffuse and dissipate exterior evils. Bitter, warm apricot kernel (*xìng rén*) is used to disinhibit lung qì. By diffusing and downbearing the lung qì, the exterior evil is coursed and dissipated. Forsythia (*lián qiáo*) and catalpa bark (*zǐ bái pí*) are bitter and cold. They clear and disinhibit damp-heat. Rice bean (*chì xiǎo dòu*) clears heat, eliminates dampness, and disinhibits the urine. Used together, these three agents abate yellow by clearing heat and disinhibiting dampness. In modern formulae many people substitute mulberry root bark (*sāng bái pí*) for catalpa bark (*zǐ bái pí*). Licorice (*gān cǎo*) and jujube (*dà zǎo*) harmonize and boost the center burner, thereby improving movement and transformation, which helps to eliminate dampness and redistribute the fluids.

LINE 259

㈠ 伤寒发汗已，身目为黄，所以然者，以寒湿在里不解故也。㈡ 以为不可下也， 于寒湿中求之。

(1) *Shāng hán fā hàn yǐ, shēn mù wéi huáng, suǒ yǐ rán zhě, yǐ hán shī zài lǐ bù jiě gù yě.* (2) *Yǐ wéi bù kě xià yě, yú hán shī zhōng qiú zhī.*

(1) In cold damage, sweating has been promoted and [there is] generalized yellowing, including the eyes. Why [this] is so is because [there is] unresolved cold-damp in the interior. (2) It is assumed that [in this siutation] one cannot precipitate, [but should] seek [to treat the disease by addressing] cold and dampness.

Synopsis

The signs, treatment, and contraindications for damp-cold yellowing.

Commentary

In cold damage the promotion of sweating often resolves the disease. In this line it does not resolve the disease and generalized yellowing occurs. Zhāng Jī explains that it occurs because of unresolved cold-damp in the interior that may be the result of the inappropriate use of sweating damaging the center burner or it may reflect a constitutional weakness. In either case cold-damp is present in the greater yīn and produces generalized yellowing. This pattern is considered yīn yellow and the color is not the bright yellow seen in yáng brightness disease with damp-heat. It is instead a dark yellow or dusky yellow color. Yīn yellow patterns are generally not accompanied by heat effusion, vexation, or thirst.

Because this is a pattern of cold-damp in the interior, one must not use precipitation because its use would further damage the spleen and stomach, which are already weak in this pattern. Zhāng Jī suggests that one should instead treat this pattern by addressing the cold and dampness. Although Zhāng Jī does not give an indication of a formula here, it is likely that the treatment would involve warming the center, dissipating cold, and eliminating dampness to abate yellow.

Line 195

㈠ 阳明病，脉迟，食难用饱，饱则微烦头眩，必小便难，此欲作谷瘅。㈡ 虽下之，腹满如故，所以然者，脉迟故也。

(1) *Yáng míng bìng, mài chí, shí nán yòng bǎo, bǎo zé wēi fán tóu xuàn, bì xiǎo biàn nán, cǐ yù zuò gǔ dǎn.* (2) *Suī xià zhī, fù mǎn rú gù, suǒ yǐ rán zhě, mài chí gù yě.*

(1) When in yáng brightness disease the pulse is slow, [there is] difficulty eating to satiation,[1] and after satiation [there is] mild vexation and dizzy head, there will be difficult urination; this means grain jaundice[2] is about to occur. (2) Although precipitation [has been used], [there is] abdominal fullness as before, and it is this way because the pulse is slow.

Text Notes

1. Difficulty eating to satiation, 食难用饱 *shí nán yòng bǎo*: Here, 用 *yòng* means to eat and 饱 *bǎo* refers to satiation. Thus, although the patient is able to eat, he/she has difficulty satisfying the appetite and reaching satiation.
2. Grain jaundice, 谷瘅 *gǔ dǎn*: In this phrase 瘅 *dǎn* is equivalent to 疸 *dǎn*. This term means jaundice that is the result of improper dietary intake.

Synopsis

The signs and contraindications for yáng brightness disease with cold in the center burner when grain jaundice is about to occur.

Commentary

In yáng brightness disease, the pulse may be slow in two different patterns. In bowel repletion patterns, as described in line 208, p. 356, severe stagnation of dry stool can impede the flow of qì and make the pulse slow. In that situation tidal heat effusion, delirious speech, fullness and pain in the abdomen, and bound stool should also be present and precipitation is the appropriate treatment. In the present line, the pulse is also slow. Here, however, abdominal fullness reflects cold-damp congesting the center burner, which precipitation would naturally fail to resolve; consequently, we may assume that the pulse is not only slow, but probably also forceless.

In a yáng brightness disease with cold-damp in the interior, a pulse that is slow indicates yáng vacuity of the spleen and stomach. The patient is unable to eat to a point of feeling satisfied. If in an attempt to reach satiation the patient continues to eat, vexation and dizziness occur because the stomach and spleen are unable to rot and ripen the food, as well as to move and transform the digestate. The presence of non-transformed food gives rise to cold turbidity, which impairs normal upbearing and downbearing. The clear and the turbid are not separated, and the clear yáng cannot ascend. Yīn evils exploit this vacuity and cause dizziness and vexation. Because downbearing is also impaired, turbid yīn remains in the center, causing abdominal fullness. Fullness that is the result of collected turbid yīn in the center is generally not hard, only full. When the center burner is congested and movement and transformation is impaired, fluids do not move correctly and urination becomes difficult. Zhāng Jī writes that in this pattern, with cold-damp congested in the center burner, grain jaundice will occur if no treatment is given. That is, the conditions for jaundice already exist, but if one treats properly and quickly it may be avoided.

4.2 Blood Heat Patterns

Yáng brightness disease generally belongs to dryness-heat, but because yáng brightness has copious qì and blood, patterns involving the blood may also be observed. Blood-aspect patterns are the result of one of the following processes: dryness-heat entering the blood aspect, enduring static blood combining with heat, or dryness-heat entering the blood chamber. Each of these processes results in different patterns, as described above.

Line 202

阳明病，口燥，但欲漱水，不欲咽者，此必衄。

Yáng míng bìng, kǒu zào, dàn yù shù shuǐ, bù yù yān zhě, cǐ bì nǜ.

When in yáng brightness disease [there is] dry mouth and only a desire to rinse the mouth with water, [but] no desire to swallow, there will be spontaneous external bleeding.

Synopsis

A spontaneous external bleeding pattern that is the result of a yáng brightness heat evil entering the blood aspect.

Commentary

Generally, in yáng brightness disease, exuberant internal dryness-heat damages the fluids and causes great thirst, which is often unquenchable. That is considered a pattern of qì-aspect heat. In this case the mouth is dry, but the patient only desires to rinse the mouth with water and does not desire to swallow or to drink large amounts of water. When the heat enters the blood aspect, it steams the blood, forcing the construction-yīn to spread outwards. This movement does not represent the normal movement of yīn humor, but through it some fluids reach the mouth and the severity of the thirst is reduced. One should be careful not to misjudge the severity of the internal heat simply because the thirst is not severe.

When heat enters the blood aspect it may cause spontaneous external bleeding, because the heat causes reckless movement of the blood and damages the channels and network vessels. Spontaneous external bleeding may manifest as blood ejection, bloody stool, macular eruptions, disturbances of the menstrual cycle, or as other types of bleeding.

Line 227

脉浮发热，口干鼻燥，能食者则衄。

Mài fú fā rè, kǒu gān bí zào, néng shí zhě zé nǜ.

When the pulse is floating and [there is] heat effusion, dry mouth and nose, and [the person] can eat, [there will be] spontaneous external bleeding.

Synopsis

Spontaneous external bleeding that is the result of yáng brightness qì aspect exuberant heat stirring the blood.

Commentary

In greater yáng disease one may see a pulse that is floating and heat effusion, but one would also expect aversion to cold. In this pattern, although the pulse is floating and heat effusion is observed, aversion to cold is absent, and one may instead see aversion to heat, reflecting the presence of heat in the yáng brightness qì aspect. Because the yáng brightness channel is distributed to the nose and mouth, when the heat rises (as heat has a tendency to do) it follows the channel upward and causes dryness in the nose and mouth.

This patient is able to eat, indicating that the qì-aspect heat, although exuberant, has not entered the yáng brightness bowel and formed repletion bind. The patient can eat normally because food intake is not impaired by a replete evil in the bowel. In qì-aspect heat patterns, spontaneous external bleeding is generally absent, but here bleeding is observed, indicating that although qì-aspect heat is still present, the heat has entered the blood aspect, causing frenetic movement of the blood. The presence of heat effusion and a pulse that is floating means that the yáng brightness qì-aspect heat has not been eliminated and heat exists in both the qì and blood aspects. If the heat completely enters the blood aspect, the pulse should not be floating and no heat effusion should be present.

Line 216

阳明病，下血谵语者，此为热入血室，但头汗出者，刺期门，随其实而写之，濈然汗出则愈。

Yáng míng bìng, xià xuè zhān yǔ zhě, cǐ wéi rè rù xuè shì, dàn tóu hàn chū zhě, cì qī mén, suí qí shí ér xiè zhī, jí rán hàn chū zé yù.

When in yáng brightness disease [there is] blood descent and delirious speech, this means that heat has entered the blood chamber;[1] if sweat issues only from the head, needle Cycle Gate (*qī mén,* LR-14) to address the repletion by draining.[2] Streaming sweat will bring recovery.

Text Notes

1. Blood chamber, 血室 *xuè shì*:
   a) Zhāng Jǐng-Yuè (张景岳) suggests that the uterus is the blood chamber, but he also writes, "The blood chamber [includes] the thoroughfare vessel, the controlling vessel, the sea of blood, and the blood aspect." (From *Shāng Hán Lùn Yán Jiū Dà Cí Diǎn.*)
   b) Kē Qín writes, "The liver is the blood chamber. The liver is the viscus that stores the blood; hence it is called the blood chamber."
   c) Chéng Wú-Jǐ writes, "The blood chamber of the body is the thoroughfare vessel."

   Although these definitions may seem contradictory and confusing, they perhaps offer a perspective in which one can see the blood chamber as a reference to all of the places in the body involved in the movement and storage of blood. As Shěn Jīn-Áo (沈金鳌, style 芊绿 Qiān-Lǜ) writes, "So with regards to theories of the blood chamber, Chéng [Wú-Jǐ] indicates the thoroughfare vessel, [while] Kē [Qín] indicates the liver. Although there is a difference [between these] two theories, in reality they are similar. In indicating the thoroughfare vessel [Chéng] refers to the source. In indicating the liver [Kē] refers to the storehouse. Blood must exit from the source. Without the source, [there is] no root. Blood must gather in the storehouse. If it does not gather, it becomes dissipated." This perspective allows one to reconcile these views and create a broad definition.
2. Draining, 写 *xiè*: Same as 泻 *xiè*.

Synopsis

The signs and treatment of heat entering the blood chamber in yáng brightness disease.

Commentary

In some cases, delirious speech in yáng brightness disease indicates bowel repletion. In this case not only is delirious speech observed, but also blood descent. Delirious speech, when accompanied by uterine bleeding or rectal bleeding, indicates heat has entered the blood chamber. Delirious speech in bowel repletion is generally accompanied by abdominal fullness and pain, absence of defecation, tidal heat effusion, or other typical signs. When yáng brightness heat is exuberant and it enters the blood aspect, it may cause spontaneous external bleeding. In this case it enters the blood chamber (i.e., the liver, thoroughfare vessel, or the uterus) because of a pre-existing vacuity condition. When the blood is sufficient, the heat may damage the vessels, but it is not said to enter the blood chamber. If vacuity exists, as a result of irregular menstruation, bleeding hemorrhoids, or some other condition of bleeding, the heat may exploit the vacuity and enter the blood chamber. Heat in the blood aspect rises and disturbs the spirit, causing delirious speech. As the heat rises it steams the fluids, forcing them upward and resulting in sweating on the head.

The use of Cycle Gate (*qī mén,* LR-14) to drain the repletion heat in the blood aspect may be viewed in several ways. If one considers that the blood chamber is the liver, then the use of a liver channel point offers a direct way to drain blood heat. If, however, one considers the thoroughfare vessel or the uterus as the blood chamber, one must use a different logic to understand the point selection. Because the liver governs the storage of blood, liver channel points can be used to influence the blood, even if the problem is not in the liver itself. Furthermore, as will be seen in later lines, heat in the blood chamber is often accompanied by tense, hard, binding pain in the lesser abdomen or chest and under the rib-side. The liver channel passes through these regions; therefore, Cycle Gate (*qī mén,* LR-14) can be used for these accompanying signs as well.

Heat entering the blood chamber occurs in three other places in the text. In all of those it refers to women whose menstrual cycles are disturbed after contraction of an exterior evil. Commentators disagree as to whether this line refers only to women or includes men, because it is not clearly stated. Yù Chāng makes the point that because in the other three lines, it is clearly specified through the use of the word "women," 妇人 *fù rén*, that the disease primarily affects women, this line may refer only to men. Zhāng Zhì-Cōng suggests that this line includes diseases of both men and women.

Line 237

㈠ 阳明证，其人喜忘者，必有蓄血。㈡ 所以然者，本有久瘀血，故令喜忘，屎虽硬，大便反易，其色必黑者，宜抵当汤下之。

(1) *Yáng míng zhèng, qí rén xǐ wàng zhě, bì yǒu xù xuè.* (2) *Suǒ yǐ rán zhě, běn yǒu jiǔ yū xuè, gù lìng xǐ wàng, shǐ suī yìng, dà biàn fǎn yì, qí sè bì hēi zhě, yí dǐ dàng tāng xià zhī.*

(1) When in a yáng brightness disease the person is forgetful, there will be blood amassment. (2) Why [this is] so is because originally there was enduring blood amassment, thus causing forgetfulness and stool, that although hard, is nevertheless easy to pass, and that will be black in color. It is appropriate to precipitate with Dead-On Decoction (*dǐ dàng tāng*).

SYNOPSIS

The signs and treatment of yáng brightness blood amassment.

COMMENTARY

In this case of yáng brightness blood amassment, heat evil binds with old static blood. The principal signs are forgetfulness, and hard black stool that is easy to expel. The heart governs the blood and the vessels, as well as the spirit. When static blood and heat contend, it affects the heart spirit and in this case causes forgetfulness. A basis for this can be found in the *Sù Wèn*, in which it is written, "[When] the blood and qì are not gathered [in any one area], the five viscera are quiet and stable. [When] blood gathers in the upper [body] and qì gathers in the lower body, [there will be] heart vexation, oppression, and frequent anger. [When] blood gathers in the lower [body] and qì gathers in the upper body, [there will be] derangement and forgetfulness." In this case the blood, gathered in the lower body, affects the stool and causes forgetfulness.

The combination of static blood and internal heat causes the stool to become hard and black. Internal heat damages the fluids, making the stool hard and darkening the blood through its steaming action. This static dark blood turns the stool black. It should be noted that black stool can be seen in patterns without blood heat. When bowel repletion with bound stool is present over a long period of time, the stool may become black from the scorching action of the internal heat; but it will be hard to expel because the intestines will have been dried by the heat. In this case the stool is hard, but easy to expel, because it is moistened by wasted static blood that has left the proper channels. Because the pathomechanism of this pattern involves static blood, Dead-On Decoction (*dǐ dàng tāng*) is used to precipitate the blood.

Blood amassment patterns are also seen in greater yáng disease. Greater yáng blood amassment is characterized by mania, by uninhibited urination, and by hardness, fullness, and pain in the lesser abdomen. In that pattern heat evil enters the interior and contends with the blood, creating stasis; it does not involve enduring static blood. Nonetheless, both involve blood amassment; therefore, Dead-On Decoction (*dǐ dàng tāng*) is used for both. In greater yáng disease the differentiation of blood amassment is made on the basis of whether the urine is uninhibited and whether the patient is manic. In yáng brightness patterns the differentiation is made on the basis of whether the stool is black and easy to expel.

LINE 257

(一) 病人无表里证，发热七八日，虽脉浮数者，可下之。(二) 假令已下，脉数不解，合热则消谷善饥，至六七日，不大便者，有瘀血，宜抵当汤。

(1) *Bìng rén wú biǎo lǐ zhèng, fā rè qī bā rì, suī mài fú shuò zhě, kě xià zhī.* (2) *Jiǎ lìng yǐ xià, mài shuò bù jiě, hé rè zé xiāo gǔ shàn jī, zhì liù qì rì, bù dà biàn zhě, yǒu yū xuè, yí dǐ dàng tāng.*

(1) When the person has neither an exterior nor an interior pattern and has heat effusion for seven or eight days, although the pulse is floating and rapid, one can precipitate. (2) If precipitation has already [been used] and the pulse is [still] rapid, having not resolved, the heat has combined [with the blood], so [there is] swift digestion and rapid hungering, and inability to defecate for six or seven days, [which means that there is] static blood; [therefore,] Dead-On Decoction (*dǐ dàng tāng*) is appropriate.

SYNOPSIS

a) The differentiation of yáng brightness organ repletion and static blood patterns.

b) The signs and treatment of static blood patterns.

COMMENTARY

This patient has neither the aversion to cold, headache, and stiff neck characteristic of greater yáng exterior patterns, nor the tidal heat effusion, delirious speech, and abdominal fullness characteristic of yáng brightness internal repletion patterns. Heat effusion and a pulse that is rapid and floating are observed. Because Zhāng Jī writes that one can precipitate, it would appear that, although clear signs of an interior pattern are absent, the stool is bound. If the stool is bound in a yáng brightness disease one may safely use precipitation (even if the pulse is floating and rapid) as long as greater yáng signs are absent. The pulse can be interpreted as a yáng brightness pulse, indicating exuberant internal heat steaming toward the exterior and producing heat effusion.

Precipitation generally brings recovery in yáng brightness internal repletion patterns, but not in static blood patterns such as the one described in this line. In this case, after the use of precipitation, the pulse remains rapid and the disease has not resolved. The pulse is no longer floating, which means that the qì aspect heat has been eliminated; but it is still rapid, indicating that heat has entered the blood aspect and has not been eliminated through the use of cold precipitation. The heat contends with static blood and defecation does not occur for six or seven days. This disturbance of bowel function is the result not of dry stool blocking the intestines, but of the contention between static blood and heat; hence the patient is still able to eat and because of the internal heat, swift digestion and rapid hungering occur. Blood stasis causes congestion and when there is stoppage there is pain;

consequently, abdominal fullness, hardness, and pain may also be present. These signs may be accompanied by forgetfulness, mania, uninhibited urination, or other signs of blood amassment. Dead-On Decoction (*dǐ dàng tāng*) is used to precipitate the blood.

In the preceding line, the stool was hard, but easy to expel because of the moistening effect of vanquished blood as it left the proper channels and moved into the intestines. In this case of static blood, no stool passes for six or seven days because the blood has not left the vessels and moistened the stool. Static blood may remain in the vessels or leave the vessels. If it leaves the vessels, it can moisten the stool and allow for easy defecation. If the static blood remains in the vessels, the stool is not moistened and remains in the intestines.

Line 258

若脉数不解，而下不止，必协热便脓血也。

Ruò mài shuò bù jiě, ér xià bù zhǐ, bì xié rè biàn nóng xuè yě.

If the pulse is rapid, [the disease] has not resolved; [there is] incessant diarrhea, [and] there will be complex diarrhea with pus and blood.

Synopsis

Continuing from the preceding line, the signs and treatment of pus and blood in the stool following precipitation.

Commentary

In the preceding line, following the use of precipitation, the stool is bound and digestion is swift and accompanied by rapid hungering, indicating blood aspect heat and static blood. In this line, the pulse is also rapid, but instead of bound stool, incessant diarrhea is observed, indicating that heat has descended into the lower body. It scorches the channels, causing frenetic movement of the blood. The blood heat also steams putrid matter in the intestines with the result that pus and blood are present in the diarrhea.

5 YÁNG BRIGHTNESS DISEASE PATTERN IDENTIFICATION

5.1 Differentiation of Wind Strike and Cold Strike Patterns

Line 190

阳明病，若能食，名中风；不能食，名中寒。

Yáng míng bìng, ruò néng shí, míng zhòng fēng; bù néng shí, míng zhòng hán.

In yáng brightness disease, if [the person] is able to eat, it is called wind strike; if unable to eat, it is called cold strike.

SYNOPSIS

Using the ability to eat or inability to eat to differentiate yáng brightness wind strike and cold strike.

COMMENTARY

Yáng brightness disease may be categorized into wind strike and cold strike. The state of stomach and intestinal function often helps to determine which of these patterns is present. When these functions are normal, food intake and digestion are both normal; hence ability or inability to eat may be used to evaluate the exuberance or debilitation of the stomach and intestinal yáng, the presence of heat or cold in the stomach and intestines, and the strength or weakness of the stomach and intestinal qì.

Wind is a yáng evil and governs movement. When wind attacks the yáng brightness, the stomach yáng is roused and the patient is able to eat. This effect may be seen in three different situations. When the wind evil is mild, food intake may be normal. When the wind evil is severe, the patient eats less than a normal patient, but more than a patient with cold in the stomach. When an evil transforms to heat, swift digestion and rapid hungering occur. Often the patient eats large amounts of food, but remains thin or even loses weight. This pattern, known as dispersion-thirst, belongs to miscellaneous diseases, not externally contracted diseases. On the other hand, cold, a yīn evil, governs stillness; hence cold in the stomach and intestines causes debilitation of the yáng qì, loss of appetite, and inability to eat.

This line describes the basic differences between wind and cold patterns. However, both wind and cold patterns vary considerably. Patterns may be observed in which a patient with an exuberant yáng evil in the stomach cannot eat owing to congestion of the stomach and intestinal qì. Conversely, when the stomach yáng is debilitated, the patient may still able to eat, indicating that the yáng qì is not completely vacuous.

LINE 191

㈠ 阳明病，若中寒者，不能食，小便不利，手足濈然汗出，此欲作固瘕，必大便初硬后溏。㈡ 所以然者，以胃中冷，水谷不别故也。

(1) *Yáng míng bìng, ruò zhòng hán zhě, bù néng shí, xiǎo biàn bù lì, shǒu zú jí rán hàn chū, cǐ yù zuò gù jiǎ, bì dà biàn chū yìng hòu táng.* (2) *Suǒ yǐ rán zhě, yǐ wèi zhōng lěng, shuǐ gǔ bù bié gù yě.*

(1) In yáng brightness disease, if it is cold strike and [there is] inability to eat, uninhibited urination, and sweat streaming from the extremities, this means that [there is] about to be a firm conglomeration[1] and there will be stool that is first hard and then sloppy. (2) Why [this is] so is

because [there is] cold in the stomach and no separation of water and grain.[2]

TEXT NOTES

1. [There is] about to be a firm conglomeration, 欲作固瘕 *yù zuò gù jiǎ*: The preconditions for this pattern exist and it will soon follow. A firm conglomeration is an abdominal mass of indefinite form and one of four kinds of abdominal masses associated with pain and distention. Conglomerations are masses of indefinite form that gather and dissipate at irregular intervals and are attended by pain of unfixed location. They are attributed to disease in the bowels and qì aspect. The other types are concretions, accumulations, and gatherings.
2. No separation of water and grain, 水谷不别 *shuǐ gǔ bù bié*: Food and water are not being clearly separated in the stool, so non-transformed food is mixed with water in the stool.

SYNOPSIS

A yáng brightness disease with cold strike, in which a firm conglomeration is about to occur.

COMMENTARY

In yáng brightness disease, constitutional yáng vacuity or attack by cold evil may manifest as cold strike. When the center burner is cold, the yáng qì of the spleen and stomach becomes weak, food intake and transformation are disturbed, and the patient is unable to eat. When the spleen and stomach are weak, water enters the stomach, but cannot be properly transformed and moved to other areas of the body. Because the spleen and stomach govern the extremities, when the spleen is unable to move and transform fluids properly, streaming sweat may issue from the extremities while fluid that should be distributed throughout the body instead moves to the limbs. Fluid is also not transported properly to the bladder, so urination becomes inhibited. In cases where the spleen and stomach functions are disturbed by cold, food is not transformed, cold congeals in the center burner, and a firm conglomeration may form. If the stool continues to be expelled, the mass will not form; but if the stool becomes blocked, it is likely that a firm conglomeration will form. The stool is hard at first and then sloppy, indicating that the stomach is cold. The functions of the spleen and stomach are abnormal, and the clear and turbid are no longer separated, but mixed in the stool; therefore, water and non-transformed food are present in the stool.

LINE 197

阳明病，反无汗而小便利，二三日呕而咳，手足厥者，必苦头痛；若不咳，不呕，手足不厥者，头不痛。

Yáng míng bìng, fǎn wú hàn ér xiǎo biàn lì, èr sān rì ǒu ér ké, shǒu zú jué zhě, bì kǔ tóu tòng; ruò bù ké, bù ǒu, shǒu zú bù jué zhě, tóu bù tòng.

When [there is] yáng brightness disease, but sweating is absent and the urine is uninhibited, and [there have been] two or three days of retching and coughing and reversal of the extremities, [the person] will suffer from a headache. If cough, retching, [and] reversal of the limbs are absent, headache [will also be] absent.

Synopsis

Yáng brightness cold strike with counterflow ascent of cold-rheum.

Commentary

Generally, in yáng brightness disease the patient sweats copiously as a result of exuberant internal dryness-heat. In the condition described in the present line, however, sweating is absent. This pattern is thefore not heat but cold-rheum amassed in the interior. Cold-rheum attacks the center, disturbs the function of the stomach and spleen, and congests the qì dynamic. Fluids cannot be transformed and no sweat issues. One might expect urination to be inhibited, but here the rheum mainly affects the center burner; consequently, although fluid transformation has been affected, the bladder still functions normally and urination is uninhibited.

As the disease continues, the damage to the stomach qì results in abnormal upbearing and downbearing. The turbid ascends and the clear descends, causing retching. Ascending turbid qì and cold-rheum may attack the lung and cause coughing, too. Damage to the stomach yáng qì can affect the limbs. The stomach governs the extremities and it is through the warming action of the yáng that the extremities remain warm and flexible. When cold-rheum damages the stomach yáng qì and causes congestion in the center burner, the clear yáng qì cannot flow out to the extremities and they become cold. In the present line, this sign is called "reversal of the extremities." When the clear yáng qì cannot flow normally, the clear orifices may also be affected, resulting in a headache.

If retching, cough, and reversal are absent, it means that although cold-rheum is present in the center burner, the flow of the yáng qì has not yet been completely disturbed. Because the evil does not ascend counterflow to attack the upper body, headache is absent.

Line 198

阳明病，但头眩，不恶寒，故能食而咳，其人咽必痛；若不咳者，咽不痛。

Yáng míng bìng, dàn tóu xuàn, bù wù hán, gù néng shí ér ké, qí rén yān bì tòng; ruò bù ké zhě, yān bù tòng.

When in yáng brightness disease, [there is] a dizzy head only without aversion to cold, [and] consequently, [the person] is able to eat, and coughs, there will be sore throat. If cough is absent, the throat will not be sore.

Synopsis

Yáng brightness wind strike with upward harassment of heat evil.

Commentary

In yáng brightness disease the absence of aversion to cold means that an exterior evil is absent and that aversion to heat is likely to be present owing to internal heat. When the patient is able to eat, the pattern belongs to wind strike. When heat in the yáng brightness rises, it may affect the stomach, heart, lungs, and head. In the pattern described in this line, only dizziness occurs and aversion to cold is absent, indicating that the heat is harassing the clear orifices of the head. Yáng brightness heat that rises may also attack the lungs. If it does, it will cause cough. The throat is the gate of the breath and if heat harasses the lung, the throat will be painful. If, however, the heat does not attack the lung and cause cough, sore throat will be absent.

Line 226

若胃中虚冷，不能食者，饮水则哕。

Ruò wèi zhōng xū lěng, bù néng shí zhě, yǐn shuǐ zé yuē.

If [there is] vacuity cold in the stomach and inability to eat, drinking water will result in hiccup.

Synopsis

A hiccup pattern as the result of vacuity cold in the stomach and water-rheum.

Commentary

The stomach governs the ingestion of food and all food and drink enters the stomach. When the stomach yáng is effulgent, normal decomposition as well as steaming and transformation can occur. The essence is then shifted to the spleen and transported to the rest of the body. In this case the stomach is vacuous and cold, and the yáng qì cannot transform food; consequently, the patient is unable to eat. If fluids are ingested, the stomach is unable to process them normally and they collect in the center burner and cause further damage to the stomach yáng, exacerbating the vacuity cold and causing abnormal upbearing and downbearing. The result of this process is hiccups.

Line 243

食谷欲呕，属阳明也，吴茱萸汤主之；得汤反剧者，属上焦也。

Shí gǔ yù ǒu, shǔ yáng míng yě, wú zhū yú tāng zhǔ zhī; dé tāng fǎn jù zhě, shǔ shàng jiāo yě.

A desire to retch [after] eating belongs to yáng brightness; Evodia Decoction (*wú zhū yú tāng*) governs. But when taking the decoction [makes the retching more] severe, this [pattern] belongs to the upper burner.

Formula

Evodia Decoction (*wú zhū yú tāng*)

∘ Warm the center and harmonize the stomach; downbear counterflow and check retching.

吴茱萸一升（洗） 人参三两 生姜六两（切） 大枣十二枚（擘）

右四味，以水七升，煮取二升，去滓，温服七合，日三服。

Wú zhū yú yī shēng (*xǐ*) *rén shēn sān liǎng* *shēng jiāng liù liǎng* (*qiē*) *dà zǎo shí èr méi* (*bò*)

Yòu sì wèi, yǐ shuǐ qī shēng, zhǔ qǔ èr shēng, qù zǐ, wēn fú qī gě, rì sān fú.

evodia (吴茱萸 *wú zhū yú*, Evodiae Fructus) 1 shēng (washed)*
ginseng (人参 *rén shēn*, Ginseng Radix) 3 liǎng
fresh ginger (生姜 *shēng jiāng*, Zingiberis Rhizoma Recens) 6 liǎng (cut)
jujube (大枣 *dà zǎo*, Ziziphi Fructus) 12 pieces (split)

[For] the above four ingredients use seven shēng of water. Boil to get two shēng, remove the dregs and take seven gě warm, three times a day.

Text Note

* Evodia (*wú zhū yú*)(washed): This medicinal is washed to reduce toxicity.

Synopsis

The differentiation of heat and cold retching counterflow.

Commentary

In many cases, a desire to retch after eating indicates heat counterflow, but on the basis of the formula used in this case, it is clear that here it does not. Evodia Decoction (*wú zhū yú tāng*) warms the center and harmonizes the stomach, it does not clear heat. This pattern is cold counterflow. When cold is present in the stomach, the yáng qì becomes vacuous and is unable to steam and transform water and food. As a result, the patient cannot eat normally since the center burner is congested and blocked. If food is ingested, it will not be properly transformed, but will meet the congestion already present and ascend counterflow, causing counterflow retching. When retching belongs to a cold turbidity pattern, as it does here, the odor or taste in the mouth is generally not rancid or putrefied, and the tongue is usually pale with a white fur. Evodia Decoction (*wú zhū yú tāng*) warms the stomach, dissipates cold, and checks retching.

If the ingestion of Evodia Decoction (*wú zhū yú tāng*) causes an exacerbation of the signs, then the pattern does not belong to the center burner, but belongs to the upper burner, and is likely a heat pattern. Heat in the upper burner can involve the upper portion of the stomach and cause a loss of normal upbearing and downbearing. This disturbance results in retching that is characterized by a sour, putrefied odor or taste in the mouth, and a red tongue with yellow fur. In this situation the use of Evodia Decoction (*wú zhū yú tāng*) constitutes using heat to treat heat, which fortifies the evil and exacerbates the retching. The appropriate treatment would be to clear heat and check retching.

Evodia Decoction (*wú zhū yú tāng*) warms and harmonizes the stomach, and downbears counterflow to check retching. Acrid, bitter, warm evodia (*wú zhū yú*) warms the stomach and dissipates cold, and downbears counterflow and checks retching; consequently, it is used in the largest amount and is considered the sovereign. The minister, fresh ginger (*shēng jiāng*), is also used in a large amount, since it diffuses and dissipates cold qì, harmonizes the stomach, and checks retching. Ginseng (*rén shēn*) and jujube (*dà zǎo*) supplement the qì of the center burner to help restore normal upbearing and downbearing.

5.2 Differentiation of Vacuity and Repletion Patterns

Line 210

㈠ 夫实则谵语，虚则郑声。㈡ 郑声者，重语也。㈢ 直视谵语，喘满者死，下利者亦死。

(1) *Fū shí zé zhān yǔ, xū zé zhèng shēng.* (2) *Zhèng shēng zhě, chóng yǔ yě.* (3) *Zhí shì zhān yǔ, chuǎn mǎn zhě sǐ, xià lì zhě yì sǐ.*

(1) Now, [as we know,] in repletion, [there is] delirious speech and in vacuity, [there is] muttering.* (2) Muttering means repetitious speech. (3) Forward-staring eyes, delirious speech, panting, and fullness [bodes] death. [If there is] diarrhea, [this] also [bodes] death.

Text Note

* Muttering, 郑声 *zhèng shēng*: Mumbling to oneself haltingly and with frequent repetitions. Muttering is a sign of dissipation of essence-spirit and is observed in yīn or yáng collapse patterns.

Synopsis

The differentiation of delirious speech occurring as muttering and delirious speech when it is a critical sign.

Commentary

Speech disorders can be seen in both repletion and vacuity patterns. Delirious speech is generally considered to be a sign of repletion because it is marked by a strident voice and deranged speech. Delirious speech is the result of exuberant heat harassing the heart spirit and it is seen in repletion heat patterns, such as yáng brightness disease or heat entering the heart construction.

Muttering is similar to delirious speech, but it is marked by a low voice and repetition, and it occurs in severe conditions in the latter stages of disease. Generally thought to be a sign of vacuity cold, muttering is often accompanied by shortness of breath, lassitude of spirit, and withered-yellow complexion. In these patterns, right qì is vacuous, the spirit is despoliated, and the heart spirit loses governance.

Delirious speech indicates exuberant internal heat harassing the heart spirit. When accompanied by forward-staring eyes, it means that severe heat has damaged yīn humor, and as a result, the essence qì is unable to ascend and nourish the eyes—a severe and dangerous disease pattern. Panting and fullness are indications that the lung and the spleen have become vacuous. Debilitated yīn humor cannot root the yáng qì. It rises up and is preparing to desert; hence these signs indicate a fatal condition. If delirious speech and forward-staring eyes are accompanied by diarrhea, it means the qì of the center burner is wasted. Yīn is debilitated and the yáng qì is deserting through the bowels; therefore, this pattern is also fatal.

Line 211

发汗多，若重发汗者，亡其阳，谵语，脉短者死，脉自和者不死。

Fā hàn duō, ruò chóng fā hàn zhě, wáng qí yáng, zhān yǔ, mài duǎn zhě sǐ, mài zì hé zhě bù sǐ.

When copious sweating is promoted, if sweating is again promoted, there will be yáng collapse and delirious speech. If the pulse is short, [the person] will die, and if the pulse spontaneously harmonizes, [the person] will live.

Synopsis

The differentiation of favorable and adverse outcomes in yáng collapse delirious speech patterns.

Commentary

When sweating is promoted, the goal is to have the patient sweat a small amount over the whole body; copious sweating is generally inappropriate because it damages yīn humor and yáng qì. If after copious sweating is induced, sweating is again promoted it will, in some cases, result in yáng collapse. When yáng collapses, the yáng qì of the heart is dissipated and becomes chaotic, causing delirious speech. Previously Zhāng Jī wrote that in vacuity patterns one often sees muttering, not delirious speech, and delirious speech in a vacuity pattern is an indication that the disease is severe and possibly life-threatening.

In the present line, the pulse is used as an indication of a positive or a negative outcome. If the pulse is short, it means that the yáng qì has collapsed, yīn humor is exhausted, and the pulse qì is unable to continue; consequently, the pulse becomes short. The interior damage is severe and it is likely that the patient will die. If the pulse is able to harmonize, it means that although the yáng qì has collapsed, yīn and blood are still not exhausted. Spontaneous harmonization of the pulse means not that the pulse spontaneously becomes moderate but that it is no longer short and rough. One should be able to feel the three positions of the pulse clearly. The pulse is not short and rough, indicating that although yīn and blood may be vacuous, they are not exhausted, and the pulse feels relatively harmonized. If this pulse is felt, it means that the patient will live.

Line 201

㈠阳明病，脉浮而紧者，必潮热，发作有时。㈡但浮者，必盗汗出。

(1) *Yáng míng bìng, mài fú ér jǐn zhě, bì cháo rè, fā zuò yǒu shí.* (2) *Dàn fú zhě, bì dào hàn chū.*

(1) When in yáng brightness disease the pulse is floating and tight, there will be tidal heat effusion that occurs periodically. (2) If [the pulse is] only floating, there will be night sweating.

Synopsis

The differentiation of signs in yáng brightness disease when the pulse is either floating and tight or only floating.

Commentary

A pulse that is floating and tight is often seen in greater yáng disease, but in the condition described in the present line, it occurs in a yáng brightness disease. It does not indicate the presence of an exterior cold evil, but is an expression of yáng brightness internal heat. Exuberant internal heat flows throughout the interior and the exterior with the result that the pulse is floating. The tightness of the pulse is an indication of a replete evil in the interior. When the pulse is floating and tight, it indicates exuberant yáng brightness heat throughout the body and a repletion evil in the interior. Yáng brightness bowel repletion with dryness bind is this type of pattern. Tidal heat effusion is generally seen in yáng brightness repletion patterns. The periodicity of the heat effusion occurs because of the periods of the day in which the yáng brightness is exuberant.

If the pulse is not tight, but only floating, it indicates exuberant yáng brightness heat without interior repletion bind. With exuberant heat in the interior, but no repletion, night sweating occurs instead of tidal heat effusion. Night sweating, although generally associated with yīn vacuity, can also be a sign of exuberant internal heat forcing the fluids out to the exterior. See also line 268, p. 448, for another example of night sweating that occurs as the result of exuberant internal heat.

Line 245

㈠脉阳微而汗出少者，为自和也；汗出多者，为太过。㈡阳脉实，因发其汗，出多者，亦为太过。㈢太过者，为阳绝于里，亡津液，大便因硬也。

(1) *Mài yáng wēi ér hàn chū shǎo zhě, wéi zì hé yě; hàn chū duō zhě, wéi tài guò.* (2) *Yáng mài shí, yīn fā qí hàn, chū duō zhě, yì wéi tài guò.* (3) *Tài guò zhě, wéi yáng jué yú lǐ, wáng jīn yè, dà biàn yīn yìng yě.*

(1) When the yáng pulse is faint[1] and scanty sweat issues, [the exterior] spontaneously harmonizes; when copious sweat issues, this is excess. (2) When the yáng pulse is replete,[2] it is because sweating was promoted and issued copiously and that is excess. (3) Excess means cut-off yáng[3] in the interior and liquid and humor collapse, and accordingly, the stool is hard.

TEXT NOTES

1. Yáng pulse is faint, 脉阳微 *mài yáng wēi*: The pulse is floating, vacuous, and forceless. In the original text, this pulse description appears as 脉阳微 *mài yáng wēi*, but it is generally accepted that it should read 阳脉微 *yáng mài wēi*, especially in view of the presence in the same line of 阳脉实 *yáng mài shí*.
2. Yáng pulse is replete, 阳脉实 *yáng mài shí*: The pulse is floating, exuberant, and forceful.
3. Cut-off yáng, 阳绝 *yáng jué*: Yáng is separated from yīn because yīn is exhausted. 绝 *jué*, often used to mean expiry, here does not mean yáng exhaustion, but the separation of yáng as a result of yīn exhaustion.

SYNOPSIS

The mechanism and distinguishing signs of liquid damage and cut-off yáng in the interior.

COMMENTARY

When the yáng pulse is floating and vacuous, it indicates that right qì is vacuous and evil qì is not severe. This represents a pattern of exterior vacuity in which the exterior harmonizes when mild sweat issues, and the disease resolves, but if sweating is copious, the yáng qì will be damaged, and therefore it is considered excessive. Zhāng Jī repeatedly stresses the point that sweat should only issue slightly, making the entire surface of the body moist.

When the yáng pulse is floating and exuberant, it indicates a greater yáng exterior repletion. In this pattern the promotion of sweating is appropriate, but if sweat issues copiously and a large amount of fluid is discharged from the exterior of the body, the fluids may collapse. When the fluids collapse, the intestines are not moistened and the stool becomes hard. Furthermore, when yīn fluids collapse, yáng is isolated in the interior, a situation described in the text as "cut-off yáng in the interior." This pattern should not be understood as yáng collapse or yáng expiry, but as the separation of yáng from yīn that occurs in the absence of sufficient yīn.

LINE 246

脉浮而芤，浮为阳，芤为阴，浮芤相搏，胃气生热，其阳则绝。

Mài fú ér kōu, fú wéi yáng, kōu wéi yīn, fú kōu xiāng bó, wèi qì shēng rè, qí yáng zé jué.

When the pulse is floating and scallion-stalk,* floating is yáng and scallion-stalk is yīn. The floating and scallion-stalk [qualities] are [indicative of heat and vacuity] in mutual contention; the stomach qì engenders heat and yáng will then be cut off.

Text Note

* The pulse is floating and scallion-stalk, 脉浮而芤 *mài fú ér kōu*: Floating means that the pulse can be felt with light pressure and scallion-stalk means that it feels empty inside.

Synopsis

Continuing from the preceding line, another analysis of the pulse and signs of stomach heat with debilitation of liquid.

Commentary

In greater yáng disease a floating quality in the pulse indicates an exterior pattern, but in yáng brightness disease it can indicate exuberant internal heat. A scallion-stalk quality generally indicates loss of blood or yīn-blood vacuity. Qián Huáng writes, "Floating indicates an exuberant yáng evil. Scallion-stalk indicates vacuity of yīn and blood." This line presents yáng brightness disease with a pulse that is floating and scallion-stalk. When exuberant yáng brightness heat is present, as indicated by the floating quality, heat is engendered in the stomach. Vacuity of yīn and blood is also present, as indicated by the scallion-stalk quality. The heat and the vacuity are in contention, just as the qualities of the pulse are said to be in contention. When yáng heat is exuberant and yīn is vacuous, yīn humor is insufficient to harmonize the yáng, which becomes isolated in the interior.

This line presents an exuberant yáng evil heat contending with vacuous yīn. Yáng is exuberant and cannot be balanced by yīn; hence it is said to be cut off from yīn. In the preceding line, excessive sweating depleted yīn, and yáng was then relatively exuberant compared to yīn. In that situation yáng is also considered to be isolated from yīn.

In both this line and the preceding line, the term "cut-off yáng," 阳绝 *yáng jué*, can be understood in two ways. When yīn is exhausted, yáng is no longer balanced by yīn and it is cut off or isolated. Nonetheless, one can take this one step further and conclude that when yáng is cut off from yīn, yáng expiry will follow because when the yīn is exhausted, yáng has no root and may then expire.

Line 196

阳明病，法多汗，反无汗，其身如虫行皮中状者，此以久虚故也。

Yáng míng bìng, fǎ duō hàn, fǎn wú hàn, qí shēn rú chóng xíng pí zhōng zhuàng zhě, cǐ yǐ jiǔ xū gù yě.

In yáng brightness disease, there should be copious sweating; but sweating is absent and the person has a feeling of worms moving in the skin,* because of enduring vacuity.

Text Note

* Feeling of worms moving in the skin, 身如虫行皮中状 *shēn rú chóng xíng pí zhōng zhuàng*: A generalized feeling of itching, as if small insects are scratching under the skin.

Synopsis

A yáng brightness disease in which sweating is absent because the person has enduring fluid vacuity.

Commentary

When a person who is generally healthy contracts yáng brightness disease, copious sweat will issue because of the copious blood and qì in the yáng brightness. Exuberant dryness-heat in the yáng brightness steams the fluids and forces them to the exterior, resulting in copious sweating. If, however, the qì and blood are vacuous, the fluids will be insufficient to allow sweating. Dryness-heat steams in the interior, but if the source of transformation is insufficient, no sweat issues, as in the case presented in this line. When the heat evil cannot outthrust and instead becomes depressed in the fleshy exterior, it causes generalized itching, which here is described as like a feeling of insects scratching in the skin.

Line 23, p. 122, presents a pattern of greater yáng disease with generalized itching. Sweating is promoted, but issues incompletely. The evil becomes depressed in the fleshy exterior, giving rise to generalized itching. Because the itching is the result of incomplete sweating, the treatment is to promote mild sweating. In this pattern, greater yáng signs are absent. Sweating does not occur not because it was promoted incompletely, but because of enduring vacuity. One cannot promote sweating further because the fluids are insufficient. Here, the appropriate treatment is to clear heat, boost the qì, and engender liquid.

It should be noted that yáng brightness patterns without sweating may result from an unresolved greater yáng disease or damp-heat, and the absence of sweating should not be considered an unequivocal indication of enduring vacuity.

6 CHAPTER APPENDIX

Line 192

阳明病，初欲食，小便反不利，大便自调，其人骨节疼，翕翕如有热状，奄然发狂，濈然汗出而解者，此水不胜谷气，与汗共并，脉紧则愈。

Yáng míng bìng, chū yù shí, xiǎo biàn fǎn bù lì, dà biàn zì tiáo, qí rén gǔ jié téng, xì xì rú yǒu rè zhuàng, yān rán fā kuáng, jí rán hàn chū ér jiě zhě, cǐ shuǐ bù shèng gǔ qì, yǔ hàn gòng bìng, mài jǐn zé yù.

When in yáng brightness disease [there is] initially desire to eat, but urination is inhibited and defecation is regulated, the person will have joint pain, feather-warmth as if there were heat, sudden mania, streaming sweat, and then [the disease will] resolve. The water [evil] cannot overcome grain qì, and combines with sweat [and issues outward]. [When] the pulse is tight, [there will be] recovery.

SYNOPSIS

The pulse and signs of yáng brightness disease in which dampness is depressed in the exterior and struggle between the right and evil leads to recovery.

COMMENTARY

The background for this line may be found in line 190, p. 382, and line 191, p. 383. According to line 190, when a patient with yáng brightness disease can eat, it is called wind strike and when the patient cannot eat it is called cold strike. In line 191, a patient with cold strike disease develops a firm conglomeration. Here, at the beginning of a yáng brightness disease, the patient can eat; therefore, this pattern belongs to wind strike and the stomach qì is still strong. Defecation is well-regulated; hence internal repletion bind is absent. If urination were uninhibited, dampness would be expelled through the urine; but here, urination is inhibited and dampness collects in the interior. Because damp evil is stimulated by wind evil, it becomes depressed in the exterior and pours into the fleshy exterior and the joints, causing joint pain. According to *Sù Wèn*, "Yáng brightness is the sea of the five viscera and six bowels. It governs the moistening of the ancestral sinews, which leash the bones and keep the joints [moving] freely." In the present case, joint pain is explained by the presence of dampness with an inhibition of the ancestral sinews.

Dampness collected in the interior that is neither discharged to the exterior nor expelled through the urine becomes depressed in the exterior. It transforms into heat and produces a heat effusion pattern similar to feather-warm heat effusion. This pattern is different from feather-warm heat effusion that occurs in greater yáng disease, which is the result of wind-cold fettering the exterior and causing defense and construction to become unregulated. In greater yáng disease the pulse is generally floating, and other signs such as headache and neck pain may also be observed. Here, the heat effusion is the result of depressed damp evil in the fleshy exterior; consequently, the pulse may not be floating and aversion to cold is absent.

The patient's stomach qì is still strong and no internal bind exists. The right and evil qì contend fiercely and the heart spirit becomes chaotic, leading to mania. This mania is different from that which occurs in blood amassment or dryness bind patterns. In those patterns, mania is accompanied by other signs indicating the internal condition. Blood amassment and dryness bind patterns do not generally resolve spontaneously, whereas in this line, mania is a positive transmutation. Following a short period of mania, sweat issues and the disease resolves. Sweating means that right qì overcomes the damp evil, which is diffused and discharged through the mechanism of sweating. A pulse that is tight reflects the contention between the right and evil qì. It is a sign that the right qì has been roused and has the strength to expel evil qì. This pulse is an indication that the patient is moving toward recovery, and once the disease resolves the pulse should become moderate and harmonious.

Line 218

伤寒四五日，脉沉而喘满，沉为在里，而反发其汗，津液越出，大便为难，表虚里实，久则谵语。

Shāng hán sì wǔ rì, mài chén ér chuǎn mǎn, chén wéi zài lǐ, ér fǎn fā qí hàn, jīn yè yuè chū, dà biàn wéi nán, biǎo xū lǐ shí, jiǔ zé zhān yǔ.

When in cold damage for four or five days the pulse is sunken and [there is] panting and fullness, sunken means the [disease] is in the interior, but sweating is promoted [so] liquid and humor stray outward and defecation is difficult, [creating] exterior vacuity and interior repletion, [which when] persisting, [give rise to] delirious speech.

Synopsis

A pattern of interior repletion in which sweating is inappropriately promoted and causes difficult stool and delirious speech.

Commentary

Panting and fullness may be the result of an evil fettering the exterior or congested qì in the interior. Typically, in exterior patterns, it is accompanied by aversion to cold and heat effusion, whereas in interior patterns it is accompanied by aversion to heat and bound stool. When panting occurs with fullness in exterior patterns, the fullness is generally in the chest, and the pulse should be floating. When panting occurs with fullness in interior patterns, the fullness is generally in the abdomen and the pulse should be sunken. In this line, panting and fullness are observed and the pulse is sunken, indicating an interior disease. The promotion of sweating is inappropriate for interior patterns, yet that treatment is used. The fluids issue outward with the sweat, and the stool becomes dry and difficult. "Exterior vacuity" means that the fleshy exterior is open and the fluids have strayed. "Interior repletion" means that defecation is difficult and dryness bind is present in the interior. The interior bind is not severe; consequently, it is only after a period of time passes and the disease has not resolved that the speech becomes delirious.

This line may be compared with line 217, p. 349, in which the phrase "exterior vacuity and interior repletion" is also used. In that line, an exterior pattern exists simultaneously with an interior pattern. Once the exterior pattern has ceased, precipitation is suggested. In the present line, no exterior pattern exists, only interior repletion. "Exterior vacuity" does not mean an exterior pattern, but means that the fleshy exterior is open and the fluids have strayed.

Line 225

脉浮而迟，表热里寒，下利清谷者，四逆汤主之。

Mài fú ér chí, biǎo rè lǐ hán, xià lì qīng gǔ zhě, sì nì tāng zhǔ zhī.

When the pulse is floating and slow, [and there is] exterior heat and interior cold [with] clear food diarrhea, Counterflow Cold Decoction (*sì nì tāng*) governs.

Synopsis

The signs and treatment of exterior heat and interior cold.

Commentary

In patterns with exuberant yīn cold and debilitated yáng qì, movement and transformation becomes impaired and clear-food diarrhea occurs. In this line, the presence of clear-food diarrhea indicates yáng vacuity interior cold, even in the presence of exterior heat. This pattern can be considered a simultaneous exterior-interior disease, in which the interior pattern is more severe. The first treatment is to warm the interior; therefore Counterflow Cold Decoction (*sì nì tāng*) is suggested. Not only is clear-food diarrhea present, but the pulse is slow, confirming that this pattern is one of interior vacuity cold. The use of Counterflow Cold Decoction (*sì nì tāng*) in this line reflects the idea presented in line 91, p. 140, "incessant clear-food diarrhea... one should urgently relieve the interior [disease]."

Another interpretation of this line is that the pulse is floating, and exterior heat is present because of false heat. The authors of *Gāo Děng Cóng Shū* explain this as follows: "A pulse [that is] slow governs yīn cold in the interior. A pulse [that is] floating governs false heat in the exterior.... The interior cold is true and the exterior heat is false.... Use Counterflow Cold Decoction (*sì nì tāng*) to expel yīn cold and invigorate true yáng."

Line 231

㈠阳明中风，脉弦浮大，而短气，腹都满，胁下及心痛，久按之，气不通，鼻干，不得汗，嗜卧，一身及目悉黄，小便难，有潮热，时时哕，耳前后肿。㈡刺之小差，外不解，病过十日，脉续浮者，与小柴胡汤。

(1) *Yáng míng zhòng fēng, mài xián fú dà, ér duǎn qì, fù dōu mǎn, xié xià jí xīn tòng, jiǔ àn zhī, qì bù tōng, bí gān, bù dé hàn, shì wò, yī shēn jí mù xī huáng, xiǎo biàn nán, yǒu cháo rè, shí shí yuē, ěr qián hòu zhǒng.* (2) *Cì zhī xiǎo chài, wài bù jiě, bìng guò shí rì, mài xù fú zhě, yǔ xiǎo chái hú tāng.*

(1) In yáng brightness wind strike, the pulse is stringlike, floating, and large, and [there is] shortness of breath, fullness of the entire abdomen,

[and] pain under the rib-side and in the heart, which [gives rise to] qì blockage* when pressed for a long time, dry nose, inability to sweat, somnolence, yellowing of the entire body including the eyes, difficult urination, tidal heat effusion, frequent hiccup, and swelling in front of and behind the ear. (2) When needling [brings] slight recovery, [but] the exterior has not resolved, [and] the disease has [lasted] more than ten days and the pulse is still floating, one should give Minor Bupleurum Decoction (*xiǎo chái hú tāng*).

Text Note

* Qì blockage, 气不通 *qì bù tōng*: A feeling of oppression.

Synopsis

The signs and treatment of yáng brightness wind strike.

Commentary

This pattern is complicated and much of the commentary is conflicting. The line begins with yáng brightness wind strike, but most commentators view this pattern as either yáng brightness and lesser yáng combination disease or combination disease of the three yáng. Yóu Yí writes, "Although this line belongs to yáng brightness, [it is] already combined with lesser yáng.... [This is a] pattern of lesser yáng and yáng brightness evil qì depressed in the channels...." Qián Huáng represents the perhaps more accepted point of view that this pattern is combination disease of the three yáng on the basis of the pulse. He writes, "A stringlike pulse [indicates] lesser yáng wind wood evil. A floating [pulse indicates] wind evil in the exterior. A large [pulse indicates] yáng brightness heat in the interior."

If one follows this logic, without debating the issue that these pulse qualities do not necessarily indicate the given disease patterns, the signs can be categorized according to the three yáng channels. A pulse that is floating and absence of sweating indicate a greater yáng exterior pattern. Shortness of breath, abdominal fullness, dry nose, generalized yellowing, tidal heat effusion, somnolence, and hiccup all belong to yáng brightness. Congestion of yáng brightness heat qì leads to dry nose, abdominal fullness, shortness of breath, and tidal heat effusion. Generalized yellowing is an indication of the effect of heat congestion on the center burner. Heat from the center burner ascends and harasses the heart spirit, leading to somnolence. When heat ascends counterflow it impairs normal upbearing and downbearing and can cause hiccups. This pattern is similar to the one described in line 381, p. 568, with hiccup and abdominal fullness. Pain under the rib-side and below the heart, difficult urination, and swelling around the ears belong to the lesser yáng. The lesser yáng channel follows outward along the rib-side and inward to the region below the heart. Heat evil congestion blocks the movement of qì in the channel and causes pain. The area around the ears is also part of the lesser yáng channel pathway. Heat evil in the channel causes congestion and swelling around the ears. Exuberant heat in the lesser yáng not only inhibits the pivot dynamic, but also causes a loss of regulation in the triple burner waterways. As a result, urination is inhibited. Yáng brightness disease is generally characterized by copious sweating, but here the presence of an unresolved greater yáng evil fetters the exterior and no sweat issues.

Because in combination disease one must be cautious about resolving the exterior or attacking the interior, needling is suggested instead, in order to drain heat, to diffuse and open depressed yáng qì, and to course and disinhibit channel qì. If after needling the patient has improved slightly, but the exterior pattern has not resolved and the pulse is still is floating, it means that the interior heat has already resolved. Given the fact that Minor Bupleurum Decoction (*xiǎo chái hú tāng*) is suggested, we can assume that lesser yáng signs have appeared and therefore harmonizing treatment is appropriate.

Line 232

㈠脉但浮，无余证者，与麻黄汤。㈡若不尿，腹满加哕者，不治。

(1) *Mài dàn fú, wú yú zhèng zhě, yǔ má huáng tāng.* (2) *Ruò bù niào, fù mǎn jiā yuē zhě, bù zhì.*

(1) When only the pulse is floating and no other signs [are present], one can give Ephedra Decoction (*má huáng tāng*). (2) If [there is] no urination and [there is] abdominal fullness and hiccup, no treatment [is possible].

Synopsis

a) Continuing from the preceding line, the signs and treatment of a pattern in which the interior signs have ceased and the exterior has not yet resolved.

b) The prognosis for this pattern.

Commentary

This pattern is a continuing commentary on the preceding line. Following the use of acupuncture, and after ten days of disease, the interior signs are absent. The pulse, however, is still floating, which suggests that the exterior pattern is still present. Given that the exterior pattern is unresolved and no sweat has issued, Ephedra Decoction (*má huáng tāng*) is used to promote sweating and resolve the exterior. This logic is similar to that used in line 37, p. 95: "When in greater yáng disease, after ten days have passed, the pulse is floating and fine, and [there is] somnolence, the outer body has already resolved. If [there is] fullness in the chest and rib-side pain, give Minor Bupleurum Decoction (*xiǎo chái hú tāng*); if the pulse is floating only, give Ephedra Decoction (*má huáng tāng*)."

The second part of this line refers to the preceding line prior to treatment. That is, if the pulse is floating, stringlike, and large, and all of the previous signs are present, but urinary difficulty gives way to absence of urination and the abdominal fullness and hiccup become worse (one can assume that they become worse because of their repetition) it means that the stomach qì has been wasted, the triple burner is congested, and the qì dynamic is blocked. The evil has no outward path, and consequently, treatment is not possible or at least very difficult.

Line 234

阳明病，脉迟，汗出多，微恶寒者，表未解也，可发汗，宜桂枝汤。

Yáng míng bìng, mài chí, hàn chū duō, wēi wù hán zhě, biǎo wèi jiě yě, kě fā fàn, yí guì zhī tāng.

When in yáng brightness disease the pulse is slow, and [there is] copious sweating and mild aversion to cold, the exterior has not resolved; sweating can be promoted and [therefore,] Cinnamon Twig Decoction (*guì zhī tāng*) is appropriate.

Synopsis

The signs and treatment of a yáng brightness disease with greater yáng exterior vacuity.

Commentary

Not all yáng brightness disease is characterized by heat and repletion; patterns of vacuity and cold may also be seen. In this yáng brightness pattern the pulse is slow, suggesting that this is a cold pattern. Copious sweating and slight aversion to cold indicate greater yáng exterior vacuity and disharmony of the construction and defense. In unresolved exterior patterns one should promote sweating and resolve the exterior, but in this case copious sweat has already issued. Therefore, Cinnamon Twig Decoction (*guì zhī tāng*), which promotes mild sweating and harmonizes the construction and defense, is suggested instead of Ephedra Decoction (*má huáng tāng*).

A pulse that is slow appears in several yáng brightness patterns. In line 208, p. 356, the pulse is slow and forceful. It is the result of an inhibition of the movement of qì and blood caused by severe congestion from dry stool in a repletion pattern. In line 195, p. 375, a pulse that is slow appears in a pattern of stomach cold and spleen damp with dietary irregularity yellowing. In line 225, p. 396, a cold evil enters the stomach and intestines and, as a result, the true yáng is insufficient and the pulse becomes slow.

Line 235

阳明病，脉浮，无汗而喘者，发汗则愈，宜麻黄汤。

Yáng míng bìng, mài fú, wú hàn ér chuǎn zhě, fā hàn zé yù, yí má huáng tāng.

When in yáng brightness disease, the pulse is floating, sweating is absent, and [there is] panting, the promotion of sweating will bring about recovery; [therefore,] Ephedra Decoction (*má huáng tāng*) is appropriate.

SYNOPSIS

The signs and treatment of a yáng brightness disease with greater yáng exterior repletion.

COMMENTARY

In this line, which is described as a yáng brightness disease, signs of a greater yáng exterior repletion pattern are present. The pulse is floating, sweating is absent, and it is likely that one would also observe heat effusion and aversion to cold. Wind cold fetters the exterior, the defense is blocked, and the construction is depressed. When the skin and hair are blocked, the lung qì becomes inhibited and the patient pants. Ephedra Decoction (*má huáng tāng*) promotes sweating, diffuses the lung, and calms panting. This line is similar to line 36, p. 99, in which greater yáng and yáng brightness combination disease with panting and chest fullness is treated with Ephedra Decoction (*má huáng tāng*). If the pattern involves abdominal fullness and panting, this formula is not appropriate.

In the pattern described in this line, Ephedra Decoction (*má huáng tāng*) is used because the primary signs relate to greater yáng exterior repletion. If yáng brightness signs, such as red tongue, thirst, and vexation and agitation were evident, one might consider instead using Major Bupleurum Decoction (*dà chái hú tāng*). If the exterior pattern had already resolved and the heat evil were congesting, causing panting and sweating, one would use Ephedra, Apricot Kernel, Licorice, and Gypsum Decoction (*má huáng xìng rén gān cǎo shí gāo tāng*).

LINE 240

㈠ 病人烦热，汗出则解，又如疟状，日晡所发热者，属阳明也。㈡ 脉实者，宜下之；脉浮虚者，宜发汗。㈢ 下之与大承气汤；发汗宜桂枝汤。

(1) *Bìng rén fán rè, hàn chū zé jiě, yòu rú nüè zhuàng, rì bū suǒ fā rè zhě, shǔ yáng míng yě.* (2) *Mài shí zhě, yí xià zhī; mài fú xū zhě, yí fā hàn.* (3) *Xià zhī yǔ dà chéng qì tāng; fā hàn yí guì zhī tāng.*

(1) When the patient has heat vexation that resolves after sweating and then has signs like malaria, [such as] late afternoon heat effusion, this [pattern] belongs to yáng brightness. (2) If the pulse is replete, it is appropriate to precipitate, and if the pulse is floating and vacuous, it is appropriate to promote sweating. (3) For precipitation, give Major Qì-Coordinating Decoction (*dà chéng qì tāng*). To promote sweating, Cinnamon Twig Decoction (*guì zhī tāng*) is appropriate.

SYNOPSIS

According to the vacuity or repletion of the pulse and signs, one can determine whether the promotion of sweating or use of precipitation is appropriate.

Commentary

Heart vexation and heat effusion are the only signs that appear prior to sweating. The disease resolves after sweat issues, but further signs (described as being similar to malaria) appear. Late afternoon heat effusion is said to belong to yáng brightness and one can use the pulse to identify the type of yáng brightness disease. If the pulse is replete and forceful, it suggests that repletion dryness bind is already present in the bowel, and precipitation may be used. If the pulse is floating, vacuous, and forceless, it suggests that the interior heat is not yet replete and the exterior evil has not yet been eliminated; hence one should promote sweating.

The pattern in this line is similar to greater yáng and yáng brightness combination disease, where in one case the exterior pattern is predominant and in the other the interior pattern is primary. The primary criterion used in the differentiation of these patterns is the pulse. When the pulse is replete, Major Qì-Coordinating Decoction (*dà chéng qì tāng*) is used to attack interior repletion. When the pulse is vacuous, Cinnamon Twig Decoction (*guì zhī tāng*) is used to harmonize the construction and resolve the exterior. The present line may also be viewed as describing a pattern of simultaneous exterior-interior disease. The basic treatment principle is to first resolve the exterior and then attack the interior. From this perspective, the suggested formulae are simply examples of what may be used for exterior resolution and interior precipitation. One should understand the principles involved, observe a specific pattern, then make a decision about the appropriate formula.

Line 244

太阳病，寸缓、关浮、尺弱，其人发热汗出，复恶寒，不呕，但心下痞者，此以医下之也，如其不下者，病人不恶寒而渴者，此转属阳明也，小便数者，大便必硬，不更衣十日无所苦也，渴欲饮水，少少与之，但以法救之，渴者，宜五苓散。

Tài yáng bìng, cùn huǎn、 guān fú、 chǐ ruò, qí rén fā rè hàn chū, fù wù hán, bù ǒu, dàn xīn xià pǐ zhě, cǐ yǐ yī xià zhī yě, rú qí bù xià zhě, bìng rén bù wù hán ér kě zhě, cǐ zhuǎn shǔ yáng míng yě, xiǎo biàn shuò zhě, dà biàn bì yìng, bù gēng yī shí rì wú suǒ kǔ yě, kě yù yǐn shuǐ, shǎo shǎo yǔ zhī, dàn yǐ fǎ jiù zhī, kě zhě, yí wǔ líng sǎn.

When in greater yáng disease the inch pulse is moderate, the bar pulse is floating, the cubit pulse is weak, and the patient has heat effusion and sweating, followed by aversion to cold and absence of retching, [but there is] glomus below the heart, this is because the physician used precipitation. If [he] has not used precipitation, the person [feels] no aversion to cold and is thirsty, this being [because the disease] has shifted to the yáng brightness. When urination is frequent, the stool will be hard and [the person will] not change clothes for ten days, [but] will have no discomfort. [When there is] thirst with a desire to drink water, give a small amount [of water]. Only by this method [will the disease be] eliminated. When [there is] thirst, Poria (Hoelen) Five Powder (*wǔ líng sǎn*) is appropriate.

SYNOPSIS

a) A greater yáng wind strike pattern in which inappropriate precipitation causes a glomus to form.

b) Identification of the signs that indicate that this pattern is passing to the yáng brightness.

COMMENTARY

The pulse in this line is moderate, floating, and weak, and is classified as a greater yáng wind strike pulse. Upon examination, however, it appears that this pulse description is problematic. The primary problem is that Zhāng Jī does not generally refer to the bar pulse in this way, 关 *guān*, preferring to write 关上 *guān shàng*. This consideration and the fact that Zhāng Jī seldom describes the qualities of the pulse at each position have led some commentators to believe that this may have been added by later authors. Consequently, this line is placed in this Chapter Appendix.

If we continue on the assumption that this pulse indicates a greater yáng wind strike pattern, we can observe the corroborating signs of heat effusion, sweating, and aversion to cold. The absence of retching means that lesser yáng and yáng brightness signs are absent. Glomus below the heart, however, is not a sign generally seen in greater yáng disease. We are told that it is the result of precipitation used prior to the resolution of the exterior pattern. The evil falls inward and congests the qì dynamic, causing the glomus. Although Zhāng Jī does not suggest any treatment, we might assume that he would first resolve the exterior with a formula like Cinnamon Twig Decoction (*guì zhī tāng*) and then treat the glomus with one of the Heart-Draining Decoctions (*xiè xīn tāng*).

If precipitation is not used and the aversion to cold changes to aversion to heat and the patient becomes thirsty, the disease may be assumed to have shifted into the yáng brightness. Because many different yáng brightness patterns exist, one must investigate further. If urination is frequent, not only is there heat in the yáng brightness, but the fluids have percolated into the bladder. The stomach and intestines are depleted of fluids and the stool becomes hard. Although more than ten days pass without defecation, the patient does not feel abdominal pain and discomfort. This pattern is straitened spleen and should be treated with Hemp Seed Pill (*má zǐ rén wán*) to precipitate with moistness. This pattern should be differentiated from the one in which the stool is bound and accompanied by signs such as abdominal hardness, fullness, and pain, tidal heat effusion, and delirious speech and which is treated with one of the Qì-Coordinating Decoctions (*chéng qì tāng*).

Chapter Three
Lesser Yáng Disease
Pulses and Signs; Treatment
辨少阳病脉证并治

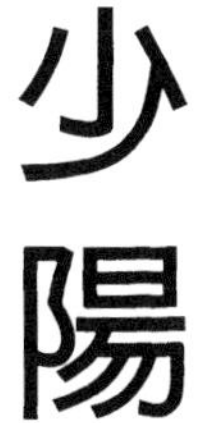

1 OVERVIEW

The lesser yáng is the middle of the three yáng channels. Greater yáng lies next to it on the outside and yáng brightness on the inside. Lesser yáng disease is therefore the stage of progression from exterior to interior and the transformation of cold into heat. At this stage the disease has left the greater yáng exterior, but has not yet entered the yáng brightness interior. Lesser yáng disease is neither an exterior cold pattern nor an interior heat pattern, but is a half exterior half interior heat pattern. The term half exterior half interior introduced by Chéng Wú-Jǐ (it does not appear in the original text) is potentially confusing because it gives the false impression that lesser yáng disease in nature is partly exterior and partly interior. Lesser yáng disease is *neither* exterior *nor* interior; rather, it is a disease pattern arising *halfway* between the exterior and interior. The terms exterior and interior are relative. By comparison with the greater yáng, the lesser yáng is relatively interior, and by comparison with yáng brightness is comparatively exterior.

Because lesser yáng is located between the exterior and interior, the mechanisms of lesser yáng disease can shift out to the greater yáng and into the yáng brightness. For this reason, it is considered to be like the pivot on which a door swings. Because "lesser yáng is the pivot" (少阳为枢 *shào yáng wéi shū*), lesser yáng disease is often associated with concurrent greater yáng exterior or yáng brightness interior patterns. Both the gallbladder and the triple burner belong to the lesser yáng, and impairment of gallbladder free coursing and/or impairment of the triple burner's regulation of the waterways are often described in terms of inhibition of the "pivot mechanism."

The content of the *Shāng Hán Lùn* lines suggests that greater yáng is the exterior, while yáng brightness is the interior, and that lesser yáng lies between the two. According to this schema, the three yáng include both exterior and interior. However, according to the order in which the channel diseases are discussed in the

Shāng Hán Lùn, the chapter on lesser yáng comes after yáng brightness and before greater yīn. Because of this, it has been suggested that the three yáng are the exterior, while the three yīn are the interior, and that since lesser yáng lies at the junction of the yáng and yīn channels, therefore in the normal progression of cold damage, lesser yáng disease lies between yáng brightness and greater yīn. Although this point of view is not entirely unjustified, it nevertheless does not conform with the way by which the diseases of the six channels develop.

1.1 PULSES AND SIGNS

The basic signs of lesser yáng disease are bitter taste in the mouth, dry throat, and dizzy vision. Other signs include alternating aversion to cold and heat effusion, chest and rib-side fullness, taciturnity with no desire to eat, and heart vexation and frequent retching. The pulse associated with lesser yáng disease is one that is stringlike and fine.

Bitter taste in the mouth, 口苦 *kǒu kǔ*; **dry throat**, 咽干 *gān gān*; **dizzy vision**, 目眩 *mù xuàn*: The lesser yáng homes to the gallbladder, which governs free coursing. When disease is in lesser yáng, the free coursing action of the gallbladder is inhibited. Depressed qì becomes heat and gallbladder heat ascends to cause bitter taste in the mouth. The lesser yáng vessel clasps the throat, so gallbladder heat also scorches liquid and humor, causing dry throat. Because the lesser yáng vessel starts at the outer canthus, and the gallbladder stands in exterior-interior relationship with the liver (which opens at the eyes), gallbladder heat can cause dizzy vision. These three signs indicate that the evil has already transformed into heat and entered the interior, but the interior heat is still not exuberant. Bitter taste in the mouth, dry throat, and dizzy vision are sufficient basis for diagnosing lesser yáng disease; hence they are the essential features of lesser yáng disease. Although some have suggested that bitter taste in the mouth and dry throat are observed in yáng brightness wind strike, it must be borne in mind that the heat in yáng brightness is much stronger than in lesser yáng. Therefore, bitter taste and dry throat may be observed, but there should be other signs of intense evil heat that enable differentiation. It therefore still makes sense to consider bitter taste in the mouth, dry throat, and dizzy vision as the main features of lesser yáng disease.

Alternating aversion to cold and heat effusion, 往来寒热 *wǎng lái hán rè*: This sign reflects evil half in the exterior and half in the interior (or more correctly, halfway between the two). The evil qì is trying to advance, but at the same time right qì is trying to repel it. Thus, right and evil fight in turns, and when right overcomes evil there is heat effusion, and when evil overcomes right, there is aversion to cold. Alternating aversion to cold and heat effusion is only observed in lesser yáng disease. It differs from the simultaneous occurrence of aversion to cold and heat effusion in greater yáng disease, and from the heat effusion without aversion to cold that is observed in yáng brightness heat repletion patterns.

Chest and rib-side fullness, 胸胁苦满 *xiōng xié kǔ mǎn*: The chest and rib-side lie on the path of the lesser yáng channel, which passes down into the chest, and crosses the diaphragm before netting the liver and homing to the gallbladder. When evil is depressed in the lesser yáng, the channel qì is disinhibited, so there is distention and fullness in the chest and rib-side.

Taciturnity with no desire to eat or drink, 嘿嘿不欲饮食 *mò mò bù yù yǐn shí*: When gallbladder fire is internally depressed and the qì dynamic stagnates, the patient will be taciturn with a glum expression. When the gallbladder free coursing is impaired, this affects the stomach, causing torpor of the digestive function; hence no desire to eat or drink. No desire to eat or drink means a relative lack of appetite; it is not as severe as "inability to eat."

Heart vexation, 心烦 *xīn fán*; **frequent retching,** 喜呕 *xīn fán*: Lesser yáng wood fire depressed in the inner body is reflected in a feeling of unrest or irritability centered in the heart, and described as "heart vexation." When gallbladder and stomach qì move counterflow, there is "frequent retching."

A pulse that is fine and stringlike, 脉弦细 *mài xián xì*: A pulse that is fine and stringlike is the main pulse of lesser yáng disease. The pulse tends to become stringlike whenever liver and gallbladder qì become depressed and stagnant. This is different from the floating quality that reflects right qì resisting evil in the outer body; it is also different from the surging and large qualities associated with exuberant yáng brightness heat.

1.2 Treatment

The representative pattern in lesser yáng disease is half exterior half interior. This pattern is often referred to as a Minor Bupleurum Decoction (*xiǎo chái hú tāng*) pattern, in reference to the principal formula used in its treatment. Minor Bupleurum Decoction (*xiǎo chái hú tāng*) harmonizes the lesser yáng. Although the text includes a detailed description of the pattern for which Minor Bupleurum Decoction (*xiǎo chái hú tāng*) is suggested, we should remember that the therapeutic range of this formula is quite broad, as will be seen in the lines below. Harmonization is the main treatment principle in lesser yáng patterns, while the promotion of sweating and the use of vomiting or precipitation are generally contraindicated.

Although the promotion of sweating and the use of precipitation are generally contraindicated in lesser yáng patterns, there are exceptions, particularly in combination disease where signs of more than one channel may simultaneously be observed. In line 146, p. 429, Bupleurum and Cinnamon Twig Decoction (*chái hú guì zhī tāng*), a formula that promotes sweating and harmonizes, is used to treat greater yáng and lesser yáng combination disease. Then, in line 103, p. 431, in a pattern of lesser yáng and yáng brightness combination disease, Major Bupleurum Decoction (*dà chái hú tāng*) is used to harmonize and precipitate. Furthermore, in mild patterns of lesser yáng and yáng brightness combination disease in which the interior repletion is mild, Bupleurum Decoction Plus Mirabilite (*chái hú jiā máng xiāo tāng*) may be used.

The triple burner and gallbladder belong to lesser yáng. In patterns of lesser yáng disease the ministerial fire can become depressed, allowing water-rheum to collect in the interior. This pattern, presented in line 147, p. 437, is treated by harmonizing the lesser yáng and warming and transforming water-rheum with Bupleurum, Cinnamon Twig, and Dried Ginger Decoction (*chái hú guì zhī gān jiāng tāng*). When a lesser yáng disease is treated inappropriately or not treated and when there are both interior and exterior patterns with simultaneous vacuity and repletion, as in line 107, p. 439, the appropriate formula is Bupleurum Decoction

Plus Dragon Bone and Oyster Shell (*chái hú jiā lóng gǔ mǔ lì tāng*), which harmonizes the lesser yáng, supports the right and dispels evil, frees yáng and discharges heat, and quiets the spirit with heavy settlers.

Because of the half exterior and half interior position of the lesser yáng, movement of evils outward or inward through the lesser yáng is frequently discussed. In the text we find: greater yáng disease shifting into the lesser yáng; patterns in which this shift occurs but exterior symptoms are still present; lesser yáng disease shifting into the yáng brightness; lesser yáng disease shifting into the three yīn; persistent lesser yáng disease that has not shifted after many days; chest-bind patterns that are the result of the inappropriate use of precipitation in a lesser yáng disease; and aggravated disease that is the result of mistreatment of a lesser yáng pattern.

This section also includes lines describing heat entering the blood chamber. These lines originally appeared in the greater yáng chapter, but because their treatment relates to the lesser yáng, they have been placed in this chapter.

1.3 SCHEMATIC OVERVIEW

Lesser Yáng Disease Patterns

- **Basic Lesser Yáng Disease Pattern (Half interior half exterior pattern)** with bitter taste in the mouth, dry throat, dizzy vision, alternating aversion to cold and heat effusion, chest and rib-side fullness, taciturnity with no desire to eat, heart vexation, frequent retching, and a pulse that is fine and stringlike: Minor Bupleurum Decoction (*xiǎo chái hú tāng*)

- **Transmuted Patterns**

  - Unresolved exterior pattern with heat effusion and aversion to cold, joint pain, retching, and vexation: Bupleurum and Cinnamon Twig Decoction (*chái hú guì zhī tāng*)

  - Concurrent interior repletion with alternating aversion to cold and heat effusion, fullness in the chest and rib-side, retching, depression and vexation, distress below the heart, and hard glomus: Major Bupleurum Decoction (*dà chái hú tāng*)

  - Concurrent interior repletion after precipitation with fullness in the chest and rib-side retching counterflow, tidal heat effusion, and diarrhea: Bupleurum Decoction Plus Mirabilite (*chái hú jiā máng xiāo tāng*)

  - Concurrent water-rheum bound in the interior with fullness in the chest and rib-side, alternating aversion to cold and heat effusion, heart vexation, thirst, and inhibited urination: Bupleurum, Cinnamon Twig, and Dried Ginger Decoction (*chái hú guì zhī gān jiāng tāng*)

  - Vexation fright and delirious speech with heat effusion, fullness in the chest and rib-side, vexation and agitation, delirious speech, and inhibited urination: Bupleurum Decoction Plus Dragon Bone and Oyster Shell (*chái hú jiā lóng gǔ mǔ lì tāng*)

2 ESSENTIAL FEATURES OF LESSER YÁNG DISEASE

Line 263

少阳之为病，口苦，咽干，目眩也。

Shào yáng zhī wéi bìng, kǒu kǔ, yān gān, mù xuàn yě.

In disease of the lesser yáng, [there is] a bitter taste in the mouth, dry throat, and dizzy vision.*

Text Note

* Dizzy vision, 目眩 *mù xuàn*: Visual distortion with a whirling sensation in the head that in severe cases can upset the sense of balance.

Synopsis

The essential features of lesser yáng disease.

Commentary

An evil in the lesser yáng is considered to have left the greater yáng, but not yet entered the yáng brightness; therefore, it is described as half exterior half interior. One may regard an evil in the lesser yáng as being in the interior when compared with the greater yáng, and in the exterior when compared with the yáng brightness. The lesser yáng governs the ministerial fire and the pivot mechanism. The ministerial fire is a fire in the body inhabiting the life gate, liver, gallbladder, and triple burner. It is thought to come essentially from the life gate (to which extent it is indissociable from kidney yáng). It stands in complementary opposition to the sovereign fire, which is the heart fire. The sovereign and ministerial fires together warm the bowels and viscera and power activity in the body. The pivot refers to the position of the lesser yáng between the greater yáng and the yáng brightness. The lesser yáng governs the pivot, and its functions are crucial in the movement of qì between the different regions of the body. When the gallbladder is coursed and discharging normally, the ministerial fire moves normally, warming the organs and powering activity. In this state, it is unseen. If the movement of the ministerial fire becomes frenetic, it will manifest in observable disease signs.

In this line an evil has entered the lesser yáng. It congests the pivot and impairs qì movement. The gallbladder functions of coursing and discharging become abnormal and the ministerial fire becomes depressed. In this state it flames upward and gives rise to observable signs. Flaming ministerial fire can scorch the fluids, causing a bitter taste in the mouth and a dry throat. The foot lesser yáng channel starts from the outer canthus, the gallbladder and the liver stand in exterior-interior relationship, and the liver opens into the eyes; therefore, when gallbladder fire flames upward, it may attack the clear orifices in the head, particularly the eyes, so that there is clouded head and dizzy vision.

This line provides a simple outline of the primary signs seen in lesser yáng disease. Nonetheless, when an evil enters the lesser yáng and the pivot becomes inhibited, right qì and evil qì struggle by turns, and in severe cases the spleen and stomach are affected, so that in addition to the signs explicitly mentioned in the line there will also be alternating aversion to cold and heat effusion, fullness in the chest and rib-side, taciturnity and lack of desire for food, and heart vexation and frequent retching. See line 96, p. 410.

LINE 264

少阳中风，两耳无所闻，目赤，胸中满而烦者，不可吐下，吐下则悸而惊。

Shào yáng zhòng fēng, liǎng ěr wú suǒ wén, mù chì, xiōng zhōng mǎn ér fán zhě, bù kě tù xià, tù xià zé jì ér jīng.

When in lesser yáng wind strike, [there is] no hearing in either ear, the eyes are red, [and there is] fullness in the chest and vexation, one cannot [use] vomiting or precipitation, as vomiting and precipitation will [lead to] palpitations and fright.

SYNOPSIS

1) Contraindications for lesser yáng wind strike.
2) A transmuted pattern following inappropriate treatment.

COMMENTARY

The term "lesser yáng wind strike" refers to a wind evil assailing the lesser yáng. Wind by nature is swift and changeable; hence wind encountering water results in cold, and wind encountering fire results in heat. The lesser yáng governs ministerial fire, and when wind invades, wind and fire fan each other. The two evils inevitably rise to assault the clear orifices of the head, affecting the channels and network vessels. The eyes and the ears are two of the clear orifices, and when assaulted by wind and fire they become congested and inhibited. Hearing is impaired and the eyes become red. Red eyes generally belong to a repletion pattern of wind fire, but hearing loss may also be seen in vacuity patterns. In repletion patterns the ears will feel blocked and distended, or even painful, whereas in vacuity patterns the level of discomfort should be less.

Vexation and fullness in the chest can be explained in two ways. In the *Gāo Děng Cóng Shū* these signs are directly attributed to wind-fire running through the channel vessel and becoming bound in the chest and rib-side. A slightly different interpretation is offered by *Shāng Hán Lùn Yì Shì*, in which the evil enters the lesser yáng channel causing depression and stagnation of qì that results in fullness and vexation. In this pattern the appropriate treatment is to harmonize and resolve, thereby restoring the normal movement of the pivot, which in turn will allow the wind-fire to dissipate.

If one sees fullness in the chest and vexation, yet erroneously assumes that a repletion evil is causing internal obstruction, one might commit the error of using vomiting or precipitating treatment. However, because the evil is in the lesser yáng, these treatments cannot resolve the disease and will only damage the qì and blood, deprive the heart of nourishment, and leave the heart-spirit ungoverned, resulting in palpitations and fright. For this reason, vomiting and precipitation is contraindicated in lesser yáng disease.

LINE 265

(一) 伤寒，脉弦细，头痛发热者，属少阳。(二) 少阳不可发汗，发汗则谵语，此属胃，胃和则愈，胃不和，烦而悸。

(1) *Shāng hán, mài xián xì, tóu tòng fā rè zhě, shǔ shào yáng.* (2) *Shào yáng bù kě fā hàn, fā hàn zé zhān yǔ, cǐ shǔ wèi, wèi hé zé yù, wèi bù hé, fán ér jì.*

(1) When in cold damage the pulse is stringlike and fine and [there is] headache and heat effusion, this belongs to lesser yáng. (2) [In] lesser yáng [patterns] one cannot promote sweating, as promoting sweating will [lead to] delirious speech, which belongs to the stomach. [If] the stomach is harmonized [there will be] recovery, [and if] the stomach is not harmonized, [there will be] vexation and palpitations.

SYNOPSIS

1) The promotion of sweating is contraindicated in lesser yáng cold damage patterns.

2) A transmuted pattern following inappropriate promotion of sweating and two scenarios.

COMMENTARY

The pulse most closely associated with lesser yáng disease is a stringlike pulse. In externally contracted diseases, headache and heat effusion can appear in any disease of the three yáng. Headache and heat effusion with a pulse that is floating indicates greater yáng exterior disease, and therefore sweating should be promoted. Headache and heat effusion with a pulse that is surging, large, slippery, and rapid may indicate yáng brightness interior disease, for which clearing and precipitation would be appropriate. In this line, headache and heat effusion are accompanied by a pulse that is stringlike and fine. A pulse that is stringlike is the governing pulse of the lesser yáng and is usually fine. The combination of headache and heat effusion with a pulse that is stringlike and fine indicates half exterior half interior disease in which the pivot mechanism is inhibited and gallbladder fire is flaming upward. This disease should be treated by harmonizing and resolving the lesser yáng to restore the pivot mechanism and the free coursing of the liver and gallbladder. Once this occurs, the upward flaming of gallbladder fire will spontaneously resolve.

The promotion of sweating is contraindicated in lesser yáng disease for two reasons: First, the disease is half exterior and half exterior, that is, not wholly in the exterior. Second, the formulae used in the promotion of sweating are acrid and warm. If an acrid warm formula is used, the heat from the formula will assist the lesser yáng fire. The fluids will be discharged through the exterior and the stomach will become dry. Because the lesser yáng is considered to be between the greater yáng and the yáng brightness, when inappropriate treatment is used, it easily affects the yáng brightness. Heat is engendered in the stomach because of the fluid damage; the heat ascends, harassing the heart and causing delirious speech. Following this mistreatment the disease course depends on whether the stomach can be harmonized. If stomach qì can be harmonized, that is, the heat can be eliminated and the fluids restored, the delirious speech will stop and the patient will recover. Because "yáng brightness resides in the center and governs earth. All things converge [here and] nothing passes further" (line 184, p. 310), the stomach heat and damage to liquid spontaneously harmonize only with difficulty. Normally, harmonization must be brought about by treatment to clear and discharge the heat evil, and to enrich the fluids. If harmonization does not occur (either because treatment was not given on time, or because the treatment failed to produce the desired effect) the stomach heat and damage to liquid are further aggravated, resulting in a transmuted pattern of heart vexation and palpitations.

3 BASIC LESSER YÁNG DISEASE PATTERNS

3.1 MINOR BUPLEURUM DECOCTION PATTERNS

Here we discuss lesser yáng half exterior half interior patterns and the signs associated with them. The main signs are alternating aversion to cold and heat effusion, fullness in the chest and rib-side, taciturnity and no desire to eat, and heart vexation and retching. When an evil enters the lesser yáng, it inhibits the pivot mechanism and the right and evil qì struggle without either being able to overcome the other, which produces the signs described above. The appropriate treatment is to harmonize using Minor Bupleurum Decoction (*xiăo chái hú tāng*) or a variation that addresses other signs that may occur.

LINE 96

伤寒五六日，中风，往来寒热，胸胁苦满，嘿嘿不欲饮食，心烦喜呕，或胸中烦而不呕，或渴，或腹中痛，或胁下痞硬，或心下悸、小便不利，或不渴、身有微热，或咳者，小柴胡汤主之。

Shāng hán wŭ liù rì, zhòng fēng, wăng lái hán rè, xiōng xié kŭ măn, mò mò bù yù yĭn shí, xīn fán xĭ ŏu, huò xiōng zhōng fán ér bù ŏu, huò kĕ, huò fù zhōng tòng, huò xié xià pĭ yìng, huò xīn xià jì, xiăo biàn bù lì, huò bù kĕ、 shēn yŏu wēi rè, huò ké zhĕ, xiăo chái hú tāng zhŭ zhī.

When in cold damage [that has lasted for] five or six days [or] wind strike,[1] [there is] alternating [aversion to] cold and heat [effusion];[2] [the person] suffers from fullness in the chest and rib-side,[3] taciturnity[4] with no desire for food or drink, heart vexation and frequent retching, or possibly [there is] vexation in the chest and no retching, or thirst or pain in the abdomen, or a hard glomus under the rib-side, or palpitations below the heart with inhibited urination, or absence of thirst with mild generalized heat, or cough; [then] Minor Bupleurum Decoction (*xiǎo chái hú tāng*) governs.

TEXT NOTES

1. When in cold damage [that has lasted for] five or six days [or] wind strike, 伤寒五六日，中风 *shāng hán wǔ liù rì, zhòng fēng*: Although the Chinese suggests, "When, after cold damage [that has lasted for] five or six days, [the patient contracts] wind strike," the authors of *Gāo Děng Cóng Shū* write that this is incorrect, and that we should take this line to mean, "When in cold damage or wind strike that has lasted for five or six days...."
2. Alternating [aversion to] cold and heat [effusion], 往来寒热 *wáng lái hán rè*: Alternation of heat effusion and aversion to cold.
3. [The person] suffers from fullness in the chest and rib-side, 胸胁苦满 *xiōng xié kǔ mǎn*: The region of the chest and rib-side is afflicted with fullness. The word 苦 *kǔ* acts as a verb and means "to suffer."
4. Taciturnity, 嘿嘿 *mò mò*: The patient has a taciturn demeanor and does not wish to speak.

FORMULA

Minor Bupleurum Decoction (*xiǎo chái hú tāng*)

○ Harmonize the lesser yáng.

柴胡半斤　黄芩三两　人参三两　半夏半升（洗）　甘草（炙）　生姜（切）各三两　大枣十二枚（擘）

(一) 右七味，以水一斗二升，煮取六升，去滓，再煎取三升，温服一升，日三服。(二) 若胸中烦而不呕者，去半夏、人参，加栝楼实一枚。(三) 若渴，去半夏，加人参合前成四两半，栝楼根四两。(四) 若腹中痛者，去黄芩，加芍药三两。(五) 若胁下痞硬，去大枣，加牡蛎四两。(六) 若心下悸，小便不利者，去黄芩，加茯苓四两。(七) 若不渴、外有微热者，去人参，加桂枝三两，温覆微汗愈。(八) 若咳者，去人参、大枣、生姜，加五味子半升，干姜二两。

Chái hú bàn jīn　huáng qín sān liǎng　rén shēn sān liǎng　bàn xià bàn shēng (xǐ)　gān cǎo (zhì)　shēng jiāng (qiē) gè sān liǎng　dà zǎo shí èr méi (bò)

(1) *Yòu qī wèi, yǐ shuǐ yī dǒu èr shēng, zhǔ qǔ liù shēng, qù zǐ, zài jiān qǔ sān shēng, wēn fú yī shēng, rì sān fú.* (2) *Ruò xiōng zhōng fán ér bù ǒu zhě, qù bàn xià、rén shēn, jiā guā lóu shí yī méi.* (3) *Ruò kě, qù bàn xià, jiā rén shēn hé qián chéng sì liǎng bàn, guā lóu gēn sì liǎng.* (4) *Ruò fù zhōng tòng zhě, qù huáng qín, jiā sháo yào sān liǎng.* (5) *Ruò xié xià pǐ yìng, qù dà zǎo, jiā mǔ lì sì liǎng.* (6) *Ruò xīn xià jì, xiǎo biàn bù lì zhě, qù huáng qín, jiā fú líng sì liǎng.* (7) *Ruò bù kě、wài yǒu wēi rè zhě, qù rén shēn, jiā guì zhī sān liǎng, wēn fù wēi hàn yù.*

(8) *Ruò ké zhě, qù rén shēn、 dà zǎo、 shēng jiāng, jiā wǔ wèi zǐ bàn shēng, gān jiāng èr liǎng.*

bupleurum (柴胡 *chái hú*, Bupleuri Radix) half jīn
scutellaria (黄芩 *huáng qín*, Scutellariae Radix) 3 liǎng
ginseng (人参 *rén shēn*, Ginseng Radix) 3 liǎng
pinellia (半夏 *bàn xià*, Pinelliae Tuber) half shēng (washed)
mix-fried licorice (甘草 *gān cǎo*, Glycyrrhizae Radix) 3 liǎng
fresh ginger (生姜 *shēng jiāng*, Zingiberis Rhizoma Recens) 3 liǎng (cut)
jujube (大枣 *dà zǎo*, Ziziphi Fructus) 12 pieces (broken)

(1) [For] the above seven ingredients use one dǒu and two shēng of water. Boil to get six shēng, remove the dregs, and decoct again to get three shēng. Take one shēng warm, three times a day. (2) If [there is] vexation in the chest without retching, remove pinellia (*bàn xià*) and ginseng (*rén shēn*) and add one piece of trichosanthes fruit (*guā lóu shí*). (3) If [there is] thirst, remove pinellia (*bàn xià*) and add ginseng (*rén shēn*), so the combined total is four and a half liǎng, and four liǎng of trichosanthes root (*guā lóu gēn*). (4) If [there is] pain in the abdomen, remove scutellaria (*huáng qín*) and add three liǎng of peony (*sháo yào*). (5) If [there is] a hard glomus under the rib-side, remove jujube (*dà zǎo*) and add four liǎng of oyster shell (*mǔ lì*). (6) If there are palpitations below the heart with inhibited urination, remove scutellaria (*huáng qín*) and add four liǎng of poria (*fú líng*). (7) If [there is] no thirst and mild generalized heat, remove ginseng (*rén shēn*) and add three liǎng of cinnamon twig (*guì zhī*), and take the decoction warm to obtain slight sweating for recovery. (8) If [there is] cough, remove ginseng (*rén shēn*), jujube (*dà zǎo*), and fresh ginger (*shēng jiāng*), and add a half shēng of schisandra (*wǔ wèi zǐ*) and two liǎng of dried ginger (*gān jiāng*).

Synopsis

The signs and treatment of lesser yáng disease.

Commentary

In either cold damage or wind strike externally contracted diseases, after a period of time the evil may shift into the lesser yáng and the greater yáng signs may cease. Lesser yáng patterns are considered half exterior half interior, since the evil is midway between the greater yáng exterior and the yáng brightness interior. From the lesser yáng, the pivot, an evil can be outthrust to the exterior or fall inward. One of the characteristic signs of lesser yáng disease is alternating aversion to cold and heat effusion. When an evil is in the lesser yáng, it contends with right qì. When the right qì prevails, heat effuses and when evil qì prevails, the patient feels aversion to cold. In lesser yáng disease, these two signs appear separately; that is, when heat effusion is observed, aversion to cold is absent and vice versa. Alternating aversion to cold and heat effusion is unique to lesser yáng disease. In greater yáng patterns, aversion to cold and heat effusion appear simultaneously. In yáng brightness patterns, heat effusion occurs without aversion to cold. In malaria or malaria-like disease, alternating aversion to cold and heat effusion may be observed, but generally only occurring once every other day, at set intervals. In lesser yáng disease, the alternation is more frequent and without a set periodicity. In the three yīn patterns, aversion to cold is observed without heat effusion.

Patients with lesser yáng disease commonly have fullness in the chest and rib-side because evil lies depressed in the lesser yáng, inhibiting channel qì. The foot lesser yáng channel descends into the chest, goes through the diaphragm, nets the liver and homes to the gallbladder, and passes along the inside of the rib-side at the border between the chest and rib-side. When evil is depressed in this part of the channel there is fullness in the chest and rib-side.

When gallbladder fire becomes internally depressed, it can influence the spleen and stomach. Wood restrains earth and stomach and spleen function is impaired; consequently, the patient has no desire for food and drink. Normal upbearing and downbearing are disturbed and the patient may retch. "Taciturnity," 嘿嘿 *mò mò*, is here caused by depressed gallbladder qì. When liver-gallbladder qì is depressed and free coursing is impaired, it causes heart qì to become constrained, which in turn affects the heart's function of governing the spirit. The result is a heart sign, "taciturnity," but the root of the problem is in the lesser yáng.

A further sign mentioned in the present line is heart vexation. Because the lesser yáng and reverting yīn stand in external-internal relationship with each other, when depressed gallbladder fire flames up, it surges up through the triple burner and harasses the pericardium, causing heart vexation. Although the disease involves the spleen-stomach, the pericardium, and the heart spirit, the cause is nevertheless evil qì in the lesser yáng disturbing the pivot mechanism. The appropriate treatment is to harmonize and resolve, allowing the pivot mechanism to return to normal and evil qì to be outthrust.

In the second sentence of this line, a list of possible signs seen in lesser yáng disease is presented. These are only possibilities; one can make a diagnosis of lesser yáng disease without seeing any of them. They are all related to evil in the lesser yáng and a disturbance of the pivot mechanism. If the evil becomes depressed in the chest and rib-side without disturbing the stomach, it may cause vexation in the chest without retching. If the lesser yáng heat involves the yáng brightness, and liquid and humor are damaged, there is thirst. Abdominal pain is the result of gallbladder wood assailing spleen earth and causing disharmony in the center burner. If the qì and blood of the liver and gallbladder are stagnant and depressed, a hard glomus may be felt under the rib-side. When the gallbladder loses its normal functions of coursing and discharging, it can influence the function of the triple burner to open and regulate the water pathways. Water-rheum may then collect and the urine may become inhibited. If the water-rheum intimidates the heart, it can cause palpitations. If water-rheum assails the lung, it can cause cough. If the disease evil has not involved the yáng brightness interior, but is associated with the greater yáng exterior, the greater yáng exterior pattern has not ceased, so there is no thirst and still mild heat in the exterior. Since only the heat is "mild," we know that the greater yáng exterior pattern is also mild. Again, all these possible variations are related to the basic pathomechanism which is inhibition of the lesser yáng pivot mechanism. Therefore, the method of treatment is still harmonization; Minor Bupleurum Decoction (*xiǎo chái hú tāng*) is used, but varied according to need.

Slightly bitter, slightly cold bupleurum (*chái hú*) is the chief agent in Minor Bupleurum Decoction (*xiǎo chái hú tāng*). Because its nature is light and clearing, bupleurum (*chái hú*) courses and dissipates, resolving lesser yáng depression and stagnation. Cold and bitter, the qì and flavor of scutellaria (*huáng qín*) is heavier and it is able to clear lesser yáng heat and eliminate vexation and fullness in the chest and abdomen. Used together, they course and resolve exterior stagnation and depression while clearing and discharging interior heat. When heat and stagnation are resolved, the pivot mechanism will return to normal. Fresh ginger (*shēng jiāng*) and pinellia (*bàn xià*) regulate the spleen and stomach, downbear counterflow, and check retching. Ginseng (*rén shēn*), licorice (*gān cǎo*), and jujube (*dà zǎo*) boost the qì and harmonize the center. These assistant medicinals support right qì in order to expel the evil. They fortify earth so that wood cannot harm it. After the dregs are removed from the decoction, it is cooked again; this method is specifically used for harmonizing formulae.

Vexation in the chest without retching indicates heat evil gathered in the chest which has not disturbed the stomach. Ginseng (*rén shēn*) is removed because of concern that it may assist the heat. Because retching counterflow is absent, pinellia (*bàn xià*) is removed. Trichosanthes fruit (*guā lóu shí*) is added to eliminate heat, flush repletion, and relieve vexation. Thirst from fluid damage is a result of depressed gallbladder fire. Acrid, drying pinellia (*bàn xià*) is therefore removed. Additional ginseng (*rén shēn*) is added, as is sweet, cool, bitter trichosanthes root (*guā lóu gēn*), to clear heat and engender liquid. Abdominal pain from wood assailing earth is treated by removing bitter, cold scutellaria (*huáng qín*) because it may further damage the center burner. White peony (*bái sháo*) is added to drain wood evil from earth, harmonize the spleen, and relieve pain. When hard glomus is present under the rib-side as a result of stagnation and depression of qì and blood, jujube (*dà zǎo*) is removed to prevent its sweet, supplementing nature from causing further congestion. Oyster shell (*mǔ lì*), which can soften hardness, is added to disperse the glomus. For inhibited urination and palpitations from collected water-rheum, scutellaria (*huáng qín*) is removed because of fear that its cold nature might cause further congealing of the rheum. Poria (*fú líng*) is added to percolate downward and disinhibit the urine. If thirst is absent but mild generalized heat is present, ginseng (*rén shēn*) is removed to prevent it from congesting the interior and not allowing the exterior evil to dissipate. Cinnamon twig (*guì zhī*) is added to resolve the exterior evil. If rheum assails the lung, producing cough, warm dried ginger (*gān jiāng*) is added to dispel interior cold and sour schisandra (*wǔ wèi zǐ*) is added to contract counterflowing qì. Ginseng (*rén shēn*) and jujube (*dà zǎo*) are removed to avoid their causing congestion. Fresh ginger (*shēng jiāng*) is removed because the warming action of dried ginger (*gān jiāng*) is considered necessary in this pattern, not the diffusing and dissipating action of fresh ginger (*shēng jiāng*).

Line 97

㈠ 血弱气尽，腠理开，邪气因入，与正气相搏，结于胁下。㈡ 正邪分争，往来寒热，休作有时，嘿嘿不欲饮食。㈢ 藏府相连，其痛必下，邪高痛下，故使呕也，小柴胡汤主之。㈣ 服柴胡汤已，渴者属阳明，以法治之。

(1) *Xuè ruò qì jìn, còu lǐ kāi, xié qì yīn rù, yǔ zhèng qí xiāng bó, jié yú xié xià.* (2) *Zhèng xié fēn zhēng, wǎng lái hán rè, xiū zuò yǒu shí, mò mò bù yù yǐn shí.* (3) *Zàng fǔ xiāng lián, qí tòng bì xià, xié gāo tòng xià, gù shǐ ǒu yě, xiǎo chái hú tāng zhǔ zhī.* (4) *Fú chái hú tāng yǐ, kě zhě shǔ yáng míng, yǐ fǎ zhì zhī.*

(1) When the blood is weak and the qì is exhausted, the interstices are open, and because evil qì enters [the body] and contends with right qì, [there is] binding under the rib-side. (2) The right and the evil struggle by turns,[1] [so there is] alternating [aversion to] cold and heat [effusion] that stops and starts periodically,[2] and taciturnity with no desire for food or drink. (3) The viscera and bowels are interconnected,[3] and [so] the pain will be low [down]; the evil is high [up] and the pain is [low] down, hence [there is] retching, and Minor Bupleurum Decoction (*xiǎo chái hú tāng*) governs. (4) When after taking [Minor] Bupleurum Decoction (*xiǎo chái hú tāng*) [there is] thirst, this belongs to yáng brightness and one [should use the appropriate] method to treat it.

Text Notes

1. The right and the evil struggle by turns, 正邪分争 *zhèng xié fēn zhēng*: The right and evil struggle, but neither is able to overcome the other. When right qì prevails, heat effusion is observed, and when evil qì prevails, aversion to cold is observed.
2. Alternating [aversion to] cold and heat [effusion] that stops and starts periodically, 往来寒热，休作有时 *wǎng lái hán rè, xiū zuò yǒu shí*: Alternation of aversion to cold and heat effusion, which occurs and stops in cycles.
3. The viscera and bowels are interconnected, 藏府相连 *zàng fǔ xiāng lián*: The interior-exterior relationship between the liver and gallbladder and the spleen and stomach, as well as the restraining relationship between wood (liver-gallbladder) and earth (spleen-stomach). The viscera and bowels means the five viscera: heart, lung, spleen, liver, and kidney (plus the pericardium) and the six bowels (paired by functional relationship with the viscera, respectively): small intestine, large intestine, stomach, gallbladder, bladder, and triple burner. Note: 藏府 *zàng fǔ* is equivalent to 脏腑 *zàng fǔ*.

Synopsis

1) The pathomechanism of lesser yáng disease.

2) The signs and treatment of lesser yáng disease that shifts into the yáng brightness.

Commentary

When qì and blood are vacuous, the construction and defense easily lose regulation and harmony. The defense qì becomes insecure and the interstices become loose and slack. In this condition an evil may exploit the vacuity, enter the body, and contend with right qì. The evil may directly enter the lesser yáng—the pattern Zhāng Jī describes in this line. If the evil enters the lesser yáng, it may inhibit channel qì. Because the lesser yáng channel passes through the rib-side, this qì congestion manifests as a bind under the rib-side, which may be accompanied by fullness.

The lesser yáng is considered half exterior half interior. When an evil is present in the lesser yáng, right qì struggles against it, which causes the sign of alternating aversion to cold and heat effusion. Aversion to cold occurs when the evil is prevailing in the struggle; when right qì is prevailing, heat effusion is observed. Zhāng Jī describes this pattern of alternation as "stopping and starting periodically," 休作有时 *xiū zuò yǒu shí*. According to *Gāo Děng Cóng Shū*, this is not the same as alternating aversion to cold and heat effusion that has a set periodicity. The definition of lesser yáng alternating aversion to cold and heat effusion is that it does not have a set periodicity, thereby differentiating it from the sign seen in malarial patterns. However, 休作有时 *xiū zuò yǒu shí* seems to suggest a set periodicity (c.f., 圆缺有时 *yuán quē yǒu shí*, describing the moon, "full and crescented at (set) times"). Traditional commentaries fail to give clear guidance on the matter. For this reason it is not entirely clear whether Zhāng Jī observed a distinction between the alternating aversion to cold and heat effusion of lesser yáng and that of malaria.

When an evil is present in the lesser yáng, it may influence other organs, particularly the spleen and stomach because of the close relationship between the organs. The gallbladder and the liver belong to wood, while the spleen and stomach belong to earth. Wood restrains earth and in lesser yáng disease the spleen and stomach may be invaded. Normal spleen and stomach function becomes impaired and the patient does not desire food. As in the previous line, taciturnity is the result of depressed gallbladder qì influencing heart qì.

Zhāng Jī writes, "the evil is high [up] and the pain is [low] down," referring to the relative positions in the body of the affected regions. The region of the liver and gallbladder, the two rib-sides where the evil resides, is said to be high. This evil influences the spleen and stomach causing, among other signs, pain in the abdomen, which is considered low. An evil in the lesser yáng affects the spleen and stomach, causing the patient to retch, another sign of the disharmony of the center burner. Minor Bupleurum Decoction (*xiǎo chái hú tāng*) is used to harmonize.

After the formula is taken, the lesser yáng disease should resolve, but if the patient normally has effulgent stomach yáng, it is possible that the evil will not be eliminated and will instead shift to the yáng brightness. If this shift occurs, the evil transforms to heat and dryness, damaging the fluids and causing thirst. This is not a case of inappropriate use of Minor Bupleurum Decoction (*xiǎo chái hú tāng*). Rather, the disease has shifted into another channel because of the patient's constitution, and one must observe changes in the pulse and signs, and treat accordingly. (The main treatment of yáng brightness heat is clearing or precipitating.)

Line 266

本太阳病，不解，转入少阳者，胁下硬满，干呕不能食，往来寒热，尚未吐下，脉沉紧者，与小柴胡汤。

Běn tài yáng bìng, bù jiě, zhuǎn rù shào yáng zhě, xié xià yìng mǎn, gān ǒu bù néng shí, wǎng lái hán rè, shàng wèi tù xià, mài chén jǐn zhě, yǔ xiǎo chái hú tāng.

When originally [there was] greater yáng disease that was unresolved and [thereby] shifted into the lesser yáng, [there is] hardness and fullness under the rib-side, dry retching and inability to eat, and alternating [aversion to] cold and heat [effusion]. When [neither] vomiting [treatment nor] precipitation has yet [been used] and the pulse is sunken and tight, [one should] give Minor Bupleurum Decoction (*xiǎo chái hú tāng*).

Synopsis

The pulse, signs, and treatment of greater yáng disease that has shifted into the lesser yáng from greater yáng.

Commentary

If greater yáng disease does not resolve spontaneously or resolve through treatment, the evil may shift into the lesser yáng. When this occurs, signs of the lesser yáng, such as rib-side fullness, dry retching, inability to eat, and alternating aversion to cold and heat effusion may be observed. In this pattern, lesser yáng signs appear, but the pulse is sunken and tight, not stringlike. Generally, a pulse that is sunken and tight indicates lesser yīn interior cold. Zhāng Jī writes, prior to the pulse description, that neither vomiting nor precipitation has been used, suggesting that if these inappropriate treatments had been used and the pulse was sunken and tight, it would indicate damage to right qì that allowed the evil to falls inward and cause a lesser yīn disease. In this line, however, Zhāng Jī reminds us that no mistreatment has occurred.

Qián Huáng writes, "When the evil passes to the lesser yáng, promotion of sweating, vomiting, and precipitation are all contraindicated. Provided that vomiting and precipitating treatment has not been given, there has been no adverse treatment. Although the pulse is sunken and tight, similar to when cold evil has entered the interior, the half exterior half interior signs of alternating [aversion to] cold and heat [effusion] and rib-side hard glomus are still present. Although the pulse is sunken and tight, the evil qì is still in the lesser yáng; it has not yet entered the interior." These pulse qualities reflect severe impairment of the qì dynamic, not an interior pattern. Fullness under the rib-side that is normally seen in lesser yáng patterns is present, but the area is hard as well. Furthermore, the patient suffers from dry retching and inability to eat. A pulse that is stringlike is the main pulse of lesser yáng disease. It is attributable to obstruction of the qì dynamic. When qì is severely obstructed, the pulse becomes tight. A pulse that is tight has more tension than a pulse that is stringlike. At the same time, in severe qì obstruction, when yáng qì is depressed in the interior and fails to diffuse freely, the pulse also becomes sunken. Although, as in previous lines, the pathomechanism involves qì congestion in the lesser yáng with impairment of the pivot mechanism, the pulse is described as sunken and tight, which is different from the standard lesser yáng stringlike pulse, and the hard glomus under the rib-side is different from fullness in the chest and rib-side. For this reason, the text says "give Minor Bupleurum Decoction (*xiǎo chái hú tāng*)" rather than "Minor Bupleurum Decoction (*xiǎo chái hú tāng*) governs." The suggestion is that the treatment should be modified according to the principles for varying Minor Bupleurum Decoction (*xiǎo chái hú tāng*) (see line 96, p. 410).

Line 99

伤寒四五日，身热恶风，颈项强，胁下满，手足温而渴者，小柴胡汤主之。

Shāng hán sì wǔ rì, shēn rè wù fēng, jǐng xiàng jiàng, xié xià mǎn, shǒu zú wēn ér kě zhě, xiǎo chái hú tāng zhǔ zhī.

When in cold damage [that has lasted for] four or five days, [there is] generalized heat [effusion] and aversion to wind, stiffness of the neck and nape, fullness under the rib-side, warm extremities and thirst, [then] Minor Bupleurum Decoction (*xiǎo chái hú tāng*) governs.

Synopsis

Treatment of triple-yáng signs through the lesser yáng, primarily by harmonization.

Commentary

Although this line begins with the words "cold damage," 伤寒 *shāng hán*, the pattern appears to be one of combination disease of the three yáng. Generalized heat and aversion to wind indicate a greater yáng exterior pattern. Because all three of the yáng channels pass through the neck, stiffness in the neck and nape can be indicative of any or all of them. Generally, the back of the neck corresponds to the greater yáng, the side of the neck to the lesser yáng, and the front of the neck to the yáng brightness. Fullness in the rib-side is indicative of lesser yáng disease. Thirst is an indication that yáng brightness heat has damaged the fluids. The extremities are warm because the limbs receive qì from the spleen and stomach and yáng brightness heat reaches the four extremities. When there is dryness repletion in yáng brightness, sweat streams from the extremities; when as in this case the heat is mild without repletion, the extremities are simply warm.

If this pattern is combination disease of the three yáng, why is only the lesser yáng treated, through the use of Minor Bupleurum Decoction (*xiǎo chái hú tāng*)? When lesser yáng disease is present, Zhāng Jī cautions that one must not promote sweating or use precipitation. Furthermore, it is not necessary for all the signs of a Minor Bupleurum Decoction (*xiǎo chái hú tāng*) pattern to be present for harmonization to be used. As long as the main signs are present, and the pathomechanism of lesser yáng disease can be deduced, then harmonizing treatment is appropriate (see line 101, p. 420). Even if in lesser yáng disease evidence of greater yáng or yáng brightness disease is observed, harmonizing treatment is generally recommended. This is the general rule. Under certain circumstances, sweating or precipitation may be used simultaneously with harmonization. Examples of such treatments include Bupleurum and Cinnamon Twig Decoction (*chái hú guì zhī tāng*) and Major Bupleurum Decoction (*dà chái hú tāng*). However, in this line the greater yáng and yáng brightness signs are not severe; hence the general rule applies, so treatment focuses on the lesser yáng and is varied according to the presenting signs. Once the evil is eliminated from the lesser yáng, the pivot mechanism will return to normal, allowing free communication between the upper body and lower body and between the exterior and interior. The greater yáng exterior signs and yáng brightness interior signs will then spontaneously resolve.

LINE 100

伤寒，阳脉濇，阴脉弦，法当腹中急痛，先与小建中汤，不差者，小柴胡汤主之。

Shāng hán, yáng mài sè, yīn mài xián, fǎ dāng fù zhōng jí tòng, xiān yǔ xiǎo jiàn zhōng tāng, bù chài zhě, yǔ xiǎo chái hú tāng zhǔ zhī.

When in cold damage, the yáng pulse is rough and the yīn pulse is stringlike,* as a rule, there should be acute pain in the abdomen, so one should first give Minor Center-Fortifying Decoction (*xiǎo jiàn zhōng tāng*) and if [there is] no improvement, giving Minor Bupleurum Decoction (*xiǎo chái hú tāng*) governs.

TEXT NOTE

* The yáng pulse is rough and the yīn pulse is stringlike, 阳脉濇，阴脉弦 *yáng mài sè, yīn mài xián*: Yáng means the feeling of the pulse when light pressure is applied; hence one is feeling the superficial level. Yīn means the feeling of the pulse when heavy pressure is applied; hence one is feeling the deep level. The method of feeling the different levels of the pulse and comparing the feeling at different levels is a unique aspect of the pulse analysis of Zhāng Jī and reflects concepts particular to the Chinese medicine of the Hàn Dynasty.

SYNOPSIS

The signs and treatment of lesser yáng disease with abdominal pain.

COMMENTARY

When the pulse felt at the superficial level is rough, it indicates insufficiency of the qì and blood. A stringlike quality felt at the deep level of the pulse is an indication of a lesser yáng wood evil. When blood and qì are vacuous, right qì has insufficient strength to counter the evil, so alternating aversion to cold and heat effusion is absent. From an analysis of the formula, one can assume that the root cause of the qì and blood vacuity is vacuity of the spleen preventing normal movement and transformation of essence. When qì and blood vacuity deprive the sinews of warmth and nourishment, and the wood evil exploits the earth weakness, the result is acute abdominal pain.

Minor Center-Fortifying Decoction (*xiǎo jiàn zhōng tāng*) is used to fortify the spleen and make the blood and qì sufficient. Once the earth is fortified, a mild wood evil may cease to exploit its weakness and spontaneously resolve. After taking the formula, however, if the pain does not resolve and the pulse is still stringlike, it indicates that the lesser yáng evil has not been eliminated. Minor Bupleurum Decoction (*xiǎo chái hú tāng*) should be used to address the lesser yáng evil directly. This method is called "discharging wood evil and safeguarding center earth."

Line 101

(一) 伤寒中风，有柴胡证，但见一证便是，不必悉具。(二) 凡柴胡汤病证而下之，若柴胡证不罢者，复与柴胡汤，必蒸蒸而振，却复发热汗出而解。

(1) *Shāng hán zhòng fēng, yǒu chái hú zhèng, dàn jiàn yī zhèng biàn shì, bù bì xī jù.* (2) *Fán chái hú tāng bìng zhèng ér xià zhī, ruò chái hú zhèng bù bà zhě, fù yǔ chái hú tāng, bì zhēng zhēng ér zhèn, què fù fā rè hàn chū ér jiě.*

(1) [When] in cold damage [or] wind strike, there are [Minor] Bupleurum [Decoction] ([*xiǎo*] *chái hú* [*tāng*]) signs, only one sign [means that] this is [the pattern], they do not all have to be present. (2) Whenever a [Minor] Bupleurum Decoction ([*xiǎo*] *chái hú tāng*) disease pattern [is treated by] precipitation, if the [Minor] Bupleurum [Decoction] ([*xiǎo*] *chái hú* [*tāng*]) pattern has not ceased, [one can] give [Minor] Bupleurum Decoction ([*xiǎo*] *chái hú tāng*) again. [There] will be steaming and quivering, then heat effusion and sweating again, by which [the disease] resolves.

Synopsis

1) The method for use of Minor Bupleurum Decoction (*xiǎo chái hú tāng*).

2) Changes following administration of Minor Bupleurum Decoction (*xiǎo chái hú tāng*) after misuse of precipitation.

Commentary

Regardless of whether a disease begins as cold damage or wind strike, it can shift into the lesser yáng. Once signs of a Minor Bupleurum Decoction (*xiǎo chái hú tāng*) pattern are seen, one need not see all of the lesser yáng signs to diagnose the disease as belonging to the lesser yáng. In this line Zhāng Jī reiterates and formally states a principle that is evident in lines previously discussed; many different signs may appear in lesser yáng disease because the basic pathomechanism involves the pivot mechanism. The pivot mechanism influences the flow of qì throughout the body, so when it is congested and impaired, the consequences are wide and varied.

In this line Zhāng Jī writes, "only one sign [means that] this is [the pattern], they do not all have to be present." The main point of this statement is that not all the signs have to be present. The statement should not be taken to suggest that the appearance of one sign of lesser yáng disease means that one can conclude that the pattern should be treated with Minor Bupleurum Decoction (*xiǎo chái hú tāng*). Rather, one only needs to see one or more of the main signs of lesser yáng disease to consider harmonizing with Minor Bupleurum Decoction (*xiǎo chái hú tāng*). If one waits for all the signs of lesser yáng disease to appear, one will miss the opportunity for successful treatment. When even one main sign of lesser yáng disease is present, one should be cautious about using the promotion of sweating, vomiting, or precipitation, which are contraindicated in lesser yáng disease.

Lesser yáng disease should be treated by harmonizing with Minor Bupleurum Decoction (*xiǎo chái hú tāng*). Precipitation is generally not an appropriate treatment. If precipitation is misused and lesser yáng signs are still present, this means that precipitation has not given rise to a transmuted pattern, and so one can still give Minor Bupleurum Decoction (*xiǎo chái hú tāng*). Nevertheless, although the evil has not fallen inward, the precipitation will have caused further damage to right qì, so that its resistance to the evil is lessened. Once Minor Bupleurum Decoction (*xiǎo chái hú tāng*) is taken, steaming and quivering will occur, indicating that the medicinals are assisting right qì in its struggle with evil qì and that the struggle is becoming more intense. Once right qì reaches the point at which it can overcome evil qì, the aversion to cold will cease, and heat effusion and sweating will be observed. Through this mechanism the evil will be expelled and the disease will resolve. This type of sweating was subsequently called 战汗 *zhàn hàn*, "shiver sweating."

LINE 229

阳明病，发潮热，大便溏，小便自可，胸胁满不去者，与小柴胡汤。

Yáng míng bìng, fā cháo rè, dà biàn táng, xiǎo biàn zì kě, xiōng xié mǎn bù qù zhě, yǔ xiǎo chái hú tāng.

When in yáng brightness disease, [there is] tidal heat effusion, sloppy stool, normal urination, and fullness in the chest and rib-side that will not go, give Minor Bupleurum Decoction (*xiǎo chái hú tāng*).

SYNOPSIS

The principle that when yáng brightness interior repletion is not pronounced and the main signs of lesser yáng disease are still present, the condition should be treated through lesser yáng.

COMMENTARY

Although this line begins with a reference to yáng brightness disease, the condition described is actually one of lesser yáng.

Tidal heat effusion in yáng brightness disease is usually a sign that bowel repletion has already formed. In addition to tidal heat effusion, there ought to be abdominal fullness, hardness, and pain with hard bound stool. Furthermore, if urination is frequent in yáng brightness disease, the stool should already be hard.

In this line, despite the presence of tidal heat effusion, there is no abdominal fullness and pain, urination is normal, and the stool is thin and sloppy. Although the disease has affected the yáng brightness, the dryness-heat has not yet become replete, and the bowel pattern has not formed. The presence of fullness in the chest and rib-side suggests that although the evil is entering the yáng brightness, it has not completely left the lesser yáng. Zhāng Jī writes that the fullness "will not go," 不去 *bù qù*, indicating that it was present previously, and therefore that the disease was originally in the lesser yáng. Minor Bupleurum Decoction (*xiǎo chái hú tāng*) is used in this case because when the lesser yáng signs have not yet been eliminated, one should first harmonize the lesser yáng.

In this pattern, simultaneous disease of the lesser yáng and yáng brightness is treated through the lesser yáng. However, when yáng brightness dryness repletion becomes more pronounced, one might consider using Major Bupleurum Decoction (*dà chái hú tāng*) to harmonize the lesser yáng and precipitate the yáng brightness simultaneously.

LINE 230

阳明病，胁下硬满，不大便，而呕，舌上白胎者，可与小柴胡汤，上焦得通，津液得下，胃气因和，身濈然汗出而解。

Yáng míng bìng, xié xià yìng mǎn, bù dà biàn, ér ǒu, shé shàng bái tāi zhě, kě yǔ xiǎo chái hú tāng, shàng jiāo dé tōng, jīn yè dé xià, wèi qì yīn hé, shēn jí rán hàn chū ér jiě.

When in yáng brightness disease, [there is] hardness and fullness under the rib-side, inability to defecate, retching, and white fur on the tongue, one can give Minor Bupleurum Decoction (*xiǎo chái hú tāng*). The upper burner [will] unblock, and liquid and humor will be able to descend, stomach qì will thereby become harmonious, and [there will be] generalized streaming sweat, bringing about resolution.

SYNOPSIS

1) The treatment method for yáng brightness disease when the Minor Bupleurum Decoction (*xiǎo chái hú tāng*) signs have not ceased.

2) The mechanism of the action of Minor Bupleurum Decoction (*xiǎo chái hú tāng*).

COMMENTARY

In the previous line, although tidal heat effusion (a sign of yáng brightness disease) is observed, because of the presence of lesser yáng signs and the lack of signs indicating yáng brightness bowel repletion, the pattern is treated through the lesser yáng. In this line the stool is bound, which may indicate a yáng brightness bowel repletion pattern. Nonetheless, although hard fullness is observed, it is not in the abdomen, but under the rib-side. The tongue fur is not yellow and dry, as one might expect in yáng brightness bowel repletion with pronounced dryness-heat; instead it is white. Retching is one of the main signs of lesser yáng disease, and its simultaneous appearance with rib-side hard fullness and the other presenting signs indicate that, although the evil may be shifting into the yáng brightness, it is currently still in the lesser yáng. As in the previous line the treatment should focus on harmonizing the lesser yáng.

Minor Bupleurum Decoction (*xiǎo chái hú tāng*) is the main harmonization formula. By its harmonizing action, the pivot mechanism is restored and the qì dynamic is disinhibited. The triple burner is freed and regulated, and free coursing is normalized, so that there is nowhere in the gallbladder channel for evils to settle, and the spleen and stomach will not be subject to restraining and robbing. When the upper burner is freed, the hard glomus under the rib-side will disappear; when depurative downbearing of lung qì is restored, liquid and humor can flow downward, so that defecation becomes naturally regulated; when the harmonious downbearing of stomach qì is restored, retching counterflow ceases; when the triple burner is freed, construction, defense, and the fluids are unobstructed, so that sweat can stream forth to bring about resolution.

LINE 148

㈠ 伤寒五六日，头汗出，微恶寒，手足冷，心下满，口不欲食，大便硬，脉细者，此为阳微结，必有表，复有里也。㈡ 脉沉，亦在里也。㈢ 汗出为阳微。㈣ 假令纯阴结，不得复有外证，悉入在里；此为半在里半在外也。㈤ 脉虽沉紧，不得为少阴病。㈥ 所以然者，阴不得有汗，今头汗出，故知非少阴也。㈦ 可与小柴胡汤，设不了了者，得屎而解。

(1) *Shāng hán wǔ liù rì, tóu hàn chū, wēi wù hán, shǒu zú lěng, xīn xià mǎn, kǒu bù yù shí, dà biàn yìng, mài xì zhě, cǐ wéi yáng wēi jié, bì yǒu biǎo, fù yǒu lǐ yě.* (2) *Mài chén yì zài lǐ yě.* (3) *Hàn chū wéi yáng wēi.* (4) *Jiǎ lìng chún yīn jié, bù dé fù yǒu wài zhèng, xī rù zài lǐ; cǐ wéi bàn zài lǐ bàn zài wài yě.* (5) *Mài suī chén jǐn, bù dé wéi shào yīn bìng.* (6) *Suǒ yǐ rán zhě, yīn bù dé yǒu hàn, jīn tóu hàn chū, gù zhī fēi shào yīn yě.* (7) *Kě yǔ xiǎo chái hú tāng, shè bù liǎo liǎo zhě, dé shǐ ér jiě.*

(1) When cold damage [has lasted for] five or six days, and [there is] sweating from the head, mild aversion to cold, cold extremities, fullness below the heart, absence of desire to eat, hard stool, and a pulse that is fine, this means mild yáng bind; there must be exterior [signs] as well

as interior [signs]. (2) A pulse that is sunken [means the evil] is in the interior. (3) Sweating means mild yáng [bind]. (4) If [there is] pure yīn bind, there can no longer be any exterior signs [since] everything has entered the interior, [whereas the pattern of mild yáng bind] is half in the interior and half in the exterior. (5) Although the pulse is sunken and tight, it does not indicate lesser yīn disease. (6) Why [this is] so is because with yīn [disease] there will be no sweating and now, in the present case, sweat issues from the head; therefore, one knows [this] is not lesser yīn [disease]. (7) One can give Minor Bupleurum Decoction (*xiǎo chái hú tāng*) and if [the pattern] does not clearly [resolve], [once] the stool [passes], [there will be] resolution.

SYNOPSIS

1) The pulse, signs, and treatment of mild yáng bind.

2) The differentiation of mild yáng bind and pure yīn bind.

COMMENTARY

This line is best read in three sections. The first is from the beginning to "exterior [signs] as well as interior [signs]." The second is from there to "[this] is not lesser yīn [disease]. The last is to the end of the line.

After five or six days of cold damage disease, sweat issues only from the head, indicating that heat is depressed in the interior. The heat cannot effuse outwards and instead steams the fluids in the interior to the upper regions of the body. Mild aversion to cold suggests that the exterior pattern has not yet resolved, and because this sign is mild, one knows that the exterior pattern is not severe. The presence of a heat evil depressed in the interior prevents yáng qì from reaching the limbs, causing cold in the extremities. This is a pattern of mild heat depression. The yáng qì depression further inhibits the movement of blood and qì through the channels and produces a pulse that is fine. On the basis of information in the latter part of this line, the pulse should be considered to be not only fine, but also sunken and tight. When qì is severely obstructed, the pulse becomes tight. At the same time, in severe qì obstruction when yáng qì is depressed in the interior and fails to diffuse freely, the pulse becomes sunken. Readers familiar with the modern definitions of pulse terms should note that a tight pulse now refers to one that is like a "twirled taut rope," 牵绳转索 *qiān shéng zhuǎn suǒ*, as compared with a stringlike pulse, which is described as being "like pressing a zither string," 如按琴弦 *rú àn qīn xián* or "like pressing a bowstring," 按之如弓弦状 *àn zhī rú gōng xián zhuàng*. The tight pulse is thicker (wider) than the stringlike pulse, and since a stringlike pulse is normal in width or narrower, a tight pulse cannot be fine. Nevertheless, in Zhāng Jī's understanding of the pulses, "tight" appears only to connote greater tension than "stringlike."

Fullness below the heart, no desire for food, and hard stool are further indications of an interior heat evil disturbing the qì dynamic, the harmony of the stomach, and the movement of fluids down into the bowel. This pattern is called "mild yáng bind" in the text. Whereas yáng brightness bowel repletion dryness bind is attributed to yáng brightness dry-heat qì desiccating the waste in the intestinal tract and is characterized by absence of defecation, abdominal fullness, hardness and pain, and tidal heat effusion, mild yáng bind is marked by milder heat bind with unresolved exterior signs. This arises when there are still exterior signs present and interior signs are already present, and therefore differs from the purely interior patterns of yáng brightness. The pathomechanism of mild yáng bind is heat evil binding mildly in the interior, inhibiting the pivot and the movement of qì and blood.

The second section of this line differentiates between mild yáng bind and pure yīn bind. Since mild yáng bind is marked by aversion to cold, cold extremities, and a pulse that is sunken, fine, and tight, it is similar to pure yīn bind. Thus, the two have still to be differentiated. First, in pure yīn bind, yáng is debilitated and yīn is exuberant. The pattern belongs only to the interior, and exterior signs should be absent. In mild yáng bind the exterior signs of heat effusion and slight aversion to cold appear before the interior signs of fullness below the heart, no desire to eat, and hard stool. Second, in yīn cold patterns, debilitation of yáng and exuberance of yīn prevent liquid from being transformed into sweat, so that normally sweating is absent. (However, there is also yáng collapse in which there is sweating from the head, with signs of vacuous yáng straying outward, but this condition is not described in the *Shāng Hán Lùn*.) This pattern is one of heat evil lying depressed in the inner body, causing the pivot mechanism to become inhibited. However, the depressed heat evil only steams to the head and there are no critical signs of vacuous yáng straying outward. Third, a pulse that is sunken and deep may be observed in lesser yīn disease and mild yáng bind, but in each case the pathomechanism is different. When the pulse is deep and tight in lesser yīn, there should also be sore throat as well as vomiting and diarrhea. In mild yáng bind, however, there is no sore throat and the stool is hard.

In the final section Zhāng Jī describes the treatment of mild yáng bind. Because this is a half exterior half interior pattern, the lesser yáng pivot mechanism is inhibited, and therefore Minor Bupleurum Decoction (*xiǎo chái hú tāng*) is given. Once the pivot mechanism is restored, the upper burner will be freed, liquid and humor will be able to descend, stomach qì will thereby become harmonious, the stool will be freed, and there will be generalized streaming sweat that will eliminate the depressed heat, bringing about resolution of the exterior and interior patterns. If after the patient has taken the formula the disease does not resolve clearly, the reason is that interior qì has not been restored to harmony, and the movement of qì and fluids through the three burners has not completely returned to normal. The final words of the line, "[once] the stool [passes], [there will be] resolution" can be interpreted in two ways. The first is that if the disease does not resolve clearly, one should give a formula to free the stool. Once the stool moves, the disease will resolve. The second interpretation is that one should not give further treatment, but should wait for the stool to move, after which the disease will resolve.

3.2 Contraindications for Minor Bupleurum Decoction

Line 98

㈠得病六七日，脉迟浮弱，恶风寒，手足温，医二三下之，不能食，而胁下满痛，面目及身黄，颈项强，小便难者，与柴胡汤，后必下重。㈡本渴饮水而呕者，柴胡汤不中与也，食谷者哕。

(1) *Dé bìng liù qī rì, mài chí fú ruò, wù fēng hán, shǒu zú wēn, yī èr sān xià zhī, bù néng shí, ér xié xià mǎn tòng, miàn mù jí shēn huáng, jǐng xiàng jiàng, xiǎo biàn nán zhě, yǔ chái hú tāng, hòu bì xià zhòng.* (2) *Běn kě yǐn shuǐ ér ǒu zhě, chái hú bù zhōng yǔ yě, shí gǔ zhě yuē.*

(1) When in an illness [that the person has] had for six or seven days, the pulse is slow, floating, and weak, and [there is] aversion to wind and cold, and warm extremities, and the physician precipitates two or three times, [there is] inability to eat, pain and fullness under the rib-side, yellowing of the eyes, face and body, stiffness of the neck and nape, and difficult urination. After Minor Bupleurum Decoction (*xiǎo chái hú tāng*) is given, there will be rectal heaviness.* (2) When originally there was thirst with retching following water intake, [Minor] Bupleurum [Decoction] ([*xiǎo*] *chái hú* [*tāng*]) should not be given, and when food is taken [there will be] hiccup.

Text Note

* Rectal heaviness, 下重 *xià zhòng*: A feeling of heaviness in the rectum accompanied by abdominal pain and a desire to defecate. The evacuation of stool is inhibited. This is the same as abdominal urgency and rectal heaviness, 里急后重 *lǐ jí hòu zhòng*, i.e., tenesmus.

Synopsis

A transmuted pattern that occurs after inappropriate treatment of interior vacuity with an exterior pattern.

Commentary

After six or seven days of an externally contracted disease, one must observe the patient carefully to see what transmuted patterns may have developed. The pulse is floating and weak, and aversion to cold persists, indicating that the exterior pattern has not yet resolved. In exterior patterns, however, one does not expect to see a pulse that is slow. In this line a pulse that is slow as well as floating and weak indicates that this is not a pure exterior pattern, and that the evil has entered the greater yīn. A pulse that is slow may be seen in patterns associated with all the three yīn channels, but only in greater yīn disease does it coincide with warm extremities. The appearance of warm extremities in a greater yīn yáng vacuity pattern is explained in this line by the fact that the greater yīn disease is combined with an exterior pattern, rather than being a pure greater yīn disease. Despite a wind-cold exterior contraction, the interior is vacuous and powerless to resist the disease; hence there is no generalized heat effusion, but only warmth in the extremities.

If this condition is misidentified as a yáng brightness disease with warm extremities, and precipitation is used repeatedly, it will exacerbate the spleen-stomach vacuity and cause debilitation of yáng qì, giving rise to internal cold-damp. When the spleen and stomach are vacuous, food intake is impaired. When cold and dampness become bound and depressed in the liver and gallbladder channels, there is fullness and pain under the rib-side. Cold-damp obstructs the center burner, spilling out to the whole body, so that the face, eyes, and body become yellow. When this happens, spleen vacuity with impaired movement and transformation causes non-movement of water, manifesting in inhibited urination. This pathomechanism is in keeping with that described in line 187, p. 462, and line 278, p. 461: "In greater yīn [disease], there should be generalized yellowing, [but] if the urine is spontaneously uninhibited, there will be inability to yellow." In this line, urination is difficult, and the dampness has no way out of the body; consequently, yellowing of the face, eyes, and body occurs. Yellowing arising in this way subsequently came to be called "yīn yellowing." Stiffness of the nape and neck is further indication that the original exterior pattern has not yet resolved. The appropriate treatment is to warm the center, dissipate cold, and eliminate dampness. If the presence of fullness and pain under the rib-side is taken as an indication of lesser yáng disease, and Minor Bupleurum Decoction (*xiǎo chái hú tāng*) is given, the bitter, cold agents in the formula will exacerbate the interior vacuity, causing spleen vacuity and qì fall, so that the diarrhea and rectal heaviness (i.e., tenesmus) are exacerbated.

In this line thirst with intake of fluids is not due to heat or dryness; rather it arises because spleen yáng is insufficient and fails to move and transform fluids, so that water qì collects internally and qì cannot transform it into (bodily) liquid. Dryness-heat thirst is due to lack of liquid; although there is great thirst, the water can be dispersed so there is no retching counterflow. Yet in this line, qì cannot transform the water that is collecting; hence the more the patient drinks, the more water will collect, causing retching counterflow. This is treated by fortifying the spleen and moving water. If the retching in this pattern is considered to be an indication of lesser yáng disease and Minor Bupleurum Decoction (*xiǎo chái hú tāng*) is given, center qì will be ruined and there will be hiccup after taking food.

4 LESSER YÁNG DISEASE AND TRANSMUTED PATTERNS

4.1 Treatment Principles for Transmuted Patterns

Line 267

若已吐、下、发汗、温针，谵语，柴胡证罢，此为坏病，知犯何逆，以法治之。

Ruò yǐ tù、 xià、 fā hàn、 wēn zhēn, zhān yǔ, chái hú zhèng bà, cǐ wéi huài bìng, zhī fàn hé nì, yǐ fǎ zhì zhī.

If after vomiting, precipitation, promotion of sweating, or warm needling, [there is] delirious speech, and the [Minor] Bupleurum [Decoction] ([*xiǎo*] *chái hú* [*tāng*]) pattern ceases, this means [this is] an aggravated disease; [therefore, one should] be aware of what error one has committed, be aware of what adverse [treatment] has been given, and use the [appropriate] method to treat it.

Synopsis

1) A transmuted pattern that occurs after inappropriate treatment of a lesser yáng disease.

2) The principle of how to treat a transmuted pattern after an adverse treatment.

Commentary

This line follows line 266, p. 417, "When originally [there was] greater yáng disease that was unresolved and [thereby] shifted into the lesser yáng..." In that line no mistreatment occurs, so that the appropriate treatment is harmonization, generally with Minor Bupleurum Decoction (*xiǎo chái hú tāng*) or a variation of that formula. The present line, by contrast, presents the consequences of repeated mistreatment with vomiting, precipitation, sweating, or warm needling, which in lesser yáng disease are all considered inappropriate.

After repeated mistreatment, delirious speech (a sign not seen in lesser yáng disease) is observed. The appearance of delirious speech and the cessation of the Minor Bupleurum Decoction (*xiǎo chái hú tāng*) pattern indicates that the disease has already left the lesser yáng half exterior and half interior, and has completely entered the interior. For this reason the condition described here is called an "aggravated disease," indicating that it is a severe and complex condition that is difficult to name in terms of the six channels. Delirious speech in aggravated disease occurs in many different situations. It may, for example, arise from the yáng brightness or other channel diseases; it may be due to evil repletion, or to right vacuity with evil repletion, or even to yáng collapse. So, one has to observe the pulse and signs, establish what error has been committed, and treat according to the signs.

4.2 BUPLEURUM AND CINNAMON TWIG DECOCTION PATTERNS

LINE 146

伤寒六七日，发热，微恶寒，肢节烦疼，微呕，心下支结，外证未去者，柴胡桂枝汤主之。

Shāng hán liù qī rì, fā rè, wēi wù hán, zhī jié fán téng, wēi ǒu, xīn xià zhī jié, wài zhèng wèi qù zhě, chái hú guì zhī tāng zhǔ zhī.

When in cold damage [that has lasted for] six or seven days, [there is] heat effusion, mild aversion to cold, vexing pain of the limb joints,[1] mild retching, propping bind below the heart,[2] and the exterior pattern is still present, Bupleurum and Cinnamon Twig Decoction (*chái hú guì zhī tāng*) governs.

TEXT NOTES

1. Vexing pain of the limb joints, 支节烦疼 *zhī jié fán téng*: 支 *zhī* is equivalent to 肢 *zhī*; hence 支节 *zhī jié* means the limb joints. Vexing pain is considered to be pain that is severe enough to cause the person to become vexed.
2. Propping bind below the heart, 心下支结 *xīn xià zhī jié*: A bind below the heart characterized by a feeling that something is braced in the area below the heart.

FORMULA

Bupleurum and Cinnamon Twig Decoction (*chái hú guì zhī tāng*)

∘ Harmonize the lesser yáng in order to dissipate the exterior [evil].

桂枝（去皮） 黄芩一两半 人参一两半 甘草一两（炙） 半夏二合半（洗） 芍药一两半 大枣六枚（擘） 生姜一两半（切） 柴胡四两

㈠ 右九味，以水七升，煮取三升，去滓，温服一升。

Guì zhī (qù pí) huáng qín yī liǎng bàn rén shēn yī liǎng bàn gān cǎo yī liǎng (zhì) bàn xià èr gě bàn (xǐ) sháo yào yī liǎng bàn dà zǎo liù méi (bò) shēng jiāng yī liǎng bàn (qiē) chái hú sì liǎng

(1) *Yòu jiǔ wèi, yǐ shuǐ qī shēng, zhǔ qǔ sān shēng, qù zǐ, wēn fú yī shēng.*

cinnamon twig (桂枝 *guì zhī*, Cinnamomi Ramulus)* (remove bark)
scutellaria (黄芩 *huáng qín*, Scutellariae Radix) 1.5 liǎng
ginseng (人参 *rén shēn*, Ginseng Radix) 1.5 liǎng
mix-fried licorice (甘草 *gān cǎo*, Glycyrrhizae Radix) 1 liǎng
pinellia (半夏 *bàn xià*, Pinelliae Tuber) 2.5 gě (washed)
peony (芍药 *sháo yào*, Paeoniae Radix) 1.5 liǎng

jujube (大枣 *dà zǎo*, Ziziphi Fructus) 6 pieces (broken)
fresh ginger (生姜 *shēng jiāng*, Zingiberis Rhizoma Recens) 1.5 liǎng (cut)
bupleurum (柴胡 *chái hú*, Bupleuri Radix) 4 liǎng

(1) [For] the above ingredients use seven shēng of water. Boil to get three shēng, remove the dregs, and take one shēng warm.

Formula Note

* Cinnamon twig (*guì zhī*): The prescribed weight (specific indication of the weight is missing) is taken to be 1.5 liǎng.

Synopsis

The signs and treatment of lesser yáng disease with an exterior pattern.

Commentary

After six or seven days of a cold damage disease, the presence of heat effusion, mild aversion to cold, and vexing pain in the limb joints indicates that the greater yáng exterior pattern has not been eliminated. Mild retching without propping bind below the heart may occur in greater yáng disease. However, mild retching with propping bind below the heart only results from evil entering the lesser yáng and gallbladder evil invading the stomach, and is similar to the heart vexation and frequent retching we have seen in another lesser yáng line (i.e., line 96, p. 410). Propping bind below the heart is different from the commonly observed signs of lesser yáng disease: fullness in the chest and rib-side and hard glomus below the rib-side. However, because the foot lesser yáng channel descends into the chest, goes through the diaphragm, nets the liver, and homes to the gallbladder, when the channel qì becomes depressed and bound, the appearance of propping bind below the heart is entirely possible.

When an unresolved greater yáng exterior pattern exists, one should promote sweating to resolve the exterior. Nonetheless, when a lesser yáng disease is observed, the exclusive use of sweating is contraindicated. In this line, to treat the simultaneous disease of greater yáng and lesser yáng, the suggested formula is Bupleurum and Cinnamon Twig Decoction (*chái hú guì zhī tāng*), which combines the harmonizing formula, Minor Bupleurum Decoction (*xiǎo chái hú tāng*), with the exterior-resolving formula, Cinnamon Twig Decoction (*guì zhī tāng*). This formula harmonizes and regulates construction and defense and dissipates the exterior evil, while simultaneously harmonizing and resolving the pivot mechanism and eliminating the lesser yáng evil.

However, the amounts of the ingredients are reduced by half from the original formulae, indicating that the signs in this line are mild. The aversion to cold and retching are explicitly described as mild; generalized pain, headache, and painful stiff nape, which are typically seen in greater yáng disease, are replaced by the milder sign of vexing pain in the limbs and joints. Furthermore, the propping bind below the heart is milder than fullness in the chest and rib-side or hard glomus below the rib-side. A mild formula is used to harmonize construction and defense and dissipate the exterior evil, while simultaneously harmonizing the pivot mechanism and eliminating the lesser yáng evil.

4.3 Major Bupleurum Decoction Patterns

Line 103

㈠ 太阳病，过经十余日，反二三下之，后四五日，柴胡证仍在者，先与小柴胡。㈡ 呕不止，心下急，郁郁微烦者，为未解也，与大柴胡汤下之则愈。

(1) *Tài yáng bìng, guò jīng shí yú rì, fǎn èr sān xià zhī, hòu sì wǔ rì, chái hú zhèng réng zài zhě, xiān yǔ xiǎo chái hú.* (2) *Oǔ bù zhǐ, xīn xià jí, yù yù wēi fán zhě, wéi wèi jiě yě, yǔ dà chái hú tāng xià zhī zé yù.*

(1) When in greater yáng disease, ten or more days after channel passage, precipitation [has] instead [been used] two or three times, after four or five days, [if] the [Minor] Bupleurum [Decoction] ([*xiǎo*] *chái hú* [*tāng*]) pattern is still present, first give Minor Bupleurum [Decoction] (*xiǎo chái hú* [*tāng*]). (2) If [there is] incessant retching, distress below the heart,[1] and depression and mild vexation,[2] it means [that the disease] has not yet resolved; giving Major Bupleurum Decoction (*dà chái hú tāng*) to precipitate will lead to recovery.

Text Notes

1. Distress below the heart, 心下急 *xīn xià jí*: A feeling of hypertonicity and/or pain in the region of the stomach duct below the heart.
2. Depression and mild vexation, 郁郁微烦 *yù yù wēi fán*: See line 123, p. 279, for a discussion of this sign.

Formula

Major Bupleurum Decoction (*dà chái hú tāng*)

○ Harmonize the lesser yáng; free and precipitate interior repletion.

柴胡半斤　黄芩三两　芍药三两　半夏半升（洗）　生姜五两（切）　枳实四枚（炙）　大枣十二枚（擘）

㈠ 右七味，以水一斗二升，煮取六升，去滓，再煎，温服一升，日三服。㈡ 一方，加大黄二两。㈢ 若不加，恐不为大柴胡汤。

Chái hú bàn jīn　huáng qín sān liǎng　sháo yào sān liǎng　bàn xià bàn shēng (xǐ)　shēng jiāng wǔ liǎng (qiē)　zhǐ shí sì méi (zhì)　dà zǎo shí èr méi (bò)

(1) *Yòu qī wèi, yǐ shuǐ yī dǒu èr shēng, zhǔ qǔ liù shēng, qù zǐ, zài jiān, wēn fú yī shēng, rì sān fú.* (2) *Yī fāng, jiā dà huáng èr liǎng.* (3) *Ruò bù jiā, kǒng bù wéi dà chái hú tāng.*

bupleurum (柴胡 *chái hú*, Bupleuri Radix) half jīn

scutellaria (黄芩 *huáng qín*, Scutellariae Radix) 3 liǎng
peony (芍药 *sháo yào*, Paeoniae Radix) 3 liǎng
pinellia (半夏 *bàn xià*, Pinelliae Tuber) half shēng (washed)
fresh ginger (生姜 *shēng jiāng*, Zingiberis Rhizoma Recens) 5 liǎng (cut)
processed unripe bitter orange (枳实 *zhǐ shí*, Aurantii Fructus Immaturus) 4 pieces
jujube (大枣 *dà zǎo*, Ziziphi Fructus) 12 pieces (broken)

(1) [For] the above seven ingredients use one dǒu two shēng of water. Boil to get six shēng, remove the dregs, and decoct again. Take one shēng warm, three times a day. (2) Another [version of the] formula adds two liǎng of rhubarb (*dà huáng*). (3) If it is not added, this is not Major Bupleurum Decoction (*dà chái hú tāng*).*

Formula Note

* Another [version of the] formula adds two liǎng of rhubarb (*dà huáng*). If it is not added, this is not Major Bupleurum Decoction (*dà chái hú tāng*), 一方，加大黄二两，若不加，恐不为大柴胡汤 *yī fāng, jiā dà huáng èr liáng, ruò bù jiā, kǒng bù wéi dá chái hú tāng*: These sentences were evidently added at the end of the formula section by the editors of the Sòng version to explain that although the Sòng version does not include rhubarb (*dà huáng*), another version of the formula did include it. In fact, we know that *Jīn Guì Yào Lüè*, *Qiān Jīn Yì Fāng*, *Zhǒu Hòu Fāng* (肘后方 "Standby Remedies") and, *Wài Tái Mì Yào* all include rhubarb (*dà huáng*); only the Sòng version of the *Shāng Hán Lùn* omits it. For this reason, rhubarb (*dà huáng*) is generally included in the formula.

Synopsis

The signs and treatment of lesser yáng disease with interior repletion.

Commentary

The present line describes a condition arising when disease has completely passed from greater yáng to lesser yáng leaving no greater yáng signs, and has been in the lesser yáng for ten days or more. Although in lesser yáng disease the exclusive use of precipitation (as that of vomiting and promotion of sweating) is inappropriate, it has been used two or three times in this case. However, after four or five days, because right qì has remained effulgent the lesser yáng signs are still present and no transmuted pattern has developed. For this reason the disease can still be treated with Minor Bupleurum Decoction (*xiǎo chái hú tāng*).

If after taking the formula the pivot mechanism is restored, the patient will recover. However, if there is no improvement in the condition and if incessant retching, distress below the heart, and depression and mild vexation are observed, it means that inappropriate precipitation before taking Minor Bupleurum Decoction (*xiǎo chái hú tāng*) has caused the disease evil to partly enter the yáng brightness, so that the pathomechanism has turned into that of inhibition of the lesser yáng pivot mechanism with yáng brightness dryness formation creating repletion. In this situation, therefore, Minor Bupleurum Decoction (*xiǎo chái hú tāng*) not only fails to bring about recovery, but exacerbates the condition. Lesser yáng disease cannot be treated exclusively by precipitation; yáng brightness interior repletion must be treated by precipitation. Therefore, harmonization and precipitation are combined in Major Bupleurum Decoction (*dà chái hú tāng*) to simultaneously resolve disease evil in the lesser yáng and yáng brightness.

Major Bupleurum Decoction (*dà chái hú tāng*) is Minor Bupleurum Decoction (*xiǎo chái hú tāng*) without ginseng (*rén shēn*) and licorice (*gān cǎo*) and with the addition of peony (*sháo yào*), unripe bitter orange (*zhǐ shí*), and rhubarb (*dà huáng*). Bupleurum (*chái hú*) and scutellaria (*huáng qín*) course and discharge depressed heat in the lesser yáng, diffusing and outthrusting the half exterior half interior heat evil. Fresh ginger (*shēng jiāng*) and pinellia (*bàn xià*) downbear counterflow and suppress retching, and harmonize the stomach qì. Slightly cold, acrid, and bitter, unripe bitter orange (*zhǐ shí*) breaks binds and descends the qì. Often used for glomus and bind, it is used here to resolve the distress below the heart. Unripe bitter orange (*zhǐ shí*) and rhubarb (*dà huáng*) used together can unblock repletion in the yáng brightness bowel, as in Minor Qì-Coordinating Decoction (*xiǎo chéng qì tāng*). Because signs of abdominal distention and fullness are absent, magnolia bark (*hòu pò*) is not added. Peony (*sháo yào*) harmonizes the construction-yīn, relaxes tension, and relieves pain. Jujube (*dà zǎo*) is used to supplement the spleen and stomach because, given that the disease is affecting not only wood but also earth, a center-supplementing action should be included in formulae that primarily drain evil.

This line, line 149, p. 234, and line 264, p. 408, discuss the five developments that may occur following the inappropriate, exclusive use of precipitation in lesser yáng disease. (1) After precipitation, the Minor Bupleurum Decoction (*xiǎo chái hú tāng*) pattern may still be present. (2) The pattern may change into a major chest bind pattern. (3) The pattern may turn into a Pinellia Heart-Draining Decoction (*bàn xià xiè xīn tāng*) pattern. (4) The pattern can change into a Major Bupleurum Decoction (*dà chái hú tāng*) pattern. (5) Damage to qì and blood may cause palpitations and fright. Which of these five developments occurs depends on the patient's constitution, the strength of the evil, and the severity of the mistreatment. Furthermore, it should also be noted that any of these developments may occur spontaneously, not as a result of inappropriate precipitation.

LINE 165

伤寒发热，汗出不解，心中痞硬，呕吐而下利者，大柴胡主之。

Shāng hán fā rè, hàn chū bù jiě, xīn zhōng pǐ yìng, ǒu tù ér xià lì zhě, dà chái hú tāng zhǔ zhī.

When in cold damage [there is] heat effusion and sweating [that brings] no resolution, hard glomus in [below] the heart,* retching, vomiting, and diarrhea, [then] Major Bupleurum Decoction (*dà chái hú tāng*) governs.

Text Note

* Hard glomus in [below] the heart, 心中痞硬 *xīn zhōng pǐ yìng*: Although "in the heart," 心中, *xīn zhōng* appears in the text, Chéng Wú-Jǐ in the Jīn Dynasty and most modern commentators replace "in," 中 *zhōng*, with "below," 下 *xià*. In the *Jīn Guì Yào Lüè* the following line appears: "Pain below the heart when pressed indicates repletion. It should be precipitated, and Major Bupleurum Decoction (*dà chái hú tāng*) is appropriate." Line 103, p. 431, states that "distress below the heart" is treated with Major Bupleurum Decoction (*dà chái hú tāng*). Line 142, p. 284, mentions "hard glomus below the heart" in greater yáng and lesser yáng dragover disease, and line 172, p. 159, mentions "hardness below the heart." These examples show that when evil binds in lesser yáng, it gives rise to hard glomus below the heart. For this reason, "below" would appear to make greater sense than "in."

Synopsis

The treatment of another form of lesser yáng disease with interior repletion.

Commentary

In the present line, cold damage with heat effusion and sweating that brings "no resolution" does not mean that the greater yáng exterior pattern has not resolved. Rather it means that the evil has left the greater yáng and entered the lesser yáng and the yáng brightness. The evil in the lesser yáng inhibits the pivot mechanism, causes stagnation of the qì, and binds in the channels, causing a hard glomus below the heart. Wood evil restrains earth, so that gallbladder and stomach qì stagnate, giving rise to retching and vomiting.

Major Bupleurum Decoction (*dà chái hú tāng*) is used to harmonize the lesser yáng and unblock the yáng brightness interior repletion. It is not generally used to treat patterns involving diarrhea, but here the diarrhea is from heat bind with circumfluence. Even though the yáng brightness dryness bind has already formed, exuberant heat forces the fluids to move around the blockage and downward, causing diarrhea. Despite the diarrhea, all the other yáng brightness bowel signs are present. The use of a freeing formula to treat diarrhea is called "treating the unstopped by unstopping," 通因通用 *tōng yīn tōng yòng*.

4.4 Bupleurum Decoction Plus Mirabilite Patterns

Line 104

㈠ 伤寒十三日不解，胸胁满而呕，日晡所发潮热，已而微利。㈡ 此本柴胡证，下之以不得利，今反利者，知医以丸药下之，此非其治也。㈢ 潮热者，实也。㈣ 先宜服小柴胡汤以解外，后以柴胡加芒消汤主之。

(1) *Shāng hán shí sān rì bù jiě, xiōng xié mǎn ér ǒu, rì bū suǒ fā cháo rè, yǐ ér wēi lì.* (2) *Cǐ běn chái hú zhèng, xià zhī yǐ bù dé lì, jīn fǎn lì zhě, zhī yī yǐ wán yào xià zhī, cǐ fēi qí zhì yě.* (3) *Cháo rè*

zhě, shí yě. (4) *Xiān yí fú xiǎo chái hú tāng yǐ jiě wài, hòu yǐ chái hú jiā máng xiāo tāng zhǔ zhī.*

(1) [Here, in] cold damage [the disease] has not resolved in thirteen days, [and there is] fullness in the chest and rib-side, retching, late afternoon tidal heat effusion, and shortly afterward[1] mild diarrhea. (2) This was originally a [Major] Bupleurum [Decoction] ([*dà*] *chái hú* [*tāng*]) pattern in which precipitation should not cause diarrhea; yet now [in the present case there is] diarrhea, so [one] knows a pill medicine[2] was used to precipitate, and this is not the [appropriate] treatment. (3) Tidal heat effusion means repletion. (4) It is appropriate to first take Minor Bupleurum Decoction (*xiǎo chái hú tāng*) in order to resolve the external [aspect]. Afterward, Bupleurum Decoction Plus Mirabilite (*chái hú jiā máng xiāo tāng*) governs.

TEXT NOTES

1. Shortly afterward, 已而 *yǐ ér*: One action occurs not long after another.
2. Pill medicinal, 丸药 *wán yào*: A harsh precipitant in pill form. See line 80, p. 152, for a more complete discussion.

FORMULA

Bupleurum Decoction Plus Mirabilite (*chái hú jiā máng xiāo tāng*)

○ Harmonize the lesser yáng; drain heat and moisten dryness.

柴胡二两十六铢　黄芩一两　人参一两　甘草一两（炙）　生姜一两（切）　半夏二十铢（本云五枚，洗）　大枣四枚（擘）　芒消二两

㈠ 右八味，以水四升，煮取二升，去滓，内芒消，更煮微沸，分温再服。㈡ 不解，更作。

Chái hú èr liǎng shí liù zhū　huáng qín yī liǎng　rén shēn yī liǎng　gān cǎo yī liǎng (zhì)　shēng jiāng yī liǎng (qiē)　bàn xià èr shí zhū (běn yún wǔ méi, xǐ)　dà zǎo sì méi (bò)　máng xiāo èr liǎng

(1) *Yòu bā wèi, yǐ shuǐ sì shēng, zhǔ qǔ èr shēng, qù zǐ, nà máng xiāo, gèng zhǔ wēi fèi, fēn wēn zài fú.* (2) *Bù jiě, gèng zuò.*

bupleurum (柴胡 *chái hú*, Bupleuri Radix) 2 liǎng 16 zhū
scutellaria (黄芩 *huáng qín*, Scutellariae Radix) 1 liǎng
ginseng (人参 *rén shēn*, Ginseng Radix) 1 liǎng
mix-fried licorice (甘草 *gān cǎo*, Glycyrrhizae Radix) 1 liǎng
fresh ginger (生姜 *shēng jiāng*, Zingiberis Rhizoma Recens) 1 liǎng (cut)
pinellia (半夏 *bàn xià*, Pinelliae Tuber) 20 zhū (originally 5 pieces, washed)*
jujube (大枣 *dà zǎo*, Ziziphi Fructus) 4 pieces (broken)
mirabilite (芒硝 *máng xiāo*, Mirabilitum) 2 liǎng

(1) [For] the above eight ingredients use four shēng of water. Boil [the first seven ingredients] to get two shēng and remove the dregs. Add mirabilite (*máng xiāo*) and again boil slightly. Divide [into two parts], and take warm twice a day. (2) [If there is] no resolution, take again.

FORMULA NOTE

* Originally 5 pieces, washed, 本云五枚，洗 *běn yún wǔ méi, xǐ*: It is not clear if this appeared in the original text or was a later additon by another author.

SYNOPSIS

The signs and treatment of lesser yáng disease with interior repletion following inappropriate precipitation.

COMMENTARY

The first section of this line runs from the beginning to "shortly afterward mild diarrhea." Cold damage of thirteen days" duration is a long disease course for an externally contracted illness. That the disease has not resolved means that it has entered the interior, not that the greater yáng disease has not resolved. Chest and rib-side fullness and retching are indication that the evil has already entered the lesser yáng, inhibiting the pivot mechanism and resulting in gallbladder and stomach qì stagnation, and disturbance of normal upbearing and downbearing. The presence of late afternoon tidal heat effusion means that the evil has also entered the yáng brightness, causing dryness repletion to form. In patterns of lesser yáng with yáng brightness interior repletion, the stool is usually hard and bound, so one may use Major Bupleurum Decoction (*dà chái hú tāng*) to harmonize the lesser yáng, unblock the bowel and eliminate the disease completely. However, in the present line, the patient continues to have mild diarrhea, which is not in keeping with normal development.

The second part of the line, up to "this is not the [appropriate] treatment," explains why mild diarrhea occurs. Because this is a pattern of lesser yáng disease and yáng brightness bowel repletion, harmonization and precipitation with a formula like Major Bupleurum Decoction (*dà chái hú tāng*) should not cause continuing diarrhea. Here, diarrhea occurs and Zhāng Jī attributes this to the inappropriate use of a precipitating formula. He refers to proprietary pill medicines (see line 80, p. 152), which are harsh precipitants.

The final section of the line discusses how the unresolved disease pattern resulting from the inappropriate treatment should be dealt with. The continued presence of tidal heat effusion (which indicates interior repletion) and the presence of mild diarrhea show that neither the lesser yáng evil nor the yáng brightness evil has been eliminated. However, because inappropriate precipitation has resulted in mild diarrhea and damage to right qì, a formula such as Major Bupleurum Decoction (*dà chái hú tāng*) can no longer be used. The treatment is therefore to use Minor Bupleurum Decoction (*xiǎo chái hú tāng*), which harmonizes the lesser yáng, so that the upper burner will unblock and liquid and humor will be able to descend; stomach qì will thereby become harmonious and there will be generalized streaming sweat, bringing about resolution. If Minor Bupleurum Decoction (*xiǎo chái hú tāng*) fails to resolve the disease satisfactorily, it is because the dryness-heat is pronounced. In this case, Bupleurum Decoction Plus Mirabilite (*chái hú jiā máng xiāo tāng*) should be given to harmonize the lesser yáng and to drain heat and moisten dryness.

Bupleurum Decoction Plus Mirabilite (*chái hú jiā máng xiāo tāng*) contains Minor Bupleurum Decoction (*xiǎo chái hú tāng*), which harmonizes the lesser yáng. Mirabilite (*máng xiāo*) is added to drain heat and moisten dryness. Following inappropriate precipitation, the spleen and stomach have been damaged and right qì has been weakened, and although dryness-heat is present in the interior, the repletion bind is not severe. Therefore, the qì-moving and flushing action of rhubarb (*dà huáng*) and unripe bitter orange (*zhǐ shí*) is not necessary and the milder cold salty moist precipitation caused by mirabilite (*máng xiāo*) is sufficient. It should be noted that the dosages in this formula are one-third those in the original Minor Bupleurum Decoction (*xiǎo chái hú tāng*), and the dosage of mirabilite (*máng xiāo*) is also relatively low. Therefore, it is a mild harmonizing and precipitating formula.

4.5 BUPLEURUM, CINNAMON TWIG AND DRIED GINGER DECOCTION PATTERNS

LINE 147

伤寒五六日，已发汗而复下之，胸胁满微结，小便不利，渴而不呕，但头汗出，往来寒热，心烦者，此为未解也，柴胡桂枝干姜汤主之。

Shāng hán wǔ liù rì, yǐ fā hàn ér fù xià zhī, xiōng xié mǎn wēi jié, xiǎo biàn bù lì, kě ér bù ǒu, dàn tóu hàn chū, wǎng lái hán rè, xīn fán zhě, cī wéi wèi jiě yě, chái hú guì zhī gān jiāng tāng zhǔ zhī.

When cold damage [has lasted] five or six days, and sweating has been promoted and then precipitation has been used and [there is] fullness in the chest and rib-side and mild bind, inhibited urination, thirst without retching, sweating only from the head, alternating [aversion to] cold and heat [effusion], and heart vexation, it means [that the disease] has not yet resolved; [therefore,] Bupleurum, Cinnamon Twig, and Dried Ginger Decoction (*chái hú guì zhī gān jiāng tāng*) governs.

FORMULA

Bupleurum, Cinnamon Twig, and Dried Ginger Decoction (*chái hú guì zhī gān jiāng tāng*)

- Harmonize the lesser yáng; warm and transform water-rheum.

柴胡半斤　桂枝三两（去皮）　干姜二两　栝楼根四两　黄芩三两　牡蛎二两（熬）　甘草二两（炙）

㈠ 右七味，以水一斗二升，煮取六升。㈡ 去滓，再煎取三升，温服一升，日三服。㈢ 初服微烦，复服，汗出便愈。

Chái hú bàn jīn guì zhī sān liǎng (qù pí) gān jiāng èr liǎng guā lóu gēn sì liǎng huáng qín sān liǎng mǔ lì èr liǎng (áo) gān cǎo èr liǎng (zhì)

(1) *Yòu qī wèi, yǐ shuǐ yī dǒu èr shēng, zhǔ qǔ liù shēng.* (2) *Qù zǐ, zài jiān qǔ sān shēng, wēn fú yī shēng, rì sān fú.* (3) *Chū fú wēi fán, fù fú, hàn chū biàn yù.*

bupleurum (柴胡 *chái hú*, Bupleuri Radix) half jīn
cinnamon twig (桂枝 *guì zhī*, Cinnamomi Ramulus) 3 liǎng (remove bark)
dried ginger (干姜 *gān jiāng*, Zingiberis Rhizoma Exsiccatum) 2 liǎng
trichosanthes root (栝楼根 *guā lóu gēn*, Trichosanthis Radix) 4 liǎng
scutellaria (黄芩 *huáng qín*, Scutellariae Radix) 3 liǎng
oyster shell (牡蛎 *mǔ lì*, Ostreae Concha) 2 liǎng (dry-fry)
mix-fried licorice (甘草 *gān cǎo*, Glycyrrhizae Radix) 2 liǎng

(1) [For] the above seven ingredients use one dǒu two shēng of water. Boil to get six shēng. (2) Remove the dregs and boil again to get three shēng. Take one shēng warm, three times per day. (3) When the decoction is first taken, if [there is] mild vexation, take it again; [when the patient] sweats, [he/she will] recover.

SYNOPSIS

The signs and treatment of lesser yáng disease with water-rheum interior bind.

COMMENTARY

After the promotion of sweating and the use of precipitation, the evil enters the lesser yáng, and the greater yáng signs such as aversion to cold and heat effusion cease. Alternating aversion to cold and heat effusion is attributable to the struggle between right qì and evil qì and to the inhibition of the pivot mechanism. The evil is depressed in the lesser yáng and inhibits the movement of channel qì; consequently, the patient feels fullness in the chest and rib-side. As the gallbladder fire flames upward, it harasses the heart spirit and causes vexation.

The signs in this line, however, do not indicate a pure Minor Bupleurum Decoction (*xiǎo chái hú tāng*) pattern. An analysis of the formula supports this conclusion and gives clues as to the nature of these signs. When an evil is depressed in the lesser yáng, it causes inhibition of the pivot mechanism, impairment of free coursing, and internal depression of gallbladder fire. As a further result of these three changes, the triple-burner fails to keep the sluices clear, since the triple burner is also a lesser yáng channel. The triple burner governs the sluices; it ensures free flow through the waterways. When these functions are impaired, water-rheum can collect in the interior. Water-rheum binding in the lesser yáng channel causes minor chest bind to appear with the fullness in the chest and rib-side associated with lesser yáng disease. When water amasses in the lower burner, this is often the result of bladder qì transformation failure, so that urine becomes inhibited. The patient is thirsty because the water-rheum collects internally and qì fails to transform it into bodily liquid. Since the stomach is still in harmony, there is no retching. Given the impaired regulation of the waterways plus the inhibition of the pivot mechanism and the presence of a heat evil depressed in the interior preventing yáng qì from reaching the exterior, the heat evil causes fluids to steam upward, so that sweat, failing to issue normally, appears only on the head. In this situation, Bupleurum,

Cinnamon Twig, and Dried Ginger Decoction (*chái hú guì zhī gān jiāng tāng*) is used to harmonize the lesser yáng and transform rheum.

In this formula, bupleurum (*chái hú*) and scutellaria (*huáng qín*) resolve lesser yáng depressed heat and restore normal movement in the pivot. Trichosanthes root (*guā lóu gēn*) and oyster shell (*mǔ lì*) expel rheum and dissipate binds. Cinnamon twig (*guì zhī*), dried ginger (*gān jiāng*), and licorice (*gān cǎo*) free yáng and transform rheum. Licorice (*gān cǎo*) supplements the spleen and boosts the qì, which helps to restore normal spleen and stomach function; dried ginger (*gān jiāng*) warms the interior; and cinnamon twig (*guì zhī*) frees yáng. Together, these three medicinals warm the interior and stimulate movement and transformation. Through this mechanism, phlegm-rheum is transformed. Because retching is absent, the fresh ginger (*shēng jiāng*) and pinellia (*bàn xià*) of Minor Bupleurum Decoction (*xiǎo chái hú tāng*) are not used; because water-rheum is binding internally, the ginseng (*rén shēn*) and jujube (*dà zǎo*) are removed out of fear that they would cause further congestion.

The last sentence of the formula states that mild vexation may occur after taking the formula. This is an indication of the struggle between the right and evil qì. The formula should be taken again. When the pivot mechanism is restored and water-rheum is transformed, then yáng qì can perfuse normally, and the patient will be able to sweat, restoring harmony between exterior and interior.

4.6 Bupleurum Decoction Plus Dragon Bone and Oyster Shell Patterns

Line 107

伤寒八九日，下之，胸满烦惊，小便不利， 谵语，一身尽重，不可转侧者，柴胡加龙骨牡蛎汤主之。

Shāng hán bā jiǔ rì, xià zhī, xiōng mǎn fán jīng, xiǎo biàn bù lì, zhān yǔ, yī shēn jìn zhòng, bù kě zhuǎn cè zhě, chái hú jiā lóng gǔ mǔ lì tāng zhǔ zhī.

When in cold damage [that has lasted for] eight or nine days, precipitation is used, and [there is] fullness in the chest, vexation and fright, inhibited urination, delirious speech, heaviness of the entire body, and inability to turn sides, Bupleurum Decoction Plus Dragon Bone and Oyster Shell (*chái hú jiā lóng gǔ mǔ lì tāng*) governs.

Formula

Bupleurum Decoction Plus Dragon Bone and Oyster Shell (*chái hú jiā lóng gǔ mǔ lì tāng*)

∘ Harmonize the lesser yáng; free yáng and discharge heat; quiet the spirit with heavy settlers.

柴胡四两　龙骨　黄芩　生姜（切）　铅丹　人参　桂枝（去皮）　茯苓各一两半　半夏二合半（洗）　大黄二两　牡蛎一两半（熬）　大枣六枚（擘）

㈠ 右十二味，以水八升，煮取四升，内大黄，切如棋子，更煮一两沸，去滓，温服一升。㈡ 本云，柴胡汤，今加龙骨等。

Chái hú sì liǎng　lóng gǔ　huáng qín　shēng jiāng (qiē)　qiān dān　rén shēn　guì zhī (qù pí)　fú líng gè yī liǎng bàn　bàn xià èr gě bàn (xǐ)　dà huáng èr liǎng　mǔ lì yī liǎng bàn (áo)　dà zǎo liù méi (bò)

(1) *Yòu shí èr wèi, yǐ shuǐ bā shēng, zhǔ qǔ sì shēng, nà dà huáng, qiē rú qí zǐ, gèng zhǔ yī liǎng fèi, qù zǐ, wēn fú yī shēng.* (2) *Běn yún, chái hú tāng, jīn jiā lóng gǔ děng.*

bupleurum (柴胡 *chái hú*, Bupleuri Radix) 4 liǎng
dragon bone (龙骨 *lóng gǔ*, Mastodi Ossis Fossilia) 1.5 liǎng
scutellaria (黄芩 *huáng qín*, Scutellariae Radix) 1.5 liǎng
fresh ginger (生姜 *shēng jiāng*, Zingiberis Rhizoma Recens) 1.5 liǎng (cut)
minium (铅丹 *qiān dān*, Minium) 1.5 liǎng
ginseng (人参 *rén shēn*, Ginseng Radix) 1.5 liǎng
cinnamon twig (桂枝 *guì zhī*, Cinnamomi Ramulus) 1.5 liǎng (remove bark)
poria (茯苓 *fú líng*, Poria) 1.5 liǎng
pinellia (半夏 *bàn xià*, Pinelliae Tuber) 2.5 gě (washed)
rhubarb (大黄 *dà huáng*, Rhei Rhizoma) 2 liǎng
oyster shell (牡蛎 *mǔ lì*, Ostreae Concha) 1.5 liǎng (dry-fry)
jujube (大枣 *dà zǎo*, Ziziphi Fructus) 6 pieces (broken)

(1) [For] the above twelve ingredients [except rhubarb (*dà huáng*)] use eight shēng of water. Boil to get four shēng and add rhubarb (*dà huáng*), cut the size of go stones[1]. Boil again, once or twice. Remove the dregs and take one shēng warm. (2) This is Bupleurum Decoction (*chái hú tāng*),[2] with the addition of dragon bone (*lóng gǔ*), etc.

Formula Notes

1. Go stone, 棋子 *qí zǐ*: In *Qiān Jīn Yì Fāng* the size of this medicinal is said to be "like a square-inch spoon." In the *Fú Shí Mén* (服食门), it is written, "A go stone is two cùn long and one cùn square." According to the *Shāng Hán Lùn Yán Jiū Dà Cí Diǎn*, this amount is between 10 and 12 grams. In line 393, p. 598, this appears as 博棋子 *bó qí zǐ*.
2. Bupleurum Decoction (*chái hú tāng*): This refers to Minor Bupleurum Decoction (*xiǎo chái hú tāng*).

Synopsis

The signs and treatment of vexation fright and delirious speech that are the result of precipitation being inappropriately used in a cold damage pattern and the evil entering the lesser yáng.

COMMENTARY

After eight or nine days of a cold damage pattern it is unclear why a physician would choose to use precipitation. The passage of a week or more does not necessarily mean the disease has shifted into the interior. Nonetheless, following the use of precipitation (which is considered a mistreatment in this case), the evil enters the lesser yáng. Fullness in the chest, vexation, and fright are all indications of a lesser yáng disease. An evil in the lesser yáng inhibits the pivot mechanism and impairs the flow of qì, causing fullness in the chest, although this sign is more typically seen manifesting under the rib-side. Qì congestion in the chest and flaming of depressed gallbladder heat give rise to vexation and fright. Delirious speech is likely the result of stomach heat arising from the influence of depressed gallbladder heat. As in the previous line, inhibited urination is the result of the loss of the triple burner's management of the sluices. The waterways lose regulation, qì transformation does not occur properly, and the urine becomes inhibited. Severe qì congestion from impairment of the qì dynamic, as well as impaired movement of the fluids, results in heaviness of the entire body with an inability to turn sides. Following the misuse of precipitation, right qì is damaged and evil qì falls inward, enters the lesser yáng, and affects the heart, stomach, and triple burner.

Bupleurum Decoction Plus Dragon Bone and Oyster Shell (*chái hú jiā lóng gǔ mǔ lì tāng*) harmonizes the lesser yáng, frees yáng and discharges heat, and settles the spirit. This formula is Minor Bupleurum Decoction (*xiǎo chái hú tāng*) without mix-fried licorice (*gān cǎo*), with the addition of cinnamon twig (*guì zhī*), dragon bone (*lóng gǔ*), oyster shell (*mǔ lì*), minium (*qiān dān*), rhubarb (*dà huáng*), and poria (*fú líng*). Because the evil has entered the lesser yáng, Minor Bupleurum Decoction (*xiǎo chái hú tāng*) is used as the basic formula. Bupleurum (*chái hú*) and scutellaria (*huáng qín*) harmonize the lesser yáng and resolve depressed heat. Cinnamon twig (*guì zhī*) is added, not to resolve an exterior pattern, but to free yáng so that the evil will be outthrust. The small amount of rhubarb (*dà huáng*) that is added later during the decoction process does not have a strong flushing action, but merely drains heat and harmonizes the stomach. Dragon bone (*lóng gǔ*), oyster shell (*mǔ lì*), and minium (*qiān dān*) are heavy settlers that quiet the spirit. Minium (*qiān dān*) is effective for quieting the spirit and settling fright, but it is toxic, and there have been reports of toxic overdoses. If this medicinal is used, it must be used with extreme caution. Minium (*qiān dān*) may be used in small amounts for short periods of time, but if it is necessary to give larger amounts or to use the formula for a longer period of time, it is best to substitute iron flakes (*shēng tiě luò*) or loadstone (*cí shí*). Poria (*fú líng*) not only percolates dampness to disinhibit the urine, it also quiets the spirit. The mix-fried licorice (*gān cǎo*) of Minor Bupleurum Decoction (*xiǎo chái hú tāng*) is omitted in this formula because heat evil has pervaded the body, and so the moderating effect of licorice (*gān cǎo*) is not desirable.

4.7 Disease Passage and Prognosis

Line 269

伤寒六七日，无大热，其人躁烦者，此为阳去入阴故也。

Shāng hán liù qī rì, wú dà rè, qí rén zào fán zhě, cǐ wéi yáng qù rù yīn gù yě.

When in cold damage [that has lasted for] six or seven days, great heat is absent and the person is agitated and vexed, this is because [the evil in the] yáng is abating and entering yīn.*

Text Note

* Yáng is abating and entering yīn, 阳去入阴 *yáng qù rù yīn*: There are several interpretations of yīn and yáng in this line. The three most important ones are presented below. Generally, the first is taken to be the most valid.

a) Chéng Wú-Jǐ writes, "The exterior is yáng and the interior is yīn. [When] the evil is in the exterior, then [there is] heat in the outer body. Absence of heat in the outer body with vexation and agitation in the inner body means the exterior evil has shifted into the interior."

b) Zhāng Zhì-Cōng writes, "This disease is a lesser yáng [evil] entering the lesser yīn."

c) Shū Zhào writes, "In lesser yáng disease of six or seven days, the addition of agitation and vexation [means] the evil is entering the yáng brightness interior."

Synopsis

The signs of cold damage exterior disease entering the interior.

Commentary

In cold damage that has lasted for several days, transmutation may or may not occur. When determining whether a transmutation has occurred, one should not be bound by the number of days stipulated here, since a transmutation is identified by its manifestation in the pulse and signs. Here, "absence of great heat" is taken to mean absence of "great exterior heat" (line 63, p. 154). It is also taken to imply that other exterior signs (such as aversion to cold, headache, and a pulse that is floating) have also ceased, and the evil has left the exterior. Furthermore, the presence of agitation and vexation mean that the evil has entered the interior.

We know that the disease evil has entered the interior. However, since agitation and vexation appears in both yīn patterns and yáng patterns, this sign in itself provides an insufficient basis to judge what channel the disease evil has passed into. We have to take the signs and the pulse as a whole. When there is no great exterior heat, and there is agitation and vexation, then the appearance of exuberant internal heat signs such as thirst, red urine, bound stool, and a pulse that is rapid means that the evil has entered the yáng brightness, while the appearance of a pulse that is faint, and reversal cold of the limbs, indicate that the disease evil has fallen from the greater yáng into the lesser yīn or the reverting yīn. The phrase, "[the evil in the] yáng is abating and entering the yīn," therefore means that exterior disease has entered the interior, irrespective of whether it has entered yáng brightness or the triple yīn.

Line 270

伤寒三日，三阳为尽，三阴当受邪，其人反能食而不呕，此为三阴不受邪也。

Shāng hán sān rì, sān yáng wéi jìn, sān yīn dāng shòu xié, qí rén fǎn néng shí ér bù ǒu, cǐ wéi sān yīn bù shòu xié yě.

[When] cold damage [has lasted] three days, the three yáng [channels] have all been run through, and the three yīn [channels] should contract the evil, [but] instead, the person is able to eat and retching is absent, which means that the three yīn will not contract the evil.

Synopsis

The signs of a cold damage pattern that is not passing into the three yīn.

Commentary

The first half of the present line appears to be a reference to the passage in the *Sù Wèn* that states, "The first day is greater yáng, the second day is yáng brightness, the third day is lesser yáng...." In actual fact, it is refuting the traditional theory of determining whether channel passage has taken place by the number of days. According to clinical experience, disease passage does not occur after a certain number of days have passed. Whether a disease passes to another channel and, if it does, to which channel, is contingent upon other factors, including the severity of the evil, the strength or weakness of right qì, and the suitability of the treatment. In general, when yáng is exuberant the evil enters the triple yáng bowels; when yīn is exuberant it enters the triple yīn viscera. For discussions about the length of time that elapses before channel passage takes place, see line 4, p. 52, and line 46, p. 96.

According to the theory contained in *Sù Wèn,* the disease will have passed through the yáng channels after three days, at which point the yīn channels should receive the evil. In the present line, however, the patient is still able to eat and is not retching after three days. In triple yīn disease, food intake is generally abnormal. In greater yīn disease, abdominal fullness, vomiting, and inability to get food down are often observed. In lesser yīn disease the patient desires to vomit but cannot. In reverting yīn disease the patient feels hungry, but does not desire to eat; if he/she eats, he/she will vomit roundworm. In the present line, however, because the patient is able to eat normally and is not retching, one can conclude that visceral qì has not become vacuous, splenic movement and transformation are unimpaired, and the evil has not moved into the triple yīn. The reverse implication of the line is that regardless of the number of days that have passed, when food intake is impaired and there is retching (or if other triple yīn signs appear) one must consider the possibility that the disease has entered the three yīn.

LINE 271

伤寒三日，少阳脉小者，欲已也。

Shāng hán sān rì, shào yáng mài xiǎo zhě, yù yǐ yě.

When cold damage [has lasted for] three days, [the disease is in] the lesser yáng, and the pulse is small, [the disease] is about to cease.

SYNOPSIS

The pulse of a lesser yáng disease in which there is about to be recovery.

COMMENTARY

The present line is understood to mean that if in lesser yáng disease the string-like pulse becomes small, it is a sign that the disease evil is abating and the disease will soon resolve. Although the line specifies no signs, it is understood that the presence of lesser yáng disease is determined by correlating the signs and pulse, not just by the pulse. Although the present line appears to allude to the notion described in the *Sù Wèn* that the third day of cold damage is lesser yáng disease, the number of days is not regarded by commentators as being crucial.

4.8 SECTION APPENDIX: HEAT ENTERING THE BLOOD CHAMBER

LINE 143

妇人中风，发热恶寒，经水适来，得之七八日，热除而脉迟身凉，胸胁下满，如结胸状，谵语者，此为热入血室也，当刺期门，随其实而取之。

Fù rén zhòng fēng, fā rè wù hán, jīng shuǐ shì lái, dé zhī qī bā rì, rè chú ér mài chí shēn liáng, xiōng xié xià mǎn, rú jié xiōng zhuàng, zhān yǔ zhě, cǐ wéi rè rù xuè shì yě, dāng cì qī mén, suí qí shí ér qǔ zhī.

When a woman with wind strike has heat effusion and aversion to cold, and the menstrual flow happens to arrive, [then] seven or eight days, [after] contracting [the illness] the heat is eliminated, the pulse is slow, and [there is] generalized coolness, fullness under the chest and rib-side, [and] signs like chest bind and delirious speech, this means that the heat has entered the blood chamber.* One should needle Cycle Gate (*qī mén*, LR-14), choosing this point in view of the repletion.

TEXT NOTE

* Blood chamber, 血室 *xuè shì*: Because this line explicitly discusses a disease of women, this is taken to mean the uterus, whereas in other places it may

have other meanings, such as liver or thoroughfare vessel. See the discussion above, line 216, p. 378.

SYNOPSIS

The signs and treatment of heat entering the blood chamber.

COMMENTARY

This line describes the situation arising in women when wind strike with heat effusion and aversion to cold coincides with the onset of menstruation. Menstruation causes empty vacuity of the blood chamber; the exterior evil exploits the vacuity, falls inward, and binds in the blood chamber. This is what is called "heat entering the blood chamber."

After seven or eight days the exterior signs cease, the exterior heat is eliminated, and there is generalized coolness. The evil has entered the interior and transformed into heat, which binds with the blood. The resulting stasis and stagnation in the vessels causes the pulse to become slow. Since the liver stores the blood and governs free coursing, when the blood chamber is obstructed by blood stasis and the movement of blood stagnates, the liver vessels falls out of harmony, so that the liver's free coursing action is inhibited. As a result, there is fullness under the chest and rib-side, similar to that of chest bind, for which reason it later became known as "blood chest bind." At the same time, blood heat ascends and harasses the heart spirit causing disquietude of the spirit, which can develop into delirious speech. The present line suggests that Cycle Gate (*qī mén,* LR-14) should be needled in order to drain the repletion evil.

Although the fullness under the chest and rib-side arising when heat enters the blood chamber is similar to that observed in chest bind, the pattern described in the present line can be distinguished from chest bind. First, heat entering the blood chamber arises when the onset or cessation of menstruation coincides with externally contracted disease. Second, heat entering the blood chamber gives rise to fullness under the chest and rib-side, while chest bind gives rise to pain below the heart that is as hard as stone, and that in severe cases may be accompanied by hard fullness and pain stretching into the lesser abdomen. Third, blood entering the blood chamber is marked by the absence of exterior heat, a pulse that is slow, and generalized coolness, with delirious speech due to blood heat, whereas chest bind is marked by heat repletion manifesting in late afternoon tidal heat.

LINE 144

妇人中风，七八日续得寒热，发作有时，经水适断者，此为热入血室，其血必结，故使如疟状，发作有时，小柴胡汤主之。

Fù rèn zhòng fēng, qī bā rì xù dé hán rè, fā zuò yǒu shí, jīng shuǐ shì duàn zhě, cǐ wéi rè rù xuè shì, qí xuè bì jié, gù shǐ rú nüè zhuàng, fā zuò yǒu shí, xiǎo chái hú tāng zhǔ zhī.

When a woman with wind strike [that has lasted for] seven or eight days, has periodic heat [effusion] and [aversion to] cold and the menstrual flow happens to stop, this means that the heat has entered the blood chamber and the blood will bind, causing a malaria-like condition that occurs at [set] times; [therefore,] Minor Bupleurum Decoction (*xiǎo chái hú tāng*) governs.

SYNOPSIS

The treatment of a pattern of alternating [aversion to] cold and heat [effusion], like malaria, when heat enters the blood chamber.

COMMENTARY

After seven or eight days of a wind strike, the simultaneous heat effusion and aversion to cold seen in greater yáng disease is replaced by periodic heat effusion and aversion to cold, which means that the exterior disease has passed into the interior. As the disease passes into the interior, the menstrual flow, which started around the onset of wind strike, ceases. This is a concurrent sign of heat entering the blood chamber because it reflects the fact that the disease evil has transformed into heat, which binds with the blood. The obstruction of the blood chamber by blood stasis inhibits the flow of qì and blood. This causes "right and evil to fight by turns" in a to-and-fro tug-of-war which manifests in periodic heat effusion and aversion to cold, described by Zhāng Jī as being like malaria. Qián Huáng offers a novel explanation of the pathomechanism of periodic heat effusion and aversion to cold: "The evil blood [bind] congeals and gathers between the channels and network vessels and the uterine vessels. Inwardly, [the disease] has not entered the bowels; outwardly, it is not in the exterior. It is between the exterior and the interior and still belongs to lesser yáng. Thus there is a condition like malaria with periodicity." This commentary rests on the notion that because the uterus is an extraordinary organ, it is not as internal as the viscera and bowels. If the channels and network vessels are considered to be exterior, as opposed to the viscera and bowels of the interior, an evil in the uterus is half interior half exterior, and so the disease belongs to the lesser yáng. The weak point of this explanation is that it rests on the channels and network vessels being considered as part of the exterior; generally they are taken to be both exterior and interior.

Solely on the basis of signs such as periodic aversion to cold, heat effusion, and cessation of the menstrual flow, it is unlikely that one could conclude that the heat had entered the blood chamber. In addition to these signs one would expect to see the other signs described in the previous line: fullness below the chest and rib-side, and delirious speech.

Heat entering the blood chamber, with malaria-like aversion to cold, and heat effusion, should be differentiated from the following three conditions in which aversion to cold and heat effusion appear. 1) In greater yáng disease, the two occur simultaneously and without periodicity. 2) In lesser yáng disease, aversion to cold and heat effusion alternate without set periodicity. 3) In malaria, shivering aversion to cold is followed by vigorous heat effusion, which abates with the appearance of splitting headache and sweating, leaving the patient free of heat and cold signs; this sequence is repeated every day, every other day, or every third day.

Line 145

妇人伤寒发热，经水适来，昼日明了，暮则谵语，如见鬼状者，此为热入血室，无犯胃气及上二焦，必自愈。

Fù rén shāng hán fā rè, jīng shuǐ shì lái, zhòu rì míng liǎo, mù zé zhān yǔ, rú jiàn guǐ zhuàng zhě, cǐ wéi rè rù xuè shì, wú fàn wèi qì jí shàng èr jiāo, bì zì yù.

When a woman [contracts] cold damage and the menstrual flow happens to arrive and she is clear[-headed] during the day and speaks deliriously in the evening, as if seeing ghosts, this means that the heat has entered the blood chamber; [but] do not assail the stomach qì and the two upper burners, [because] recovery will be spontaneous.

Synopsis

The signs, treatment, and contraindications of heat entering the blood chamber.

Commentary

If a menstrual period arrives during cold damage with heat effusion, the evil will exploit the vacuity in the blood chamber, enter the interior, and transform into heat—which then binds with the blood. The blood heat steams upward and harasses the heart spirit causing delirious speech. Because blood belongs to yìn and the disease is in the blood aspect, the delirious speech occurs during the part of day that belongs to yīn. The patient is coherent during the day, but when evening comes she talks deliriously as though seeing ghosts.

The part of the line beginning "do not assail" cautions against certain mistreatments. In this pattern, delirious speech is not caused by stomach repletion, so the use of precipitation would be inappropriate and would only damage stomach qì. The evil is not in the center or upper burners; hence neither sweating nor vomiting are appropriate treatments. The final words, "recovery will be spontaneous," suggest that the disease will resolve without treatment. While traditional commentators tended to take this statement at face value, modern commentators are more conscious that it appears to contradict previous lines in which treatments are suggested for heat entering the blood chamber. They attempt to minimize the contradiction either by explaining 必 *bì*, "must," as "may," thereby allowing the possibility that the disease can resolve spontaneously, or by explaining 自愈 *zì yù*, "recover spontaneously," as meaning that the patient will recover provided no treatment that damages stomach qì is given. Needling Cycle Gate (*qī mén,* LR-14) or giving Minor Bupleurum Decoction (*xiǎo chái hú tāng*) are treatments that may be considered.

5 CHAPTER APPENDIX

LINE 268

三阳合病，脉浮大，上关上，但欲眠睡，目合则汗。

Sān yáng hé bìng, mài fú dà, shāng guān shàng, dàn yù mián shuì, mù hé zé hàn.

In combination disease of the three yáng, the pulse is floating, large, and rises above the upper bar.[1] [There is] desire only to sleep and sweating after the eyes close.[2]

TEXT NOTES

1. Rises above the upper bar, 上关上 *shàng guān shàng*: The pulse is long and forceful. It fills the entire length of the vessel in the wrist. This phrase is difficult to interpret and has been interpreted in different ways, without a clear consensus. Chéng Wú-Jǐ writes, "The greater yáng pulse is floating, the yáng brightness pulse is large. The pulse is floating and rises above the upper bar, so one knows [this pattern] is combination disease of the three yáng." Yet he does not do an analysis of why this pulse represents that pattern, and although this idea is not rejected, it is also not fully accepted. The authors of the *Yī Zōng Jīn Jiàn* agree with Chéng Wú-Jǐ that this pattern is combination disease of the three yáng, and suggest that the second character 上 *shàng* is a mistake. They write that it should be "stringlike," 弦 *xián*, thereby supporting their view of the whole pattern.
2. Sweating after the eyes close, 目合则汗 *mù hé zé hàn*: Equivalent to night sweating, 盗汗 *dào hàn*.

SYNOPSIS

The pulse and signs of combination disease of the three yáng.

COMMENTARY

This line has been placed in the Chapter Appendix because of disagreement about the interpretation of the pulse description. We have chosen to present this as combination disease of the three yáng for purposes of clarity in the commentary, not because this interpretation is universally accepted.

Combination disease of the three yáng involves the greater yáng, yáng brightness, and lesser yáng. A pulse that is floating may indicate greater yáng disease. A pulse that is large may indicate yáng brightness disease. The pulse in the present line is also long and forceful (which is considered to be similar to stringlike) and belongs to the lesser yáng.

Heat in the three yáng easily disturbs the heart spirit, leading to a mental state in which the patient is groggy and only desires to sleep. This state should be differentiated from the desire to sleep found in lesser yīn disease. Lesser yīn disease, with vacuity cold, is characterized by heart and kidney yáng vacuity and insufficiency of the qì and blood. Sweating and heat signs are absent. The pulse is sunken, faint, and fine. Here, clouding sleep and night sweating are a result of steaming internal heat. The pulse is floating, large, and long. This pattern is one of yáng, repletion, and heat.

Sweating that occurs during sleep is called night sweating. In this line, sweating that occurs after the eyes close belongs to the category of night sweating. In general, night sweating belongs to yīn vacuity, but in this pattern it indicates yáng exuberance. This pattern involves the lesser yáng, which is the pivot between the exterior and the interior. During sleep, yáng enters the interior and defense yáng decreases. Interior heat becomes exuberant and distresses humor, which discharges outward in the form of sweat. Line 201, p. 390, also contains an example of night sweating which is the result of exuberant internal heat.

Chapter Four

Greater Yīn Disease

Pulses and Signs; Treatment

辨太阴病脉证并治

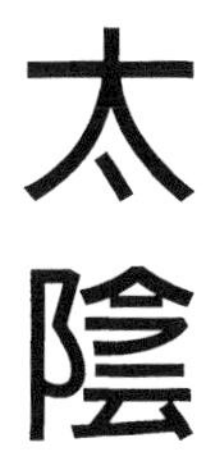

1 OVERVIEW

The spleen stands in interior-exterior relationship with the stomach. The spleen belongs to greater yīn and the stomach belongs to yáng brightness. When stomach yáng is exuberant, evil entering yáng brightness transforms into dryness and heat. When spleen yáng is insufficient, evil entering greater yīn transforms into dampness and cold. Therefore, unlike yáng brightness, which governs interior heat repletion patterns with dryness and heat damaging liquid, greater yīn governs interior vacuity cold patterns in which cold and dampness collect in the interior. The spleen and stomach are closely related; therefore disease affecting one can easily affect the other. In yáng brightness disease, if the central qì becomes vacuous, the evil may shift into greater yīn; conversely, in greater yīn disease, if center qì returns, the evil can shift into yáng brightness. Greater yīn disease is generally the result of one of two pathomechanisms. In the first, a patient with constitutional spleen yáng vacuity contracts wind-cold or experiences internal damage that engenders cold. In the second, damage to the spleen arising when a condition is not treated or treated inappropriately causes the disase to shift to the greater yīn.

1.1 Pulses and Signs

Greater yīn patterns are characterized by abdominal fullness with periodic pain, inability to get food down, no thirst, vomiting, diarrhea, and a pulse that is moderate.

Abdominal fullness with periodic pain 腹满时痛 *fù mǎn shí tòng*: When spleen yáng is insufficient, the qì dynamic becomes inhibited, giving rise to abdominal fullness. Although cold qì is stagnant, causing abdominal pain, yáng qì is still sometimes free; consequently, the pain is periodic. This should be clearly distinguished from persistent abdominal fullness and pain that refuses pressure, which is observed in yáng brightness interior repletion patterns. Here, the fullness and pain periodically decreases, and likes pressure and warmth.

Inability to get food down, 食不下 *shí bù xià*; **absence of thirst**, 不渴 *bù kě*; **vomiting**, 吐 *tù*; and **spontaneous diarrhea**, 自利 *zì lì*: In greater yīn disease, vacuity cold in the center impairs movement and transformation; consequently, the patient is unable to eat normally. Impaired movement and transformation also results in vomiting and spontaneous diarrhea because turbid qì and clear qì are not properly managed. The cold and dampness is primarily in the center and does not affect qì transformation in the lower burner; consequently, liquid and humor are able to ascend to the mouth and thirst is absent. When vomiting and diarrhea are severe, however, the patient may feel thirst, as a result of damage to liquid and humor. Nonetheless, the increase in fluid intake will be minimal and the patient will probably desire hot drinks.

A pulse that is moderate or weak, 脉缓、脉弱 *mài huǎn*、 *mài ruò*: In greater yīn disease, the pulse is usually moderate or weak, reflecting interior vacuity cold.

Yellowing, 发黄 *fā huáng*: If dampness is depressed in the interior, it can give rise to yīn yellowing.

1.2 TREATMENT

Greater yīn disease should be treated by warming the spleen and drying dampness, using formulae such as Center-Rectifying Decoction (*lǐ zhōng tāng*) and Counterflow Cold Decoction (*sì nì tāng*).

1.3 SCHEMATIC OVERVIEW

Greater Yīn Disease Patterns

- **Basic Greater Yīn Disease Pattern**
  - Spontaneous diarrhea, absence of thirst, abdominal fullness and periodic pain, vomiting, and inability to get food down: Counterflow Cold Decoction type of formula (*sì nì bèi*)
- **Concurrent and Transmuted Patterns**
  - Concurrent unresolved exterior pattern: Cinnamon Twig Decoction (*guì zhī tāng*)
  - Abdominal pain patterns
    * Abdominal fullness and periodic pain: Cinnamon Twig Decoction Plus Peony (*guì zhī jiā sháo yào tāng*)
    * Great repletion pain: Cinnamon Twig Decoction Plus Rhubarb (*guì zhī jiā dà huáng tāng*)

2 ESSENTIAL FEATURES OF GREATER YĪN DISEASE

Line 273

太阴之为病，腹满而吐，食不下，自利益甚，时腹自痛，若下之，必胸下结硬。

Tài yīn zhī wéi bìng, fù mǎn ér tù, shí bù xià, zì lì yì shèn, shí fù zì tòng, ruò xià zhī, bì xiōng xià jié yìng.

In disease of the greater yīn, [there is] abdominal fullness and vomiting, inability to get food down,* severe spontaneous diarrhea, and periodic spontaneous abdominal pain, and if precipitation [is used], there will be a hard bind below the chest.

Text Note

* Inability to get food down, 食不下 *shí bù xià*: A lack of desire for food or an inability to eat. This phrase is considered equivalent to 不能食 *bù néng shí*.

Synopsis

An outline of the signs and treatment contraindications for greater yīn vacuity cold patterns.

Commentary

The greater yīn belongs to earth and governs dampness. Among the viscera it corresponds to the spleen, and like the yáng brightness it is associated with gastrointestinal diseases. Nonetheless, the natures of the greater yīn and the yáng brightness are very different. Disease of the yáng brightness mostly takes the form of interior heat repletion patterns, whereas disease of the greater yīn mostly manifests in interior vacuity cold patterns. For this reason, it is said, "[if the condition is one of] repletion, it is yáng brightness, [if one of] vacuity, it is greater yīn," 实则阳明，虚则太阴 *shí zé yáng míng, xū zé tài yīn*. However, yáng brightness and greater yīn are mutually convertible.

The spleen governs the larger abdomen. When the spleen is vacuous, movement is impaired. Cold and dampness are not transformed, dampness congests, and qì stagnates. As a result, there is abdominal fullness. Greater yīn disease is closely associated with dampness evil. As *Sù Wèn* states, "All dampness with swelling and fullness is ascribed to the spleen."

The spleen and the stomach stand in exterior-interior relationship; diseases of the spleen invariably affect the stomach. When turbid yīn moves counterflow and invades the stomach, it causes vomiting and inability to get food down. At the same time, spleen yáng fails to bear upward, causing diarrhea. The diarrhea is described as severe because it is accompanied by an inability to get food down. Normally, when food intake is reduced, diarrhea decreases. In this pattern, reduced food intake does not decrease the diarrhea. Periodic spontaneous abdominal pain is a result of alternating blockage and free flow of yáng qì. Blockage of the yáng qì causes pain and when the qì moves, the pain abates. These signs are not necessarily the result of an externally contracted evil. Greater yīn vacuity cold patterns may also be seen in miscellaneous disease (i.e., disease that is not due to external contraction).

Abdominal fullness and pain can occur in yáng brightness bowel repletion as well as greater yīn disease. However, because these patterns are opposite in nature, differentiation is quite clear. Greater yīn abdominal fullness is a vacuity cold pattern caused by spleen yáng vacuity with stagnating cold-damp. This type of fullness is intermittent and it is not eliminated by diarrhea. The abdominal fullness of yáng míng bowel repletion is a repletion heat pattern caused by dry stool becoming bound in the intestines. It is persistent and is eliminated by freeing the stool.

Greater yīn disease should be treated by warming and moving the center yáng, fortifying the spleen, and drying dampness. Precipitation should not be used, as it will damage an already vacuous spleen yáng. If precipitation is mistakenly used, the further damage caused to center yáng will cause turbid yīn to ascend counterflow, resulting in a transmuted pattern of hard bind below the chest.

2.1 Period of Resolution for Greater Yīn Disease

Line 274

太阴中风，四肢烦疼，阳微阴濇而长者，为欲愈。

Tài yīn zhòng fēng, sì zhī fán téng, yáng wēi yīn sè ér cháng zhě, wéi yù yù.

When in greater yīn wind strike, [there is] vexing pain in the limbs,[1] and the pulse [in its] yáng [aspect] is faint and [in its] yīn [aspect] is rough, and is long,[2] this means [there is] about to be recovery.

Text Notes

1. Vexing pain in the limbs, 四肢烦疼 *sì zhī fán téng*: Pain in the limbs that is severe and consequently disturbs the heart spirit and leads to vexation.
2. The pulse [in its] yáng [aspect] is faint and [in its] yīn [aspect] is rough, and is long, 阳微阴濇而长 *yáng wēi yīn sè ér cháng*: When the pulse is felt with light pressure, it is faint and with heavy pressure, it is rough. The overall pulse is long.

Synopsis

The primary signs, and signs of imminent recovery, in greater yīn wind strike.

Commentary

Vexing pain in the four limbs is a characteristic sign of greater yīn wind strike because the spleen governs the four limbs. When spleen yáng is vacuous and the greater yīn contracts external wind evil, there is pain in the limbs that causes the patient to feel vexed. This sign is not accompanied by aversion to cold or heat effusion and it is not the same as generalized pain; it should not be confused with the pain that occurs in greater yáng exterior patterns.

The pulse permits inference about the further development of greater yīn wind strike. When, as in the present line, the pulse is found to be faint at the superficial level, this indicates that the evil is not exuberant. The pulse is found to be rough at the deep level, indicating interior vacuity and stagnation of dampness. However, the fact that the pulse is long rather than short is an indication that spleen qì is returning to normal. Because the evil is mild and right qì is regaining strength, the patient is about to recover.

3 BASIC GREATER YĪN DISEASE PATTERNS

LINE 277

自利不渴者，属太阴，以其藏有寒故也，当温之，宜服四逆辈。

Zì lì bù kě zhě, shǔ tài yīn, yǐ qí zàng yǒu hán gù yě, dāng wēn zhī, yí fú sì nì bèi.

When [there is] spontaneous diarrhea and thirst is absent, this belongs to greater yīn [disease]; because [there is] cold in the storehouse,[1] one should [use] a warming [treatment]. A Counterflow Cold [Decoction] type [of formula][2] is appropriate.

TEXT NOTES

1. Cold in the storehouse, 藏有寒 *zàng yǒu hán*: Vacuity cold in the center burner. 藏 *zàng* is equivalent to 脏 *zàng*.
2. Counterflow Cold [Decoction] type [of formula]: 四逆辈 *sì nì bèi*: Formulae that warm the interior and dissipate cold, represented by Counterflow Cold Decoction.

SYNOPSIS

The primary signs, pathomechanism, and treatment principle for greater yīn disease.

COMMENTARY

Spontaneous diarrhea without thirst is a characteristic of greater yīn disease. When the spleen yáng is vacuous, the clear yáng cannot ascend, giving rise to diarrhea. The greater yīn governs dampness and most diseases of the greater yīn involve a tendency to cold and dampness. When cold and dampness are not transformed, they spread throughout the interior and even following diarrhea, the patient is not thirsty. For this reason, Zhāng Jī attributes this to "cold in the storehouse."

Diarrhea resulting from center burner vacuity cold is usually not associated with thirst, and this point differentiates it from interior heat diarrhea and lesser yīn disease spontaneous diarrhea. In diarrhea due to internal heat, heat evil damages the fluids, and so the patient is thirsty. In diarrhea occurring in lesser yīn disease, the kidney yáng is vacuous, and cannot distill the fluids; consequently, fluid fails to ascend, so the patient is thirsty. These differences normally apply, but there are exceptions. For example, if spleen vacuity diarrhea persists for a long time, damage to fluids may, in some patients, result in thirst. Generally, this type of thirst is characterized by a desire to drink small amounts of fluids and a preference for warm fluids. Another example is seen in the Pueraria Decoction (*gé gēn tāng*) pattern of greater yáng and yáng brightness combination disease, where diarrhea may occur without thirst as the result of an exterior evil forcing its way into the yáng brightness. Both these examples illustrate the point that one must consider the main signs and accompanying signs as a whole before making a diagnosis.

The treatment principle for greater yīn vacuity cold diarrhea is to warm the interior. Zhāng Jī does not suggest a specific formula, but rather a type of formula represented by Counterflow Cold Decoction. The implication of this is that one should assess the clinical presentation and choose an appropriate formula. This type of formula includes Center-Rectifying Decoction (*lǐ zhōng tāng*), used in milder cases to warm the center and dispel cold, and Counterflow Cold Decoction (*sì nì tāng*), used in more severe cases to supplement fire and engender earth.

4 GREATER YĪN DISEASE AND TRANSMUTED PATTERNS

4.1 GREATER YĪN DISEASE AND EXTERIOR PATTERNS

LINE 276

太阴病，脉浮者，可发汗，宜桂枝汤。

Tài yīn bìng, mài fú zhě, kě fā hàn, yí guì zhī tāng.

When in greater yīn disease the pulse is floating; one can promote sweating, and [therefore,] Cinnamon Twig Decoction (*guì zhī tāng*) is appropriate.

SYNOPSIS

The treatment method for greater yīn disease with an exterior pattern.

COMMENTARY

Since greater yīn disease usually manifests in the form of interior vacuity cold patterns, one would expect to see a pulse that is sunken. However, the pulse described in the present line is floating, suggesting that this is greater yīn disease with a concurrent exterior pattern, and that one can use Cinnamon Twig Decoction (*guì zhī tāng*) to resolve the exterior. Nonetheless, the present line describes the pulse, but mentions no signs. It would be mistaken to assume that the pattern could be determined exclusively on the basis of the pulse. The reason why the present line describes greater yīn disease with a concurrent exterior pattern, and recommends treating the exterior first, rather than treating the interior before the exterior, is evidently because the interior vacuity cold is not pronounced. In more pronounced interior vacuity cold, even though there would be a concurrent exterior pattern, the appropriate treatment would not be to treat the exterior first, but to first warm the interior or simultaneously warm the interior and resolve the exterior (the latter with Cinnamon Twig and Ginseng Decoction (*guì zhī rén shēn tāng*)).

4.2 GREATER YĪN ABDOMINAL PAIN PATTERNS

LINE 279

本太阳病，医反下之，因尔腹满时痛者，属太阴也，桂枝加芍药汤主之；大实痛者，桂枝加大黄汤主之。

Běn tài yáng bìng, yī fǎn xià zhī, yīn ěr fù mǎn shí tòng zhě, shǔ tài yīn yě, guì zhī jiā sháo yào tāng zhǔ zhī; dà shí tòng zhě, guì zhī jiā dà huáng tāng zhǔ zhī.

When originally there was greater yáng disease, but the physician used precipitation, and consequently [there is] abdominal fullness with periodic pain, this belongs to greater yīn [disease]; Cinnamon Twig Decoction Plus Peony (*guì zhī jiā sháo yào tāng*) governs. If [there is] great repletion pain,* Cinnamon Twig Decoction Plus Rhubarb (*guì zhī jiā dà huáng tāng*) governs.

TEXT NOTE

* Great repletion pain, 大实痛 *dà shí tòng*: Severe distention pain in the abdominal region that is exacerbated by pressure.

FORMULAE

Cinnamon Twig Decoction Plus Peony (*guì zhī jiā sháo yào tāng*)

○ Warm yáng and boost the spleen; quicken the blood and harmonize the networks.

桂枝三两（去皮） 芍药六两 甘草二两（炙） 大枣十二枚（擘） 生姜三两（切）

(一) 右五味，以水七升，煮取三升，去滓，温分三服。(二) 本云，桂枝汤，今加芍药。

Guì zhī sān liǎng (qù pí) sháo yào liù liǎng gān cǎo èr liǎng (zhì) dà zǎo shí èr méi (bò) shēng jiāng sān liǎng (qiē)

(1) *Yòu wǔ wèi, yǐ shuǐ qī shēng, zhǔ qǔ sān shēng, qù zǐ, wēn fēn sān fú.* (2) *Běn yún, guì zhī tāng, jīn jiā sháo yào.*

cinnamon twig (桂枝 *guì zhī*, Cinnamomi Ramulus) (remove bark) 3 liǎng
peony (芍药 *sháo yào*, Paeoniae Radix) 6 liǎng
mix-fried licorice (*gān cǎo*) 2 liǎng
jujube (大枣 *dà zǎo*, Ziziphi Fructus) 12 pieces (broken)

fresh ginger (生姜 *shēng jiāng*, Zingiberis Rhizoma Recens) 3 liǎng (cut)

(1) [For] the above five ingredients use seven shēng of water. Boil to get three shēng and remove the dregs. Separate into three [doses] and take warm. (2) This is Cinnamon Twig Decoction (*guì zhī tāng*) with additional peony (*sháo yào*).

Cinnamon Twig Decoction Plus Rhubarb (*guì zhī jiā dà huáng tāng*)

○ This formula has the same effect as the preceding, but includes repletion-draining agents to treat great repletion pain.

桂枝三两（去皮） 大黄二两 芍药六两 生姜三两（切） 甘草二两（炙） 大枣十二枚（擘）

右六味，以水七升，煮取三升，去滓，温服一升，日三服。

Guì zhī sān liǎng (qù pí) dà huáng èr liǎng sháo yào liù liǎng shēng jiāng sān liǎng (qiē) gān cǎo èr liǎng (zhì) dà zǎo shí èr méi (bò)

Yòu liù wèi, yǐ shuǐ qī shēng, zhǔ qǔ sān shēng, qù zǐ, wēn fú yī shēng, rì sān fú.

cinnamon twig (桂枝 *guì zhī*, Cinnamomi Ramulus) 3 liǎng (remove bark)
rhubarb (大黄 *dà huáng*, Rhei Rhizoma) 2 liǎng
peony (芍药 *sháo yào*, Paeoniae Radix) 6 liǎng
fresh ginger (生姜 *shēng jiāng*, Zingiberis Rhizoma Recens) 3 liǎng (cut)
mix-fried licorice (*gān cǎo*) 2 liǎng
jujube (大枣 *dà zǎo*, Ziziphi Fructus) 12 pieces (broken)

[For] the above six ingredients use seven shēng of water. Boil to get three shēng and remove the dregs. Take one shēng warm, three times a day.

SYNOPSIS

The signs and treatment of an evil falling into the greater yīn, following inappropriate precipitation in a greater yáng disease.

COMMENTARY

This line describes conditions arising when greater yáng disease which should be treated by sweating is inappropriately treated by precipitation. Inappropriate precipitation in greater yáng disease can give rise to a variety of consequences, but in this case it damages the spleen and causes the exterior evil to fall inward into the greater yīn, resulting in qì stagnation and stasis of the network vessels that manifests in abdominal fullness and pain. Mild cases are characterized by abdominal fullness with periodic pain, and are treated by warming yáng and harmonizing the network vessels with Cinnamon Twig Decoction Plus Peony (*guì zhī jiā sháo yào tāng*). The more severe sign of "great repletion pain" is treated by warming yáng and harmonizing the network vessels and by draining repletion and abducting stagnation with Cinnamon Twig Decoction Plus Rhubarb (*guì zhī jiā dà huáng tāng*).

The present line and line 273, p. 453, which presents the outline of greater yīn disease, both speak of abdominal fullness with periodic pain. The nature of the two conditions is different. In line 273, there is abdominal fullness with periodic pain, accompanied by severe spontaneous diarrhea that constitutes a greater yīn vacuity cold pattern and which is treated by warming the spleen and dissipating cold with Center-Rectifying Decoction (*lǐ zhōng tāng*). In the present line diarrhea is originally absent and arises after inappropriate precipitation damages the spleen, causing qì stagnation and stasis in the network vessels. The treatment in this case is to warm yáng and harmonize the network vessels.

Cinnamon Twig Decoction Plus Peony (*guì zhī jiā sháo yào tāng*) contains all the ingredients of Cinnamon Twig Decoction (*guì zhī tāng*), but the dosage of peony (*sháo yào*) is greatly increased. This increase changes the focus of the formula from exterior resolution to warming yáng and harmonizing the network vessels. The sovereign of the formula is peony (*sháo yào*). The suggestion by some traditional commentators that this formula should be understood in terms of the exterior-resolving action of Cinnamon Twig Decoction (*guì zhī tāng*) is inappropriate, because the sovereign of this formula is cinnamon twig (*guì zhī*); the suggestion by others that it should be understood in terms of the supplementing action of Minor Center-Fortifying Decoction (*xiǎo jiàn zhōng tāng*) is inappropriate, since the sovereign of this formula is malt sugar (*yí táng*). Páng Ān-Shí (庞安时, style 安常 Ān-Cháng) writes, "[If one] does not use malt sugar (*yí táng*) in Minor Center-Fortifying Decoction (*xiǎo jiàn zhōng tāng*), then peony (*sháo yào*) is the sovereign, because [the formula] relieves pain and disinhibits evil."

In patterns with great repletion pain, Cinnamon Twig Decoction Plus Peony (*guì zhī jiā sháo yào tāng*) is ineffective to cope with the severe congestion and stagnation of qì and blood. Therefore, a small amount of rhubarb (*dà huáng*) is added to help peony (*sháo yào*) quicken the blood and drain the repletion. With this addition the formula is called Cinnamon Twig Decoction Plus Rhubarb (*guì zhī jiā dà huáng tāng*). Although peony (*sháo yào*) and rhubarb (*dà huáng*) are cold, the formula as a whole is still slightly warm, and hence differs from the cold precipitation of the Qì-Coordinating Decoctions (*chéng qì tāng*); it is therefore appropriate for use in greater yīn disease.

Traditional commentators have disagreed considerably over the interpretation of this line. Chéng Wú-Jǐ asserts that both formulae simultaneously treat the exterior and the interior. "Give Cinnamon Twig Decoction (*guì zhī tāng*) to resolve the exterior and add peony (*sháo yào*) to harmonize the interior.... Add rhubarb (*dà huáng*) in order to eliminate great repletion." According to Zhāng Zhì-Cōng, both formulae treat the interior. "Cinnamon Twig Decoction Plus Peony (*guì zhī jiā sháo yào tāng*) ... this is the concept of using Minor Center-Fortifying Decoction (*xiǎo jiàn zhōng tāng*) to treat urgent pain in the abdomen. Great repletion pain is [a result of] residual putrid foulness which cannot be eliminated; therefore, Cinnamon Twig Decoction Plus Rhubarb (*guì zhī jiā dà huáng tāng*) governs." Commentators also disagree as to whether these patterns belong to vacuity or repletion and whether the repletion for which Cinnamon Twig Decoction Plus Rhubarb (*guì zhī jiā dà huáng tāng*) is used is yīn repletion or yáng repletion. The authors of *Gāo Děng Cóng Shū* conclude their commentary as follows:

> So far, no consensus of understanding has been reached. We believe that to insist that there is concurrent exterior pattern is to get bogged down in the idea of Cinnamon Twig Decoction (*guì zhī tāng*) as a formula that resolves the exterior and promotes sweating, which neither necessarily conforms to the spirit of the original text, nor matches clinical experience. The Cinnamon

Twig Decoction Plus Rhubarb (*guì zhī jiā dà huáng tāng*) pattern is indeed a repletion pattern, but the Cinnamon Twig Decoction Plus Peony (*guì zhī jiā sháo yào tāng*) pattern cannot be said to be entirely one of vacuity. Looking at Cinnamon Twig Decoction Plus Rhubarb (*guì zhī jiā dà huáng tāng*) from the perspective of its ingredients, we can see that the warm and hot medicinals are stronger than the cold and cool ones, so that the formula is a warm precipitating formula, not a cold precipitating one. Consequently, the pattern is one of yīn repletion and not yáng repletion.

Line 280

太阴为病，脉弱，其人续自便利，设当行大黄、芍药者，宜减之，以其人胃气弱，易动故也。

Tài yīn wéi bìng, mài ruò, qí rén xù zì biàn lì, shè dāng xíng dà huáng、sháo yào zhě, yí jiǎn zhī, yǐ qí rén wèi qì ruò, yì dòng gù yě.

When in greater yīn disease, the pulse is weak and the person is about to have spontaneous diarrhea, if [one] must use rhubarb (*dà huáng*) and peony (*sháo yào*), it is appropriate to reduce [the dosage], because the person's stomach qì is weak, and [therefore] easily stirred [by these medicinals].*

Text Note

* Stomach qì is weak, and [therefore] easily stirred [by these medicinals] 胃气弱，易动 *wèi qì ruò, yì dòng*: Poor spleen-stomach function and susceptibility to diarrhea.

Synopsis

This line illustrates the need to safeguard stomach qì when using harsh medicinals in patients with vacuity of center qì.

Commentary

In greater yīn disease, a pulse that is weak indicates vacuity of the center qì. Since the spleen and stomach are vacuous, the clear yáng cannot ascend. Consequently, the patient is susceptible to diarrhea. Although the stool is normal for the time being, diarrhea can easily occur spontaneously at any moment.

When, as described in the preceding line, inappropriate precipitation in greater yáng causes the evil to fall into greater yīn, Zhāng Jī suggests adding peony (*sháo yào*) or rhubarb (*dà huáng*) to Cinnamon Twig Decoction (*guì zhī tāng*). In the present line, he emphasizes that one must take into account the patient's constitution when deciding on appropriate medication. This means that if these two ingredients, which are considered cold and attacking (especially the latter), are to be used in patients with center qì vacuity, excessive doses should be avoided since they will exacerbate the center qì vacuity and cause incessant diarrhea.

4.3 GREATER YĪN DISEASE SHIFTING TO RECOVERY AND SHIFTING INTO YÁNG BRIGHTNESS

LINE 278

伤寒脉浮而缓，手足自温者，系在太阴；太阴当发身黄，若小便自利者，不能发黄；至七八日，虽暴烦下利，日十余行，必自止，以脾家实，腐秽当去故也。

Shāng hán mài fú ér huǎn, shǒu zú zì wēn zhě, xì zài tài yīn; tài yīn dāng fā shēn huáng, ruò xiǎo biàn zì lì zhě, bù néng fā huáng; zhì qī bā rì, suī bào fán xià lì, rì shí yú xíng, bì zì zhǐ, yǐ pí jiā shí, fǔ huì dāng qù gù yě.

When in cold damage, the pulse is floating and moderate and the extremities are spontaneously warm, this is related to the greater yīn. In greater yīn [disease], there should be generalized yellowing, [but] if the urine is spontaneously uninhibited, there will be inability to yellow. At seven or eight days, although [there is] sudden vexation and diarrhea, [which] occurs ten or more [times per] day, it will spontaneously cease, because the spleen domain is replete[1] and the putrid foulness[2] should be eliminated.

TEXT NOTES

1. Spleen domain is replete, 脾家实 *pí jiā shí*: Recovery of the spleen yáng. Here, this expression is similar to the 胃家实 *wèi jiā shí*, "stomach domain is replete" of yáng brightness disease. However, in 脾家实 *pí jiā shí*, the 实 *shí* is explained as meaning "right qì repletion" rather than "evil qì repletion."
2. Putrid foulness, 腐秽 *fǔ huì*: Rotten turbid matter in the intestines.

SYNOPSIS

The clinical manifestation and mechanism of recovery in greater yīn disease.

COMMENTARY

Spontaneous warming of the extremities is a characteristic of lesser yīn disease. In triple yáng disease, heat effusion may occur, but when it does it affects the whole body (not just the hands and feet). Triple yīn disease is rarely marked by heat effusion. In particular, reverting yīn disease and lesser yīn disease usually involve severe yáng vacuity, and so in most cases there is reversal cold of the extremities. In greater yīn disease, yáng vacuity is milder and yáng qì is still able to spread to the extremities, so the hands and feet remain warm. In externally contracted disease (cold damage in the broad sense), a pulse that is floating and moderate might be taken to indicate greater yáng wind strike. However, in the present line, generalized heat effusion or other signs of greater yáng wind strike are absent; the only sign observed is spontaneous warmth of the hands and feet. Therefore this is greater yīn disease. This line shows that signs and pulses must be considered together; diagnosis should not be made solely on the basis of one or the other.

The greater yīn is the viscus of damp earth. If the spleen is vacuous, cold and dampness are not transformed and become stagnant, so yellowing is likely to occur. This type of yellowing is considered to be yīn yellowing, in which the color is a dark yellow, different from the bright yellow seen in yáng yellowing, which is caused by damp-heat lying depressed and steaming in the interior. Line 259, p. 374, offers another example of unresolved cold-damp in the interior causing yīn yellowing. If urination is uninhibited, the damp evil will be discharged through the urine; it will not become depressed in the interior and cause yellowing. Thus, by establishing whether the urine is inhibited or not, one can determine whether yellowing is likely to develop.

After seven or eight days, sudden vexation and diarrhea is considered to be a sign that the spleen yáng is recovering and the disease will soon resolve. Normally, the sudden appearance of pronounced signs such as these would be interpreted as a marked worsening in the condition, calling for prompt therapeutic action. However, it is taken in this line to be a sign of recovery, because although there is diarrhea, we are told that the "spleen domain is replete."

We should take care to distinguish the favorable and unfavorable conditions in which sudden vexation and diarrhea appear. If there is counterflow cold of the extremities, torpor of the spirit, and no change in the tongue fur, vexation and severe diarrhea are an indication that the disease is worsening and one must assess and treat quickly. By contrast, severe diarrhea and vexation are taken as a sign of recovery if accompanied by warm limbs, bright spirit, and a slimy tongue fur that is gradually transforming. In this condition, right qì and evil qì are struggling and the evil is being expelled. There is no need to treat the diarrhea, since that is the route through which the evil is being expelled. When the evil has been completely expelled, the diarrhea will stop spontaneously. "The spleen domain is replete" means that the spleen yáng is recovering and that waste in the stomach and intestines will be normally expelled.

LINE 187

(一) 伤寒脉浮而缓，手足自温者，是为系在太阴。(二) 太阴者，身当发黄，若小便自利者，不能发黄。(三) 至七八日，大便硬者，为阳明病也。

(1) *Shāng hán mài fú ér huǎn, shǒu zú zì wēn zhě, shì wéi xì zài tài yīn.* (2) *Tài yīn zhě, shēn dāng fā huáng, ruò xiǎo biàn zì lì zhě, bù néng fā huáng.* (3) *Zhì qī bā rì, dà biàn yìng zhě, wéi yáng míng bìng yě.*

(1) When in cold damage, the pulse is floating and moderate, and the limbs are spontaneously warm, this is bound to the greater yīn. (2) In greater yīn [disease], there should be generalized yellowing, [but]

if the urine is spontaneously uninhibited, there will be inability to yellow. (3) At seven or eight days, hard stool means yáng brightness disease.

Synopsis

The distinguishing evidence of a greater yīn disease shifting into the yáng brightness.

Commentary

In the Sòng version, the present line is placed under yáng brightness disease. However, the first half of the line is very similar to the preceding line. It deals with the relationship between the greater yīn disease and the yáng brightness disease, and the mutual convertibility of the two. The greater yīn and the yáng brightness both belong to center-earth. However, yáng brightness is the stomach; it belongs to yáng earth and governs dryness. Greater yīn is the spleen; it belongs to yīn earth and governs dampness. Therefore, yáng brightness disease mostly manifests in interior heat dryness repletion patterns; greater yīn disease mostly manifests in interior vacuity cold-damp patterns. Although repletion and vacuity, dryness and dampness, heat and cold are opposites, under certain conditions they are mutually convertible. As in the preceding line, when spleen yáng is recovering in greater yīn disease, sudden vexation and diarrhea means that the patient is recovering. Nonetheless, it is also possible for dampness to transform into dryness, for cold to transform into heat, for vacuity to convert into repletion, and for yīn to turn into yáng; in other words, greater yīn disease can turn into yáng brightness disease. The phrase, "vacuity is greater yīn; repletion is yáng brightness," refers to the mutual convertibility of the two.

When greater yīn disease turns into yáng brightness disease, the stool becomes hard. Hard stool is a characteristic of yáng brightness repletion pattern. Alone it does not constitute sufficient evidence to conclude that the disease is in yáng brightness; nevertheless, when other signs of yáng brightness disease are present, it is a key sign.

This line may be compared to the preceding line; the two present similar conditions in which spleen yáng is recovering, but with very different outcomes. In the preceding line, the evil is expelled, waste matter in the stomach and intestines is eliminated, and the patient recovers. In the present line, because of pronounced heat in the stomach, the evil transforms into dryness, the disease shifts to yáng brightness, and the stool becomes hard.

Chapter Five

Lesser Yīn Disease

Pulses and Signs; Treatment

辨少阴病脉证并治

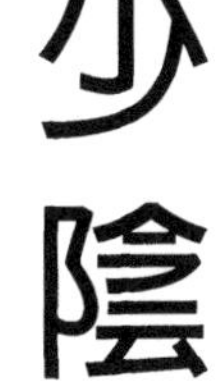

1 OVERVIEW

The lesser yīn includes the hand lesser yīn heart channel and the foot lesser yīn kidney channel. The heart holds the office of the monarch; the kidney is the root of earlier heaven. The kidney is in the lower burner and belongs to water. The yáng in the heart descends to the kidney to warm and nourish kidney yáng. The yīn of the kidney ascends to the heart and nourishes heart yīn. Under normal circumstances, heart fire and kidney water interact in this way and maintain a balance. This is often described as "interaction of the heart and kidney" (心肾相交 *xīn shèn xiāng jiāo*) or as "fire and water helping each other" (水火相济 *shuǐ huǒ xiāng jì*).

When disease is in lesser yīn, the heart and kidney are both vacuous. Because the kidney is the root of yīn and yáng of the whole body, kidney yáng vacuity manifests in general signs of vacuity cold. These constitute the main feature of lesser yīn disease. Lesser yīn vacuity cold patterns may result from the contraction of an external evil in patients constitutionally suffering from heart-kidney vacuity; they may also be a further development of greater yīn vacuity cold patterns; or they may be the result of inappropriate treatment of yáng channel disease (especially from the greater yáng, given the exterior-interior relationship between greater yīn and lesser yīn).

In addition to vacuity cold patterns, there are also heat patterns. These arise when evil heat damages yīn, and yīn vacuity transforms into heat. These patterns are completely different in nature and have to be treated differently.

1.1 Pulses and Signs

Lesser yīn cold transformation takes the form of heart-kidney yáng vacuity. It is characterized by signs of generalized vacuity cold such as absence of heat with aversion to cold, a pulse that is faint and fine, desire only to sleep, reversal cold of the limbs, and clear-food diarrhea.

Absence of heat effusion and aversion to cold, 无热恶寒 *wú rè wù hán*: When an evil initially damages the body, and right qì has not yet been weakened and can struggle to resist the evil, aversion to cold is usually accompanied by heat effusion; this is observed in greater yáng patterns. In lesser yīn patterns, yáng qì is debilitated and there is only pronounced yīn cold, giving rise to aversion to cold, but without heat effusion. At the onset of greater yáng cold damage aversion to cold may appear alone before heat effusion develops. However, in the aversion to cold of greater yáng disease, the evil in the fleshy exterior causes depression of defense yáng. Depressed yáng must struggle with the evil; hence sooner or later heat is bound to effuse. Aversion to cold without heat effusion in greater yáng is thus only a temporary condition. Aversion to cold without heat effusion in lesser yīn disease is attributable to vacuous yáng failing to warm the whole body. This is what is meant by the phrase, "when yáng is vacuous, there is external cold," 阳虚则外寒 *yáng xū zé wài hán*.

Pulse that is faint and fine, 脉微细 *mài wēi xì*: When heart and kidney yáng qì are debilitated and powerless to move the blood, then the pulse will be faint and forceless. When yáng qì is vacuous and yīn blood is weak, the vessels are not properly filled, so the pulse becomes fine and small in form. In clinical practice, a pulse that is faint is certain to be small. A pulse that is faint and fine is an external indicator of heart-kidney yáng vacuity. In externally contracted disease, no matter what the disease pattern, the appearance of a pulse that is faint and fine means that the condition can be treated as heart-kidney yáng vacuity using yáng-returning counterflow-stemming formulae.

Desire only to sleep, 但欲寐 *dàn yù mèi*: A condition in which the patient is fatigued and stuporous; not a normal desire for sleep. When yáng qì is debilitated, spirit qì is deprived of nourishment, and so the patient desires only to sleep. Desire only to sleep is usually observed together with a pulse that is faint and fine. It is essentially different from the somnolence observed in protracted greater yáng disease after the abatement of the evil. Desire only to sleep in lesser yīn disease is associated with a clear spirit-mind; hence it differs from somnolence with clouded spirit that is associated with exuberant heat patterns.

Reversal cold of the limbs, 四肢厥冷 *sì zhī jué lěng*: Also called "counterflow cold of the limbs." In mild cases the hands and feet are cold, and in severe cases there is cold up to the elbows and knees. It is mostly attributable to exuberant cold evil and heart-kidney vacuity depriving the extremities of warmth. When in greater yīn disease, vacuity cold is not severe, the reversal cold of the limbs will be mild, or the extremities will become spontaneously warm.

Clear-food diarrhea, 下利清谷 *xià lì qīng gǔ*: Diarrhea is a major sign of greater yīn disease. Hence the saying, "If the spleen is undamaged, there is no diarrhea." However, in greater yīn disease, "nontransformation of food" (完谷不化 *wán gǔ bù huà*, i.e., undigested food in the stool) is not observed. It is only when spleen vacuity affects the kidney, causing debilitation of kidney yáng, that grain and water are not decomposed properly so that there is nontransformation of food. In short, nontransformation of food is a sign not of greater yīn but of lesser yīn disease. Greater yīn disease only involves center burner vacuity that does not affect the yáng qì of the lower burner, so greater yīn disease is characterized by diarrhea that is usually without thirst. By contrast, in lesser yīn disease not only is there inability to decompose grain and water, but also liquid and humor fail to rise; hence diarrhea is usually associated with thirst.

The discussion of heat transformation patterns is significantly shorter than that of cold transformation. There are two heat transformation patterns: yīn vacuity with yáng hyperactivity, and yīn vacuity heat with inhibited water qì. The former is characterized by vexation in the heart and inability to sleep. The latter is characterized by diarrhea, cough, retching, thirst, and heart vexation with inability to sleep.

1.2 TREATMENT

Counterflow Cold Decoction (*sì nì tāng*) treats spleen and kidney yáng vacuity with cold in the center and the extremities by warming and moving yáng. When exuberant yīn in the interior repels yáng to the exterior, Vessel-Freeing Counterflow Cold Decoction (*tōng mài sì nì tāng*) is used to free and outthrust yáng qì. When exuberant yīn in the interior repels yáng upward, Scallion [Yáng-]Freeing Decoction (*bái tōng tāng*) is used to diffuse and free yáng qì so that it can descend. If yáng medicinals are repelled by yīn, then cold, salty, bitter ingredients, such as pig's bile (*zhū dǎn zhī*) and human urine (*rén niào*), can be added to the formula to allow the body to accept it. Scallion [Yáng-]Freeing Decoction Plus Pig's Bile (*bái tōng jiā zhū dǎn zhī tāng*) is an example of this method. Efflux desertion diarrhea containing pus and blood is treated with Peach Blossom Decoction (*táo huā tāng*) to warm the kidney, astringe the intestines, and stem desertion. For yáng vacuity cold with invasion of water qì, one may use Aconite Decoction (*fù zǐ tāng*) or True Warrior Decoction (*zhēn wǔ tāng*) to warm kidney yáng and transform water qì.

In heat transformation patterns, yáng hyperactivity due to yīn vacuity is treated with Coptis and Ass Hide Glue Decoction (*huáng lián ē jiāo tāng*), which fosters yīn and clears heat. If inhibited water qì is also present, one may use Polyporus Decoction (*zhū líng tāng*) to clear heat and enrich yīn.

In reversal patterns, disharmony between liver and stomach causes yáng qì to become depressed in the interior. The appropriate formula for these patterns is Counterflow Cold Powder (*sì nì sǎn*), which regulates the qì dynamic and outthrusts depressed yáng.

Pig Skin Decoction (*zhū fū tāng*), which enriches kidney yīn, moistens the lung, and supplements the spleen, is used to treat sore throat from vacuity fire flaming upward. If visiting heat attacks the throat, Licorice Decoction (*gān cǎo tāng*) or Platycodon Decoction (*jié gěng tāng*) can be used to clear heat and disinhibit the throat. In more severe patterns in which sores arise in the throat, Vinegar Decoction (*kǔ jiǔ tāng*) is used to clear heat and flush phlegm, and to constrain sores and disperse swelling. If visiting cold invades, Pinellia Powder and Decoction (*bàn xià sǎn jí tāng*) can be used to dissipate cold and free yáng, and to flush phlegm and open binds.

Because most lesser yīn disease belongs to vacuity, the promotion of sweating and the use of precipitation are generally contraindicated. Nonetheless, this contraindication is not absolute, and if a mild lesser yīn pattern occurs when an exterior pattern is still present, Ephedra, Asarum, and Aconite Decoction (*má huáng xì xīn fù zǐ tāng*) or Ephedra, Aconite, and Licorice Decoction (*má huáng fù zǐ gān cǎo tāng*) can be used to warm the channels and resolve the exterior. Finally, for lesser yīn patterns of yīn vacuity in which yáng brightness bowel repletion is also present and the true yīn is about to be exhausted, Major Qì-Coordinating Decoction (*dà chéng qì tāng*) can be used to rescue yīn.

1.3 Schematic Overview

Lesser Yīn Disease Patterns

- **Basic Lesser Yīn Disease Pattern**
  - Cold transformation patterns
    * Pattern requiring urgent warming with a pulse that is sunken, desire only to sleep, reversal cold of the limbs, clear-food diarrhea, retching and vomiting, and aversion to cold: Counterflow Cold Decoction (*sì nì tāng*)
    * Exuberant yīn repelling yáng with a pulse that is faint and verging on expiry, clear-food diarrhea, desire only to sleep, reversal cold of the limbs, vexation and agitation, and absence of aversion to cold: Vessel-Freeing Counterflow Cold Decoction (*tōng mài sì nì tāng*)
    * Exuberant yīn and upcast yáng with a pulse that is faint and verging on expiry, clear-food diarrhea, reversal cold of the limbs, dry retching, heart vexation, and aversion to cold: Scallion [Yáng-]Freeing Decoction (*bái tōng tāng*), Scallion [Yáng-]Freeing Decoction Plus Pig's Bile (*bái tōng jiā zhū dǎn zhī tāng*)
    * Yáng vacuity and water flooding with desire only to sleep, palpitations below the heart, dizzy head, inhibited urination, pain and heaviness of the limbs, and diarrhea: True Warrior Decoction (*zhēn wǔ tāng*)
    * Yáng vacuity cold dampness with generalized pain and joint pain, aversion to cold in the back, cold limbs, and a pulse that is sunken: Aconite Decoction (*fù zǐ tāng*)
    * Yáng vacuity and yīn exuberance with vomiting, diarrhea, counterflow cold of the limbs, and vexation and agitation: Evodia Decoction (*wú zhū yú tāng*)
    * Efflux desertion with intractable diarrhea containing pus and blood, inhibited urination, and abdominal pain: Peach Blossom Decoction (*táo huā tāng*)
  - Heat transformation patterns
    * Yīn vacuity and hyperactive yáng with vexation in the heart and inability to sleep: Coptis and Ass Hide Glue Decoction (*huáng lián ē jiāo tāng*)
    * Yīn vacuity with heat and inhibited water qì with diarrhea, cough, retching, thirst, heart vexation, and inability to sleep: Polyporus Decoction (*zhū líng tāng*)
- **Concurrent and Transmuted Patterns**

- Concurrent exterior pattern with heat effusion and a pulse that is sunken: Ephedra, Asarum, and Aconite Decoction (*má huáng xì xīn fù zǐ tāng*)
- Concurrent exterior pattern: Ephedra, Aconite, and Licorice Decoction (*má huáng fù zǐ gān cǎo tāng*)
- Pattern requiring urgent precipitation with dry mouth and throat, pain below the heart, and clear-water diarrhea that is a pure green-blue color: Major Qì-Coordinating Decoction (*dà chéng qì tāng*)
- Reversal from yáng depression with cold limbs, cough, palpitations, inhibited urination, pain in the abdomen, and diarrhea with rectal heaviness: Counterflow Cold Powder (*sì nì sǎn*)

- **Sore Throat Patterns**
  - Yīn vacuity fire with sore throat, diarrhea, abdominal fullness, and heart vexation: Pig Skin Decoction (*zhū fū tāng*)
  - Basic lesser yīn sore throat pattern: Licorice Decoction (*gān cǎo tāng*) and Platycodon Decoction (*jié gěng tāng*)
  - Damage in the throat with sores and difficulty speaking: Vinegar Decoction (*kǔ jiǔ tāng*)
  - Visiting cold sore throat: Pinellia Powder and Decoction (*bàn xià sǎn jí tāng*)

2 ESSENTIAL FEATURES OF LESSER YĪN DISEASE

2.1 PRIMARY PULSE AND SIGNS OF COLD TRANSFORMATION PATTERNS

LINE 281

少阴之为病，脉微细，但欲寐也。

Shào yīn zhī wéi bìng, mài wēi xì, dàn yù mèi yě.

In disease of the lesser yīn, the pulse is faint and fine and [there is] a desire only to sleep.

SYNOPSIS

The outline of the lesser yīn cold transformation pattern.

COMMENTARY

The lesser yīn includes the heart and kidney. The relationship between these two organs is complex and that fact, in conjunction with the ambiguity of some lines in the lesser yīn section, has given rise to a great deal of disagreement among commentators with regard to the interpretation of even the most basic aspects of these patterns. The heart governs the blood and belongs to fire. The kidney stores the essence and belongs to water. Heart fire is kept in balance by kidney water and kidney water is warmed by heart fire. When this relationship is disturbed, as in lesser yīn disease, a transformation to cold or heat may occur. Cold reflects yáng vacuity and exuberant yīn. Heat reflects yīn vacuity and vacuity heat.

When the heart and kidney are vacuous, as in lesser yīn disease, yáng qì is debilitated and has decreased power to move the blood; consequently, the pulse becomes faint. In these patterns the yīn is also vacuous; hence the pulse is fine as well. The faint quality is considered to be the more important of the two, just as yáng vacuity is considered to be more prominent in these patterns than yīn vacuity. In the *Mài Jīng* (脉经 "The Pulse Canon"), Wáng Shū-Hé (王叔和) writes, "A faint pulse is extremely fine and soft, or [it may be] about to expire, sometimes present, sometimes absent.... A fine pulse is small [but] bigger than a faint [pulse], [it is] usually present, only fine." This text was written after the *Shāng Hán Lùn* and the author's method of describing the pulse characteristics is different from Zhāng Jī's. Nonetheless, since Zhāng Jī did not write a clear description of these pulse qualities, and the interpretation of this line is problematic, later commentators have used this quote as a reference.

Given that heart and kidney yáng is vacuous, yīn cold in the interior becomes exuberant. The spirit is not nourished and the patient desires sleep. When the pulse is faint and fine, and the patient desires sleep, this is a lesser yīn disease of yáng vacuity cold. "Desire for sleep" does not mean that the patient is able to sleep, but is instead characterized by a listlessness of the essence-spirit, which should be differentiated from the somnolence that occurs following the resolution of disease or as the result of severe heat clouding the spirit. In line 37, p. 95, somnolence occurs following the resolution of a greater yáng disease. "When in greater yáng disease, after ten days have passed, the pulse is floating and fine, and [there is] somnolence, the outer body has already resolved." In that pattern the evil has been eliminated, right qì has prevailed, the spirit is peaceful, and the patient's sleep is tranquil. In line 231, p. 396, somnolence occurs as a result of exuberant heat clouding the spirit. In that pattern the tendency to sleep is accompanied by other signs of depressed heat, such as inability to sweat, yellowing of the entire body, difficult urination, and tidal heat effusion.

As explained above, the condition described in the present line is one of yáng vacuity cold lesser yīn disease, but it has also been variously explained as a pattern of heat and cold transformation or one of heat transformation. Shěn Yáo-Fēng (沈尧封) and Chén Píng-Bó (陈平伯) represent those commentators who believe that the pulse and signs described here can indicate a lesser yīn disease transforming to cold or heat. Shěn Yáo-Fēng writes, "Faint means thin and belongs to yáng vacuity. Fine means small and belongs to yīn vacuity. Desire only to sleep means the defense qì moves in the yīn and not in the yáng." Because he includes both yáng vacuity and yīn vacuity in his explanation, the possibility of the transformation to heat and cold is included. Chén Píng-Bó continues this idea:

> Fine and faint is the pulse of lesser yīn disease. A desire only to sleep is the lesser yīn condition. Because the lesser yīn is the viscera that stores essence and the source from which qì is engendered, when an evil enters this channel the pivot mechanism becomes inhibited and the essence does not ascend; consequently, the pulse is fine and faint. [Without] essence, the spirit

> is not bright and [there is] desire only to sleep. Regardless of whether cold evil or heat evil, diseases [of the lesser yīn] all have this sign and this pulse; therefore, this is an outline of lesser yīn disease.

Wāng Hŭ offers another perspective, suggesting that this line represents the transformation to heat. "This is a description of extreme encumbrance of heat in lesser yīn disease. [When the evil] shifts into the lesser yīn, the pulse becomes fine and faint, which means the heat evil is deep [in the interior] and the pulse is hidden in the interior. This is not true sleep, but extreme heat clouding the spirit-mind, resembling a desire to sleep."

The perspectives offered by Shěn Yáo-Fēng, Chén Píng-Bó, and Wāng Hŭ do not appear to agree with clinical reality, and consequently have not gained much acceptance.

Line 282

少阴病，欲吐不吐，心烦但欲寐，五六日，自利而渴者，属少阴也，虚故引水自救；若小便色白者，少阴病形悉具，小便白者，以下焦虚有寒，不能制水，故令色白也。

Shào yīn bìng, yù tù bù tù, xīn fán dàn yù mèi, wǔ liù rì, zì lì ér kě zhě, shǔ shào yīn yě, xū gù yǐn shuǐ zì jiù; ruò xiǎo biàn sè bái zhě, shào yīn bìng xíng xī jù, xiǎo biàn bái zhě, yǐ xià jiāo xū yǒu hán, bù néng zhì shuǐ, gù lìng sè bái yě.

When in lesser yīn disease, [there is] desire but inability to vomit, heart vexation, and desire only for sleep, and [after] five or six days, spontaneous diarrhea and thirst, this belongs to lesser yīn. [There is] vacuity; hence water intake [should] relieve [the thirst]. If the urine color is clear,* then lesser yīn signs are all present. The urine is clear because of vacuity cold in the lower burner and inability to control water; consequently, that makes the color clear.

Text Note

* The urine color is clear, 小便色白 *xiǎo biàn sè bái*: In this context, 白 *bái*, which can mean "white," means a clear appearance.

Synopsis

The essential signs of lesser yīn vacuity cold patterns.

Commentary

This line presents a lesser yīn cold transformation pattern, but contains some signs that appear to indicate heat. Heart vexation and desire to vomit are often seen in heat patterns, but here they belong to yáng vacuity with exuberant cold. Zhāng Jī explains that one knows these are cold signs because the urine is clear, which means vacuity cold is present in the lower burner.

When kidney yáng is vacuous, turbid yīn ascends counterflow, causing disharmony of the stomach qì and disturbing normal downbearing. The patient desires to vomit but is unable to because the patient's food intake is reduced; therefore, the stomach is empty. This line can be compared with line 324, p. 477, in which the patient vomits food directly after eating because of the presence of a repletion evil in the upper burner.

Vacuous kidney yáng in the lower burner struggles with exuberant yīn cold and is pushed upward, where it harasses the heart and causes vexation. Yáng vacuity in these patterns is severe; hence although vexation is present, the patient also desires to sleep. The presence of a desire to sleep allows one to differentiate this pattern from vexation patterns that are the result of yīn vacuity and hyperactive yáng, in which there is insomnia.

The lesser yīn disease above should be treated by warming yáng and expelling cold. If no treatment is given for five or six days, the yáng vacuity will increase in severity, as will yīn cold. Vacuous kidney yáng is unable to warm the spleen, and the spleen loses its ability to upbear, giving rise to diarrhea. Vacuous yáng is also unable to steam and transform fluids, which then do not ascend; therefore the patient feels thirst. Diarrhea damages the fluids and vacuous yáng is unable to steam the fluids; hence the patient is not only thirsty, but also desires to drink. The presence or absence of thirst is an important diagnostic indicator for lesser yīn patterns.

Lesser yīn and greater yīn diarrhea both occur as the result of yáng vacuity, but the patterns differ in severity. Greater yīn disease is characterized by spleen yáng vacuity with exuberant cold-damp; consequently, diarrhea is present and thirst is absent. In lesser yīn disease, the yáng vacuity is more severe, affecting both the spleen and kidney. Because kidney yáng is affected, the fluids are not distributed properly and diarrhea occurs simultaneously with thirst. Nonetheless, it should be noted that in chronic spleen vacuity diarrhea, thirst may occur as a result of enduring fluid loss.

Diarrhea and thirst in lesser yīn disease should be differentiated from similar signs that appear in reverting yīn disease as a result of heat. In reverting yīn heat patterns, the diarrhea is putrid, scorching heat is felt in the anus, and the patient desires cold fluids. He/she drinks large amounts of fluid, the tongue fur is yellow and grimy, and the urine is short and red. Generalized heat and a pulse that is rapid may also be observed. In lesser yīn disease the diarrhea is clear and thin and may contain non-transformed food. The patient desires warm fluids and does not drink much. The tongue is pale and moist and the urine is clear and long. Aversion to cold and a pulse that is faint may also be observed. These two patterns should be clearly differentiated.

Line 283

病人脉阴阳俱紧，反汗出者，亡阳也，此属少阴，法当咽痛而复吐利。

Bìng rén mài yīn yáng jù jǐn, fǎn hàn chū zhě, wáng yáng yě, cǐ shǔ shào yīn, fǎ dāng yān tòng ér fù tù lì.

When the person's yīn and yáng pulses* are both tight, but [there is] sweating, it means yáng collapse, and belongs to the lesser yīn. There should be sore throat and then vomiting and diarrhea.

Text Note

* Yīn and yáng pulses, 脉阴阳 *mài yīn yáng*: The entire pulse, not the superficial and deep levels. Here, this term does not mean superficial and deep levels because the basic pulse in lesser yīn disease in sunken. The pulse is not felt in the superficial level. See line 3, p. 44, for a similar pulse in a greater yáng disease.

Synopsis

The pulse and signs of lesser yīn yáng collapse.

Commentary

In lesser yīn cold transformation patterns, the pulse was previously described as faint and fine; but here, all three positions of the pulse are tight. Because lesser yīn disease belongs to the interior and a sunken pulse is characteristic of interior patterns, the pulse in this pattern should be considered not only tight, but also sunken. The sunken quality means an interior pattern and the tight quality means cold. In lesser yīn disease with exuberant interior cold, sweating is generally absent, but here, sweating is present; therefore, Zhāng Jī uses the word "but" 反 *fǎn*, to emphasize that this sign is unexpected. Here, exuberant yīn cold forces vacuous yáng out towards the exterior, a phenomenon known as "yáng collapse," which manifests as sweating.

The other signs described in this line (sore throat, vomiting, and diarrhea) are explained below. The lesser yīn channel ascends to the throat and when vacuous yáng strays, it can ascend and cause sore throat. This type of throat pain, however, should be clearly differentiated from repletion heat-type sore throat. When sore throat is the result of yáng collapse, it is not severe, and redness and swelling are absent. Conversely, heat repletion sore throat is characterized by severe pain and a red, swollen throat. Vacuous yáng cannot control turbid yīn; consequently, it ascends counterflow, causing the patient to vomit. Vacuous yáng cannot upbear clear yáng; hence there is diarrhea.

Although no treatment is suggested in this line, it is likely that a formula like Counterflow Cold Decoction (*sì nì tāng*) would be given to return yáng and stem counterflow.

The yīn and yáng pulses are described as "tight" in this line and in line 3, p. 44, of the greater yáng section. In the greater yáng section the pulse is floating and tight and is accompanied by heat effusion, aversion to cold, no sweating, and headache. In this pattern the pulse is sunken and tight and is accompanied by signs of vacuity cold.

2.2 Contraindications for the Treatment of Lesser Yīn Disease

Line 285

少阴病，脉细沉数，病为在里，不可发汗。

Shào yīn bìng, mài xì chén shuò, bìng wèi zài lǐ, bù kě fā hàn.

When in lesser yīn disease, the pulse is fine, sunken, and rapid, the disease is in the interior and one cannot promote sweating.

Synopsis

In lesser yīn interior patterns the promotion of sweating is contraindicated.

Commentary

In exterior diseases the promotion of sweating is appropriate to expel the evil and resolve the disease. In interior diseases the promotion of sweating is inappropriate, as it will damage the right qì and fail to resolve the evil. Nonetheless, in certain lesser yīn disease, sweating can be promoted. For example, mild lesser yīn interior vacuity occurring simultaneously with an exterior pattern can be treated with a formula like Ephedra, Asarum, and Aconite Decoction (*má huáng xì xīn fù zǐ tāng*), which supports yáng and promotes sweating. In this line, however, only an interior disease is present; therefore, the promotion of sweating is contraindicated.

The pulse is fine, sunken, and rapid. This type of pulse may appear in both lesser yīn cold and heat transformation patterns. If it is accompanied by signs of yīn vacuity heat, such as insomnia and vexation, then it is likely a sign of heat transformation. If it is accompanied by signs of exuberant yīn cold and yáng vacuity, such as aversion to cold, diarrhea without thirst, and vomiting, it is likely a sign of cold transformation. In either case, heat or cold, one must not promote sweating because this is a pure interior pattern.

Line 286

少阴病，脉微，不可发汗，亡阳故也；阳已虚，尺脉弱濇者，复不可下之。

Shào yīn bìng, mài wēi, bù kě fā hàn, wáng yáng gù yě; yáng yǐ xū, chǐ mài ruò sè zhě, fù bù kě xià zhī.

When in lesser yīn disease, the pulse is faint, one cannot promote sweating, because yáng [will] collapse. [If] yáng is already vacuous and the cubit pulse is weak and rough, then one cannot precipitate.

Synopsis

In lesser yīn disease, when yīn and yáng are both vacuous, precipitation is contraindicated.

Commentary

As described in the previous line, the promotion of sweating is generally contraindicated in lesser yīn disease, except in specific instances in which sweating is promoted and yáng is simultaneously supplemented. This line reiterates this basic principle and expands the pulse description. In a lesser yīn disease a pulse that is faint means yáng vacuity. The promotion of sweating will further damage yáng and cause yáng collapse; therefore, the promotion of sweating is contraindicated in these patterns.

If yáng is vacuous and the pulse is weak and rough, it indicates that yīn and blood are vacuous as well. In this situation one cannot precipitate, since this treatment will damage both yīn and yáng and exacerbate the disease.

In the text these two patterns are separated, and a strict reading of the text would not link them. The contraindication for the promotion of sweating applies to yáng vacuity and the contraindication for precipitation applies to yīn-yáng dual vacuity. Most commentators, however, suggest that the contraindications in this line can be broadly applied. That is, in lesser yīn disease, as a general rule, both the promotion of sweating and the use of precipitation are contraindicated.

3 BASIC LESSER YĪN DISEASE PATTERNS

3.1 Cold Transformation Patterns

3.1.1 Counterflow Cold Decoction Patterns

Line 323

少阴病，脉沉者，急温之，宜四逆汤。

Shào yīn bìng, mài chén zhě, jí wēn zhī, yí sì nì tāng.

When in lesser yīn disease the pulse is sunken, [it is necessary] to warm urgently and [therefore] Counterflow Cold Decoction (*sì nì tāng*) is appropriate.

Formula

Counterflow Cold Decoction (*sì nì tāng*)

◦ Return yáng and stem counterflow.

甘草二两（炙） 干姜一两半 附子一枚（生用，去皮，破八片）

㈠ 右三味，以水三升，煮取一升二合，去滓，分温再服。㈡ 强人可大附子一枚，干姜三两。

Gān cǎo èr liǎng (zhì) gān jiāng yī liǎng bàn fù zǐ yī méi (shēng yòng, qù pí, pò bā piàn)

(1) *Yòu sān wèi, yǐ shuǐ sān shēng, zhǔ qǔ yī shēng èr gě, qù zǐ, fēn wēn zài fú.* (2) *Qiáng rén kě dà fù zǐ yī méi, gān jiāng sān liǎng.*

mix-fried licorice (甘草 *gān cǎo*, Glycyrrhizae Radix) 2 liǎng

dried ginger (干姜 *gān jiāng*, Zingiberis Rhizoma Exsiccatum) 1.5 liǎng

aconite (附子 *fù zǐ*, Aconiti Tuber Laterale) 1 piece (use raw, remove skin, break into 8 pieces)

(1) [For] the above three ingredients use three shēng of water. Boil to get one shēng two gě and remove the dregs. Divide [into two parts], and take warm twice a day. (2) Strong people can [use] a large piece of aconite (*fù zǐ*) and 3 liǎng of dried ginger (*gān jiāng*).

Synopsis

In lesser yīn disease when the pulse is deep, urgent warming is appropriate.

Commentary

This line is very short and in order to understand its content and the clinical implications, one must consider what Zhāng Jī has not written. It is unlikely that Zhāng Jī would suggest urgent warming treatment solely on the basis of a pulse that is sunken, but when this pulse is accompanied by clear-food diarrhea, counterflow cold of the extremities, and other signs of severe yīn cold and yáng vacuity, this treatment is appropriate. In the entire lesser yīn section, this is the only line in which urgent warming is suggested. In fact, other lines that suggest stronger formulae do not specify urgent warming. No clear explanation exists for this apparent contradiction, but the authors of *Gāo Děng Cóng Shū* explain that in yáng collapse with reversal desertion the pattern is critical and the signs are very clear, but when the pattern has not reached that critical stage, it is easy to misinterpret the signs and provide ineffective treatment. It may be that Zhāng Jī suggests urgent warming in this case in order to avoid the transmutation to the more severe pattern of yáng collapse reversal desertion.

In this line the pulse is sunken, indicating an interior pattern, but its strength is not specified. If the pulse is sunken, large, and strong, one cannot use urgent warming, since this is probably an internal repletion pattern. Here, the pulse is probably not only sunken, but also faint and fine, as in the previous lines describing lesser yīn disease. The presence of this type of pulse suggests that heart and kidney yáng are vacuous; hence one can use Counterflow Cold Decoction (*sì nì tāng*) to warm urgently.

The formula name, Counterflow Cold Decoction (*sì nì tāng*), refers to the sign of counterflow cold in the four limbs, 四肢厥逆 *sì zhī jué nì*, which it treats. Aconite (*fù zǐ*) warms the kidney and returns yáng. Dried ginger (*gān jiāng*) warms the center and dissipates cold. Licorice (*gān cǎo*) regulates the center and supplements vacuity. This formula is the basic one for returning yáng and stemming counterflow. It warms both the spleen and the kidney and can be used in patterns involving spleen and kidney yáng vacuity cold, regardless of the origin of the disease.

Line 324

㈠ 少阴病，饮食入口则吐，心中温温欲吐，复不能吐，始得之，手足寒，脉弦迟者，此胸中实，不可下也，当吐之。㈡ 若膈上有寒饮， 干呕者，不可吐也，当温之，宜四逆汤。

(1) *Shào yīn bìng, yǐn shí rù kǒu zé tù, xīn zhōng yùn yùn yù tù, fù bù néng tù, shǐ dé zhī, shǒu zú hán, mài xián chí zhě, cǐ xiōng zhōng shí, bù kě xià yě, dāng tù zhī.* (2) *Ruò gé shàng yǒu hán yǐn, gān ǒu zhě, bù kě tù yě, dāng wēn zhī, yí sì nì tāng.*

(1) When in lesser yīn disease [there is] immediate vomiting of ingested food and drink, seething in the heart with desire to vomit,* yet inability to vomit, [but] at the beginning the extremities are cold, and the pulse is stringlike and slow, this indicates repletion in the chest. One cannot precipitate, [but] should [use] vomiting. (2) If [there is] cold-rheum above the diaphragm and dry retching, one cannot [use] vomiting, [but] should [use] warming. Counterflow Cold Decoction (*sì nì tāng*) is appropriate.

Text Note

* Seething in the heart with a desire to vomit, 心中温温欲吐 *xīn zhōng wēn wēn yù tù*: Vexation and oppression felt in the chest with nausea. See line 123, p. 279, for an occurrence of a similar sign.

Synopsis

The differentiation of lesser yīn disease with cold-rheum above the diaphragm and repletion evil in the chest.

Commentary

In lesser yīn disease, vomiting after eating and seething in the heart are generally considered signs of exuberant yīn cold ascending counterflow. This correlation, however, is not absolute; hence Zhāng Jī provides some information to assist in identification.

At the beginning of the disease, if the extremities are cold and the pulse is stringlike and slow, the pattern does not belong to lesser yīn, but is more likely a repletion pattern with phlegm-rheum congested in the chest. In this pattern, when an evil stagnates in the chest, right qì rises up to expel the evil, causing vomiting after food intake. The presence of phlegm-rheum in the chest causes a feeling of vexation and oppression in the chest with nausea. The patient is unable to eat and since the contents of the stomach have already been expelled, no more vomiting occurs. Because yáng qì is congested in the chest by the phlegm-rheum and cannot move out to the extremities, they become cold and the pulse becomes slow and stringlike. When the evil is in the chest, one should not use precipitation because it will damage the center burner and fail to expel the evil in the upper body. In this case one should use vomiting treatment to expel the evil from the chest. Although no formula is suggested, it is likely that a formula similar to Melon Stalk Powder (*guā dì sǎn*) would be used.

In a lesser yīn disease, when cold-rheum is present above the diaphragm with dry retching, one should not use vomiting treatment, but should warm the interior because the origin of cold-rheum lies in spleen and kidney yáng vacuity. Vacuous yáng is unable to transform qì and distribute the fluids; consequently, the fluids collect and form cold-rheum. Because the fluids are not being properly distributed, they congest in the region of the diaphragm and dry retching occurs. Since the origin of this pattern is yáng vacuity, Counterflow Cold Decoction (*sì nì tāng*), which warms and moves spleen and kidney yáng, is given in order to transform cold-rheum; vomiting treatment is not used.

For cold-rheum in the region of the diaphragm one may consider using Center-Rectifying Decoction (*lǐ zhōng tāng*), which warms the center and dissipates cold. The pattern above, however, belongs to lesser yīn disease, in which kidney yáng is vacuous. In patterns of kidney yáng vacuity, Counterflow Cold Decoction (*sì nì tāng*) should be used because it warms both kidney and spleen yáng.

3.1.2 Vessel-Freeing Counterflow Cold Decoction Patterns

LINE 317

㈠ 少阴病，下利清谷，里寒外热，手足厥逆，脉微欲绝，身反不恶寒。㈡ 其人面色赤，或腹痛，或干呕，或咽痛，或利止脉不出者，通脉四逆汤主之。

(1) *Shào yīn bìng, xià lì qīng gǔ, lǐ hán wài rè, shǒu zú jué nì, mài wēi yù jué, shēn fǎn bù wù hán.* (2) *Qí rén miàn sè chì, huò fù tòng, huò gān ǒu, huò yān tòng, huò lì zhǐ mài bù chū zhě, tōng mài sì nì tāng zhǔ zhī.*

(1) In lesser yīn disease, clear-food diarrhea [indicates] interior cold and exterior heat. [There is] reverse-flow of the extremities, the pulse is faint and verging on expiry, but generalized aversion to cold is absent. (2) When the person has a red facial complexion, or possibly abdominal pain, or dry retching, or sore throat, or the diarrhea ceases [and] the pulse does not move outward, Vessel-Freeing Counterflow Cold Decoction (*tōng mài sì nì tāng*) governs.

FORMULA

Vessel-Freeing Counterflow Cold Decoction (*tōng mài sì nì tāng*)

∘ Break yīn and return yáng; penetrate to reconnect the inner [yīn] and outer [yáng].

甘草二两（炙） 附子大者一枚（生用，去皮，破八片） 干姜三两（强人可四两）

(一) 右三味，以水三升，煮取一升二合，去滓，分温再服， 其脉即出者愈。(二) 面色赤者，加葱九茎。(三) 腹中痛者，去葱加芍药二两。(四) 呕者，加生姜二两。(五) 咽痛者，去芍药加桔梗一两。(六) 利止脉不出者，去桔梗加人参二两，病皆与方相应者，乃服之。

Gān cǎo èr liǎng (zhì) fù zǐ dà zhě yī méi (shēng yòng, qù pí, pò bā piàn) gān jiāng sān liǎng (qiáng rén kě sì liǎng)

(1) *Yòu sān wèi, yǐ shuǐ sān shēng, zhǔ qǔ yī shēng èr gě, qù zǐ, fēn wēn zài fú, qí mài jí chū zhě yù.* (2) *Miàn sè chì zhě, jiā cōng jiǔ jīng.* (3) *Fù zhōng tòng zhě, qù cōng jiā sháo yào èr liǎng.* (4) *Oǔ zhě, jiā shēng jiāng èr liǎng.* (5) *Yān tòng zhě, qù sháo yào jiā jié gěng yī liǎng.* (6) *Lì zhǐ mài bù chū zhě, qù jié gěng jiā rén shēn èr liǎng, bìng jiē yǔ fāng xiāng yìng zhě, nǎi fú zhī.*

mix-fried licorice (甘草 *gān cǎo*, Glycyrrhizae Radix) 2 liǎng
large aconite (*fù zǐ*) 1 piece (use raw, remove skin, break into 8 pieces)
dried ginger (干姜 *gān jiāng*, Zingiberis Rhizoma Exsiccatum) 3 liǎng (4 liǎng can be used for strong people)

(1) [For] the above three ingredients use three shēng of water. Boil to get one shēng two gě and remove the dregs. Divide [into two parts], and take warm twice a day. When the pulse comes out,[1] [this indicates] recovery. (2) For red facial complexion, add nine stems of scallion (*cōng*). (3) For pain in the abdomen, remove scallion (*cōng*) and add 2 liǎng of peony (*sháo yào*). (4) For retching, add 2 liǎng of fresh ginger (*shēng jiāng*). (5) For sore throat, remove peony (*sháo yào*) and add 1 liǎng of platycodon (*jié gěng*). (6) If the diarrhea ceases and the pulse does not move outward, remove platycodon (*jié gěng*) and add 2 liǎng of ginseng (*rén shēn*). [Only when] the disease corresponds to the formula [can the formula be] taken.

FORMULA NOTE

* The pulse comes out, 脉即出 *mài jí chū*: The pulse is restored.

SYNOPSIS

The signs and treatment of exuberant yīn repelling yáng.

COMMENTARY

In lesser yīn disease, "interior cold and exterior heat" refers to exuberant yīn repelling yáng. True cold in the interior repels yáng and produces false heat in the exterior. This pattern occurs when yáng qì is severely vacuous and exuberant yīn cold is present in the interior. The primary signs are clear-food diarrhea, reverse-flow of the extremities, and a pulse that is faint and about to expire. False heat in the exterior gives rise to red facial complexion; although yáng qì is vacuous, aversion to cold is absent.

The red complexion in this pattern must be differentiated from that seen in repletion heat patterns. When vacuous yáng floats to the exterior the face becomes red, but it is tender red and the color comes and goes. "Tender red," 嫩红 *nèn hóng*, means a soft pastel-red color. It is the color normally associated with a healthy young person's face, and it appears incongruous when seen in a patient who is ill. In yáng brightness disease if the complexion is red, it is a bright red color that is full and steady. If vacuous yáng floats to the surface or there is a yáng brightness disease, the patient may feel generalized heat. When vacuous yáng floats upward, however, the patient feels only mildly hot, and the heat sensation quickly dissipates. In yáng brightness heat patterns, the patient feels very hot and the heat persists.

Vessel-Freeing Counterflow Cold Decoction (*tōng mài sì nì tāng*) is Counterflow Cold Decoction (*sì nì tāng*) with dried ginger (*gān jiāng*) and a large dose of aconite (*fù zǐ*); consequently, its ability to warm yáng and expel cold is increased and it treats a pulse that is faint and about to expire. For this reason, it is named "vessel-freeing" counterflow cold decoction. For red complexion, scallion white (*cōng bái*) is added to free yáng that has been repelled upward. If abdominal pain is observed, peony (*sháo yào*), which harmonizes the vessels and relieves pain, is added. For dry retching, fresh ginger (*shēng jiāng*), which harmonizes the stomach and downbears counterflow, is added. When the throat is sore, platycodon (*jié gěng*), which disinhibits the throat and opens binds, is added. If the diarrhea ceases but the pulse does not move outward, add ginseng (*rén shēn*), which boosts qì and yīn in order to restore the pulse.

3.1.3 Scallion [Yáng-]Freeing Decoction and Scallion [Yáng-]Freeing Decoction Plus Pig's Bile Patterns

LINE 314

少阴病，下利，白通汤主之。

Shào yīn bìng, xià lì, bái tōng tāng zhǔ zhī.

When in lesser yīn disease, [there is] diarrhea, Scallion [Yáng-]Freeing Decoction (*bái tōng tāng*) governs.

FORMULA

Scallion [Yáng-]Freeing Decoction (*bái tōng tāng*)

∘ Break yīn and return yáng; diffuse and open the upper and lower [burners].

葱白四茎　干姜一两　附子一枚（生，去皮，破八片）。

右三味，以水三升，煮取一升，去滓，分温再服。

Cōng bái sì jīng　gān jiāng yī liǎng　fù zǐ yī méi (shēng, qù pí, pò bā piàn)
Yòu sān wèi, yǐ shuǐ sān shēng, zhǔ qǔ yī shēng, qù zǐ, fēn wēn zài fú.

scallion white (葱白 *cōng bái*, Allii Fistulosi Bulbus) 4 stems
dried ginger (干姜 *gān jiāng*, Zingiberis Rhizoma Exsiccatum) 1 liǎng
aconite (附子 *fù zǐ*, Aconiti Tuber Laterale) 1 piece (raw, remove the skin, break into 8 pieces)

[For] the above three ingredients use three shēng of water. Boil to get one shēng and remove the dregs. Divide [into two parts], and take warm twice a day.

SYNOPSIS

The signs and treatment of exuberant yīn and upcast yáng.

COMMENTARY

Because this line is very short, an analysis of the formula is used to understand the meaning of the text. Scallion [Yáng-]Freeing Decoction (*bái tōng tāng*) is used to break yīn, return yáng, and open the upper and lower burners. On the basis of the formula, one can conclude that exuberant yīn in the lower burner has repelled vacuous yáng upward. As a result, turbid yīn remains in the lower burner, causing diarrhea. The body is cold and the head is hot; hence this pattern is referred to as "upcast yáng," 戴阳 *dài yáng*. This line does not mention heat in the head or upcast yáng explicitly, and it is only by reference to the formula that one can differentiate the pattern in this line from a pattern of repelled yáng.

To gain information about this pattern, we can look at two other lines, line 317 and line 315. In line 317, p. 478, scallion white (*cōng bái*) is added to the formula for red facial complexion. Because this formula is also used for lesser yīn disease and scallion white (*cōng bái*) is the main ingredient, one may conclude that red facial complexion is a part of this pattern. Given that the pulse in line 315, p. 481, is faint in a lesser yīn disease with diarrhea, here the pulse is probably faint, too. In summary, the complete upcast yáng pattern includes diarrhea and a pulse that is faint (indicating exuberant yīn in the lower burner), and red facial complexion (indicating repelled yáng in the upper burner).

The pattern above is milder than that for which Vessel-Freeing Counterflow Cold Decoction (*tōng mài sì nì tāng*) is used; hence Scallion [Yáng-]Freeing Decoction (*bái tōng tāng*) is used instead. A smaller amount of aconite (*fù zǐ*) and dried ginger (*gān jiāng*) is sufficient to warm and return yáng. Scallion white (*cōng bái*) is added to free yáng. In combination these ingredients free yáng qì in the upper and lower burners, allowing repelled yáng to descend and return to the kidney. In this way, upcast yáng is eliminated and diarrhea will cease.

LINE 315

㈠ 少阴病，下利，脉微者，与白通汤。㈡ 利不止，厥逆无脉，干呕烦者，白通加猪胆汁汤主之。㈢ 服汤脉暴出者死，微续者生。

(1) *Shào yīn bìng, xià lì, mài wēi zhě, yǔ bái tōng tāng.* (2) *Lì bù zhǐ, jué nì wú mài, gān ǒu fán zhě, bái tōng jiā zhū dǎn zhī tāng zhǔ zhī.* (3) *Fú tāng mài bào chū zhě sǐ, wēi xù zhě shēng.*

(1) When in lesser yīn disease [there is] diarrhea and the pulse is faint, give Scallion [Yáng-]Freeing Decoction (*bái tōng tāng*). (2) When [there is] incessant diarrhea, reverse-flow, an absent pulse, dry retching,

and vexation, Scallion [Yáng-]Freeing Decoction Plus Pig's Bile (*bái tōng jiā zhū dǎn zhī tāng*) governs. (3) If [after] taking the decoction, the pulse suddenly moves outward, [this means] death, [but] if [the pulse] continues to be faint, [this means] life.

Formula

Scallion [Yáng-]Freeing Decoction Plus Pig's Bile (*bái tōng jiā zhū dǎn zhī tāng*)

○ Break yīn and return yáng; diffuse and open the upper and lower; paradoxically assist with salty and bitter [flavors].

葱白四茎　干姜一两　附子一枚（生，去皮，破八片）　人尿五合　猪胆汁一合。

㈠ 右五味，以水三升，煮取一升，去滓，内胆汁、人尿，和令相得，分温再服。㈡ 若无胆，亦可用。

Cōng bái sì jīng gān jiāng yī liǎng fù zǐ yī méi (shēng, qù pí, pò bā piàn) rén niào wǔ gě zhū dǎn zhī yī gě

(1) *Yòu wǔ wèi, yǐ shuǐ sān shēng, zhǔ qǔ yī shēng, qù zǐ, nà dǎn zhī、rén niào, huò lìng xiāng dé, fēn wēn zài fú.* (2) *Ruò wú dǎn, yì kě yòng.*

scallion white (葱白 *cōng bái*, Allii Fistulosi Bulbus) 4 stems

dried ginger (干姜 *gān jiāng*, Zingiberis Rhizoma Exsiccatum) 1 liǎng

aconite (附子 *fù zǐ*, Aconiti Tuber Laterale) 1 piece (raw, remove the skin, break into 8 pieces)

human urine (人尿 *rén niào*, Hominis Urina) 5 gě

pig's bile (猪胆汁 *zhū dǎn zhī*, Suis Bilis) 1 gě

(1) [For] the above five ingredients use three shēng of water. Boil [the first three ingredients] to get one shēng and remove the dregs. Add the gallbladder juice and human urine, and blend thoroughly. Divide [into two parts], and take warm twice a day. (2) If [there is] no gall, one can still use [the formula].

Synopsis

In an exuberant yīn and upcast yáng pattern, after ingesting hot medicinals there is a repelling pattern, and its signs, treatment, and prognosis are described.

Commentary

The first part of this line, from the beginning to "Scallion [Yáng-]Freeing Decoction (*bái tōng tāng*)" is similar to the previous line and reinforces the assumption made in that line that the pulse is faint, since it is stated directly here. In lesser yīn disease with diarrhea and a pulse that is faint, Scallion [Yáng-]Freeing Decoction (*bái tōng tāng*) is suggested but in this line, the diarrhea does not cease after its administration. The disease becomes more severe, and the additional signs of reverse-flow (an absent pulse, dry retching, and vexation) are observed. Nonetheless, this transmutation does not mean that the treatment principle was incorrect because a similar formula is suggested to treat the transmutation. In this line, exuberant yīn evil repels yáng medicinals. Wáng Bīng (王冰) writes, "Extreme heat or cold will contend with [medicinals] of opposite nature and repel medicinals with different qì." Therefore, it is necessary to add medicinals to the formula that have a nature similar to the evil, so that the medicinals will not be repelled. This idea comes from the *Sù Wèn*: "In milder [diseases] use counteracting [treatment]; in severe [diseases] use coacting [treatment]." Counteracting treatment is treating heat with cold and cold with heat. Coacting treatment is treating cold with cold and heat with heat. In this case, the primary treatment principle is the same, to warm and return yáng, but coacting medicinals (bitter, cold pig gall and human urine) are used to allow the body to accept the formula. This type of treatment is only suggested in extreme cases.

After the second formula is taken, the two different pulses which are presented can be used as prognostic indicators. If the pulse suddenly appears, it means that vacuous yáng has effused out to the exterior. This pulse is a negative sign that occurs prior to yáng expiry and death. If the pulse returns with a faint quality, as in the beginning of the line, it means that yáng qì is slowly returning. This pulse is a positive sign and recovery will follow.

Scallion [Yáng-]Freeing Decoction Plus Pig's Bile (*bái tōng jiā zhū dǎn zhī tāng*) is Scallion [Yáng-]Freeing Decoction (*bái tōng tāng*) with the addition of pig's bile (*zhū dǎn zhī*) and human urine (*rén niào*). Scallion [Yáng-]Freeing Decoction (*bái tōng tāng*) breaks yīn, returns yáng, and opens the upper and lower burners. Salty, bitter, and cold, pig's bile (*zhū dǎn zhī*) and human urine (*rén niào*) allow yáng medicinals to enter yīn. By using these two additional medicinals, the yáng formula is not repelled by exuberant yīn cold evil. In addition to this important action, Liú Dù-Zhōu (刘渡舟) writes that the medicinal actions of these two ingredients are also important.

> ... in counterflow vomiting and diarrhea, both yīn and yáng are damaged, [so there is] not only yáng vacuity [but] also yīn exhaustion. In incessant diarrhea yīn humor is discharged, a dynamic through which yīn is desiccated. Scallion [Yáng-]Freeing [Decoction] supplements yáng with enough to spare, [but] is unable to enrich yīn.... Human urine (*rén niào*) and pig's bile (*zhū dǎn zhī*) supplement yīn humor, enrich desiccated [yīn], conduct yáng, and supplement yīn.

From this perspective, these two medicinals not only allow the yáng medicinals to enter the yīn, but they also perform an important action in enriching yīn, so that both yáng and yīn will be restored to harmony.

3.1.4 True Warrior Decoction Patterns

LINE 316

少阴病，二三日不已，至四五日，腹痛，小便不利，四肢沉重疼痛，自下利者，此为有水气，其人或咳，或小便利，或下利，或呕者，真武汤主之。

Shào yīn bìng, èr sān rì bù yǐ, zhì sì wǔ rì, fù tòng, xiǎo biàn bù lì, sì zhī chén zhòng téng tòng, zì xià lì zhě, cǐ wéi yǒu shuǐ qì, qí rén huò ké, huò xiăo biàn lì, huò xià lì, huò ǒu zhě, zhēn wǔ tāng zhǔ zhī.

When lesser yīn disease has not ceased [after] two or three days, and at four or five days [there is] abdominal pain, inhibited urination, heaviness and pain in the limbs, and spontaneous diarrhea, it means [there is] water qì,* and the person may cough, or have uninhibited urination, or diarrhea, or retching; [therefore,] True Warrior Decoction (*zhēn wǔ tāng*) governs.

TEXT NOTE

* Water qì, 水汽 *shuǐ qì*: Pathological excesses of water in the body. This term can refer to the water swelling provoked by it or other signs related to collected water. The main cause is impairment of movement and transformation of water due to spleen-kidney yáng vacuity.

FORMULA

True Warrior Decoction (*zhēn wǔ tāng*)

○ Warm kidney yáng; disinhibit water qì.

茯苓三两　芍药三两　白术二两　生姜三两（切）　附子一枚（炮，去皮，破八片）

㈠ 右五味，以水八升，煮取三升，去滓，温服七合，日三服。㈡ 若咳者，加五味子半升，细辛一两，干姜一两。㈢ 若小便利者，去茯苓。㈣ 若下利者，去芍药加干姜二两。㈤ 若呕者，去附子加生姜，足前为半斤。

Fú líng sān liăng　sháo yào sān liăng　bái zhú èr liăng　shēng jiāng sān liăng (qiē)　fù zǐ yī méi (pào, qù pí, pò bā piàn)

(1) *Yòu wǔ wèi, yǐ shuǐ bā shēng, zhǔ qǔ sān shēng, qù zǐ, wēn fú qī gě, rì sān fú.* (2) *Ruò ké zhě, jiā wǔ wèi zǐ bàn shēng, xì xīn yī liăng, gān jiāng yī liăng.* (3) *Ruò xiăo biàn lì zhě, qù fú líng.* (4) *Ruò xià lì zhě, qù sháo yào jiā gān jiāng èr liăng.* (5) *Ruò ǒu zhě, qù fù zǐ jiā shēng jiāng, zú qián wéi bàn jīn.*

poria (茯苓 *fú líng*, Poria) 3 liǎng
peony (芍药 *sháo yào*, Paeoniae Radix) 3 liǎng
ovate atractylodes (白术 *bái zhú*, Atractylodis Ovatae Rhizoma) 2 liǎng
fresh ginger (生姜 *shēng jiāng*, Zingiberis Rhizoma Recens) 3 liǎng (cut)
aconite (附子 *fù zǐ*, Aconiti Tuber Laterale) 1 piece (blast-fry, remove skin, break into 8 pieces)

(1) [For] the above five ingredients use eight shēng of water. Boil to get three shēng and remove the dregs. Take seven gě warm, three times a day. (2) If [there is] a cough, add a half shēng of schisandra (*wǔ wèi zǐ*), one liǎng of asarum (*xì xīn*) and one liǎng of dried ginger (*gān jiāng*). (3) If the urine is uninhibited, remove poria (*fú líng*). (4) If [there is] diarrhea, remove peony (*sháo yào*) and add two liǎng of dried

ginger (*gān jiāng*). (5) If [there is] retching, remove aconite (*fù zǐ*) and add enough fresh ginger (*shēng jiāng*) to make a half jīn.*

FORMULA NOTE

* Add enough fresh ginger to make a half jīn, 加生姜，足前为半斤 *jiā shēng jiāng, zú qián wéi bàn jīn*: The original formula contains three liǎng of fresh ginger (*shēng jiāng*). A half jīn is equal to eight liǎng. Therefore, one should add five liǎng.

SYNOPSIS

The signs and treatment of lesser yīn yáng vacuity water flooding.

COMMENTARY

In lesser yīn disease, the kidney yáng is vacuous. After two to five days without resolution, the evil falls inward and yáng vacuity increases. When yáng is vacuous and yīn cold is exuberant, fluids are not properly transformed. Water qì accumulates in the interior, a condition referred to as "water flooding." The water qì in the interior is influenced by yīn cold and becomes cold water qì. This evil spreads to the limbs and causes heaviness and pain in the extremities. It also spreads into the center and lower burners, influencing the spleen, stomach, and bladder. In the center burner the collected cold water qì causes abdominal pain. It influences the ability of the spleen and stomach to move and transform food and drink, resulting in diarrhea. In the lower burner it impairs qì transformation in the bladder and urination becomes inhibited.

Once a water evil is present in the interior, it can follow the qì and be moved by the qì dynamic throughout the body, resulting in a wide range of signs. If the water qì ascends counterflow, assailing the lung, it may cause cough. If it impairs the upbearing and downbearing functions of the stomach, retching may occur. Water qì in the lower burner can cause an exacerbation of yáng vacuity, with the result that the kidney is unable to control water. Both inhibited urination and uninhibited urination can occur in kidney vacuity. The main clinical difference between these two signs is that inhibited urination is usually accompanied by water swelling, particularly in the lower body, while that is less common when the urine is uninhibited. Diarrhea is included in the group of signs that may occur in the progression of this pattern, although it is already a sign in the original pattern. This inclusion has led some commentators to suggest that the diarrhea increases in severity, but others believe this peculiarity suggests that the list of possible signs included in this line may have been a later addition to the text.

In True Warrior Decoction (*zhēn wǔ tāng*), aconite (*fù zǐ*) invigorates kidney yáng so that it will govern water properly. Ovate atractylodes (*bái zhú*) dries dampness and fortifies the spleen, so that it properly controls water. These two ingredients, used together, warm the channels and eliminate cold-damp. Fresh ginger (*shēng jiāng*) diffuses and dissipates. It helps aconite (*fù zǐ*) to assist the yáng by dissipating water, so the kidney can regain governance. Poria (*fú líng*) percolates water and helps ovate atractylodes (*bái zhú*) fortify the spleen. By using poria (*fú líng*) to disinhibit the water, the spleen can regain control of the water. Peony (*sháo yào*) quickens the blood, disinhibits the urine, constrains yīn, and harmonizes the construction. It balances the warm, dry nature of the other ingredients and avoids damage to yīn from the use of a method that warms the channels and dissipates cold.

When cough occurs it means that water qì is ascending counterflow and assailing the lung. Dried ginger (*gān jiāng*) and asarum (*xì xīn*) are added to dissipate the cold water qì. Schisandra (*wǔ wèi zǐ*) is also added to constrain the lung qì. If the urine is uninhibited, one should not disinhibit the urine, so poria (*fú líng*) is removed and the focus of the formula is simply on warming yáng. Retching is a sign that water qì is assailing the stomach. When this occurs the amount of fresh ginger (*shēng jiāng*) is increased to harmonize the stomach and downbear counterflow. In the text, aconite (*fù zǐ*) is removed in this case, but because aconite (*fù zǐ*) is considered the sovereign medicinal in this formula, modern commentators feel that it should not be removed. This instruction and the apparent contradiction it raises increase the doubts about the authorship of this section. For diarrhea, one is instructed to remove peony (*sháo yào*) and add dried ginger (*gān jiāng*). The addition of dried ginger (*gān jiāng*) to warm the interior is understandable, but in the original pattern, diarrhea is present and peony (*sháo yào*) is included in the formula. Why it is removed here is not clear. One explanation offered for this seeming contradiction is that the diarrhea is very severe. If that is the case, peony (*sháo yào*) may be removed because it is bitter and cold.

In line 82, p. 185, True Warrior Decoction (*zhēn wǔ tāng*) is used in greater yáng disease with yáng vacuity and water qì. In that pattern, following excessive sweating, the signs of palpitations below the heart, dizziness, generalized twitching, and quivering are observed. The pathomechanism in these two patterns is completely different, but both belong to yáng vacuity with water qì; therefore, the same formula may be used. These patients probably have a constitutional tendency towards kidney yáng vacuity; consequently, following excessive sweating, it is kidney yáng that is damaged, not yīn.

This formula may be compared with Poria (Hoelen), Cinnamon Twig, Ovate Atractylodes, and Licorice Decoction (*fú líng guì zhī bái zhú gān cǎo tāng*), since both are used to treat yáng vacuity water flooding. The emphasis of True Warrior Decoction (*zhēn wǔ tāng*) is on the kidney, while the emphasis of Poria (Hoelen), Cinnamon Twig, Ovate Atractylodes, and Licorice Decoction (*fú líng guì zhī bái zhú gān cǎo tāng*) is on the spleen. The first warms the kidney and disinhibits water, while the second warms the spleen and transforms rheum.

3.1.5 Aconite Decoction Patterns

LINE 305

少阴病，身体痛，手足寒，骨节痛，脉沉者，附子汤主之。

Shào yīn bìng, shēn tǐ tòng, shǒu zú hán, gǔ jié tòng, mài chén zhě, fù zǐ tāng zhǔ zhī.

When in lesser yīn disease [there is] generalized pain, cold extremities, joint pain, and a pulse that is sunken, Aconite Decoction (*fù zǐ tāng*) governs.

FORMULA

Aconite Decoction (*fù zǐ tāng*)

∘ Warm the channels, expel cold, and eliminate dampness.

附子二枚（炮，去皮，破八片） 茯苓三两 人参二两 白术四两 芍药三两

右五味，以水八升，煮取三升，去滓，温服一升，日三服。

Fù zǐ èr méi (pào, qù pí, pò bā piàn) fú líng sān liǎng rén shēn èr liǎng bái zhú sì liǎng sháo yào sān liǎng

Yòu wǔ wèi, yǐ shuǐ bā shēng, zhǔ qǔ sān shēng, qù zǐ, wēn fú yī shēng, rì sān fú.

aconite (附子 *fù zǐ*, Aconiti Tuber Laterale) 2 pieces (blast-fry, remove skin, break [each] into 8 pieces)

poria (茯苓 *fú líng*, Poria) 3 liǎng

ginseng (人参 *rén shēn*, Ginseng Radix) 2 liǎng

ovate atractylodes (白术 *bái zhú*, Atractylodis Ovatae Rhizoma) 4 liǎng

peony (芍药 *sháo yào*, Paeoniae Radix) 3 liǎng

[For] the above five ingredients use eight shēng of water. Boil to get three shēng and remove the dregs. Take one shēng warm, three times a day.

SYNOPSIS

The signs and treatment of yáng vacuity cold-damp generalized pain.

COMMENTARY

Generalized pain and joint pain, signs often seen in greater yáng exterior repletion, also occur in lesser yīn disease, but without signs of an externally contracted disease. Furthermore, heat signs are absent and the extremities are cold, while the pulse is sunken, not floating. This pattern belongs to yáng vacuity cold, not exterior heat repletion. When yáng is vacuous it cannot warm the extremities and they become cold. Cold and damp are not transformed; they collect in the fleshy exterior and the joints, resulting in generalized pain and joint pain. Insufficient yáng qì in the interior is unable to lift the qì and the pulse becomes sunken.

Generalized pain appears in many patterns throughout the *Shāng Hán Lùn*. Here, we will differentiate the type of pain according to three formulae: Ephedra Decoction (*má huáng tāng*), Cinnamon Twig Decoction Newly Supplemented With One Liǎng Each of Peony and Fresh Ginger and Three Liǎng of Ginseng (*guì zhī jiā sháo yào shēng jiāng gè yī liǎng rén shēn sān liǎng xīn jiā tāng*), and Aconite Decoction (*fù zǐ tāng*). When wind cold fetters and blocks the fleshy exterior, the construction-yīn becomes depressed and stagnant. In this pattern, generalized pain and joint pain are accompanied by heat effusion, a pulse that is floating, and absence of sweating; therefore, Ephedra Decoction (*má huáng tāng*), which promotes sweating, is suggested. Once sweat issues, the evil is expelled and the pain resolves.

When qì and yīn are both vacuous the flesh is not nourished, and after sweating, generalized pain occurs. The pulse is sunken and slow. Once qì and yīn are restored, construction and defense will be uninhibited and pain will cease; therefore Cinnamon Twig Decoction Newly Supplemented With One Liǎng Each of Peony and Fresh Ginger and Three Liǎng of Ginseng (*guì zhī jiā sháo yào shēng jiāng gè yī liǎng rén shēn sān liǎng xīn jiā tāng*), which not only supplements qì and yīn, but also courses construction and defense, is suggested.

In the pattern above, generalized pain is the result of yáng vacuity and cold-damp stagnation. It is accompanied by cold extremities and a pulse that is sunken. Aconite Decoction (*fù zǐ tāng*), which warms the channels, expels cold, and eliminates dampness, is suggested; the formula contains a large dose of blast-fried aconite (*fù zǐ*), which warms the channels, expels cold, and settles pain. Ginseng (*rén shēn*) warms and supplements original yáng. Ovate atractylodes (*bái zhú*) and poria (*fú líng*) fortify the spleen in order to eliminate damp and cold. Peony (*sháo yào*), which harmonizes the construction and blood, unblocks blood impediment and increases the efficacy of the formula for relieving pain.

Aconite Decoction (*fù zǐ tāng*) and True Warrior Decoction (*zhēn wǔ tāng*) are both used to treat kidney yáng vacuity with water evil. In Aconite Decoction (*fù zǐ tāng*) patterns, yáng vacuity is more severe; therefore, a larger dose of aconite (*fù zǐ*) is used, while ginseng (*rén shēn*) is added to warm and supplement the original yáng. In True Warrior Decoction (*zhēn wǔ tāng*), a smaller dose of aconite (*fù zǐ*) is used, while ovate atractylodes (*bái zhú*) and fresh ginger (*shēng jiāng*) are added to warm and dissipate water qì and to treat spleen yáng as well.

LINE 304

少阴病，得之一二日，口中和，其背恶寒者，当灸之，附子汤主之。

Shào yīn bìng, dé zhī yī èr rì, kǒu zhōng hé, qí bèi wù hán zhě, dāng jiǔ zhī, fù zǐ tāng zhǔ zhī.

When in lesser yīn disease [that has lasted] one or two days, [there is] harmony in the mouth* and aversion to cold in the back, [this means that one] should use moxibustion; Aconite Decoction (*fù zǐ tāng*) governs.

TEXT NOTE

* Harmony in the mouth, 口中和 *kǒu zhōng hé*: The mouth is normal and bitterness, dryness, and thirst are absent.

SYNOPSIS

The essential signs and treatment of yáng vacuity damp-cold.

COMMENTARY

This line continues the discussion of Aconite Decoction (*fù zǐ tāng*) and presents "harmony in the mouth" as an important sign to be used in the identification of lesser yīn vacuity cold-damp patterns. When there is harmony in the mouth it means that heat is absent from the interior, since internal heat produces thirst, dryness, and/or bitter taste in the mouth. Furthermore, when kidney yáng is vacuous, it cannot warm the yáng aspect of the body; consequently, aversion to cold is felt in the back.

This line should be viewed in conjunction with the previous line, line 305, p. 486, because both lines present lesser yīn disease that are treated with Aconite Decoction (*fù zǐ tāng*). Harmony in the mouth and aversion to cold in the back are signs of exuberant cold in the lesser yīn, as are generalized pain, joint pain, cold extremities, and a pulse that is sunken. Different combinations of these signs may be treated with Aconite Decoction (*fù zǐ tāng*), provided that the pattern is one of lesser yīn disease with exuberant cold and kidney yáng vacuity.

Aversion to cold in the back is also seen in greater yáng and yáng brightness disease. In greater yáng disease an exterior evil invades the fleshy exterior, depressing the defensive yáng. Aversion to cold is accompanied by heat effusion, headache, a pulse that is floating, and other signs of exterior disease. In yáng brightness White Tiger Decoction Plus Ginseng (*bái hǔ jiā rén shēn tāng*) patterns, exuberant heat in the interior causes excessive sweating, and the fleshy exterior and the interstices become loose. The qì and fluids become insufficient; hence aversion to cold is accompanied by dry mouth and thirst with fluid intake. These two patterns must be differentiated from that in which aversion to cold results from yáng vacuity.

In this line, moxibustion is also suggested. It can be used along with Aconite Decoction (*fù zǐ tāng*) to invigorate the original yáng, disperse yīn cold, and strengthen the action of the formula to warm the channels and dissipate cold. Although no points are suggested in the text, one may consider points such as Great Hammer (*dà zhuī,* GV-14), Pass Head (*guān yuán,* CV-4), and Sea of Qì (*qì hǎi,* CV-6).

3.1.6 Evodia Decoction Patterns

Line 309

少阴病，吐利，手足逆冷，烦躁欲死者，吴茱萸汤主之。

Shào yīn bìng, tù lì, shǒu zú nì lěng, fán zào yù sǐ zhě, wú zhū yú tāng zhǔ zhī.

When in lesser yīn disease [there is] vomiting and diarrhea, counterflow cold of the extremities, and vexation and agitation, [as if the person is] about to die, Evodia Decoction (*wú zhū yú tāng*) governs.

Synopsis

The signs and treatment of yáng vacuity and yīn exuberance, in which there is an intense struggle between right and evil.

Commentary

This line is problematic because it presents a pattern of lesser yīn disease in which vomiting, diarrhea, and counterflow cold of the extremities are observed, yet Counterflow Cold Decoction (*sì nì tāng*) is not used. The inclusion of "agitation and vexation" appears to be the only reason why Evodia Decoction (*wú zhū yú tāng*) is used instead. In this pattern, yīn evil is exuberant, yet yáng qì is still able to struggle against it, and this gives rise to vexation. Evodia Decoction (*wú zhū yú tāng*) warms and downbears liver and stomach qì, discharges turbid yīn, and frees yáng. When the liver and stomach qì move normally, vomiting will cease. After turbid yīn is discharged, diarrhea will cease. Finally, freeing yáng will allow it to flow out to the limbs and warm them. Yáng will be supported in its struggle against yīn and the vexation and agitation will cease. This line does not represent standard treatment for lesser yīn disease and should be thought of as a special case. One difference between Evodia Decoction (*wú zhū yú tāng*) and Counterflow Cold Decoction (*sì nì tāng*) is that the former is used primarily for vomiting patterns, while the latter is used primarily for diarrhea patterns. For further discussion of Evodia Decoction (*wú zhū yú tāng*), see line 243, p. 386.

The vexation and agitation in this pattern should be differentiated from that which occurs in patterns of extreme yīn and yáng expiry. Patterns of extreme yīn and yáng expiry are characterized by clear-food diarrhea, aversion to cold and curled-up lying posture, counterflow cold of the extremities, and a pulse that is faint and about to expire.

3.1.7 Peach Blossom Decoction Patterns

LINE 306

少阴病，下利便脓血者，桃花汤主之。

Shào yīn bìng, xià lì biàn nóng xuè zhě, táo huā tāng zhǔ zhī.

When in lesser yīn disease, [there is] diarrhea with pus and blood, Peach Blossom Decoction (*táo huā tāng*) governs.

FORMULA

Peach Blossom Decoction (*táo huā tāng*)

○ Warm and astringe; stem desertion.

赤石脂一斤（一半全用，一半筛末） 干姜一两 粳米一升

㈠ 右三味，以水七升，煮米令熟，去滓，温服七合，内赤石脂末方寸匕，日三服。㈡ 若一服愈，余勿服。

Chì shí zhī yī jīn (yī bàn quán yòng, yī bàn shāi mò) gān jiāng yī liǎng gēng mǐ yī shēng

(1) *Yòu sān wèi, yǐ shuǐ qī shēng, zhǔ mǐ lìng shú, qù zǐ, wēn fú qī gě, nà chì shí zhī mò fāng cùn bǐ, rì sān fú.* (2) *Ruò yī fú yù, yú wù fú.*

halloysite (赤石脂 *chì shí zhī*, Halloysitum Rubrum) 1 jīn (use one-half whole [in the decoction], [crush and] sieve the other half and use as a powder)

dried ginger (干姜 *gān jiāng*, Zingiberis Rhizoma Exsiccatum) 1 liǎng

rice (粳米 *gēng mǐ*, Oryzae Semen) 1 shēng

(1) [For] the above three ingredients use seven shēng of water. Boil until the rice is cooked and remove the dregs. Take seven gě warm, [after] adding a square-inch-

spoonful of halloysite (*chì shí zhī*) powder.* Take three [times a] day. (2) If recovery [occurs] after one dose, do not take [again].

FORMULA NOTE

* Take seven gě warm, [after] adding a square-inch-spoonful of halloysite (*chì shí zhī*) powder, 温服七合，内赤石脂末方寸匕 *wēn fú qī gě, nà chì shí zhī mò fāng cùn bǐ*: When the decoction is taken, a square-inch-spoonful (approximately 6-9 grams) of halloysite (*chì shí zhī*) powder should be taken with it.

SYNOPSIS

The signs and treatment of vacuity cold efflux desertion diarrhea with pus and blood.

COMMENTARY

In general, diarrhea with pus and blood constitutes a heat pattern. Nonetheless, here diarrhea with pus and blood occurs in a lesser yīn disease and belongs to vacuity cold in the lower burner with spleen and kidney vacuity. When the kidney yáng is vacuous, it cannot warm the spleen, and diarrhea occurs. If it continues, damage to kidney yáng qì increases and the anus becomes insecure, resulting in efflux desertion (uncontrollable loss of stool to a degree that is critical). Because vacuity cold diarrhea damages both yīn and yáng, qì and blood are not contained, and pus and blood appear in the stool.

The nature of diarrhea with pus and blood that occurs in yáng vacuity patterns with efflux desertion is different than that which occurs in heat patterns. The blood is dark and not fresh, unlike the fresh red blood seen in heat patterns. The stool may have a fishy odor or no odor at all, unlike the putrid odor associated with heat-type diarrhea. Furthermore, yáng vacuity diarrhea is generally not urgent, nor is it accompanied by scorching heat in the anus. It may be accompanied by abdominal pain that is relieved by warmth and pressure.

Peach Blossom Decoction (*táo huā tāng*) warms, astringes, and stems desertion. Halloysite (*chì shí zhī*), the sovereign ingredient, performs all of these actions. Dried ginger (*gān jiāng*) assists by warming the center yáng. Rice (*gēng mǐ*) boosts the qì of the spleen and stomach.

Halloysite (*chì shí zhī*) is cooked with the other medicinals to obtain its warming and astringing actions. However, a small amount of it, powdered, is taken with the decoction in order to increase its restraining action in the intestines. This formula treats efflux desertion resulting from pure vacuity in the absence of repletion evil. Pus and blood need not be present to use this formula, but because it is extremely effective for astringing, it must not be used when a repletion evil is present.

LINE 307

少阴病，二三日至四五日，腹痛，小便不利，下利不止，便脓血者，桃花汤主之。

Shào yīn bìng, èr sān rì zhì sì wǔ rì, fù tòng, xiǎo biàn bù lì, xià lì bù zhǐ, biàn nóng xuè zhě, táo huā tāng zhǔ zhī.

When in lesser yīn disease [that has lasted] two or three days, [for] up to four or five days, [there is] abdominal pain, inhibited urination, and incessant diarrhea with pus and blood in the stool, Peach Blossom Decoction (*táo huā tāng*) governs.

SYNOPSIS

Further discussion of the signs and treatment of vacuity cold diarrhea with pus and blood.

COMMENTARY

This line is a further discussion of a Peach Blossom Decoction (*táo huā tāng*) pattern in which lesser yīn disease persists for several days to a week and cold evil falls inward, exacerbating yáng vacuity. It is a pattern of efflux desertion from debility of spleen and kidney yáng. Spleen and kidney yáng debility means an inability to warm and transform. Cold congeals and causes abdominal pain. Controlling and containing are not managed properly and diarrhea is incessant. Inhibited urination is explained through two different mechanisms. When yáng qì in the lower burner is vacuous, it can influence qì transformation in the bladder and directly inhibit urination. The other possibility is that incessant diarrhea damages the fluids, leading to inhibited urination. Blood appears in the stool because vacuous yáng is unable to contain the blood within the vessels. Peach Blossom Decoction (*táo huā tāng*), which warms, astringes, and stems desertion, is therefore appropriate.

Because abdominal pain, inhibited urination, and diarrhea with pus and blood may be seen in many different patterns, it is necessary to differentiate clearly the distinguishing characteristics of each pattern. Abdominal pain may occur in yáng brightness and lesser yīn disease. In yáng brightness bowel repletion patterns, it is characterized by severe pain and a refusal of pressure. In lesser yīn disease, it is generally a continuous dull pain, which is alleviated by heat and pressure.

Inhibited urination may be seen in exuberant heat, water amassment, and lesser yīn disease. When exuberant heat damages the fluids causing inhibited urination, it is often accompanied by signs such as great heat, vexing thirst, and a dry tongue with yellow fur. In water amassment patterns, qì transformation in the bladder is impaired, causing inhibited urination and other signs such as a pulse that is floating, heat effusion, thirst, lesser abdominal urgency, and white tongue fur. In lesser yīn patterns, inhibited urination is accompanied by diarrhea and signs of heat are generally absent.

Diarrhea with pus and blood may be seen in both heat and lesser yīn vacuity cold patterns. Heat-type diarrhea is characterized by the appearance of bright red blood and the presence of a putrid odor. This is accompanied by urgency to defecate with a heavy feeling after defecation and scorching heat in the anus. In lesser yīn disease, the blood is dark red or pale and the stool (although it may smell fishy) is not strongly malodorous or urgent and other heat signs are absent.

3.1.8 Needling and Moxibustion

LINE 308

少阴病，下利便脓血者，可刺。

Shào yīn bìng, xià lì biàn nóng xuè zhě, kě cì.

When in lesser yīn disease [there is] diarrhea with pus and blood, one can needle.

SYNOPSIS

In lesser yīn diarrhea with pus and blood, one can choose acupuncture.

COMMENTARY

In this line, Zhāng Jī suggests that needling treatment may be used in lesser yīn disease with diarrhea, but it is not clear if this treatment should be used in conjunction with medicinal therapy or as an independent treatment, nor does Zhāng Jī provide suggestions as to what points should be used. It is likely that needling is suggested as a compliment to medicinal therapy. Needling can be used both to discharge evil, secure, and contain. Because needling is often used to drain repletion evils, and moxibustion is used to warm vacuity cold, many commentators suggest that the diarrhea in this line is heat type. Nonetheless, if one considers a point such as Long Strong (*cháng qiáng,* GV-1), it can be used for diarrhea that is the result of repletion or vacuity, heat or cold.

LINE 292

少阴病，吐利，手足不逆冷，反发热者，不死，脉不至者，灸少阴七壮。

Shào yīn bìng, tù lì, shǒu zú bù nì lěng, fǎn fā rè zhě, bù sǐ, mài bù zhì zhě, jiǔ shào yīn qī zhuàng.

When in lesser yīn disease [there is] vomiting and diarrhea, and counterflow cold of the extremities is absent, but heat effusion [is present], [the person will] not die. The pulse fails to arrive [normally],* so [use] seven cones of moxa on the lesser yīn.

TEXT NOTE

* Pulse fails to arrive [normally], 脉不至 *mài bù zhì*: The pulse arrives, then suddenly stops. When one presses down to find the pulse, it is absent.

SYNOPSIS

When there is sudden vomiting and diarrhea, although yáng is vacuous, the vacuity is not yet severe and if the pulse does not arrive normally one can use moxibustion.

Commentary

In lesser yīn disease, vomiting and diarrhea indicates yáng qì vacuity. Normally, one would expect the limbs to be cold, but in this pattern, counterflow cold is not observed; therefore yáng vacuity is not severe. When these signs are accompanied by heat effusion, it is not a sign of yáng straying to the exterior prior to desertion, but it means that yáng qì is able to prevail against yīn; therefore, this patient should recover.

The pulse is not able to arrive normally; it arrives then stops suddenly and cannot be felt. This type of pulse can occur when yīn and yáng are about to separate and expire, but it may also be observed when yáng vacuity is not severe and yáng qì is returning. Here, on the basis of the other signs, we can conclude that yáng qì is returning, but has not yet returned completely and is still blocked by the presence of exuberant yīn. Moxibustion is used to warm the interior and free yáng qì so that the pulse can arrive normally.

Zhāng Jī suggests that moxibustion should be used on the lesser yīn, but not which points should be treated. Zhāng Nán suggests Great Ravine (*tài xī,* KI-3). Kē Qín suggests Recover Flow (*fù liū,* KI-7) and Gushing Spring (*yǒng quán,* KI-1).

Line 325

少阴病，下利，脉微濇，呕而汗出，必数更衣，反少者，当温其上，灸之。

Shào yīn bìng, xià lì, mài wēi sè, ǒu ér hàn chū, bì shuò gēng yī, fǎn shǎo zhě, dāng wēn qí shàng, jiǔ zhī.

When in lesser yīn disease, [there is] diarrhea, a pulse that is faint and rough, retching and sweating, there will be frequent defecation but scant [stool],* so one should warm the upper [burner] with moxibustion.

Text Note

* Frequent defecation but scant [stool], 数更衣，反少 *shuò gēng yī, fǎn shào*: Two different interpretations are offered for this phrase.

a) Frequent bowel movements in which a small amount of stool is expelled each time.

b) Bowel movements should be frequent, but in this case, they are not.

The first explanation is considered the most reasonable one.

Synopsis

The distinguishing evidence and treatment of lesser yīn yáng vacuity with scant blood and diarrhea.

Commentary

In lesser yīn disease with diarrhea, yáng is vacuous; over time, yīn and blood become vacuous, too. The pulse in this line is faint and rough, indicating yáng qì vacuity, and fluid and blood vacuity, respectively. Vacuous yáng cannot warm the lower burner and yīn cold ascends counterflow, disturbing the function of the stomach, which causes retching. Yáng qì is insufficient, so the defensive exterior becomes insecure and sweat issues.

As in the note above, the diarrhea in this pattern may be interpreted in two different ways. In one, defecation is frequent and each time the amount of stool is small. This means that yáng qì is unable to contain the qì, which falls, causing frequent defecation. Because the blood and fluids are also vacuous, the source of transformation is insufficient and only a small amount of material remains in the stomach and intestines; hence the stool is scant. In the other interpretation, defecation, expected to be frequent in yáng vacuity patterns, is instead infrequent due to simultaneous vacuity of blood and fluids. For the purposes of clarity we use the first interpretation, since that is generally accepted, but the second interpretation may also be considered.

This line presents a pattern of yáng vacuity and scant blood with qì fall and counterflow ascent of exuberant yīn. This pattern is difficult to treat because when warming yáng, one must be careful not to damage the blood; when downbearing counterflow, one must be careful not to exacerbate the diarrhea; and when raising yáng, one must be careful not to increase counterflow. Thus, it is difficult to choose a formula. Assuming that yáng vacuity and qì fall is primary, moxibustion is used to warm the upper burner. This treatment upbears yáng and checks diarrhea.

3.1.9 Prognosis

3.1.9.1 Treatable Patterns of Yáng Return and Spontaneous Recovery

LINE 287

少阴病，脉紧，至七八日，自下利，脉暴微，手足反温，脉紧反去者，为欲解也，虽烦下利，必自愈。

Shào yīn bìng, mài jǐn, zhì qī bā rì, zì xià lì, mài bào wēi, shǒu zú fǎn wēn, mài jǐn fǎn qù zhě, wéi yù jiě yě, suī fán xià lì, bì zì yù.

When in lesser yīn disease the pulse is tight, and at seven or eight days [there is] spontaneous diarrhea and the pulse suddenly [becomes] faint, but the extremities are warm and the tightness in the pulse ceases, it means that the disease is about to resolve [and] although [there is] vexation and diarrhea, [the person] will spontaneously recover.

SYNOPSIS

The pulse and signs of spontaneous recovery when yáng returns in lesser yīn disease.

COMMENTARY

In lesser yīn disease when the pulse is tight it generally indicates an exuberant yīn evil. At seven or eight days, if vexation and diarrhea are observed and the pulse suddenly becomes faint, two basic transmutations are possible. One is that right qì has prevailed and the evil is being eliminated; hence the patient will soon recover. The second is that the evil has prevailed and the right has been defeated; hence the disease will become more severe. Here, the limbs (often cold in lesser yīn disease) become warm and the tight quality in the pulse (which is associated with exuberant cold) ceases; therefore, we know that yáng qì is returning and evil qì is abating.

When yáng qì returns it struggles with residual evil qì, which causes vexation. Furthermore, in this pattern diarrhea is considered to be a sign that right qì is expelling the evil through the stool. As in previous patterns where Zhāng Jī writes that "spontaneous recovery" will occur, it is generally taken to mean that one should investigate the signs and choose an appropriate treatment, not that one should do nothing.

LINE 288

少阴病，下利，若利自止，恶寒而蜷卧，手足温者，可治。

Shào yīn bìng, xià lì, ruò lì zì zhǐ, wù hán ér quán wò, shǒu zú wēn zhě, kě zhì.

In lesser yīn disease with diarrhea, if the diarrhea spontaneously ceases, and [there is] aversion to cold, a curled-up lying posture, and the extremities are warm, [this] can be treated.

SYNOPSIS

In lesser yīn vacuity cold patterns, when the extremities are warm one can treat the pattern.

COMMENTARY

In lesser yīn disease, diarrhea, aversion to cold, and curled-up lying posture are indications of exuberant yīn and vacuous yáng. If the diarrhea spontaneously ceases it can be a sign of either a positive or a negative transmutation. If the diarrhea ceases and counterflow cold of the extremities continues, it means that yáng qì has not returned and yīn has been exhausted; this is a negative transmutation, which means that the disease is becoming more severe. If the diarrhea ceases and the extremities become warm, it means that yáng qì is returning and evil qì is abating. This is a positive transmutation—even when accompanied by signs such as aversion to cold and curled-up lying posture; hence Zhāng Jī writes that this pattern can be treated. It is likely that a formula to support yáng and repress yīn, such as Counterflow Cold Decoction (*sì nì tāng*) or Scallion [Yáng-]Freeing Decoction (*bái tōng tāng*) would be used at this point.

The clinical significance of this line lies in two points. The first is that the patient's posture during sleep can be used to differentiate heat and cold patterns. When the patient is in a supine posture, lying down, and the limbs are slack, this belongs to heat. When the patient is lying down and the limbs are constrained, this belongs to cold. In lesser yīn disease the warmth or cold of the extremities is also an important indication of the disease progression. The extremities represent the farthest region that yáng qì must reach; hence they offer important information about the exuberance or debility of yáng qì. When the extremities are warm, it generally means that yáng is returning and the prognosis is positive. When counterflow cold of the extremities is observed, yáng is not returning and yīn is exuberant, suggesting a negative prognosis.

Line 289

少阴病，恶寒而蜷，时自烦，欲去衣被者，可治。

Shào yīn bìng, wù hán ér quán, shí zì fán, yù qù yī bèi zhě, kě zhì.

When in lesser yīn disease [there is] aversion to cold, a curled-up lying posture, periodic spontaneous vexation, and the person desires to remove the clothes and the bedclothes, [this] can be treated.*

Text Note

* [This] can be treated, 可治 *kě zhì*: In *Qiān Jīn Yì Fāng* this line appears as, "this cannot be treated," 不可治 *bù kě zhì*. See the commentary below for a discussion of this issue.

Synopsis

In lesser yīn disease, when yáng returns and there is vexation heat with a desire to remove the clothing and the bedclothes, the pattern is treatable.

Commentary

In lesser yīn disease, aversion to cold and a curled-up lying posture indicate yīn exuberance and yáng vacuity. When these signs are accompanied by periodic spontaneous vexation and a desire to remove the clothes, yáng qì may be returning because it struggles against yīn cold, producing a feeling of warmth in the body that manifests as vexation and a desire to remove the clothes. When yáng qì returns, the disease can be treated. If yáng qì returns, the extremities should be warm; therefore, if these same signs are accompanied by counterflow cold of the extremities, it means that yáng qì is not returning and is a negative sign. The presence or absence of warm extremities is an essential piece of information when making a prognosis.

In the version of the *Shāng Hán Lùn* contained in the *Qiān Jīn Yì Fāng*, this line ends with, "this cannot be treated," 不可治 *bù kě zhì*. Because that text is considered the most important edition of the *Shāng Hán Lùn* prior to the Sòng dynasty version, modern commentators have been forced to attempt to reconcile this seeming contradiction. Most attempts have focused on the terms "agitation" and "vexation," and their meaning when used separately and in combination. Further on in this text, one can find examples of "vexation and agitation" as an indication of a critical condition, "no vexation but agitation," as an indication of a critical condition, and "inability to sleep with vexation and agitation," as an indication of a critical condition. "Vexation," 烦 *fán*, means an irritated or vexed state of mind or mood. "Agitation," 躁 *zào*, means restless movement and is the opposite of tranquility. Comparing the two, vexation is a subjective feeling of heat and disquietude, whereas agitation is objective fidgetiness of the limbs. Vexation often occurs without agitation, but it is less common to see agitation without vexation. When agitation occurs alone, it often means a critical case. In the line above, vexation is present and the patient desires to remove his/her clothes. This level of disquiet and restlessness can be interpreted as approaching agitation. In line 344, p. 570, the presence of agitation with restlessness, which manifests as an inability to sleep, means that the patient will die. The problem of applying that interpretation to this line is that the information in this line is inadequate. One would want information about any other signs present before making a decision. If the signs in this line appear with warm extremities, it is likely that treatment would be possible. If these signs are accompanied by counterflow cold of the extremities, the prognosis is extremely poor.

3.1.9.2 Untreatable Patterns of Yáng Collapse

LINE 295

少阴病，恶寒身蜷而利，手足逆冷者，不治。

Shào yīn bìng, wù hán shēn quán ér lì, shǒu zú nì lěng zhě, bù zhì.

When in lesser yīn disease [there is] aversion to cold, a curled-up body [posture], diarrhea, and counterflow cold of the extremities, [this] cannot be treated.

SYNOPSIS

Critical signs of pure yīn without yáng.

COMMENTARY

When making a prognosis in lesser yīn disease it is essential to identify whether it appears that yáng qì is returning or expiring, not just any one sign. Line 289, p. 497, presents a pattern in which the presence of aversion to cold, curled-up body, vexation, and a desire to remove the clothes, indicates that yáng qì is returning and treatment is possible. In the pattern characterized by diarrhea, aversion to cold, a curled-up body posture, and warm extremities, as in line 288, p. 496, yáng is returning; hence treatment is possible. Here, aversion to cold, a curled-up body posture, and diarrhea are accompanied by cold limbs. The warmth or cold of the extremities is an important indication of the state of the yáng qì; hence coldness in the limbs suggests that yáng qì is not returning and this pattern cannot be treated.

"Cannot be treated" is now generally understood to mean that this is an extremely critical pattern that is difficult to treat. It does not necessarily mean that the patient will die; hence treatment can be attempted. In this case, a formula such as Counterflow Cold Decoction (*sì nì tāng*) or Scallion [Yáng-]Freeing Decoction (*bái tōng tāng*) may be used.

LINE 296

少阴病，吐利躁烦，四逆者，死。

Shào yīn bìng, tù lì zào fán, sì nì zhě, sǐ.

When in lesser yīn disease [there is] vomiting and diarrhea, agitation and vexation, and counterflow cold of the limbs, [this bodes] death.

Synopsis

Critical signs of yáng unable to overcome yīn.

Commentary

In lesser yīn disease when agitation and vexation appear with vomiting and diarrhea, it generally indicates that yáng qì, though debilitated, is struggling against yīn evil. If yáng qì is able to prevail, the diarrhea and vomiting will cease, the limbs will become warm, and the patient will recover. In the pattern presented here, counterflow cold of the extremities is observed, suggesting that yáng qì is already exhausted and does not have the power to prevail against yīn evil; consequently, this case cannot be treated and the patient will probably die.

This pattern, which is untreatable, is considered the result of mistreatment or inappropriately timed treatment and is very similar to the one presented in line 309, p. 489. "When in lesser yīn disease [there is] vomiting and diarrhea, counterflow cold of the extremities, and vexation and agitation, [as if the person is] about to die, Evodia Decoction (*wú zhū yú tāng*) governs." The signs are the same, but one pattern is treated with Evodia Decoction (*wú zhū yú tāng*) and the other is untreatable. In the pattern that is treated with Evodia Decoction (*wú zhū yú tāng*), the patient's extremities become cold prior to the occurrence of severe vexation and agitation. The primary sign is vexation, suggesting that although yīn evil is exuberant, yáng qì is still able to struggle against it; therefore, the decoction can be used to discharge turbidity and free yáng. In the pattern presented directly above, the appearance of cold extremities is preceded by vomiting, diarrhea, and agitation and vexation. The agitation is considered to be a primary sign, suggesting that vacuous yáng is struggling with yīn evil, but is unable to overcome the evil. Yáng is about to expire and the prognosis is poor. Yóu Yí writes the following, "In lesser yīn disease, vomiting and diarrhea, agitation and vexation, and counterflow cold of the limbs, [bode] death. This again [presents the pattern that] Evodia Decoction (*wú zhū yú tāng*) governs. One is extreme yīn with yáng about to expire, the other is exuberant yīn with yáng struggling. The signs are the same, the differentiation is between struggling and expiry." These two lines represent different stages in a disease process. In one, yáng can still struggle with yīn and Evodia Decoction (*wú zhū yú tāng*) can be used to assist yáng. In the other, yáng is no longer able to struggle and treatment is no longer possible.

Line 297

少阴病，下利止而头眩，时时自冒者，死。

Shào yīn bìng, xià lì zhǐ ér tóu xuàn, shí shí zì mào zhě, sǐ.

When in lesser yīn disease diarrhea ceases, and the head is dizzy, [and] [there is] frequent spontaneous veiling,* [this bodes] death.

TEXT NOTE

* Frequent spontaneous veiling, 时时自冒 *shí shí zì mào*: A feeling of cloudiness and dizziness in the head and eyes, as if something is obscuring them.

SYNOPSIS

Critical signs of exhausted yīn below and deserting yáng above.

COMMENTARY

In lesser yīn disease, if diarrhea spontaneously ceases, yáng qì may be returning and evil qì may be abating. Conversely, yīn may also be exhausted to the point at which no more material can be expelled. If yáng qì is returning, one would expect to see other signs of recovery, such as warm extremities, but here only dizziness and veiling are present. These signs indicate that yīn has been exhausted and yáng is deserting upward. Yīn and yáng are about to separate completely; therefore this patient will probably die.

This line may be compared with line 288, p. 496, in which lesser yīn diarrhea also spontaneously ceases. In that line, when diarrhea ceases the limbs become warm, yáng qì returns, and treatment is possible. In the present line, the limbs are not mentioned and only dizziness and veiling is observed; this indicates that yīn has been exhausted and yáng qì has lost its attachment. It strays upward causing dizziness and veiling prior to complete desertion and separation of yīn and yáng; therefore, it is untreatable.

LINE 298

少阴病，四逆恶寒而身蜷，脉不至，不烦而躁者死。

Shào yīn bìng, sì nì wù hán ér shēn quán, mài bù zhì, bù fán ér zào zhě sǐ.

When in lesser yīn disease [there is] counterflow cold of the limbs, aversion to cold, curled-up body posture, the pulse fails to arrive [normally], and [there is] agitation without vexation, [this bodes] death.

SYNOPSIS

Critical signs of yáng expiry and spirit collapse.

COMMENTARY

In lesser yīn disease, counterflow cold of the extremities, aversion to cold, and curled-up body posture are all signs of yáng vacuity and yīn exuberance. When the pulse does not arrive normally, but is felt and then ceases, it means that true yáng is extremely vacuous. The absence of vexation suggests that yáng qì has no strength to struggle against yīn evil; hence only restless movement occurs. Yóu Yí writes, "'Vexation' means heat and vexation. 'Agitation' means derangement and there need not be heat. 'Vexation and agitation' means yáng anger and struggle with yīn.... 'Agitation without vexation' means yáng cannot fight, is unable to be quiet, and is about to dissipate." In summary, these signs indicate severe yáng vacuity and extreme yīn exuberance; hence this pattern cannot be treated and the patient will die.

The phrase, "the pulse fails to arrive [normally]," also appears in line 292, p. 493, but in that line treatment is possible. Vomiting and diarrhea occur without counterflow cold of the extremities, and the presence of heat effusion means that although yáng qì has been blocked by yīn evil, causing an abnormal pulse, yáng is not at the point of expiry. Moxibustion is used to warm and free yáng. Here, the pulse does not arrive normally and this sign is accompanied by counterflow cold of the extremities, aversion to cold, curled-up body posture, and agitation. Yáng qì has been vanquished and only yīn remains. Treatment to restore yáng is extremely difficult at this stage and the patient will probably die.

Vexation and agitation may occur in both yáng and yīn patterns. In general, vexation belongs to yáng and agitation belongs to yīn. Vexation without agitation is often seen in mild patterns. It is less common to see agitation without vexation and this generally occurs in very severe patterns. This information is used in the commentary on line 344, p. 570, to explain why that pattern cannot be treated.

Line 299

少阴病，六七日，息高者死。

Shào yīn bìng, liù qì rì, xī gāo zhě sǐ.

When in lesser yīn disease [that has lasted] six or seven days, [there is] high breathing,* [this bodes] death.

Text Note

* High breathing, 息高 *xī gāo*: The breathing is shallow and the breath qì floats in the upper burner. This type of breathing is characterized by decreased inhalation and increased exhalation.

Synopsis

A critical sign of kidney qì expiry below.

Commentary

When high breathing is observed after six or seven days of lesser yīn disease, it means that kidney qì is expiring. The lung governs inhalation of qì and the kidney governs absorption of qì. Here, the kidney is vacuous so it fails to absorb the qì, and the breath remains in the upper burner. The kidney qì is expiring in the lower burner and the lung qì is deserting in the upper burner; consequently, the patient will probably die.

Line 300

少阴病，脉微细沉，但欲卧，汗出不烦，自欲吐，至五六日，自利，复烦躁不得卧寐者死。

Shào yīn bìng, mài wēi xì chén, dàn yù wò, hàn chū bù fán, zì yù tù, zhì wǔ liù rì, zì lì, fù fán zào bù dé wò mèi zhě sǐ.

[When] in lesser yīn disease the pulse is faint, fine, and sunken, [there is] desire only to sleep, sweating, [and] vexation is absent, [and there is] a spontaneous desire to vomit, [and then] at five or six days, [there is] spontaneous diarrhea, a relapse of vexation and agitation, and inability to sleep, [this bodes] death.

Synopsis

Critical signs of yīn and yáng separation.

Commentary

Lesser yīn cold transformation patterns are characterized by a pulse that is sunken, fine, and faint, desire to sleep, and vomiting, but sweating is not generally seen in these patterns. Its presence in this case, along with the lack of vexation, means that yáng is unable to struggle with yīn and is collapsing outwards. At this point yáng qì has already been severely damaged and is at the point of expiry; therefore, it must be warmed urgently. If this treatment is given and after five or six days there is diarrhea, vexation and agitation, and inability to sleep, this is a negative transmutation, which confirms that yáng qì has become more vacuous and yīn cold evil has become more exuberant. Yáng vacuity and yīn exuberance in the lower burner causes diarrhea. Vacuous yáng cannot enter yīn so there is vexation and agitation, and an inability to sleep. In this pattern, right cannot overcome evil and yīn and yáng are separating. This patient will probably die, even if treatment is continued.

It should be noted that in the description in this line the patient initially desires only to sleep, but after five or six days he/she is unable to sleep. A desire only to sleep indicates yáng vacuity and yīn exuberance with spirit debility. Nonetheless, as yáng vacuity increases and yáng begins to desert, it is unable to enter yīn, and the patient becomes vexed and is unable to sleep.

3.2 Heat Transformation Patterns

3.2.1 Coptis and Ass Hide Glue Decoction Patterns

Line 303

少阴病，得之二三日以上，心中烦，不得卧，黄连阿胶汤主之。

Shào yīn bìng, dé zhī èr sān rì yǐ shàng, xīn zhōng fán, bù dé wò, huáng lián ē jiāo tāng zhǔ zhī.

When in lesser yīn disease [that has lasted] more than two or three days, [there is] vexation in the heart and inability to sleep, Coptis and Ass Hide Glue Decoction (*huáng lián ē jiāo tāng*) governs.

Formula

Coptis and Ass Hide Glue Decoction (*huáng lián ē jiāo tāng*)

○ Clear heart fire; enrich kidney yīn.

黄连四两　黄芩二两　芍药二两　鸡子黄二枚　阿胶三两

右五味，以水六升，先煮三物，取二升，去滓，内胶烊尽，小冷，内鸡子黄，搅令相得，温服七合，日三服。

Huáng lián sì liǎng huáng qín èr liǎng sháo yào èr liǎng jī zǐ huáng èr méi ē jiāo sān liǎng

Yòu wǔ wèi, yǐ shuǐ liù shēng, xiān zhǔ sān wù, qǔ èr shēng, qù zǐ, nà jiāo yáng jìn, xiǎo lěng, nà jī zǐ huáng, jiǎo lìng xiāng dé, wēn fú qī gě, rì sān fú.

coptis (黄连 *huáng lián*, Coptidis Rhizoma) 4 liǎng
scutellaria (黄芩 *huáng qín*, Scutellariae Radix) 2 liǎng
peony (芍药 *sháo yào*, Paeoniae Radix) 2 liǎng
egg yolk (鸡子黄 *jī zǐ huáng*, Galli Vitellus) 2 [raw] yolks
ass hide glue (阿胶 *ē jiāo*, Asini Corii Gelatinum) 3 liǎng*

[For] the above five ingredients use six shēng of water. First boil [the first] three ingredients to get two shēng. Remove the dregs, add ass hide glue (*ē jiāo*) and dissolve completely. Cool a little. Add egg yolk (*jī zǐ huáng*) and mix thoroughly. Take seven gě warm, three times a day.

Formula Note

* Ass hide glue (*ē jiāo*) 3 liǎng: In the *Qiān Jīn Yì Fāng* the amount is recorded as 3 blocks.

Synopsis

The signs and treatment of yīn vacuity and hyperactive yáng in lesser yīn disease.

Commentary

In lesser yīn disease, cold transformation can occur if the patient has yáng vacuity or an existing cold pattern. If the patient has yīn vacuity or an existing heat pattern, a heat transformation pattern is more likely. The patient's constitution, however, is not the only factor that can influence the progression of a lesser yīn disease. Yáng brightness heat can scorch and damage the true yīn and lead to a heat transformation pattern. A warm heat evil in the interior may also scorch the true yīn and cause this pattern. Regardless of the origin, when true yīn is damaged and intense heat evil is present, one can diagnosis a lesser yīn heat transformation pattern.

In lesser yīn disease after two days or more, the presence of heart vexation and inability to sleep means that there is a constitutional kidney water depletion and the evil has transformed to heat. When kidney water is insufficient, heart fire becomes hyperactive and the heart and kidney do not interact properly, leading to vexation and insomnia. It is likely that along with these signs, dry throat and mouth, red tongue with yellow fur, and a pulse that is sunken, fine, and rapid will also be present. The vexation and inability to sleep in this pattern should be clearly differentiated from that which occurs in patterns of exuberant yīn and vacuous yáng where yáng strays prior to the separation of yīn and yáng, as in the previous line.

In this pattern yīn vacuity is accompanied by heat evil; hence Coptis and Ass Hide Glue Decoction (*huáng lián ē jiāo tāng*), which clears heart fire and enriches kidney yīn, is suggested. Scutellaria (*huáng qín*) and coptis (*huáng lián*) drain heart fire and eliminate heat vexation. Ass hide glue (*ē jiāo*) enriches kidney yīn. Egg yolk (*jī zǐ huáng*) nourishes heart blood and stabilizes the spirit. Peony (*sháo yào*) harmonizes the blood and constrains yın. Peony (*sháo yào*), scutellaria (*huáng qín*), and coptis (*huáng lián*) are sour and bitter so they drain fire. Egg yolk (*jī zǐ huáng*) and ass hide glue (*ē jiāo*) are sour and sweet; they transform fluids in order to enrich yīn, while also constraining heat and quieting the spirit in order to harmonize yīn and yáng. The formula is particularly effective for insomnia that is caused by a lack of proper interaction between the heart and kidney. It is important that ass hide glue (*ē jiāo*) and egg yolk (*jī zǐ huáng*) be added to the decoction after it has been cooked. Ass hide glue (*ē jiāo*) is dissolved in the hot decoction and egg yolk (*jī zǐ huáng*) is added after the decoction has cooled slightly.

Heart vexation and insomnia in lesser yīn disease should be differentiated from the pattern for which Gardenia and Fermented Soybean Decoction (*zhī zǐ chǐ tāng*) is used. In that pattern, residual heat harasses the region of the chest and diaphragm, but the kidney is not vacuous; hence vexation and insomnia are generally accompanied by anguish in the heart, binding pain in the heart, and other signs of heat in the upper burner, not signs of kidney yīn vacuity.

3.2.2 Polyporous Decoction Patterns

LINE 319

少阴病，下利，六七日，咳而呕渴，心烦不得眠者，猪苓汤主之。

Shào yīn bìng, xià lì, liù qī rì, ké ér ǒu kě, xīn fán bù dé mián zhě, zhū líng tāng zhǔ zhī.

When in lesser yīn disease [there is] diarrhea for six or seven days, cough, retching, thirst, heart vexation, and inability to sleep, Polyporus Decoction (*zhū líng tāng*) governs.

SYNOPSIS

The signs and treatment of yīn vacuity with heat and inhibited water qì.

COMMENTARY

In lesser yīn disease, generally, and in lesser yīn diarrhea patterns, specifically, one must differentiate between heat and cold transformation patterns. Because both lines suggest Polyporus Decoction (*zhū líng tāng*), this line may be compared with line 223, p. 324, to aid with this differentiation. "If the pulse is floating and [there is] heat effusion, thirst with a desire to drink water, and inhibited urination, Polyporus Decoction (*zhū líng tāng*) governs." On the basis of this comparison we may assume that inhibited urination, not explicitly stated in the text, is also present in this pattern. This is a pattern of yīn vacuity with heat and inhibited water qì. Impaired water movement produces the signs observed in this pattern. Water qì percolates into the large intestine, causing diarrhea. It ascends counterflow and assails the lung, causing cough. When water qì assails the stomach, the patient retches. Collected water qì in the interior impairs normal water movement, giving rise to thirst. Vexation and insomnia, however, are unrelated to water qì, but are a result of vacuity heat harassing the heart spirit. Although the signs in this line are different from that in line 223, p. 324, the pathomechanism is the same; hence the same treatment is used in both cases. Polyporus Decoction (*zhū líng tāng*), which clears heat, enriches yīn, and disinhibits urination, is suggested for both patterns.

Line 282, p. 471, presents a pattern of diarrhea, heart vexation, and thirst, belonging to yáng vacuity with exuberant cold, whereas here these same signs belong to yīn vacuity with heat and inhibited water qì. In that line, although there is heart vexation and desire to sleep, urination is clear and long "because of vacuity cold in the lower burner and inability to control water." In this pattern there is heart vexation, inability to sleep, and inhibited urination; therefore, we can conclude that this pattern belongs to heat, while the other belongs to cold.

Line 316, p. 483, presents a pattern of water qì with cough, retching, and diarrhea. "... [I]nhibited urination... spontaneous diarrhea, it means [there is] water qì and the person may cough, or have uninhibited urination... or retching; [therefore] True Warrior Decoction (*zhēn wǔ tāng*) governs." True Warrior Decoction (*zhēn wǔ tāng*) is used to treat yáng vacuity with exuberant cold, whereas in the pattern above, inhibited water qì, cough, retching, and diarrhea is treated with Polyporus Decoction (*zhū líng tāng*), which clears heat, enriches yīn, and disinhibits urination. In line 316, heaviness and pain in the limbs indicate the presence of vacuity cold and water. Here, heart vexation and insomnia indicate the presence of vacuity heat. The pathomechanisms in these two lines are different; therefore, the treatment principles are different.

Finally, this pattern of heart vexation and insomnia appears similar to that for which Coptis and Ass Hide Glue Decoction (*huáng lián ē jiāo tāng*) is used. Nonetheless, in that pattern, yīn vacuity and heat are present, and water qì is absent. Furthermore, the heat in that pattern is more severe than in this pattern. It should be noted that in patterns with fluid exhaustion and thirst, Polyporus Decoction (*zhū líng tāng*) is contraindicated. This contraindication is stated in line 224, p. 326, "When in yáng brightness disease, [there is] copious sweating and thirst, one cannot give Polyporus Decoction (*zhū líng tāng*) because with copious sweat the stomach is dry and Polyporus Decoction (*zhū líng tāng*) disinhibits the urine." Polyporus Decoction (*zhū líng tāng*) can be used here because this pattern is a combination of inhibited water qì, mild heat, and yīn vacuity. (See line 223, p. 324, for a complete discussion of Polyporus Decoction (*zhū líng tāng*).)

4 LESSER YĪN DISEASE AND TRANSMUTED PATTERNS

4.1 EPHEDRA, ACONITE, AND ASARUM DECOCTION PATTERNS

LINE 301

少阴病，始得之，反发热，脉沉者，麻黄细辛附子汤主之。
Shào yīn bìng, shǐ dé zhī, fǎn fā rè, mài chén zhě, má huáng xì xīn fù zǐ tāng zhǔ zhī.

When greater yīn disease has just started, but [there is] heat effusion and the pulse is sunken, Ephedra, Asarum, and Aconite Decoction (*má huáng xì xīn fù zǐ tāng*) governs.

FORMULA
Ephedra, Asarum, and Aconite Decoction (*má huáng xì xīn fù zǐ tāng*),

∘ Warm the channels; effuse the exterior.

麻黄二两（去节） 细辛二两 附子一枚（炮，去皮，破八片）

右三味，以水一斗，先煮麻黄，减二升，去上沫，内诸药，煮取三升，去滓，温服一升，日三服。

Má huáng èr liǎng (qù jié) xì xīn èr liǎng fù zǐ yī méi (pào, qù pí, pò bā piàn)

Yòu sān wèi, yǐ shuǐ yī dǒu, xiān zhǔ má huáng, jiǎn èr shēng, qù shàng mò, nà zhū yào, zhǔ qǔ sān shēng, qù zǐ, wēn fú yī shēng, rì sān fú.

ephedra (麻黄 *má huáng*, Ephedrae Herba) 2 liǎng (remove the nodes)
asarum (细辛 *xì xīn*, Asiasari Herba cum Radice) 2 liǎng
aconite (附子 *fù zǐ*, Aconiti Tuber Laterale) 1 piece (blast-fry, remove the skin, break into 8 pieces)

[For] the above three ingredients use one dǒu of water. First, boil ephedra (*má huáng*) and reduce by two shēng. Remove the foam [collecting] on top. Add all [the other] ingredients and boil to get three shēng. Remove the dregs. Take one shēng warm, three times a day.

SYNOPSIS
The signs and treatment of lesser yīn disease with an exterior pattern.

COMMENTARY
In lesser yīn vacuity cold patterns, heat signs are generally absent and aversion to cold may be present. Here, although heat effusion (which is commonly seen in exterior patterns) is present, the pulse is sunken, which is characteristic of lesser yīn yáng vacuity patterns. Heat effusion suggests an exterior evil and a pulse that

is sunken indicates interior disease; therefore, this pattern belongs to simultaneous exterior-interior disease. Ephedra, Asarum, and Aconite Decoction (*má huáng xì xīn fù zǐ tāng*), which resolves both exterior and interior patterns, is suggested.

In most cases of simultaneous exterior-interior disease, the interior is replete, not vacuous. When the interior is replete and an exterior evil is present, one should first resolve the exterior pattern and then address the interior disease. When the interior is vacuous and an exterior evil is present, one should first address the interior disease and then resolve the exterior. An example of this is found in line 372, p. 563, "When [there is] diarrhea with abdominal distention and pain, and generalized pain, first warm the interior, then attack the exterior. To warm the interior, Counterflow Cold Decoction (*sì nì tāng*) is appropriate. [For] attacking the exterior, Cinnamon Twig Decoction (*guì zhī tāng*) is appropriate." In the present line, although vacuity cold exists, neither the vacuity nor the cold is severe. The absence of clear-food diarrhea or other signs of severe interior vacuity cold suggests that simultaneous treatment can be used.

Heat effusion in lesser yīn disease should be differentiated from that which occurs in patterns of exuberant yīn and repelled yáng. Here, heat effusion is probably generalized and accompanied by aversion to cold. When heat effusion is a manifestation of repelled yáng, counterflow cold occurs and aversion to cold is absent. Furthermore, in repelled yáng patterns, these signs may be accompanied by clear-food diarrhea and a pulse that is fine and about to expire.

Ephedra, Asarum, and Aconite Decoction (*má huáng xì xīn fù zǐ tāng*) resolves the exterior and warms yáng. Ephedra (*má huáng*) resolves exterior cold. Aconite (*fù zǐ*) warms the kidney yáng. Acrid, warm asarum (*xì xīn*) assists ephedra (*má huáng*) in resolving the exterior and aconite (*fù zǐ*) in warming the channels.

Line 302

少阴病，得之二三日，麻黄附子甘草汤微发汗，以二三日无证，故微发汗也。

Shào yīn bìng, dé zhī èr sān rì, má huáng fù zǐ gān cǎo tāng wēi fā hàn, yǐ èr sān rì wú zhèng, gù wēi fā hàn yě.

In lesser yīn disease [that has lasted] two or three days, promote sweating mildly with Ephedra, Aconite, and Licorice Decoction (*má huáng fù zǐ gān cǎo tāng*). In two or three days, [if there are] no [interior] signs* then [one should] promote sweating mildly.

Text Note

* No [interior] signs, 无证 *wú zhèng*: In the *Jīn Guì Yù Hán Jīng* and Chéng Wú-Jǐ's *Zhù Jiě Shāng Hán Lùn*, this is written as, 无里证 *wú lǐ zhèng*, indicating that vomiting, diarrhea, or other signs of severe interior vacuity cold are absent.

Formula

Ephedra, Aconite, and Licorice Decoction (*má huáng fù zǐ gān cǎo tāng*)

○ Warm the channels; resolve the exterior.

麻黄二两（去节） 甘草二两（炙） 附子一枚（炮，去皮，破八片）

右三味，以水七升，先煮麻黄一两沸，去上沫，内诸药，煮取二升，去滓，温服一升，日三服。

Má huáng èr liǎng (qù jié) gān cǎo èr liǎng (zhì) fù zǐ yī méi (pào, qù pí, pò bā piàn)

Yòu sān wèi, yǐ shuǐ qī shēng, xiān zhǔ má huáng yī liǎng fèi, qù shàng mò, nà zhū yào, zhǔ qǔ sān shēng, qù zǐ, wēn fú yī shēng, rì sān fú.

ephedra (麻黄 *má huáng*, Ephedrae Herba) 2 liǎng (remove the nodes)

licorice (甘草 *gān cǎo*, Glycyrrhizae Radix) 2 liǎng

aconite (附子 *fù zǐ*, Aconiti Tuber Laterale) 1 piece (blast-fry, remove the skin, break into 8 pieces)

[For] the above three ingredients use seven shēng of water. First boil ephedra (*má huáng*) once or twice and remove the foam [collecting] on top. Add all [the other] ingredients and boil to get three shēng. Remove the dregs and take one shēng warm, three times a day.

SYNOPSIS

Further discussion of the signs and treatment of lesser yīn disease with an exterior pattern.

COMMENTARY

This line continues the discussion of simultaneous exterior-interior disease begun in the previous line. The formulae for both these lines contain ephedra (*má huáng*) and aconite (*fù zǐ*); hence they simultaneously treat interior and exterior disease. Heat effusion is probably present in this pattern and the pulse is sunken, as in the previous line. "No [interior] signs," can be applied to both this line and the previous one, indicating the absence of signs of severe interior vacuity cold. One need not urgently warm the interior, but can treat the exterior and the interior simultaneously. In this line, however, the disease has proceeded for several days and although the pattern is moderate, right qì is more vacuous than in the previous line, which describes the pattern at the beginning of the disease.

In Ephedra, Aconite, and Licorice Decoction (*má huáng fù zǐ gān cǎo tāng*), the warm, acrid asarum (*xì xīn*) of Ephedra, Asarum, and Aconite Decoction (*má huáng xì xīn fù zǐ tāng*), is replaced with licorice (*gān cǎo*), which is mildly supplementing. The pattern is more moderate; hence the acrid nature of asarum (*xì xīn*) is not necessary. Most importantly, the addition of licorice (*gān cǎo*) balances the nature of ephedra (*má huáng*), and does not further assist the promotion of sweating, whereas the acrid nature of asarum (*xì xīn*) assists ephedra (*má huáng*) in the promotion of sweating. Aconite (*fù zǐ*), which warms and secures yáng, is still considered necessary.

4.2 Urgent Precipitation

Line 320

少阴病，得之二三日，口燥咽干者，急下之，宜大承气汤。

Shào yīn bìng, dé zhī èr sān rì, kǒu zào yān gān zhě, jí xià zhī, yí dà chéng qì tāng.

When in lesser yīn disease [that has lasted] two or three days, [there is] a dry mouth and throat, precipitate urgently; [therefore,] Major Qì-Coordinating Decoction (*dà chéng qì tāng*) is appropriate.

Synopsis

In dryness repletion liquid damage, when the true yīn is going to be exhausted, one should urgently precipitate.

Commentary

In this line a dry mouth and throat represent a yáng brightness repletion pattern for which Major Qì-Coordinating Decoction (*dà chéng qì tāng*) is used. Dryness indicates that a hyperactive heat evil has exhausted water, and yīn humor must be rescued. The text in this line is extremely terse; hence in cases of internal repletion dryness bind with heat, in addition to dry mouth and throat, one would expect to see other corroborating signs such as difficult bound stool, delirious speech, and streaming sweat (which support the hypothesis that the fluids have been scorched and the kidney yīn has been damaged). If enough of these signs are observed, Major Qì-Coordinating Decoction (*dà chéng qì tāng*) can be used. It should not be inferred from this line that the presence of dry mouth and throat is a sufficient indication for the use of a harsh precipitating formula, such as Major Qì-Coordinating Decoction (*dà chéng qì tāng*).

Line 321

少阴病，自利清水，色纯青，心下必痛，口干燥者，可下之，宜大承气汤。

Shào yīn bìng, zì lì qīng shuǐ, sè chún qīng, xīn xià bì tòng, kǒu gān zào zhě, kě xià zhī, yǐ dà chéng qì tāng.

When in lesser yīn disease [there is] spontaneous clear-water diarrhea [that is] a pure green-blue color,[1] pain below the heart, and a dry mouth, one can precipitate;[2] [therefore,] Major Qì-Coordinating Decoction (*dà chéng qì tāng*) is appropriate.

Text Notes

1. A pure green-blue color, 色纯青 *sè chún qīng*: This description of the color of the diarrhea has been interpreted in many different ways by different authors

and no general consensus has been reached. The authors of the *Gāo Děng Cóng Shū* write, "With regard to 'a pure green color,' Zhōu Yáng-Jùn thinks [it means] wood evil exploiting earth; Chéng Wú-Jǐ believes [it means] a liver evil shifting to the kidney; and Fāng Yǒu-Zhí believes [it means] a kidney evil shifting to the liver. Although the three writers' statements are different, they are all without solid theoretical [basis]. If this is a wood evil exploiting earth, why is Qì-Coordinating [Decoction] used to attack the center burner? [Regardless of] whether it is a liver evil shifting to the kidney or a kidney evil shifting to the liver, on the basis of all that [we] know, Qì-Coordinating [Decoction] is not a formula used to treat the liver and kidney. Spontaneous diarrhea with a blue-green color is no doubt a clinical reality, but it is not necessarily a sign of heat bind with circumfluence. Thus, the goal of using Major Qì-Coordinating Decoction (*dà chéng qì tāng*) is to attack the dry stool, not to treat the blue-green colored diarrhea."

2. One can precipitate, 可下 *kě xià*: In the *Jīn Guì Yù Hán Jīng*, this is written as, "urgent precipitation," 急下 *jí xià*.

SYNOPSIS

In heat bind with circumfluence, when fire is desiccating liquid, one should urgently precipitate.

COMMENTARY

As in the preceding line, one must conclude on the basis of the formula that this is a pattern of yáng brightness internal heat dryness bind. In the previous line, we assumed that the stool was bound and dry, while in this line, clear-water diarrhea with a blue-green color is observed. In yáng brightness repletion patterns, diarrhea is generally thought to be heat bind with circumfluence, in which exuberant heat forces watery stool to be expelled around the stool blockage.

Heat bind with circumfluence producing clear-water diarrhea is clearly different from the clear-food diarrhea present in lesser yīn vacuity cold patterns. In heat bind with circumfluence, the diarrhea is thin, watery, and malodorous, and no fecal residue is intermixed. Dryness and heat bind in the interior, forcing the fluids to be expelled around the dry stool blocking the bowel. Dryness-heat repletion congested in the interior causes stagnation and blockage of the stomach qì and a feeling of pain below the heart. Because the dryness-heat scorches the yīn humor, the mouth is dry.

As in the previous line, in order to justify the use of a harsh precipitating formula such as Major Qì-Coordinating Decoction (*dà chéng qì tāng*), particularly when diarrhea is observed, one should also see accompanying signs of repletion bind, such as abdominal fullness that is exacerbated by pressure, peri-umbilical pain, and a grimy, yellow tongue fur. Urgent precipitation is used in order to rescue the true yīn, which is about to expire. One must be extremely cautious when using this type of treatment.

Line 322

少阴病，六七日，腹胀，不大便者，急下之，宜大承气汤。

Shào yīn bìng, liù qī rì, fù zhàng, bù dà biàn zhě, jí xià zhī, yí dà chéng qì tāng.

When in lesser yīn disease [that has lasted] six or seven days, [there is] abdominal fullness and inability to defecate, precipitate urgently; [therefore,] Major Qì-Coordinating Decoction (*dà chéng qì tāng*) is appropriate.

Synopsis

For stagnation in the intestines, earth repletion, and water exhaustion, urgent precipitation is appropriate.

Commentary

As in the previous lines, this line presents a pattern that is described as a lesser yīn disease, but is actually yáng brightness dryness repletion bind damaging yīn fluids. The abdominal fullness in this pattern is likely to be severe and persistent. Along with bound stool, other likely accompanying signs include tidal heat effusion, peri-umbilical pain, and refusal of pressure on the abdomen. Only if one is certain that this represents repletion bind can Major Qì-Coordinating Decoction (*dà chéng qì tāng*) be used.

4.3 Counterflow Cold Powder Patterns

Line 318

少阴病，四逆，其人或咳，或悸，或小便不利，或腹中痛，或泄利下重者，四逆散主之。

Shào yīn bìng, sì nì, qí rén huò ké, huò jì, huò xiǎo biàn bù lì, huò fù zhōng tòng, huò xiè lì xià zhòng zhě, sì nì sǎn zhǔ zhī.

When in lesser yīn disease [there is] counterflow cold of the limbs, the person may cough, or have palpitations, or inhibited urination, or pain in the abdomen, or diarrhea with rectal heaviness;* Counterflow Cold Powder (*sì nì sǎn*) governs.

Text Note

* Diarrhea with rectal heaviness, 泄利下重 *xiè lì xià zhòng*: Diarrhea accompanied by abdominal urgency and rectal heaviness, 里急后重 *lǐ jí hòu zhòng*.

Formula

Counterflow Cold Powder (*sì nì sǎn*)

- Course the liver and harmonize the stomach; outthrust depressed yáng.

甘草（炙） 枳实（破，水渍，炙干） 柴胡 芍药

㈠ 右四味，各十分，捣筛，白饮和，服方寸匕，日三服。㈡ 咳者，加五味子、干姜各五分，并主下利。㈢ 悸者，加桂枝五分。㈣ 小便不利者，加茯苓五分。㈤ 腹中痛者，加附子一枚，炮令坼。㈥ 泄利下重者，先以水五升，煮薤白三升，煮取三升，去滓，以散三方寸匕，内汤中，煮取一升半，分温再服。

Gan cǎo (zhì) zhǐ shí (pò, shuǐ zì, zhì gān) chái hú sháo yào

(1) *Yòu sì wèi, gè shí fēn, dǎo shāi, bái yǐn huò, fú fāng cùn bǐ, rì sān fú.* (2) *Ké zhě, jiā wǔ wèi zǐ、gān jiāng gè wǔ fēn, bìng zhǔ xià lì.* (3) *Jì zhě, jiā guì zhī wǔ fēn.* (4) *Xiǎo biàn bù lì zhě, jiā fú líng wǔ fēn.* (5) *Fù zhōng tòng zhě, jiā fù zǐ yī méi, pào lìng chè.* (6) *Xiè lì xià zhòng zhě, xiān yǐ shuǐ wǔ shēng, zhǔ xiè bái sān shēng, zhǔ qǔ sān shēng, qù zǐ, yǐ sǎn sān fāng cùn bǐ, nà tāng zhōng, zhǔ qǔ yī shēng bàn, fēn wēn zài fú.*

mix-fried licorice (甘草 *gān cǎo*, Glycyrrhizae Radix)

unripe bitter orange (枳实 *zhǐ shí*, Aurantii Fructus Immaturus) (break, soak in water, and fry [until] dry)

bupleurum (柴胡 *chái hú*, Bupleuri Radix)

peony (芍药 *sháo yào*, Paeoniae Radix)

(1) [For] the above four ingredients, use ten fēn of each. Pound and sieve [all four ingredients]. Mix a square-inch-spoonful into a white [rice] cool decoction and take three times a day. (2) [If there is a] cough, add five fēn each of schisandra (*wǔ wèi zǐ*) and dried ginger (*gān jiāng*). [This] also governs diarrhea. (3) [For] palpitations, add five fēn of cinnamon twig (*guì zhī*). (4) [For] inhibited urination, add five fēn of poria (*fú líng*). (5) [For] pain in the abdomen, add one piece of aconite (*fù zǐ*), [that is] blast-fried and made to crack. (6) [For] diarrhea with rectal heaviness, place three shēng of scallion white (*cōng bái*) in five shēng of water, boil to get three shēng, and remove the dregs. Use three square-inch-spoonfuls of the powder in the decoction. Boil to get one and a half shēng. Divide [into two parts], and take warm twice a day.

SYNOPSIS

The signs and treatment of reversal from depressed yáng, when the liver and stomach qì is stagnant.

COMMENTARY

Counterflow cold of the limbs can be the result of different pathomechanisms. In lesser yīn disease, with yáng vacuity and exuberant yīn, yáng is unable to warm the extremities and they become cold. In those patterns, formulae such as Counterflow Cold Decoction (*sì nì tāng*) are used to return yáng and stem counterflow. In this line, signs of yáng vacuity cold are absent. Furthermore, the formula used, Counterflow Cold Powder (*sì nì sǎn*), courses the liver and outthrusts depressed yáng. Stagnation of liver and stomach qì inhibits the qì dynamic and yáng qì becomes depressed in the interior. It is unable to flow out to the extremities and they become cold.

When wood qì becomes stagnant, it rebels against earth. In this line, wood evil exploits earth, causing abdominal pain and diarrhea with abdominal urgency and rectal heaviness. Stagnation of the liver and stomach qì impairs the qì dynamic. Qì counterflow disturbs the lung and causes cough. Considering that dried ginger (*gān jiāng*) is added to the formula, cold is thought to be present in the upper burner. When the qì dynamic is impaired, and particularly if cold is present in the upper burner, the yáng qì in the chest is unable to flow and diffuse normally, the result is palpitations. Impairment of the qì dynamic also causes a loss of normal management of the sluices resulting in inhibited urination.

Counterflow Cold Powder (*sì nì sǎn*) is used to course the liver, resolve depression, disinhibit and harmonize the qì dynamic, and outthrust depressed yáng. Unripe bitter orange (*zhǐ shí*) moves the qì and dissipates binds. Peony (*sháo yào*) emolliates the liver, harmonizes construction, and regulates the liver and the spleen. Licorice (*gān cǎo*) harmonizes the center and relaxes tension. Once the liver qì is regulated, the depressed yáng will be able to move outward and the cold extremities will become warm. Once the liver and the spleen are harmonized, the abdominal pain and diarrhea will cease. For cough, schisandra (*wǔ wèi zǐ*) and dried ginger (*gān jiāng*) are added to warm and constrain the lung qì. Because of their ability to warm and restrain, they are also used for cold diarrhea. Impairment of the qì dynamic may cause stagnation of the yáng qì in the chest, giving rise to palpitations; this can be treated with cinnamon twig (*guì zhī*) because it frees yáng qì in the chest. Congestion of the qì dynamic may cause impairment of qì transformation, giving rise to inhibited urination; this can be treated with poria (*fú líng*) because it disinhibits the water. The use of aconite (*fù zǐ*), which we know to warm the center and settle pain, suggests that the abdominal pain in this line is likely caused by congealed cold in the interior. Abdominal urgency and rectal heaviness is a sign of qì depression and constrained liver qì. Scallion white (*cōng bái*) is added to move stagnant qì. The additions to the formula are based on changing signs and should not be seen as representative of the basic treatment principles of the main formula.

4.4 Patterns of Heat Shifting into the Bladder

Line 293

少阴病，八九日，一身手足尽热者，以热在膀胱，必便血也。

Shào yīn bìng, bā jiǔ rì, yī shēn shǒu zú jìn rè zhě, yǐ rè zài páng guāng, bì biàn xuè yě.

When in lesser yīn disease [that has lasted] eight or nine days, the body and extremities are completely hot, it is because the heat is in the bladder, and there will be bloody excretions.*

Text Note

* Bloody excretions, 便血 *biàn xuè*: Because of the description of heat in the bladder, here, this term means blood in the urine.

Synopsis

A transmuted pattern of lesser yīn disease in which heat enters the blood aspect of the bladder.

Commentary

If a lesser yīn heat pattern continues for an extended period of time, the heat can spread to the bladder blood aspect and cause bloody urine. The only sign in the text prior to the appearance of blood in the urine is that the body and extremities are completely hot. This important sign should be differentiated from the heat that occurs in lesser yīn disease with exuberant yīn and repelled yáng. When yáng is repelled, the body is hot, but aversion to cold and cold extremities are also observed. In this pattern, the whole body is hot, including the extremities, and aversion to cold is absent. Heat throughout the external body is a manifestation of the heat in the bladder, since the urinary bladder governs the exterior.

No treatment is offered in this line, but Kē Qín suggests Polyporus Decoction (*zhū líng tāng*) for mild cases and Coptis and Ass Hide Glue Decoction (*huáng lián ē jiāo tāng*) for severe cases. Cháng Qì-Zhī (常器之) suggests using Peach Kernel Qì-Coordinating Decoction (*táo hé chéng qì tāng*) or Rhinoceros Horn and Rehmannia Decoction (*xī jiăo dì huáng tāng*).

4.5 Patterns of Fluid Damage and Blood Stirring

Line 284

少阴病，咳而下利，谵语者，被火气劫故也，小便必难，以强责少阴汗也。

Shào yīn bìng, ké ér xià lì, zhān yŭ zhě, bèi huŏ qì jié gù yě, xiăo biàn bì nán, yĭ qiăng zé shào yīn hàn yě.

When in lesser yīn disease [there is] cough, diarrhea, and delirious speech, [it is] because [the person] was plundered by fire qì.* Urination will be difficult because sweating was mistakenly forced in a lesser yīn [disease].

Text Note

* Plundered by fire qì, 被火气劫 *bèi huŏ qì jié*: Inappropriate use of a fire method to force sweating.

Synopsis

A transmuted pattern of lesser yīn disease in which fire plundering damages yīn.

Commentary

In lesser yīn disease, the use of fire treatments is inappropriate and here it damages yīn and fluids. In most lesser yīn disease, the promotion of sweating is contraindicated, since this method easily damages yīn and yáng. Cough and diarrhea are signs often seen in lesser yīn disease, but delirious speech is not commonly observed. If cough and diarrhea are the result of yáng vacuity and exuberant yīn with water qì, one can use True Warrior Decoction (*zhēn wǔ tāng*). If they are the result of yīn vacuity with heat and water qì, one can use Polyporus Decoction (*zhū líng tāng*). In this case, delirious speech is also observed during the asking examination. Because this sign is not normally seen in lesser yīn patterns, Zhāng Jī asks the patient and determines that a fire method was used previously by another physician to force sweating. The use of a fire method not only does not resolve the disease, but also damages yīn fluids (causing dryness in the stomach and delirious speech); hence Zhāng Jī indicates that this will be followed by difficult urination. When the kidney yīn is damaged through the inappropriate promotion of sweating, the source of transformation is insufficient and urination becomes difficult.

LINE 294

少阴病，但厥无汗，而强发之，必动其血，未知从何道出，或从口鼻，或从目出者，是名下厥上竭，为难治。

Shào yīn bìng, dàn jué wú hàn, ér qiǎng fā zhī, bì dòng qí xuè, wèi zhī cóng hé dào chū, huò cóng kǒu bì, huò cóng mù chū zhě, shì míng xià jué shàng jié, wéi nán zhì.

When in lesser yīn disease [there is] only reversal and no sweating, and promotion [of sweating] is forced, this will stir the blood and [one] does not know from where [the blood] will issue; it may [come] from the nose and mouth or from the eyes. This is called lower reversal and upper exhaustion* and it is difficult to treat.

TEXT NOTE

* Lower reversal and upper exhaustion, 下厥上竭 *xià jué shàng jié*: Yáng debilitation in the lower burner and yīn debilitation in the upper burner. Severe weakness of both yīn and yáng.

SYNOPSIS

A transmuted pattern of lesser yīn disease in which the blood is stirred.

COMMENTARY

In this lesser yīn pattern, reversal is observed and the patient is not sweating. This is a pattern of kidney yáng vacuity, but it has not reached the point of yáng collapse. The correct treatment principle is to warm the kidney and return the yáng, not promote sweating. If sweating is promoted, it is clearly an inappropriate treatment; hence it is described in the text as being "forced." The promotion of sweating not only further damages both the yīn and yáng, but it harasses and stirs the construction and blood. The blood follows the vacuous yáng and ascends. It then issues from one of the clear orifices of the head—the eyes, nose, or mouth.

This is a pattern of yáng debilitation below and yīn debilitation above. The causal relationship in this line can be interpreted in two ways. The main question is whether yīn debilitation above is the result of the mistreatment or the result of blood loss. That is, inappropriate promotion of sweating can directly exhaust yīn, but it is also possible that the yīn debilitation did not occur until after the blood loss. Yóu Yí writes, "distressing the blood and [causing] frenetic stirring. As a consequence, [there is] upper exhaustion."

This pattern is difficult to treat because yáng debilitation should be treated by warming yáng, which would further injure the exhausted yīn, and yīn debilitation should be treated by clearing heat and boosting yīn, which would injure debilitated yáng.

5 SORE THROAT PATTERNS

5.1 Pig Skin Decoction Patterns

Line 310

少阴病，下利，咽痛，胸满，心烦，猪肤汤主之。
Shào yīn bìng, xià lì, yān tòng, xiōng mǎn, xīn fán, zhū fū tāng zhǔ zhī.

When in lesser yīn disease [there is] diarrhea, sore throat, fullness in the chest, and heart vexation, Pig Skin Decoction (*zhū fū tāng*) governs.

Formula

Pig Skin Decoction (*zhū fū tāng*)

∘ Enrich the kidney, moisten the lung, and supplement the spleen.

猪肤一斤。

右一味，以水一斗，煮取五升，去滓，加白蜜一升，白粉五合，熬香，和令相得，温分六服。

Zhū fū yī jīn

Yòu yī wèi, yǐ shuǐ yī dǒu, zhǔ qǔ wǔ shēng, qù zǐ, jiā bái mì yī shēng, bái fěn wǔ gě, áo xiāng, huò lìng xiāng dé, wēn fēn liù fú.

pig skin (猪肤 *zhū fū*, Suis Corium) 1 jīn

[For] the above one ingredient use one dǒu of water. Boil to get five shēng and remove the dregs. Add one shēng of honey (*bái mì*), and five gě of rice flour (*bái fěn*). Dry-fry until the aroma [comes out] and blend thoroughly. Divide into six [doses] and take warm.*

Formula Note

* Divide into six [doses] and take warm, 温分六服 *wēn fēn liù fú*: Because this formula is taken for a sore throat, it is likely that it is divided into more doses in order to provide topical relief each time a dose is taken.

Synopsis

The signs and treatment of sore throat from lesser yīn yīn vacuity fire flaming.

Commentary

In lesser yīn disease with yīn vacuity and heat, the heat evil can flow downward and cause diarrhea. Diarrhea damages the fluids and vacuity fire flames upward. It pours into the chest, damages lung yīn, and scorches the throat, causing sore throat, chest fullness, and heart vexation. Because the root of this disease is yīn vacuity, scutellaria (*huáng qín*) and coptis (*huáng lián*) are not used to clear heat. Instead, Pig Skin Decoction (*zhū fū tāng*) is used to enrich yīn and moisten dryness.

Sore throat from yīn vacuity heat should be distinguished from that which is the result of repletion heat. In vacuity patterns, the pain is generally not severe, the local region is not very red or swollen, and the throat is dry. This pattern is quite different from the pain, redness, and swelling seen in heat repletion patterns. Sore throat in lesser yīn disease has a special relation to the lung. As Qín Zhī-Zhēn (秦之桢, style 皇士 Huáng-Shì) writes, "Lesser yīn sore throat [occurs] because the kidney water is insufficient. [From] out of the water, fire effuses, upwardly tormenting the lung metal."

Pig Skin Decoction (*zhū fū tāng*) enriches, moistens, and supplements. Pig skin (*zhū fū*) is the skin of a pig that has had the inner layer of fatty meat removed. Salty and cold, it enters the kidney and enriches kidney water, clears heat, and moistens dryness. Sweet and cold, honey (*bái mì*) moistens the lung, clears vacuity fire flaming in the upper burner, and disinhibits the throat. Sweet and moderate, rice flour (*bái fěn*) harmonizes the center and supports earth to check diarrhea. In combination, these ingredients enrich the kidney, moisten the lung, and supplement the spleen.

5.2 Licorice Decoction and Platycodon Decoction Patterns

Line 311

少阴病，二三日，咽痛者，可与甘草汤；不差，与桔梗汤。

Shào yīn bìng, èr sān rì, yān tòng zhě, kě yǔ gān cǎo tāng; bù chài, yǔ jié gěng tāng.

When in lesser yīn disease [that has lasted for] two or three days, [there is] sore throat, one can give Licorice Decoction (*gān cǎo tāng*); [if the person] does not recover, give Platycodon Decoction (*jié gěng tāng*).

Formulae

Licorice Decoction (*gān cǎo tāng*)

◦ Clear heat and disinhibit the throat.

甘草二两

右一味，以水三升，煮取一升半，去滓，温服七合，日二服。

Gān cǎo èr liǎng

Yòu yī wèi, yǐ shuǐ sān shēng, zhǔ qǔ yī shēng bàn, qù zǐ, wēn fú qī gě, rì èr fú.

licorice (甘草 *gān cǎo*, Glycyrrhizae Radix) 2 liǎng

[For] the above one ingredient use three shēng of water. Boil to get one and a half shēng and remove the dregs. Take seven gě warm, two times a day.

Platycodon Decoction (*jié gěng tāng*)

桔梗一两　甘草二两

右二味，以水三升，煮取一升，去滓，温分再服。

jié gěng yī liǎng　gān cǎo èr liǎng
Yòu èr wèi, yǐ shuǐ sān shēng, zhǔ qǔ yī shēng, qù zǐ, wēn fēn zài fú.

platycodon (桔梗 *jié gěng*, Platycodonis Radix) 1 liǎng
licorice (甘草 *gān cǎo*, Glycyrrhizae Radix) 2 liǎng

[For] the above two ingredients use three shēng of water. Boil to get one shēng and remove the dregs. Divide [into two parts], and take warm twice a day.

SYNOPSIS

The signs and treatment of sore throat from lesser yīn visiting heat.

COMMENTARY

Because of the brevity of this line, it is understood by analyzing the formulae. The sore throat in this line is not severe and the local region is probably not very red or swollen. This sign is described as "lesser yīn sore throat from visiting heat." The idea of "visiting heat" is introduced because a mild heat evil enters the lesser yīn channel and invades the throat. Licorice Decoction (*gān cǎo tāng*) clears heat and resolves toxin. If it is not sufficient to relieve the pain, platycodon (*jié gěng*) may be added to open the lung and disinhibit the throat.

In Licorice Decoction (*gān cǎo tāng*), licorice (*gān cǎo*), the sole ingredient, is used raw because in that form it clears heat and resolves toxin. In Platycodon Decoction (*jié gěng tāng*), acrid platycodon (*jié gěng*) is used with licorice (*gān cǎo*) to open the lung and dissipate bind. Platycodon Decoction (*jié gěng tāng*), which has come to be known as Licorice and Platycodon Decoction (*gān jié tāng*), is the basis of many formulae that are used to treat sore throat. For example, in Sagacious Decoction (*rú shèng tāng*), schizonepeta (*jīng jiè*), ledebouriella (*fáng fēng*), and forsythia (*lián qiáo*) are added to the base formula Licorice and Platycodon Decoction (*gān jié tāng*).

5.3 VINEGAR DECOCTION PATTERNS

LINE 312

少阴病，咽中伤，生疮，不能语言，声不出者，苦酒汤主之。

Shào yīn bìng, yān zhōng shāng, shēng chuāng, bù néng yǔ yán, shēng bù chū zhě, kǔ jiǔ tāng zhǔ zhī.

When in lesser yīn disease, [there is] damage in the throat, sores* are engendered, [there is] an inability to speak, [and] no sound issues, Vinegar Decoction (*kǔ jiǔ tāng*) governs.

TEXT NOTE

* Sores, 疮 *chuāng*: A generic term for diseases of external medicine, such as welling-abscess (痈 *yōng*), flat-abscess (疽 *jū*), clove sore (疔 *dīng*), boil (疖 *jié*), streaming sore (流注 *liú zhù*), flowing phlegm (流痰 *liú tán*), and scrofula (瘰疬 *luǒ lì*). Here, the sore is in the throat.

FORMULA

Vinegar Decoction (*kǔ jiǔ tāng*)

∘ Clear fire and flush phlegm; close sores and disperse swelling.

半夏十四枚（洗，破如枣核） 鸡子一枚（去黄，内上苦酒，着鸡子壳中）。

(一) 右二味，内半夏，著苦酒中，以鸡子壳置刀环中，安火上，令三沸，去滓，少少含咽之。(二) 不差，更作三剂。

Bàn xià shí sì méi (xǐ, pò rú zǎo hé) jī zǐ yī méi (qù huáng, nà shàng kǔ jiǔ, zháo jī zǐ ké zhōng)

(1) *Yòu èr wèi, nà bàn xià, zháo kǔ jiǔ zhōng, yǐ jī zǐ ké zhì dāo huán zhōng, ān huǒ shàng, lìng sān fèi, qù zǐ, shǎo shǎo hán yàn zhī.* (2) *Bù chài, gèng zuò sān jì.*

pinellia (半夏 *bàn xià*, Pinelliae Tuber) 14 pieces (wash, break into pieces [the size of] jujube kernels)

chicken's egg (鸡子 *jī zǐ*, Galli Ovum) one piece (remove yolk and add vinegar (*kǔ jiǔ*) into the egg shell)

(1) [For] the above two ingredients, add pinellia (*bàn xià*) to the vinegar (*kǔ jiǔ*).[1] Place the egg shell in the ring of a knife [handle][2] over a flame. Boil three times and remove the dregs. Hold a little in the mouth, then swallow. (2) [If there is] no recovery, make three more formulae.

FORMULA NOTES

1. Vinegar, 苦酒 *kǔ jiǔ*: Rice vinegar, 米醋 *mǐ cù*. The rice vinegar should be added to the egg shell containing the egg white. The amount is not specified, because it depends on the size of the egg shell and the amount of egg white.
2. Place the egg shell in the ring of a knife [handle], 鸡子壳置刀环中 *jī zǐ ké zhì dāo huán zhōng*: In the Hàn dynasty, knife handles often had small holes. The egg shell was placed in the hole and then it could be comfortably held over a low flame without burning the hand.

SYNOPSIS

The signs and treatment of sores from throat damage and loss of voice.

COMMENTARY

The throat may develop sores as the result of a wound or from an internal process in which ulceration occurs. In either case, the throat disorder in this line is not the typical sore throat seen in other lesser yīn disease. Here, the throat is likely to be red, swollen, and ulcerated with discharge. This is a case of severe sore throat, in which the patient is unable to speak and no sound issues from the mouth. Neither Licorice Decoction (*gān cǎo tāng*) nor Platycodon Decoction (*jié gěng tāng*) is strong enough to treat this pattern, and Vinegar Decoction (*kǔ jiǔ tāng*), which closes sores, disperses swelling, disinhibits the clear orifices, and frees the voice, should be given.

In Vinegar Decoction (*kǔ jiǔ tāng*), pinellia (*bàn xià*) flushes phlegm and dissipates binds. Sweet, cold chicken's egg (*jī zǐ*) clears heat, moistens dryness, and relieves pain. Vinegar (*kǔ jiǔ*) disperses swelling and closes sores. The directions for ingesting the formula should be noted. The decoction is held in the mouth so that it can directly affect the local region. After that, it is swallowed, since the ingredients also work systemically.

5.4 PINELLIA POWDER AND DECOCTION PATTERNS

LINE 313

少阴病，咽中痛，半夏散及汤主之。

Shào yīn bìng, yān zhōng tòng, bàn xià sǎn jí tāng zhǔ zhī.

When in lesser yīn disease, [there is] soreness in the throat, Pinellia Powder and Decoction (*bàn xià sǎn jí tāng*) governs.

FORMULA

Pinellia Powder and Decoction (*bàn xià sǎn jí tāng*)

∘ Dissipate cold and free the throat; flush phlegm and open binds.

半夏（洗） 桂枝（去皮） 甘草（炙）

㈠ 右三味，等分，各别捣筛已，合治之。㈡ 白饮和，服方寸匕，日三服。㈢ 若不能散服者，以水一升，煎七沸，内散两方寸匕，更煮三沸，下火令小冷，少少咽之。㈣ 半夏有毒， 不当散服。

Bàn xià (xǐ) guì zhī (qù pí) gān cǎo (zhì)

(1) *Yòu sān wèi, děng fēn, gè bié dǎo shāi yǐ, hé zhì zhī.* (2) *Bái yǐn huò, fú fāng cùn bǐ, rì sān fú.* (3) *Ruò bù néng sǎn fú zhě, yǐ shuǐ yī shēng, jiān qī fèi, nà sǎn liǎng fāng cùn bǐ, gèng zhǔ sān fèi, xià huǒ lìng xiǎo lěng, shǎo shǎo yān zhī.* (4) *Bàn xià yǒu dú, bù dāng sǎn fú.*

pinellia (半夏 *bàn xià*, Pinelliae Tuber) (washed)
cinnamon twig (桂枝 *guì zhī*, Cinnamomi Ramulus) (remove the bark)
mix-fried licorice (甘草 *gān cǎo*, Glycyrrhizae Radix)

(1) For the above three ingredients use equal parts. Pound and sieve each separately, and combine. (2) Mix with a white [rice] cool decoction and take a square-inch-spoonful

three times a day. (3) If one cannot take the powder, boil one shēng of water seven times and add two square-inch-spoonfuls of powder. Boil three more times, remove from the flame, and allow to cool slightly. Swallow a small amount. (4) Pinellia (*bàn xià*) has toxin, and should not be taken in powdered [form].*

Formula Note

* Pinellia (*bàn xià*) has toxin, and should not be taken in powdered [form], 半夏有毒，不当散服 *bàn xià yǒu dú, bù dāng sǎn fú*: This line is thought to be a later addition to the text because if Zhāng Jī had been concerned with this problem here, he would not have suggested that this formula be used as a powder.

Synopsis

The signs and treatment of sore throat from lesser yīn visiting cold.

Commentary

It is difficult to determine from the text whether this is a pattern of lesser yīn heat transformation or cold transformation. Yet it is clear from the formula that this is a pattern involving cold and phlegm. In patterns with visiting cold and phlegm evil congesting the throat, the pain is severe and accompanied by aversion to cold, phlegm-drool congestion, cough, and possibly vomiting.

Pinellia Powder and Decoction (*bàn xià sǎn jí tāng*) can be used as a powder or a decoction. Cinnamon twig (*guì zhī*) unblocks yáng and dissipates cold. Pinellia (*bàn xià*) flushes phlegm and opens binds. Mix-fried licorice (*gān cǎo*) harmonizes the center, relaxes tension, and relieves pain. By taking the powder with a white rice cool decoction, the stomach fluids are protected and the dry, acrid ingredients are less likely to damage yīn. The final sentence in the directions for the formula, in which it is suggested that pinellia (*bàn xià*) should not be taken powdered because of its toxicity, is considered to be a later addition to the text and is generally disregarded.

6 CHAPTER APPENDIX

Line 290

少阴中风，脉阳微阴浮者，为欲愈。

Shào yīn zhòng fēng, mài yáng wēi yīn fú zhě, wéi yù yù.

When in lesser yīn disease the yáng [aspect of the] pulse is faint and the yīn [aspect of the] pulse is floating, it means [that the person] is about to recover.

Synopsis

The pulse of lesser yīn disease when recovery is about to occur.

Commentary

In lesser yīn disease the pulse is generally sunken and fine. In this line, the yīn pulse (represented in the cubit pulse) is floating, and the yáng pulse (represented in the inch pulse) is faint. When the inch pulse is faint, it means that the evil is faint.

When the cubit pulse is floating, it means that the yáng qì is returning. This type of pulse indicates that yáng qì is prevailing, the evil is debilitated, and recovery will soon occur. The presence of this type of pulse does not ensure recovery, but must be considered along with the other signs.

Chapter Six

Reverting Yīn Disease

Pulses and Signs; Treatment

辨厥阴病脉证并治

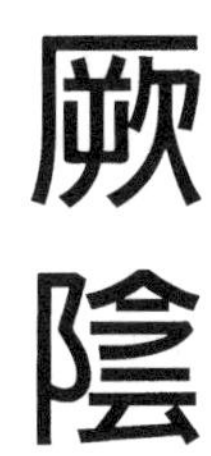

1 OVERVIEW

The primary pattern in the reverting yīn section is cold-heat complex, although patterns of pure heat or cold are also described. This pattern is upper heat and lower cold with signs such as thirst, qì surging up to the heart, pain and vexation in the heart, hunger with no desire to eat, and vomiting of roundworms. Alternation of reversal and heat effusion is commonly observed in reverting yīn disease, reflecting the struggle between yīn and yáng: When yīn evil prevails, reversal cold is observed; when right yáng returns, heat effusion is observed. In reverting yīn disease, the respective periods of reversal and heat effusion can be used to determine whether the disease is abating or advancing. Because these patterns involve the reverting yīn liver channel, signs of the liver invading the stomach or exploiting the spleen may also be observed.

1.1 Treatment

The three main formulae used in upper heat and lower cold patterns are Mume Pill (*wū méi wán*), which is the representative formula for this section; Dried Ginger, Scutellaria, Coptis, and Ginseng Decoction (*gān jiāng huáng qín huáng lián rén shēn tāng*), which is used in patterns with stomach heat, repelled cold, and retching; and Ephedra and Cimicifuga Decoction (*má huáng shēng má tāng*), which is used for lung heat and spleen cold. This final formula treats a pattern that is not reverting yīn disease, but is included in this section for comparison.

Reversal, diarrhea, retching, and hiccup are observed in reverting yīn disease, reflecting that yīn and yáng are not connecting favorably. Loss of regulation between the liver and spleen gives rise to diarrhea. If liver qì and stomach qì ascend counterflow, retching or hiccup may be observed. Differentiation of these signs is described below.

Reversal patterns can be divided into cold, heat, phlegm, water, and roundworm types. Roundworm reversal is characterized by upper heat and lower cold, and vomiting of roundworms. It is treated with Mume Pill (*wū méi wán*). Cold reversal patterns can be divided into three types: blood vacuity and congealing cold; yáng vacuity and yīn exuberance; and cold bind. These different types of cold reversal are treated with Tangkuei Counterflow Cold Decoction (*dāng guī sì nì tāng*), Tangkuei Counterflow Cold Decoction Plus Evodia and Fresh Ginger (*dāng guī sì nì jiā wú zhū yú shēng jiāng tāng*), and Counterflow Cold Decoction (*sì nì tāng*). Heat reversal is divided into patterns with formed repletion and with formless heat. The former is treated with one of the Qì-Coordinating Decoctions (*chéng qì tāng*). The latter can be treated with either White Tiger Decoction (*bái hǔ tāng*) for severe heat and severe reversal, or Counterflow Cold Powder (*sì nì sǎn*) when these signs are mild. Phlegm reversal is treated with Melon Stalk Powder (*guā dì sǎn*). Water reversal is treated with Poria (Hoelen) and Licorice Decoction (*fú líng gān cǎo tāng*).

Many diarrhea patterns are discussed in the reverting yīn section, as described below. Liver heat descending and distressing the intestines manifests as blood and pus in the stool, abdominal urgency and rectal heaviness, and thirst with a desire to drink. The main formula suggested for this pattern is Pulsatilla Decoction (*bái tóu wēng tāng*). Heat bind with circumfluence produces signs of diarrhea, delirious speech, and abdominal fullness and distention. It is treated with Minor Qì-Coordinating Decoction (*xiǎo chéng qì tāng*). Formless evil harassing the chest and diaphragm causing vacuity vexation is treated with Gardenia and Fermented Soybean Decoction (*zhī zǐ chǐ tāng*). Exuberant yīn in the interior and vacuous yáng floating to the exterior manifest as clear-food diarrhea, sweating, and reversal. This pattern is treated with Vessel-Freeing Counterflow Cold Decoction (*tōng mài sì nì tāng*). Vacuity cold diarrhea that occurs simultaneously with an exterior pattern is treated by first warming the interior and then resolving the exterior.

Retching patterns may also be differentiated, as follows. When cold invades the stomach and turbid yīn ascends counterflow, signs such as retching, ejection of drool and foam, and headache may be observed; Evodia Decoction (*wú zhū yú tāng*) is suggested for this pattern. In patterns of yīn exuberance and yáng vacuity, retching may be accompanied by a pulse that is weak, uninhibited urination, mild generalized heat, and reversal cold; these patterns are treated with Counterflow Cold Decoction (*sì nì tāng*). Patterns in which counterflow ascent of liver and stomach qì causes retching and heat effusion can be treated with Minor Bupleurum Decoction (*xiǎo chái hú tāng*).

1.2 SCHEMATIC OVERVIEW

Reverting Yīn Disease Patterns

- **Upper body heat and lower body cold patterns**
  - Roundworm reversal with retching, vomiting of roundworms, vexation, and chronic diarrhea: Mume Pill (*wū méi wán*)
  - Mutual repulsion of cold and heat with immediate vomiting of ingested food and diarrhea: Dried Ginger, Scutellaria, Coptis, and Ginseng Decoction (*gān jiāng huáng qín huáng lián rén shēn tāng*)

- Evil fall and yáng depression with incessant diarrhea, reverse-flow of the limbs, inhibited throat, and spitting of pus and blood: Ephedra and Cimicifuga Decoction (*má huáng shēng má tāng*)

- **Reversal patterns**
  - Heat reversal with a pulse that is slippery and interior heat: White Tiger Decoction (*bái hǔ tāng*)
  - Cold reversal
    * Yáng vacuity and yīn exuberance with great sweating, pain in the limbs, diarrhea, and aversion to cold: Counterflow Cold Decoction (*sì nì tāng*)
    * Blood vacuity and congealing cold with a pulse that is fine and verging on expiry: Tangkuei Counterflow Cold Decoction (*dāng guī sì nì tāng*)
    * Blood vacuity and congealing cold with enduring cold: Tangkuei Counterflow Cold Decoction Plus Evodia and Fresh Ginger (*dāng guī sì nì jiā wú zhū yú shēng jiāng tāng*)
  - Other reversal patterns
    * Phlegm repletion in the chest with fullness below the heart, vexation, hunger, and inability to eat: Melon Stalk Powder (*guā dì sǎn*)
    * Stomach vacuity and collected water with palpitations below the heart: Poria (Hoelen) and Licorice Decoction (*fú líng gān cǎo tāng*)

- **Diarrhea patterns**
  - Heat diarrhea with rectal heaviness and desire to drink water: Pulsatilla Decoction (*bái tóu wēng tāng*)
  - Heat bind with circumfluence with delirious speech: Minor Qì-Coordinating Decoction (*xiǎo chéng qì tāng*)
  - Vacuity vexation after diarrhea with sogginess below the heart: Gardenia and Fermented Soybean Decoction (*zhī zǐ chǐ tāng*)
  - True cold and false heat with clear-food diarrhea, sweating, and reversal: Vessel-Freeing Counterflow Cold Decoction (*tōng mài sì nì tāng*)

- **Retching and hiccup patterns**
  - Counterflow ascent of turbid yīn with ejection of drool and foam, and headache: Evodia Decoction (*wú zhū yú tāng*)
  - Yīn exuberance and yáng vacuity with a pulse that is weak, uninhibited urination, generalized heat, and reversal: Counterflow Cold Decoction (*sì nì tāng*).
  - Lesser yáng pattern with heat effusion: Minor Bupleurum Decoction (*xiǎo chái hú tāng*).

2 ESSENTIAL FEATURES OF REVERTING YĪN DISEASE

Line 326

厥阴之为病，消渴，气上撞心，心中疼热，饥而不欲食，食则吐蚘，下之利不止。

Jué yīn zhī wéi bìng, xiāo kě, qì shàng zhuàng xīn, xīn zhōng téng rè, jī ér bù yù shí, shí zé tù huí, xià zhī lì bù zhǐ.

In disease of the reverting yīn, [there is] dispersion-thirst,[1] qì surging upward to the heart,[2] pain and heat in the heart,[3] hunger with no desire to eat, vomiting of roundworms after eating, and [if] precipitation [is used], [there will be] incessant diarrhea.

Text Notes

1. Dispersion-thirst, 消渴 *xiāo ké*: A condition in which the patient drinks copious amounts of water, but is unable to allay the thirst. See line 71, p. 195.
2. Qì surging upward to the heart, 气上撞心 *qì shàng zhuàng xīn*: A subjective feeling of qì ascending counterflow into the region of the heart and chest. This term is equivalent to 气上冲心 *qì shàng chōng xīn*.
3. Pain and heat in the heart, 心中疼热 *xīn zhōng téng rè*: Pain in the region of the chest or the upper stomach accompanied by a feeling of scorching heat.

Synopsis

The outline of upper heat and lower cold in reverting yīn disease.

Commentary

This line describes a pattern of upper heat and lower cold, the analysis of which is based not only on the text itself, but also on the formulae that are suggested in the next several lines. It presents a pattern in which liver evil exploits the spleen and invades the stomach, giving rise to spleen cold and stomach heat. The pathomechanism can be understood as follows. The liver is the viscus of wind and wood, and the ministerial fire resides within it. During disease, wood fire burns and damages stomach fluids, giving rise to dispersion-thirst. Liver qì ascends counterflow toward the heart, resulting in pain in the chest region and a feeling of heat. These signs represent an upper burner heat pattern.

The liver evil exploits the spleen, causing spleen vacuity and a loss of normal movement and transformation. As a result, the patient is hungry, but unable to eat. Spleen vacuity is accompanied by cold in the intestines. In this case, if roundworms are present in the intestines, food intake will stimulate the worms. The movement of the worms may result in a disturbance of the stomach and intestines and vomiting of roundworms. These signs represent a pattern of lower burner cold. Because vacuity cold exists in the lower burner, if precipitation is used it will damage the spleen yáng and exacerbate the vacuity, causing a pattern of incessant diarrhea.

Considering this pattern from a six-channel perspective, we know that reverting yīn is the final channel in the sequence. It is the viscus where yīn ends and yáng is engendered; therefore, disease of reverting yīn results in a loss of the normal regulation of yīn and yáng with yīn and yáng hastening toward their mutual extremes. Reverting yīn disease is often characterized by heat in the upper burner and cold in the lower burner, but patterns may appear that are characterized by only heat or only cold. In general, disease of reverting yīn is characterized by yīn and yáng exuberance and retaliation, in which yīn evil and right qì alternately retaliate against each other. In this contention between yīn evil and right qì, reversal cold, a sign of yīn exuberance, alternates with heat signs, a sign of returning yáng.

3 UPPER HEAT AND LOWER COLD PATTERNS

3.1 Mume Pill Patterns

Line 338

㈠ 伤寒，脉微而厥，至七八日，肤冷，其人躁无暂安时者，此为藏厥，非蚘厥也。㈡ 蚘厥者，其人当吐蚘。㈢ 令病者静，而复时烦者，此为藏寒。㈣ 蚘上入其膈，故烦，须臾复止，得食而呕，又烦者，蚘闻食臭出，其人常自吐蚘。㈤ 蚘厥者，乌梅丸主之。㈥ 又主久利。

(1) *Shāng hán, mài wēi ér jué, zhì qī bā rì, fū lěng, qí rén zào wú zhàn ān shí zhě, cǐ wéi zàng jué, fēi huí jué yě.* (2) *Huí jué zhě, qí rén dāng tù huí.* (3) *Lìng bìng zhě jìng, ér fù shí fán zhě, cǐ wéi zàng hán.* (4) *Huí shàng rù qí gé, gù fán, xī yú fù zhǐ, dé shí ér ǒu, yòu fán zhě, huí wén shí chòu chū, qí rén cháng zì tù huí.* (5) *Huí jué zhě, wū méi wán zhǔ zhī.* (6) *Yòu zhǔ jiǔ lì.*

(1) When in cold damage the pulse is faint and [there is] reversal, and at seven or eight days, [there is] cold skin and the person is agitated without temporary [periods of] quiet, this indicates visceral reversal,[1] not roundworm reversal.[2] (2) In roundworm reversal, the person should vomit roundworms. (3) Now, the person is still, and then has periodic vexation, which indicates visceral cold.[3] (4) Roundworms ascend and enter the diaphragm; hence [there is] vexation, [but] wait a moment and it will cease. After eating there is retching and again vexation, when the roundworms smell malodor of food. The person often spontaneously vomits roundworms. (5) For roundworm reversal, Mume Pill (*wū méi wán*) governs. (6) It also governs enduring diarrhea.

TEXT NOTES

1. Visceral reversal, 藏厥 *zàng jué*: Reversal cold of the limbs that results from extreme yáng vacuity in the viscera. 藏 *zàng* is equivalent to 脏 *zàng*.
2. Roundworm reversal, 蚘厥 *huí jué*: Reversal cold of the limbs that results from roundworms penetrating into and harassing the body. Note that 蚘 *huí* is the same as 蛔 *huí*.
3. Visceral cold, 藏寒 *zàng hán*: Vacuity cold of the stomach and intestines.

FORMULA

Mume Pill (*wū méi wán*)

○ Support the right and control roundworms.

乌梅三百枚　细辛六两　干姜十两　黄连十六两　当归四两　附子六两（炮，去皮）　蜀椒四两（出汗）　桂枝六两（去皮）　人参六两　黄蘖六两

(一) 右十味，异捣筛，合治之。(二) 以苦酒渍乌梅一宿，去核，蒸之五斗米下，饭熟捣成泥，和药令相得，内臼中，与蜜杵二千下，丸如梧桐子大，先食饮服十丸，日三服，稍加至二十丸。(三) 禁生冷、滑物、臭食等。

Wū méi sān bǎi méi　xì xīn liù liǎng　gān jiāng shí liǎng　huáng lián shí liù liǎng　dāng guī sì liǎng　fù zǐ liù liǎng (pào, qù pí)　shǔ jiāo sì liǎng (chū hàn) guì zhī (qù pí) liù liǎng　rén shēn liù liǎng　huáng bǎi liù liǎng

(1) *Yòu shí wèi, yì dǎo shāi, hé zhì zhī.* (2) *Yǐ kǔ jiǔ zì wū méi yī xiǔ, qù hé, zhēng zhī wǔ dǒu mǐ xià, fàn shú dǎo chéng ní, huò yào lìng xiāng dé, nà jiù zhōng, yǐ mì chǔ èr qiān xià, wán rú wú tóng zǐ dà, xiān shí yǐn fú shí wán, rì sān fú, shāo jiā zhì èr shí wán.* (3) *Jìn shēng lěng, huá wù, chòu shí děng.*

mume (乌梅 *wu mei*, Mume Fructus) 300 pieces
asarum (细辛 *xì xīn*, Asiasari Herba cum Radice) 6 liǎng
dried ginger (干姜 *gān jiāng*, Zingiberis Rhizoma Exsiccatum) 10 liǎng
coptis (黄连 *huáng lián*, Coptidis Rhizoma) 16 liǎng
tangkuei (当归 *dāng guī*, Angelicae Sinensis Radix) 4 liǎng
aconite (附子 *fù zǐ*, Aconiti Tuber Laterale) 6 liǎng (blast-fry, remove the skin)
zanthoxylum (蜀椒 *shǔ jiāo*, Zanthoxyli Pericarpium) 4 liǎng (sweated*)
cinnamon twig (桂枝 *guì zhī*, Cinnamomi Ramulus) 6 liǎng (remove bark)
ginseng (人参 *rén shēn*, Ginseng Radix) 6 liǎng
phellodendron (黄蘖 *huáng bǎi*, Phellodendri Cortex) 6 liǎng

(1) [For] the above ten ingredients separately pound and sieve, then combine for treatment. (2) Use vinegar (*kǔ jiǔ*) to soak mume (*wu mei*) for one night. Remove the kernels and steam with five dǒu of rice. [When] the rice is cooked, pound to a paste. Blend the medicinals thoroughly. Place in a mortar with honey and [pound] two thousand [times]. Make pills the size of firmiana seeds. (See line 247, p. 351.) Take ten pills before eating, three times a day. Gradually increase to twenty pills. (3) Raw

and cold [foods], slimy foods, and malodorous foods, etc., are contraindicated [while taking the pills].

Formula Note

* Zanthoxyli Pericarpium (sweated),蜀椒 (出汗) *shǔ jiāo (chū hàn)*: Use a very low flame to fry the medicinal until water and oil begin to effuse outwards.

Synopsis

a) The distinguishing signs for the differentiation of visceral reversal and roundworm reversal.

b) The primary formula for the treatment of roundworm reversal.

Commentary

In both visceral reversal and roundworm reversal, one may observe reversal cold and a pulse that is faint, but the prognosis for the two patterns is different. Visceral reversal is considered a critical pattern with a poor prognosis, whereas roundworm reversal is considered a milder pattern with a better prognosis.

In visceral reversal patterns, reversal cold is severe and not only are the limbs cold, but the body and skin are also cold. True yáng is extremely vacuous and visceral qì is about to expire; therefore, the patient is continuously in a state of agitation.

In roundworm reversal, the reversal cold is less severe and the skin and body are not cold. In this pattern there is lower burner cold and upper burner heat. The roundworms ascend and harass so the patient experiences periods of quiet and periods of vexation, depending on the activity of the worms. After eating, retching and vexation are a sign of the worms becoming stimulated by the food. Patients with roundworm reversal may also have a history of vomiting of roundworms. Because this pattern is considered to be one of upper heat and lower cold, Mume Pill (*wū méi wán*), the main formula used, contains both hot and cold ingredients. This formula is useful not only for cold-heat complex roundworm reversal, but also for chronic diarrhea, with a mixture of cold and heat signs.

Mume Pill (*wū méi wán*), which contains both hot and cold ingredients to address the cold-heat complex, also includes ingredients that are sour, bitter, and acrid. Sour flavors quiet worms, bitter flavors cause worms to descend, and acrid flavors cause worms to subside. The formula contains sour mume (*wu mei*) and vinegar (*kǔ jiǔ*); bitter coptis (*huáng lián*) and phellodendron (*huáng bǎi*); and acrid asarum (*xì xīn*), dried ginger (*gān jiāng*), aconite (*fù zǐ*), cinnamon twig (*guì zhī*), and zanthoxylum (*shǔ jiāo*). When worms penetrate and harass the interior, right qì becomes vacuous. Thus, the formula also contains ginseng (*rén shēn*) and tangkuei (*dāng guī*), which boost qì and nourish blood. The sour, astringent flavor of the formula is very strong and it simultaneously warms and clears heat; therefore, it can be also be used for chronic diarrhea with a mixture of heat and cold signs.

Looking at this formula without considering the pattern presented in the text allows one to gain a broader perspective. The formula is sour, bitter, and acrid but it also contains honey and rice. These sweet ingredients, when combined with the sour flavors in the formula, can enrich yīn. The combination of sour and bitter ingredients can drain heat. Acrid and sweet ingredients together can warm yáng. Acrid and bitter ingredients together can open and downbear. This formula should not only be considered a formula for roundworm reversal, but should be considered the primary formula for treating reverting yīn cold-heat complex patterns.

3.2 Dried Ginger, Scutellaria, Coptis, and Ginseng Decoction Patterns

Line 359

伤寒本自寒下，医复吐下之，寒格更逆吐下， 若食入口即吐， 干姜黄芩黄连人参汤主之。

Shāng hán běn zì hán xià, yī fù tù xià zhī, hán gé gèng nì tù xià, ruò shí rù kǒu jí tù, gān jiāng huáng qín huáng lián rén shēn tāng zhǔ zhī.

In cold damage originally there was spontaneous cold diarrhea, yet the physician [used] vomiting and precipitation so [there is] repelling cold.* [After] further adverse [treatment] [through] vomiting and precipitation, if [there is] immediate vomiting after food enters the mouth, Dried Ginger, Scutellaria, Coptis, and Ginseng Decoction (*gān jiāng huáng qín huáng lián rén shēn tāng*) governs.

Text Note

* Repelling cold, 寒格 *hán gé*: Mutual repulsion between lower burner cold and upper burner heat.

Formula

Dried Ginger, Scutellaria, Coptis, and Ginseng Decoction (*gān jiāng huáng qín huáng lián rén shēn tāng*)

∘ Discharge and downbear with bitter and cold [flavors]; free yáng with acrid and warm [flavors].

干姜 黄芩 黄连 人参各三两

右四味，以水六升，煮取二升，去滓，分温再服。

Gān jiāng huáng qín huáng lián rén shēn gè sān liǎng

Yòu sì wèi, yǐ shuǐ liù shēng, zhǔ qǔ èr shēng, qù zǐ, fēn wēn zài fú.

dried ginger (干姜 *gān jiāng*, Zingiberis Rhizoma Exsiccatum)
scutellaria (黄芩 *huáng qín*, Scutellariae Radix)
coptis (黄连 *huáng lián*, Coptidis Rhizoma)
ginseng (人参 *rén shēn*, Ginseng Radix)
each 3 liǎng

[For] the above four ingredients use six shēng of water. Boil to get two shēng and remove the dregs. Divide [into two parts], and take warm twice a day.

Synopsis

The signs and treatment of cold-heat repulsion.

Commentary

The paucity of information in this line makes its interpretation problematic. Two main interpretations have been offered. In the first, lower burner cold is present with an exterior evil. Mistreatment of this pattern causes the exterior evil to fall inward and transform to heat, which gives rise to a pattern of mutual repulsion of lower burner cold and upper burner heat. The second interpretation is that the original pattern is characterized by lower burner cold with upper burner heat. The physician uses vomiting and precipitation to address both these problems.

The first interpretation is explained in *Shāng Hán Lùn Jiǎng Yì* as follows. In a cold damage pattern, spontaneous cold diarrhea is observed, suggesting that the patient has vacuity cold in the spleen and stomach. After the patient contracts an external evil, the physician misdiagnoses the pattern, and instead of using a formula to treat both the exterior and interior patterns, uses vomiting and precipitation. This mistreatment exacerbates the spleen and stomach vacuity cold and causes the evil to fall inward. The evil transforms to heat as it enters the interior and is repelled by the lower burner cold, resulting in a pattern of mutual repulsion of lower burner cold and upper burner heat. The physician perceives this pattern as one of repletion, and uses vomiting and precipitation again, exacerbating the illness. Heat in the upper burner disturbs the stomach qì, which then does not downbear properly, and the patient vomits after eating. Because of vacuity cold in the lower burner, the spleen yáng cannot ascend, causing diarrhea. Dried Ginger, Scutellaria, Coptis, and Ginseng Decoction (*gān jiāng huáng qín huáng lián rén shēn tāng*) contains hot and cold ingredients to address the cold-heat complex, but it also contains acrid flavors, which open, and bitter flavors, which downbear. This formula harmonizes the spleen and stomach to eliminate mutual repulsion of heat and cold.

The second interpretation, explained in *Gāo Děng Cóng Shū* describes the pattern in a slightly different way. The diarrhea in the beginning of the line is traced back to the treatment of a previous disease pattern involving upper burner heat and lower burner cold. The physician misdiagnoses this cold-heat complex and uses vomiting and precipitating treatment. The first instance of mistreatment causes repelling cold and does not resolve the illness. The second use of these inappropriate treatments further exacerbates the disharmony. Vomiting after eating is a key point for pattern identification and it indicates the presence of severe heat in the stomach and qì counterflow. Bitter, cold medicinals, which clear heat and drain fire, are used to clear upper burner heat; warm, acrid medicinals, which dissipate cold, are used to address cold in the lower burner.

In terms of pattern presentation, these signs are similar to upcast yáng, which is also characterized by upper heat and lower cold, but the pathomechanism is completely different in the two patterns. In upcast yáng and repelling cold, true cold exists in the lower burner. But in upcast yáng patterns, false heat exists in the upper burner, whereas in repelling cold patterns true heat exists in the upper burner.

In the pattern above, the upper burner heat is severe and results in retching counterflow. Thus, Dried Ginger, Scutellaria, Coptis, and Ginseng Decoction (*gān jiāng huáng qín huáng lián rén shēn tāng*) contains scutellaria (*huáng qín*) and coptis (*huáng lián*). These bitter, cold medicinals clear upper burner heat and when the heat is cleared, the stomach qì will downbear normally and vomiting will cease. Acrid, warm dried ginger (*gān jiang*) dispels cold from the lower burner. Once cold is dispelled, the spleen yáng will be able to ascend normally and the diarrhea will cease. This restorative process is assisted through the inclusion of ginseng (*rén shēn*), which supplements the center and boosts the qì. In summary, this formula opens with acrid flavors and downbears with bitter flavors. It clears upper heat and warms lower cold and regulates the spleen and stomach. Chén Niàn-Zǔ writes that whenever retching is complicated by heat, "it is not appropriate to use tangerine [peel] (*jú [pí]*), pinellia (*bàn [xià]*), and licorice (*gān cǎo*). Dried Ginger, Scutellaria, Coptis, and Ginseng Decoction (*gān jiāng huáng qín huáng lián rén shēn tāng*) governs."

3.3 EPHEDRA AND CIMICIFUGA DECOCTION PATTERNS

LINE 357

伤寒六七日，大下后，寸脉沉而迟，手足厥逆，下部脉不至，喉咽不利，唾脓血，泄利不止者，为难治，麻黄升麻汤主之。

Shāng hán liù qī rì, dà xià hòu, cùn mài chén ér chí, shǒu zú jué nì, xià bù mài bù zhì, hóu yān bù lì, tuò nóng xuè, xiè lì bù zhǐ zhě, wéi nán zhì, má huáng shēng má tāng zhǔ zhī.

When in cold damage [that has lasted] six or seven days, after great precipitation, the inch pulse is sunken and slow, [there is] reverse-flow of the extremities, the lower portion of the pulse* fails to arrive normally, the throat is inhibited, [there is] spitting of pus and blood, and incessant diarrhea, this is difficult to treat. Ephedra and Cimicifuga Decoction (*má huáng shēng má tāng*) governs.

TEXT NOTE

* Lower portion of the pulse, 下部脉 *xià bù mài*: The cubit pulse, 尺脉 *chǐ mài*.

FORMULA

Ephedra and Cimicifuga Decoction (*má huáng shēng má tāng*)

∘ Effuse depressed yáng, clear the lung, and move the spleen.

麻黄二两半（去节） 升麻一两一分 当归一两一分 知母十八铢 黄芩十八铢 萎蕤十八铢 芍药六铢 天门冬六铢（去心） 桂枝六铢（去皮） 茯苓六铢 甘草六铢（炙） 石膏六铢（碎，绵裹） 白术六铢 干姜六铢

(一) 右十四味，以水一斗，先煮麻黄一两沸，去上沫，内诸药，煮取三升，去滓，分温三服。(二) 相去如炊三斗米顷，令尽，汗出愈。

Má huáng èr liǎng bàn (qù jié) shēng má yī liǎng yī fēn dāng guī yī liǎng yī fēn zhī mǔ shí bā zhū huáng qín shí bā zhū wěi ruí shí bā zhū sháo yào liù zhū tiān mén dōng liù zhū (qù xīn) guì zhī liù zhū (qù pí) fú líng liù zhū gān cǎo liù zhū (zhì) shí gāo liù zhū (suì, mián guǒ) bái zhú liù zhū gān jiāng liù zhū

(1) *Yòu shí sì wèi, yǐ shuǐ yī dǒu, xiān zhǔ má huáng yī liǎng fèi, qù shàng mò, nà zhū yào, zhǔ qǔ sān shēng, qù zǐ, fēn wēn sān fú.* (2) *Xiāng qù rú chuī sān dǒu mǐ qǐng, lìng jìn, hàn chū yù.*

ephedra (麻黄 *má huáng*, Ephedrae Herba) 2.5 liǎng (remove nodes)
cimicifuga (升麻 *shēng má*, Cimicifugae Rhizoma) 1 liǎng 1 fēn
tangkuei (当归 *dāng guī*, Angelicae Sinensis Radix) 1 liǎng 1 fēn
anemarrhena (知母 *zhī mǔ*, Anemarrhenae Rhizoma) 18 zhū (12 grams)
scutellaria (黄芩 *huáng qín*, Scutellariae Radix) 18 zhū
Solomon's seal (萎蕤 *wēi ruí*, Polygonati Yuzhu Rhizoma) 18 zhū
peony (芍药 *sháo yào*, Paeoniae Radix) 6 zhū
asparagus (天门冬 *tiān mén dōng*, Asparagi Tuber) 6 zhū (remove hearts)
cinnamon twig (桂枝 *guì zhī*, Cinnamomi Ramulus) 6 zhū (remove bark)
poria (茯苓 *fú líng*, Poria) 6 zhū
mix-fried licorice (*gān cǎo*) 6 zhū
gypsum (石膏 *shí gāo*, Gypsum) 6 zhū (crushed, wrapped in cloth)
ovate atractylodes (白术 *bái zhú*, Atractylodis Ovatae Rhizoma) 6 zhū
dried ginger (干姜 *gān jiāng*, Zingiberis Rhizoma Exsiccatum) 6 zhū

(1) [For] the above fourteen ingredients use one dǒu of water. First boil ephedra (*má huáng*) once or twice, then remove the foam [collecting] on top. Add all the ingredients and boil to get three shēng. Remove the dregs, separate [into] three [parts], and take warm. (2) The time between [doses should be] as little as [the time] to cook three dōu of rice. Completely finish [the decoction] and when sweat issues, [the patient will] recover.

SYNOPSIS

The signs and treatment of a cold-heat complex in which an evil falls [inward] and yáng is depressed.

COMMENTARY

Following the use of precipitation in a cold damage pattern, counterflow cold of the limbs is observed, the inch pulse is sunken and slow, and the cubit pulse does not arrive. This pattern appears as if it might be yáng vacuity with exuberant yīn, but in yáng vacuity patterns one would not expect to see an inhibited throat and spitting of pus and blood. We may conclude that the inappropriate use of precipitation caused the evil to fall inward and yáng qì to become depressed. When yáng qì is depressed in the interior, it is unable to outthrust to the limbs and they become cold. Furthermore, inappropriate use of precipitation damages both yīn and yáng. In this pattern, damage to yīn results in lung heat and network vessel impediment. This causes inhibition of the throat and spitting of pus and blood. Damage to yáng results in cold spleen and qì fall; consequently, incessant diarrhea is observed.

The reason this pattern is difficult to treat is that if one uses cold medicinals to address lung heat, it will exacerbate spleen cold. Conversely, warm medicinals used to treat spleen cold will exacerbate lung heat. In this type of complex pattern the formula must also reflect the mixture of heat and cold. The crucial aspect of this pathomechanism is that the evil falls inward and depresses the yáng qì; therefore, the formula's main goal is to effuse the depressed yáng, although it also enriches and nourishes the construction-yīn and blood.

The main ingredient in Ephedra and Cimicifuga Decoction (*má huáng shēng má tāng*) is ephedra (*má huáng*), which is used because it strongly effuses outwards. The combination of ephedra (*má huáng*), gypsum (*shí gāo*), and mix-fried licorice (*gān cǎo*) is similar to Spleen-Effusing Decoction (*yuè bì tāng*), which clears interior heat and effuses depressed yáng. Cimicifuga (*shēng má*), added to assist ephedra (*má huáng*) in dissipating depression and upbearing the clear, also clears heat and resolves toxin. Its combination with scutellaria (*huáng qín*) and asparagus (*tiān mén dōng*) effectively clears lung heat and resolves toxins. Tangkuei (*dāng guī*) and Solomon's seal (*wēi ruí*) enrich yīn, nourish the blood, and help to prevent the effusing medicinals from damaging yīn. Cinnamon twig (*guì zhī*) and peony (*sháo yào*) harmonize the construction and resolve the fleshy exterior. Ovate atractylodes (*bái zhú*) and poria (*fú líng*) move the spleen and open yáng. Dried ginger (*gān jiāng*) and mix-fried licorice (*gān cǎo*) warm the center and dispel cold. It should be noted that except for ephedra (*má huáng*), cimicifuga (*sheng ma*), and tangkuei (*dāng guī*), all the other ingredients are used in very small amounts. This method is used to obtain the actions of these medicinals, while still maintaining the primary focus of the formula. This formula is to be taken in short intervals of time so that the entire decoction is ingested in a shorter period of time than is recommended for many other formulae. This decrease in time between doses increases the efficacy of the formula. The therapeutic goal is to cause sweat to issue, a sign that depressed heat has begun to outthrust to the exterior.

4 DIFFERENTIATION OF OVERCOMING OR RELAPSE IN REVERSAL HEAT PATTERNS

The characteristic clinical presentation of prevailing heat reversal is alternating reversal cold of the extremities and heat effusion, caused by the struggle between right and evil qì. When yīn evil prevails, there is reversal cold; when yáng qì returns, there is heat effusion. On the basis of the relative times of heat effusion and reversal cold, and the severity of the signs, one can assess the dynamic of the disease process and decide if it is abating or advancing. This pattern manifests in four primary types.

a) When the period of heat effusion equals the period of reversal, spontaneous recovery can occur.

b) When the period of reversal is longer than the period of heat effusion, yīn is prevailing and yáng has returned insufficiently; hence the disease is advancing.

c) When the period of heat effusion is longer than the period of reversal, right can prevail over evil; hence the disease is abating.

d) When heat effusion persists after yīn evil has abated, yáng has returned excessively and the disease is advancing.

Excessive return of yáng can damage the qì, the blood, and the channels. When heat damages the upper burner qì aspect, sore throat and throat impediment occur. When heat damages the lower burner blood aspect, pus and blood appear in the stool. When heat damages the channels, suppurating abscesses appear.

If cold medicinals are erroneously given in patterns of exuberant yīn and vacuous yáng, a critical pattern of eliminated center can result (see line 332, p 539).

In patterns with reversal and diarrhea, if the patient is able to eat, an eliminated center pattern may be present or stomach qì may be returning. One can feed the patient a small amount of food and observe the reaction. If heat effusion is absent, stomach qì is returning and recovery will follow. If sudden heat effusion is observed, stomach qì has been vanquished and an eliminated center pattern is present.

LINE 331

伤寒先厥， 后发热而利者，必自止； 见厥复利。

Shāng hán xiān jué, hòu fā rè ér lì zhě, bì zì zhǐ; jiàn jué fù lì.

When in cold damage, first [there is] reversal* and then heat effusion and diarrhea, it will cease spontaneously; [if one again] sees reversal, [there will be] diarrhea again.

TEXT NOTE

* Reversal, 厥 *jué*: Reversal cold of the extremities.

SYNOPSIS

The relationship between diarrhea and reversal heat.

COMMENTARY

Reverting yīn disease is often characterized by contention between right and evil qì, described as yīn and yáng exuberance and retaliation (阴阳胜复 *yīn yáng shèng fù*). In this line, when cold evil prevails, reversal cold of the extremities is observed, and when yáng qì returns, it manifests as heat effusion. Thus, the appearance of reversal cold and heat effusion in reverting yīn disease can be used to determine the disease progression and prognosis.

In reversal cold patterns, yáng qì is vacuous, qì falls, and diarrhea often occurs. Heat effusion means that yáng qì is returning, and when it does, yīn will abate and diarrhea will cease. If yáng qì is restored, but not sufficiently, abatement of yīn evil may not be complete and reversal cold may occur again. When this happens, one knows that yīn evil has returned and that diarrhea will also recur.

Line 336

㈠ 伤寒病，厥五日，热亦五日，设六日，当复厥，不厥者自愈。㈡ 厥终不过五日，以热五日，故知自愈。

(1) *Shāng hán bìng, jué wǔ rì, rè yì wǔ rì, shè liù rì, dāng fù jué, bù jué zhě zì yù.* (2) *Jué zhōng bù guò wǔ rì, yǐ rè wǔ rì, gù zhī zì yù.*

(1) When in cold damage disease, [there is] reversal for five days and heat for five days, if [there is] a sixth day [of disease], there should again be reversal, and if [there is] no reversal, [the person] will spontaneously recover. (2) The [duration of] reversal [from beginning to] end [will] not surpass five days. Because there were five days of heat, one knows there will be spontaneous recovery.

Synopsis

When heat and reversal are equal, this is a sign of spontaneous recovery.

Commentary

If reversal cold is followed by heat effusion, it means right qì is returning and evil qì is being eliminated. If the period of time for each of these signs is the same, and yáng qì returns neither excessively nor insufficiently, then recovery will occur. Here, five days of reversal is followed by five days of heat, and according to the text, on the sixth day reversal should occur again. If it does not occur, then recovery is likely.

The period of time for reversal cold should not exceed five days, according to the text, but the principle of determining the progress of a disease based on the number of days since its contraction does not seem to correlate with clinical experience. The lines in which this numerological theory is used reflect the influence of *Sù Wèn* and may well have been the additions of a later author.

Line 342

㈠ 伤寒，厥四日，热反三日，复厥五日，其病为进。㈡ 寒多热少，阳气退，故为进也。

(1) *Shāng hán, jué sì rì, rè fǎn sān rì, fù jué wǔ rì, qí bìng wéi jìn.* (2) *Hán duō rè shǎo, yáng qì tuì, gù wéi jìn yě.*

(1) [When] in cold damage, [there is] reversal for four days, but [then] heat for three days, then again reversal for five days, [it] means the disease is advancing. (2) [There is] more cold and less heat and yáng qì is abating; hence [the disease] is advancing.

SYNOPSIS

When reversal is greater than heat, there is yáng vacuity and the disease will progress.

COMMENTARY

The four days of reversal cold mentioned at the start of this line are followed by only three days of heat, indicating that yáng qì has returned insufficiently. Another five days of reversal cold follow. The period of reversal cold greatly exceeds that of heat effusion, indicating yáng qì vacuity. The disease continues to advance because yáng qì is insufficient to contend with yīn evil effectively; consequently, yáng qì abates and yīn evil advances.

LINE 334

㈠ 伤寒，先厥后发热，下利必自止。㈡ 而反汗出，咽中痛者，其喉为痹。㈢ 发热无汗，而利必自止，若不止，必便脓血。㈣ 便脓血者，其喉不痹。

(1) *Shāng hán, xiān jué hòu fā rè, xià lì bì zì zhǐ.* (2) *Ér fǎn hàn chū, yān zhōng tòng zhě, qí hóu wéi bì.* (3) *Fā rè wú hàn, ér lì bì zì zhǐ, ruò bù zhǐ, bì biàn nóng xuè.* (4) *Biàn nóng xuè zhě, qí hóu bù bì.*

(1) [When in] cold damage, [if there is] reversal first and then heat effusion, diarrhea will spontaneously cease. (2) But if [there is] sweating and soreness in the throat, this is throat impediment.* (3) [When there is] heat effusion and sweating is absent, diarrhea will spontaneously cease. If it does not cease, there will be pus and blood in the stool. (4) If [there is] pus and blood in the stool, throat impediment is absent.

TEXT NOTE

* Throat impediment, 喉为痹 *hóu wéi bì*: Swelling and pain in the throat region with a feeling of congestion and inhibition.

SYNOPSIS

Two transmuted patterns that can occur when yáng returns excessively.

COMMENTARY

Reversal cold, in this line, is an indication of exuberant cold evil and yáng vacuity. (In other lines it can be an indication of yáng qì depression and congestion in the interior.) Reversal cold is generally accompanied by diarrhea. When it is followed by heat effusion, this means that yáng qì is returning, and reversal cold and diarrhea should resolve.

Heat effusion in patterns that begin with reversal cold indicates that yáng is returning and that the patient is moving toward recovery. If the yáng qì returns insufficiently, as in line 331, p. 535, a relapse of reversal cold and diarrhea can occur.

Furthermore, if the yáng qì returns excessively, a pattern of cold may change to one of heat. In this line, two heat transmutations that are the result of excessive yáng are presented. In the first, heat evil in the qì aspect steams the fluids and forces them outward, which causes sweating. The heat scorches upward and causes throat impediment. In the second, the heat falls inward and distresses the blood aspect. Sweat does not issue and the heat damages the blood network vessels, resulting in pus and blood in the stool.

In the first transmutation, heat remains in the qì aspect and causes sweating and throat impediment. In the second, heat enters the blood aspect and causes blood and pus to appear in the stool. The last line of the text indicates that these two transmutations do not generally appear together. If the heat remains in the qì aspect, the blood aspect will not be affected, and pus and blood will not enter the stool. Conversely, if the heat enters the blood aspect, the qì aspect will not be affected, and sweating and throat impediment will be absent.

LINE 341

㈠ 伤寒发热四日，厥反三日，复热四日，厥少热多者，其病当愈。㈡ 四日至七日，热不除者，必便脓血。

(1) *Shāng hán fā rè sì rì, jué fǎn sān rì, fù rè sì rì, jué shǎo rè duō zhě, qí bìng dāng yù.* (2) *Sì rì zhì qī rì, rè bù chú zhě, bì biàn nóng xuè.*

(1) When in cold damage, [there is] heat effusion for four days, but then reversal for three days, then again heat for four days, this is less reversal and more heat, [and a person with] this disease should recover. (2) In four days to seven days, [if] the heat is not eliminated, pus and blood will [appear] in the stool.

SYNOPSIS

The dynamic of disease in reverting yīn disease in which yáng returns or yáng returns excessively.

COMMENTARY

In this line the period of heat effusion is greater than that of reversal cold. This is yīn and yáng exuberance and retaliation in which yáng qì is returning and yīn evil is abating. Yáng qì should prevail and the patient should recover.

After yáng qì returns, heat effusion should spontaneously cease and if it continues for about four or five days, or up to seven days or more, it means that yáng qì has returned excessively and heat remains even after yīn evil has already fully abated. In this case the heat will damage the blood network vessels, and pus and blood will appear in the stool.

LINE 332

㈠ 伤寒始发热六日，厥反九日而利。㈡ 凡厥利者，当不能食，今反能食者，恐为除中。㈢ 食以索饼，不发热者，知胃气尚在，必愈。㈣ 恐暴热来出而复去也。㈤ 后日脉之，其热续在者，期之旦日夜半愈。㈥ 所以然者，本发热六日，厥反九日，复发热三日，并前六日，亦为九日，与厥相应，故期之旦日夜半愈。㈦ 后三日脉之而脉数，其热不罢者，此为热气有余，必发痈脓也。

(1) *Shāng hán shǐ fā rè liù rì, jué fǎn jiǔ rì ér lì.* (2) *Fán jué lì zhě, dāng bù néng shí, jīn fǎn néng shí zhě, kǒng wéi chú zhōng.* (3) *Sì yǐ suǒ bǐng, bù fā rè zhě, zhī wèi qì shàng zài, bì yù.* (4) *Kǒng bào rè lái chū ér fù qù yě.* (5) *Hòu rì mài zhī, qí rè xù zài zhě, qí zhī dàn rì yè bàn yù.* (6) *Suǒ yǐ rán zhě, běn fā rè liù rì, jué fǎn jiǔ rì, fù fā rè sān rì, bìng qián liù rì, yì wéi jiǔ rì, yǔ jué xiāng yìng, gù qī zhī dàn rì yè bàn yù.* (7) *Hòu sān rì mài zhī ér mài shuò, qí rè bù bà zhě, cǐ wéi rè qì yǒu yú, bì fā yōng nóng yě.*

(1) [In this case] at the onset of cold damage, [there is] heat effusion for six days, but then reversal and diarrhea for nine days. (2) In all [cases of] reversal and diarrhea, there should be inability to eat; but today [the patient is] able to eat [and one] fears [this is] an indication of eliminated center.[1] (3) If [one] feeds[2] [the person] string noodles[3] [and] heat effusion is absent, one knows the stomach qì is still present and there will be recovery. (4) [There is] fear that sudden heat will come and then go again. (5) The next day [if one] investigates[4] and the heat is still present, expect recovery at midnight of the next day. (6) Why [this is] so is because originally [there was] heat effusion for six days, then, instead, reversal for nine days, then again heat effusion for three days. Together with the previous six days this is nine days [of heat effusion], [which] corresponds to the [nine days] of reversal. Thus, expect recovery at midnight of the next day. (7) After three days, [if one] investigates [and] the pulse is rapid, the heat has not ceased and this means heat qì is superabundant and a suppurating welling-abscess[5] will erupt.

TEXT NOTES

1. Eliminated center, 除中 *chú zhōng*: Dispersion of the qì in the center burner. When this occurs, the stomach qì has been vanquished but the patient is still able to eat. It is a sign that the stomach qì is about to expire completely.
2. If [one] feeds, 食以 *sì yǐ*: Food is given to the patient. In this line, 食 *shí* is read as 食 *sì*, which is the verb form "to feed."
3. String noodles, 索饼 *suǒ bǐng*: This is generally thought to be regular ribbon-shaped noodles. In modern Chinese, 饼 *bǐng* generally means a flat cake, but in the Hàn Dynasty it also referred to noodles.
4. [If one] investigates, 脉之 *mài zhī*: Here, 脉 *mài* is a verb, meaning to investigate.
5. Suppurating welling-abscess, 痈脓 *yōng nóng*: A painful swelling of the flesh that produces pus and is red and clearly circumscribed. Before rupturing, these soft abscesses are characterized by a thin, shiny skin. Before suppuration begins, they can be easily dispersed; when pus has formed, they easily rupture; after rupture, they easily close and heal.

SYNOPSIS

a) A method for identifying an eliminated center pattern.

b) The prognosis for several different situations that may occur when reverting heat overcomes again.

COMMENTARY

When the period of reversal cold is greater than that of heat effusion, and diarrhea occurs, it indicates yīn exuberance and yáng vacuity. In these patterns the patient is generally unable to eat. If the patient is able to eat, one must consider whether stomach qì is still present or if an eliminated center pattern is occurring in which stomach qì is about to expire.

Two possible outcomes for a vacuity cold pattern in which the patient is able to eat are presented here. One is that stomach qì is restored and the patient recovers. The other is that stomach qì is vanquished and the patient dies. The method used to determine which of these outcomes will occur is to give the patient some food. If, after eating, heat effusion is absent or mild, it means that stomach qì is returning and is a sign of recovery. The next day, if one finds evidence of heat, then the patient will recover on the following day. Here, the period of heat effusion is equal to the period of reversal cold, yīn and yáng are balanced, and the patient will recover. If after eating, heat effusion suddenly occurs, the stomach qì is exhausted and the heat is considered the "last radiance of the setting sun," 回光返照 *huí guāng fǎn zhào*. Sudden heat will then give way to an eliminated center pattern and death.

The final possibility presented in this line is that yáng qì returns, but is excessive. After three days, when yīn and yáng should be balanced and recovery should occur, if the pulse is still rapid, it means that the heat has not ceased. Yáng heat damages the channels and the network vessels and causes stagnation of the qì and blood. One possible transmutation is that interior heat will cause the eruption of an abscess.

Line 333

伤寒脉迟，六七日，而反与黄芩汤彻其热，脉迟为寒，今与黄芩汤复除其热，腹中应冷，当不能食，今反能食，此名除中，必死。

Shāng hán mài chí, liù qī rì, ér fǎn yǔ huáng qín tāng chè qí rè, mài chí wéi hán, jīn yǔ huáng qín tāng fù chú qí rè, fù zhōng yīng lěng, dāng bù néng shí, jīn fǎn néng shí, cǐ míng chú zhōng, bì sǐ.

[When in] cold damage the pulse is slow for six or seven days, but one gives Scutellaria Decoction (*huáng qín tāng*) to eradicate heat, a pulse that is slow indicates cold. Now [when] Scutellaria Decoction (*huáng qín tāng*) is given to eliminate heat, the abdomen should be cold and and [the patient] should be unable to eat. Today, instead [the patient is] able to eat. [This pattern] is called eliminated center and [the person] will die.

Synopsis

In a cold pattern, if cold medicinals are used inappropriately they can cause an eliminated center pattern.

Commentary

A pulse that is slow is indicative of cold, although it may also be seen in other patterns. After six or seven days of a cold pattern (perhaps with reversal cold), it is possible that yáng qì is returning, at which point heat effusion may occur along with the diarrhea seen in cold patterns. Here, the physician misdiagnoses the return of yáng qì as heat repletion, and uses Scutellaria Decoction (*huáng qín tāng*) to clear heat. The use of a bitter, cold formula in a cold pattern causes severe damage to yáng qì. The abdomen becomes cold and we anticipate that the patient will be unable to eat. That this patient is able to eat is not a sign of harmonized stomach qì, but is a sign of stomach qì expiration. This pattern is known as "eliminated center" and because of its severe nature the prognosis is death.

5 IDENTIFICATION OF REVERSAL PATTERNS

Counterflow cold of the extremities is common to all reversal patterns. It means that yīn and yáng are not connecting favorably.

Although many reversal patterns are discussed in the reverting yīn section of the text, only a small number of these are actually reverting yīn patterns. Many of the lines discussing reversal patterns are provided for comparison. The previously discussed patterns of roundworm reversal and visceral reversal belong to reverting yīn. Blood vacuity and congealed cold can cause reversal in a pattern characterized by reversal cold of the extremities and a pulse that is fine and about to expire. This pattern, which belongs to reverting yīn, can be treated with Tangkuei Counterflow Cold Decoction (*dāng guī sì nì tāng*), which warms the channels and dissipates cold, and nourishes the blood and opens the channels. Cold bind reversal, also seen in reverting yīn patterns, is characterized by smaller abdomen fullness that is painful when pressed. It is treated with Tangkuei Counterflow Cold Decoction Plus Evodia and Fresh Ginger (*dāng guī sì nì jiā wú zhū yú shēng jiāng tāng*). The remaining reversal patterns do not belong to reverting yīn disease, although they appear in this section: exuberant yīn with yáng vacuity, which is treated with Counterflow Cold [Decoction] type [of formula] (*sì nì bèi*); severe heat and depressed yáng with substantial repletion, which is treated by precipitation; formless heat, which is treated with White Tiger Decoction (*bái hǔ tāng*); phlegm repletion in the chest, which is treated with Melon Stalk Powder (*guā dì sǎn*); and stomach yáng vacuity and collected water, which is treated with Poria (Hoelen) and Licorice Decoction (*fú líng gān cǎo tāng*).

Vacuity cold reversal should be treated by warming and moxibustion is appropriate. Offensive precipitation is contraindicated. Precipitation and clearing methods can be used in heat reversal patterns.

5.1 Pathomechanism and Special Signs of Reversal Patterns

Line 337

㈠ 凡厥者，阴阳气不相顺接，便为厥。㈡ 厥者，手足逆冷者是也。

(1) *Fán jué zhě, yīn yáng qì bù xiāng shùn jiē, biàn wéi jué.* (2) *Jué zhě, shǒu zú nì lěng zhě shì yě.*

(1) In all reversal [patterns], yīn and yáng qì are not connecting smoothly, which means reversal. (2) Reversal means counterflow cold of the extremities.

Synopsis

The pathomechanism and distinguishing clinical evidence of reversal patterns.

Commentary

Many different types of reversal are described throughout the literature, including cold reversal, heat reversal, roundworm reversal, phlegm reversal, water reversal, and cold bind reversal. Although differences in the presentation of these patterns exist, the basic pathomechanism always involves yīn and yáng not connecting favorably, which gives rise to reversal cold of the extremities. Because reversal cold of the extremities is the manifestation of movement in an improper direction or counterflow, it is also referred to as counterflow cold of the extremities.

The terms "yīn" and "yáng" have broad meanings, and in this line, "yīn and yáng qì" has been given several different interpretations. Fāng Yǒu-Zhí and Chéng Wú-Jǐ write that this term means the movement of qì within the channels. The three yīn channels and the three yáng channels connect at the fingertips. If yīn and yáng do not connect normally at the fingertips, the qì will be unable to flow from yīn to yáng and counterflow cold in the limbs will occur. Shěn Míng-Zōng writes that yīn refers to the reverting yīn liver and yáng refers to the yáng brightness stomach.

When the liver contracts disease, wood qì may counterflow and adversely affect earth. This counterflow depresses stomach yáng, which is then unable to outthrust to the limbs, so they become cold. Huáng Yuán-Yù writes that yīn and yáng means spleen yīn and stomach yáng. Yīn and yáng qì not connecting favorably means stomach yáng qì counterflow and spleen yīn qì fall. Finally, Chén Píng-Bó writes, "the yáng [channels] receive qì from the four limbs, the yīn [channels] receive qì from the viscera; the qì of the yīn and yáng [channels] connect like a circle without end." Thus, an unfavorable connection between the yīn and yáng [channels] means that the qì of the extremities and of the viscera has lost harmony. This disharmony results in reversal cold of the limbs.

If one accepts the interpretation that this phrase means the movement of qì at the fingertips, it appears difficult to rationalize why in reversal cold all the fingers and toes are cold, not just certain ones corresponding to a given channel. Furthermore, reversal cold may occur in patterns when the liver is affected, but it also may occur when the spleen and stomach are the primary affected organs. To interpret yīn and yáng in terms of only the liver or only the spleen and stomach is incomplete. The fourth interpretation, that yīn and yáng qì refers to the connection between the viscera qì and the qì of the extremities, is the most acceptable.

Reversal cold is frequently observed in lesser yīn disease, but as in the line above, many different types of reversal exist and may appear in reverting yīn disease, lesser yáng disease, yáng brightness disease, or even greater yáng exterior patterns.

5.2 Heat Reversal

Line 335

㈠ 伤寒一二日，至四五日，厥者，必发热，前热者，后必厥。㈡ 厥深者热亦深，厥微者，热亦微。㈢ 厥应下之，而反发汗者，必口伤烂赤。

(1) *Shāng hán yī èr rì, zhì sì wǔ rì, jué zhě, bì fā rè, qián rè zhě, hòu bì jué.* (2) *Jué shēn zhě, rè yì shēn, jué wēi zhě, rè yì wēi.* (3) *Jué yīng xià zhī, ér fǎn fā hàn zhě, bì kǒu shāng làn chì.*

(1) When in cold damage [that has lasted] one or two days, up to four or five days, [there is] reversal, there will be heat effusion. First [there will be] heat, [then] later, reversal. (2) If the reversal is severe, the heat is severe. If the reversal is mild, the heat is mild. (3) In reversal, one should precipitate, but [if] sweating is promoted instead, there will be mouth damage with putrefaction and redness.*

Text Note

* Mouth damage with putrefaction and redness, 口伤烂赤 *kǒu shāng làn chì*: The presence of sores in the mouth and on the tongue with redness, swelling, and eroded flesh.

Synopsis

The distinguishing signs, treatment principles, and transmuted patterns after mistreatment of heat reversal.

Commentary

This line presents a pattern of heat reversal in which a deep-lying heat evil prevents yáng qì from outthrusting to the extremities, giving rise to reversal cold. Although the limbs are cold, it is likely that in this pattern, heat signs, such as heat effusion, would be observed. In fact, the presence of heat signs is critical for identifying heat reversal patterns. The mildness or severity of reversal cold can be used to evaluate the internal heat. When reversal is severe, it means severe depression of heat in the interior; if reversal is mild, the interior heat is also mild.

Zhāng Jī writes that in this reversal pattern one should use precipitation. Because it is not the typical pattern in which he suggests the use of precipitation, commentators have differed on their interpretations of this suggestion. Shěn Míng-Zōng suggests using a bitter, cold formula to downbear heat, but adds that true precipitating formulae, such as one of the Qì-Coordinating Decoctions (*chéng qì tāng*), should not be used. Conversely, Gāo Xué-Shān writes that one of the Qì-Coordinating Decoctions (*chéng qì tāng*) should be used. In *Gāo Děng Cóng Shū*, the authors write that this suggestion should be taken more broadly to include simple precipitation and heat-clearing methods as well. One may use one of the Qì-Coordinating Decoctions (*chéng qì tāng*), or a formula like White Tiger Decoction (*bái hǔ tāng*), according to the signs.

In heat reversal, heat is depressed in the interior; therefore, one should not promote sweating because it will damage the fluids and assist heat, which will then flame upward and engender sores, erosion, redness, and swelling in the mouth.

Line 339

㈠ 伤寒，热少微厥，指头寒，嘿嘿不欲食，烦躁。㈡ 数日，小便利，色白者，此热除也，欲得食，其病为愈。㈢ 若厥而呕，胸胁烦满者，其后必便血。

(1) *Shāng hán, rè shǎo wēi jué, zhǐ tóu hán, mò mò bù yù shí, fán zào.* (2) *Shù rì, xiǎo biàn lì, sè bái zhě, cǐ rè chú yě, yù dé shí, qí bìng wéi yù.* (3) *Ruò jué ér ǒu, xiōng xié fán mǎn zhě, qí hòu bì biàn xuè.*

(1) In cold damage [there is] scant heat and mild reversal, cold fingers, taciturnity with no desire for food, and vexation and agitation. (2) When [after] several days the urine is uninhibited and clear, it means that the heat [has been] eliminated, [and] a desire for food means [that a patient with] this disease [will] recover. (3) If [there is] reversal, and retching, [as well as] vexation and fullness in the chest and rib-side, after this, there will be bloody excretions.*

TEXT NOTE

* Bloody excretions, 便血 *biàn xuè*: Blood in the urine or the stool.

SYNOPSIS

Two scenarios in the mild heat reversal pattern.

COMMENTARY

In this line, scant heat and mild reversal constitute a mild heat reversal pattern; consequently, only the fingers are cold. Yet heat depressed in the interior has caused qì stagnation. The stomach qì is not revived, the patient is reticent, and has no desire to eat. The heat evil also harasses the spirit, causing vexation and agitation.

After a couple of days the disease may shift toward recovery or it may become more severe. If the urine is uninhibited and clear, and the patient's appetite returns, it means that heat is abating and the stomach qì is returning to harmony. Recovery will follow these positive transmutations. If, however, reversal cold continues and it is accompanied by retching and vexation fullness in the chest and rib-side, yáng qì depression has become more severe and the heat is not abating. If heat damages the blood network vessels in the lower burner, blood may appear in the stool or the urine.

LINE 350

伤寒，脉滑而厥者，里有热，白虎汤主之。

Shāng hán, mài huá ér jué zhě, lǐ yǒu rè, bái hǔ tāng zhǔ zhī.

When in cold damage, the pulse is slippery and [there is] reversal, [there is] heat in the interior, and White Tiger Decoction (*bái hǔ tāng*) governs.

SYNOPSIS

The signs and treatment of reversal that is caused by formless heat depression.

COMMENTARY

Reversal cold, when accompanied by a pulse that is slippery, is generally not a sign of vacuity cold, but a sign of repletion heat; therefore, it is likely that other signs of heat would also be observed in this pattern. To treat interior heat, one may consider using one of the Qì-Coordinating Decoctions (*chéng qì tāng*) or White Tiger Decoction (*bái hǔ tāng*). Referring back to line 335, p. 543, we know that reversal can be mild or severe. The decision to use one of these formulae is made on the basis of the severity of the depressed heat. Here, the pulse is described as slippery, indicating that it is flowing and uninhibited. The pulse is not stagnant or rough, as it would be if interior heat bind were present. Therefore, White Tiger Decoction (*bái hǔ tāng*) is used to clear heat and the Qì-Coordinating Decoctions (*chéng qì tāng*), which are used to precipitate interior heat bind, are not suggested.

5.3 Cold Reversal

5.3.1 Reversal from Yáng Vacuity and Exuberant Cold

Line 353

大汗出，热不去，内拘急，四肢疼，又下利，厥逆而恶寒者，四逆汤主之。

Dà hàn chū, rè bù qù, nèi jū jí, sì zhī téng, yòu xià lì, jué nì ér wù hán zhě, sì nì tāng zhǔ zhī.

When great sweat issues, the heat has not gone, and [there is] internal hypertonicity,* pain in the limbs, diarrhea, reverse-flow, and aversion to cold, Counterflow Cold Decoction (*sì nì tāng*) governs.

Text Note

* Internal hypertonicity, 内拘急 *nèi jū jí*: Hypertonicity in the abdomen that causes discomfort and pain.

Synopsis

The signs and treatment of cold reversal from yáng vacuity and exuberant yīn.

Commentary

This line is frequently interpreted as presenting a pattern of interior yīn exuberance and exterior yáng collapse. Following great sweating, the heat is not eliminated, indicating that the evil has not resolved through the sweating process. Instead, the yáng qì is damaged by the use of sweating, and collapses. When yáng collapses it cannot warm the channels, causing interior hypertonicity and pain in the limbs, reverse-flow cold, and aversion to cold. Yáng vacuity and exuberant cold also give rise to diarrhea. One should break yīn and return yáng using Counterflow Cold Decoction (*sì nì tāng*).

A careful analysis of the text suggests that this interpretation is faulty. The fact that sweating does not resolve the heat suggests that heat was part of the original pattern; this does not represent a new pattern. Although it is true that a pattern can transform during the disease process, aversion to cold does not generally appear in patterns in which vacuous yáng qì floats to the exterior. This information, considered together with the presence of heat effusion, suggests that this is an unresolved exterior pattern. The exterior pattern was not resolved through the promotion of sweating because sweat issued copiously, which is inappropriate. Inappropriate sweating not only fails to resolve the disease, but also damages yáng qì. Following damage to yáng qì, internal hypertonicity, pain in the limbs, diarrhea, and counterflow cold occur. Furthermore, if this were a pattern of exuberant yīn and floating yáng, it is likely that Zhāng Jī would have suggested a formula such as Vessel-Freeing Counterflow Cold Decoction (*tōng mài sì nì tāng*), not Counterflow Cold Decoction (*sì nì tāng*).

If one accepts the interpretation that these signs do not mean vacuous yáng floating to the exterior, but instead mean an unresolved exterior pattern, why is

Counterflow Cold Decoction (*sì nì tāng*) used and not a formula to resolve the exterior? This continues the precedent set in line 92, p. 141, "[When] in illness [there is] heat effusion and headache, but the pulse is sunken, and if (after taking Ephedra, Asarum, and Aconite Decoction (*má huáng xì xīn fù zǐ tāng*)) [there is] no recovery and [there is] generalized pain, one should relieve the interior. Counterflow Cold Decoction (*sì nì tāng*) [is appropriate]." This idea is also evident in line 225, p. 396, "When the pulse is floating and slow, [and there is] exterior heat and interior cold, [with] clear food diarrhea, Counterflow Cold Decoction (*sì nì tāng*) governs," in which urgent interior patterns are treated prior to mild exterior patterns.

Line 354

大汗，若大下利而厥冷者，四逆汤主之。

Dà hàn, ruò dà xià lì ér jué lěng zhě, sì nì tāng zhǔ zhī.

[After] great sweating, if [there is] severe diarrhea and counterflow cold, Counterflow Cold Decoction (*sì nì tāng*) governs.

Synopsis

The treatment method for reversal from yáng debility and exuberant yīn when yáng has been damaged by inappropriate treatment.

Commentary

With or without great sweating, severe diarrhea damages both the fluids and the yáng qì. When reversal cold follows severe diarrhea, it means that the yáng qì has been damaged severely. Counterflow Cold Decoction (*sì nì tāng*) is appropriate to return yáng and stem counterflow. Because it is not specified in the text as being the result of treatment, commentators disagree as to whether or not the sweating is the result of inappropriate treatment or some other disease process. This point, however, is not critical to the understanding of the line. As long as one can determine that a pattern of reversal cold belongs to yáng vacuity, it is appropriate to use Counterflow Cold Decoction (*sì nì tāng*), regardless of the pathomechanism.

5.3.2 Reversal from Blood Vacuity and Congealed Cold

Line 351

手足厥寒，脉细欲绝者，当归四逆汤主之。

Shǒu zú jué hán, mài xì yù jué zhě, dāng guī sì nì tāng zhǔ zhī.

When [there is] reversal cold of the limbs and the pulse is fine and verging on expiry, Tangkuei Counterflow Cold Decoction (*dāng guī sì nì tāng*) governs.

Formula

Tangkuei Counterflow Cold Decoction (*dāng guī sì nì tāng*)

∘ Nourish the blood and free the vessels; warm the channels and dissipate cold.

当归三两 桂枝三两（去皮） 芍药三两 细辛三两 甘草二两（炙） 通草二两 大枣二十五枚（擘，一法，十二枚）

右七味，以水八升，煮取三升，去滓，温服一升，日三服。

Dāng guī sān liǎng guì zhī sān liǎng (qù pí) sháo yào sān liǎng xì xīn sān liǎng gān cǎo èr liǎng (zhì) tōng cǎo èr liǎng dà zǎo èr shí wǔ méi (bò, yī fǎ, shí èr méi)

Yòu qī wèi, yǐ shuǐ bā shēng, zhǔ qǔ sān shēng, qù zǐ, wēn fú yī shēng, rì sān fú.

tangkuei (当归 *dāng guī*, Angelicae Sinensis Radix) 3 liǎng
cinnamon twig (桂枝 *guì zhī*, Cinnamomi Ramulus) 3 liǎng (remove bark)
peony (芍药 *sháo yào*, Paeoniae Radix) 3 liǎng
asarum (细辛 *xì xīn*, Asiasari Herba cum Radice) 3 liǎng
mix-fried licorice (*gān cǎo*) 2 liǎng
rice-paper plant pith (通草 *tōng cǎo*, Tetrapanacis Medulla) 2 liǎng
jujube (大枣 *dà zǎo*, Ziziphi Fructus) 25 pieces (broken)

[For] the above seven ingredients use eight shēng of water. Boil to get three shēng and remove the dregs. Take one shēng warm, three times a day.

SYNOPSIS

The signs and treatment of reversal from blood vacuity and congealing cold.

COMMENTARY

In this pattern, because not only reversal cold of the extremities is observed, but the pulse is fine and verging on expiry, this pattern belongs to blood vacuity and depressed cold. In blood vacuity patterns, the pulse loses normal nourishment and becomes fine, and if the vacuity is severe, about to expire. The extremities are not warmed and nourished by vacuous yáng qì, and reversal cold is observed.

This pattern is generally seen in patients who have constitutional blood insufficiency and then contract an exterior cold evil. The qì and blood are obstructed by the cold evil, and normal movement becomes inhibited. Tangkuei Counterflow Cold Decoction (*dāng guī sì nì tāng*) warms and opens the channels, nourishes the blood, and dissipates cold.

Tangkuei Counterflow Cold Decoction (*dāng guī sì nì tāng*) is a modification of Cinnamon Twig Decoction (*guì zhī tāng*). Fresh ginger (*shēng jiāng*) is removed; tangkuei (*dāng guī*), asarum (*xì xīn*), and rice-paper plant pith (*tōng cǎo*) are added; and the amount of jujube (*dà zǎo*) is increased. Acrid, warm tangkuei (*dāng guī*) nourishes and harmonizes the blood. It is the primary medicinal for nourishing liver blood. Peony (*sháo yào*), which boosts yīn and harmonizes the construction, increases the ability of tangkuei (*dāng guī*) to nourish the blood. Cinnamon twig (*guì zhī*) when combined with tangkuei (*dāng guī*) has a greater ability to warm the channels and free yáng. The combination of cinnamon twig (*guì zhī*) and peony (*sháo yào*) courses the reverting yīn and harmonizes the construction and defense. Asarum (*xì xīn*) warms the channels, dissipates cold, and frees the blood vessels.

Mix-fried licorice (*gān cǎo*) and jujube (*dà zǎo*) boost the qì, fortify the spleen, and promote the source of transformation, to support the production of new blood.

The formula also contains rice-paper plant pith (*tōng cǎo*), which has been the subject of some disagreement. Lǐ Shí-Zhēn (李时珍, sobriquet 滨湖 Bīn Hú) in his *Běn Cǎo Gāng Mù* writes,

> [通草 *Tōng cǎo*] is fine and hollow, with openings at both ends; hence it is called 通草 *tōng cǎo* [open grass]. This is what is today called mutong (*mù tōng*). Today's rice-paper plant pith (*tōng cǎo*) in ancient times was called 通脱木 *tōng tuō mù*. The Sòng [Dynasty] Materia Medica mixed these up as one, with the names in chaos. Today's mutong (*mù tōng*) is of two colors, purple and white. The purple [one] has a thick skin and acrid flavor and the white [one] has a thin skin and a bland flavor.... Both are able to open and disinhibit. Mutong (*mù tōng*)... in the upper body is able to open the heart and clear the lungs for treating headache and disinhibiting the nine orifices. In the lower body, it is able to discharge damp-heat, disinhibit the urine, open the large intestine and treat one-sided hypertonicity and pain.... Mutong (*mù tōng*) is appropriate for opening the orifices of the heart; it allows the channels and network vessels to flow and move [freely]. Rice-paper plant pith (*tōng cǎo*) is white and has a bland flavor.... It abducts heat downward and disinhibits urine... [and it] frees the qì [so that it may] ascend and outthrust, and it promotes lactation.

As a result of this analysis, many people are of the opinion that rice-paper plant pith (*tōng cǎo*) in the formula actually is mutong (*mù tōng*). Bitter and cold, it not only disinhibits urination, frees strangury, and discharges heat, it also opens the blood vessels and disinhibits the joints. Here, it not only assists in opening the channels and network vessels, but also helps prevent the warm, drying medicinals from damaging yīn.

LINE 352

若其人内有久寒者，宜当归四逆加吴茱萸生姜汤。

Ruò qí rén nèi yǒu jiǔ hán zhě, yí dāng guī sì nì jiā wú zhū yú shēng jiāng tāng.

If the person has enduring internal cold, Tangkuei Counterflow Cold Decoction Plus Evodia and Fresh Ginger (*dāng guī sì nì jiā wú zhū yú shēng jiāng tāng*) is appropriate.

FORMULA

Tangkuei Counterflow Cold Decoction Plus Evodia and Fresh Ginger (*dāng guī sì nì jiā wú zhū yú shēng jiāng tāng*)

∘ Nourish the blood and free the vessels; warm and downbear the liver and stomach.

当归三两　芍药三两　甘草二两（炙）　通草二两　桂枝三两（去皮）　细辛三两　生姜半斤（切）　吴茱萸二升　大枣二十五枚（擘）

右九味，以水六升，清酒六升和，煮取五升，去滓，温分五服。

Dāng guī sān liǎng sháo yào sān liǎng gān cǎo èr liǎng (zhì) tōng cǎo èr liǎng guì zhī sān liǎng (qù pí) xì xīn sān liǎng shēng jiāng bàn jīn (qiē) wú zhū yú èr shēng dà zǎo èr shí wǔ méi (bò)

Yòu jiǔ wèi, yǐ shuǐ liù shēng, qīng jiǔ liù shēng huò, zhǔ qǔ wǔ shēng, qù zǐ, wēn fēn wǔ fú.

tangkuei (当归 *dāng guī*, Angelicae Sinensis Radix) 3 liǎng
peony (芍药 *sháo yào*, Paeoniae Radix) 3 liǎng
mix-fried licorice (甘草 *gān cǎo*, Glycyrrhizae Radix) 2 liǎng
rice-paper plant pith (通草 *tōng cǎo*, Tetrapanacis Medulla) 2 liǎng
cinnamon twig (桂枝 *guì zhī*, Cinnamomi Ramulus) 3 liǎng (remove bark)
asarum (细辛 *xì xīn*, Asiasari Herba cum Radice) 3 liǎng
fresh ginger (生姜 *shēng jiāng*, Zingiberis Rhizoma Recens) half jīn (cut)
evodia (吴茱萸 *wú zhū yú*, Evodiae Fructus) 2 shēng
jujube (大枣 *dà zǎo*, Ziziphi Fructus) 25 pieces (broken)

[For] the above nine ingredients use six shēng of water mixed with six shēng of clear wine (*qīng jiǔ*). Boil to get five shēng and remove the dregs. Divide into five [parts] and take warm.

SYNOPSIS

The treatment method for blood vacuity and congealing cold with enduring intractable cold.

COMMENTARY

This line is a continuation of the previous one. When a patient with a cold constitution and enduring cold disease has signs for which Tangkuei Counterflow Cold Decoction (*dāng guī sì nì tāng*) would be appropriate, one can add evodia (*wú zhū yú*) and fresh ginger (*shēng jiāng*). These additions address enduring cold by increasing the formula's action to dissipate cold by warming the liver and harmonizing the stomach, by freeing yáng and dissipating cold. The addition of clear wine (*qīng jiǔ*) during the preparation process further strengthens the action of Tangkuei Counterflow Cold Decoction Plus Evodia and Fresh Ginger (*dāng guī sì nì jiā wú zhū yú shēng jiāng tāng*) to free yáng and dissipate cold.

5.3.3 Reversal from Cold Bind in the Lower Burner

LINE 340

病者手足厥冷，言我不结胸，小腹满，按之痛者，此冷结在膀胱关元也。

Bìng zhě shǒu zú jué lěng, yán wǒ bù jié xiōng, xiǎo fù mǎn, àn zhī tòng zhě, cǐ lěng jié zài páng guāng guān yuán yě.

The patient has reversal cold of the extremities and says, "I have no chest bind." If [there is] smaller abdominal fullness that is painful when pressed, this is cold bind in the bladder and Pass Head (*guān yuán*, CV-4).*

TEXT NOTE

* Bladder and Pass Head (*guān yuán*, CV-4), 膀胱关元 *páng guāng guān yuán*: The region of the smaller abdomen corresponding to the location of the urinary bladder and CV-4. CV-4 is located three cùn below the umbilicus.

SYNOPSIS

The pattern of limb reversal from cold bind in the lower burner.

COMMENTARY

Reversal cold of the limbs can be the result of many different causes including heat, cold, vacuity, and repletion. Cold reversal, aside from being the result of exuberant yīn and vacuous yáng, or blood vacuity and depressed cold, may also be the result of cold evil bound in the interior. This bound cold results in the yáng qì being unable to move out to the limbs where it provides warmth. This line presents a pattern of bound cold in the interior, specifically bound in the lower burner.

The diagnosis in this line is made following both questioning and palpation. Through questioning, one can determine that the location of the disease is in the lower burner, and through palpation, one can determine that it is replete. It should be noted that this information is not enough to make a conclusive diagnosis, but that other signs of lower burner bound cold, such as a liking for warmth and fear of cold in the smaller abdomen, urine that is clear and long, a pulse that is slow, and a tongue that is white, should also be present.

Although no treatment is suggested in the text, one may consider using moxibustion on points in the smaller abdomen, such as CV-4 and CV-6. A formula such as Tangkuei Counterflow Cold Decoction Plus Evodia and Fresh Ginger (*dāng guī sì nì jiā wú zhū yú shēng jiāng tāng*) may also be considered.

5.3.4 Reversal Patterns and Moxibustion

LINE 349

伤寒脉促，手足厥逆，可灸之。

Shāng hán mài cù, shǒu zú jué nì, kě jiǔ zhī.

When in cold damage the pulse is skipping and [there is] reverse-flow of the extremities, one can [apply] moxibustion.

SYNOPSIS

When exuberant yīn with yáng vacuity causes reverse flow, moxibustion can be used.

COMMENTARY

When the pulse is skipping, it is rapid and this is often considered a sign of heat and yáng exuberance. Based on this interpretation, the reverse-flow in the line above may be seen as heat reversal. Nonetheless, in patterns with exuberant yáng heat, the use of moxibustion is contraindicated. Considering just the pulse, in line 122, p. 138, a pulse that is rapid indicates yáng vacuity. Therefore, a pulse that is skipping or rapid need not necessarily indicate heat. It may indicate yáng exuberance or yáng vacuity. This differentiation should be made on the basis of the strength of the pulse, in addition to the other accompanying signs. If the pulse is skipping and strong, it is likely an indication of yáng exuberance. If it is skipping and has no strength, it is likely an indication of yáng vacuity.

Here, the skipping quality of the pulse indicates yáng vacuity; consequently, moxibustion is appropriate. No formula is suggested in this line, but one may consider Cinnamon Twig Decoction Minus Peony (*guì zhī qù sháo yào tāng*), which is suggested for a similar pattern in line 21, p. 85.

Several lines in the text provide clear and direct contraindication for the use of moxibustion in heat patterns. Two such examples are line 115, p. 255, in which the use of moxibustion in a heat pattern causes dryness of the throat and blood ejection and line 116, p. 256, in which the use of moxibustion boosts fire, causing vexation counterflow and dissipation of the blood from the pulse.

5.4 OTHER REVERSAL PATTERNS

5.4.1 Phlegm Reversal

LINE 355

病人手足厥冷，脉乍紧者，邪结在胸中，心下满而烦，饥不能食者，病在胸中，当须吐之，宜瓜蒂散。

Bìng rén shǒu zú jué lěng, mài zhà jǐn zhě, xié jié zài xiōng zhōng, xīn xià mǎn ér fán, jī bù néng shí zhě, bìng zài xiōng zhōng, dāng xū tù zhī, yí guā dì sǎn.

When the patient has reversal cold of the extremities and the pulse is suddenly tight, the evil is bound in the chest. Fullness below the heart, vexation, and hunger with inability to eat [means that] the disease is in the chest and one should use vomiting; [therefore,] Melon Stalk Powder (*guā dì sǎn*) is appropriate.

SYNOPSIS

The signs and treatment of reversal from phlegm repletion in the chest.

COMMENTARY

Reversal cold of the extremities can be differentiated through reference to the pulse. In line 350, p. 545, the pulse is slippery, indicating the presence of heat in the interior, and White Tiger Decoction (*bái hǔ tāng*) is used. When the pulse is fine and about to expire, as in line 351, p. 547, it indicates blood vacuity and cold; therefore Tangkuei Counterflow Cold Decoction (*dāng guī sì nì tāng*) is suggested. Vessel-Freeing Counterflow Cold Decoction (*tōng mài sì nì tāng*), from line 317, p. 478, is used when exuberant yīn repels yáng, as indicated by a pulse that is faint and about to expire.

In the line above, reversal cold is the result of a repletion evil causing congestion and stagnation in the chest. Yáng qì is unable to move out to the extremities and reversal cold is observed. The pulse is suddenly tight. A pulse that is tight indicates a bound evil, although it may also indicate pain. An analysis of Melon Stalk Powder (*guā dì sǎn*) indicates that a phlegm repletion evil is bound in the chest. A phlegm repletion evil bound in the chest obstructs the yáng qì, causing fullness below the heart and vexation. When a phlegm evil congests in the chest, the patient still feels hunger because the evil does not directly affect the stomach, but is unable to eat because the chest region is blocked.

The evil is located in the upper body; therefore, it is appropriate to use vomiting to expel the evil. Melon Stalk Powder (*guā dì sǎn*) is appropriate for causing vomiting. (See line 166, p. 266, for more information about this formula.)

5.4.2 Water Reversal

LINE 356

㈠伤寒，厥而心下悸，宜先治水，当服茯苓甘草汤，却治其厥。㈡不尔，水渍入胃，必作利也。

(1) *Shāng hán, jué ér xīn xià jì, yí xiān zhì shuǐ, dāng fú fú líng gān cǎo tāng, què zhì qí jué.* (2) *Bù ěr, shuǐ zì rù wèi, bì zuò lì yě.*

(1) When in cold damage [there is] reversal and palpitations below the heart, it is appropriate to first treat the water. One should take Poria (Hoelen) and Licorice Decoction (*fú líng gān cǎo tāng*) [which will] then treat reversal.[1] (2) [If] not [treated] in that way,[2] the water [will] soak into the stomach and there will be diarrhea.

TEXT NOTE

1. [Which will] then treat reversal, 却治其厥 *què zhì qí jué*: This phrase may be interpreted in two ways. In the first, the treatment will eliminate the reversal; in the second, after giving this formula one should then treat the reversal.

2. [If] not [treated] in that way, 不尔 *bù ěr*: The preceding sentence provides information to guide correct treatment. 尔 *ěr* is similar to 这样 *zhè yàng*, which means "in this way."

SYNOPSIS

The signs and treatment of reversal from stomach vacuity with collected water.

COMMENTARY

In this pattern, reversal cold occurs at the same time as palpitations below the heart. This reversal is different from that seen in patterns of exuberant yīn and yáng vacuity. It is also different from the reversal seen with exuberant heat and depressed yáng. From analyzing the formula, one may conclude that cold-rheum is present in the stomach. As a result, the yáng qì is obstructed and unable to outthrust to the limbs. The palpitations are also a result of water-rheum, as is written in the *Jīn Guì Yào Lüè*, "Water collected below the heart [when] severe results in palpitations...."

Poria (Hoelen) and Licorice Decoction (*fú líng gān cǎo tāng*) warms the stomach yáng in order to dissipate water. The signs of reversal and palpitations are addressed indirectly by treating the root of the disease. If this treatment is not followed, the water-rheum will not resolve and further transmutations may occur. The water-rheum may descend deeper into the interior and give rise to diarrhea.

The issue that is raised in this line relates to the anatomical location of evils in the interior of the body. While modern commentators infer from the formula recommended in the first part of the line that the evil is in the intestines, Zhāng Jī himself speaks of water entering the stomach and causing diarrhea. In terms of modern anatomical description, the water evil would be said to move into the intestines, not the stomach. Nonetheless, this was not Zhāng Jī's understanding of the disease process, so he did not write of the intestines, only the stomach. This is similar to line 215, p. 347, in which Zhāng Jī writes about dry stool in the stomach. That line is interpreted as meaning that the stool is in the intestines, not the stomach.

5.5 CONTRAINDICATIONS FOR THE TREATMENT OF REVERSAL PATTERNS

LINE 330

诸四逆厥者，不可下之，虚家亦然。

Zhū sì nì jué zhě, bù kě xià zhī, xū jiā yì rán.

In all counterflow cold reversal patterns, one cannot use precipitation; [in] vacuity patients* [this is] also [the case].

TEXT NOTE

* Vacuity patients, 虚家 *xū jiā*: People who have a constitutional insufficiency of blood, qì, yīn, or yáng. Yóu Yí (尤怡, style 在泾 Zài-Jīng) writes, "'Vacuity patients' means people whose constitution [is] insufficient."

Synopsis

For all patterns of reversal from vacuity cold, precipitation is contraindicated.

Commentary

The causes and pathomechanisms of reversal are varied, with the result that many different kinds of reversal patterns may be seen, including heat, cold, vacuity, and repletion. Precipitation is not contraindicated in reversal patterns associated with heat and repletion. Therefore, in the line above, "in all counterflow cold reversal patterns," cannot be understood to mean all reversal patterns, but instead should be understood to mean all vacuity cold reversal patterns. This differentiation is supported by the end of the line, in which reference is made to vacuity patients.

In healthy people, yáng is exuberant and full, reaching all the way to the ends of the extremities; hence the limbs remain warm and harmonious. A constitutional insufficiency of yáng qì encourages evil to invade and exacerbate the yáng vacuity. When yīn is exuberant and yáng is vacuous, the yáng qì is unable to warm the extremities and counterflow cold occurs. Because the patient is already vacuous, precipitation is contraindicated.

Yóu Yí concurs with this interpretation of the line.

> Counterflow cold [means that] the four limbs are not warm. Reversal [means] cold extremities.... This line speaks of yīn cold reverse-flow and [one] should warm and dissipate [cold], and warm and nourish. Thus, it says one cannot [use] precipitation.

Chén Niàn-Zǔ, however, offers a different interpretation.

> The hands and arms cold up to the elbows and the feet and legs cold up to the knees means counterflow cold. The hands and arms cold up to the wrists and the feet and legs cold up to the ankles means reversal. All counterflow cold reversal patterns belong to great vacuity of the yáng qì for the most part... but deep heat [patterns also] have [this sign]. [In] vacuity cold reverse flow, [that] one cannot [use] precipitation goes without saying. Reversal from deep heat [indicates] exuberant heat in the interior. The true yīn, contained in the interior, is scorched and collapsing, [unable] to bear further precipitation [which would] cause its exhaustion.... [In] all [these cases,] one cannot precipitate.

Line 347

伤寒五六日，不结胸，腹濡，脉虚复厥者，不可下，此亡血，下之死。

Shāng hán wǔ liù rì, bù jié xiōng, fù rú, mài xū fù jué zhě, bù kě xià, cǐ wáng xuè, xià zhī sǐ.

When in cold damage [that has lasted for] five or six days, chest bind is absent, the abdomen is soggy,[1] the pulse is vacuous, and then [there is] reversal, one cannot precipitate [because] this [is] blood collapse,[2] and precipitation [will cause] death.

TEXT NOTES

1. The abdomen is soggy, 腹濡 *fù rú*: The abdominal region feels soft when palpated.
2. Blood collapse, 亡血 *wáng xuè*: This term means blood vacuity. See line 58, p. 258, and line 87, p. 104, for other examples of this term.

SYNOPSIS

Identification of reversal from blood vacuity and treatment contraindications.

COMMENTARY

This line uses information from abdominal palpation and the pulse in order to identify the pattern. After five or six days of a cold damage disease, if the evil enters the interior and binds with a phlegm evil in the chest, it will cause chest bind. In chest bind patterns, below the heart the patient will have pain, hardness, fullness, and distention, which may extend down into the lesser abdomen. The pulse is usually sunken and tight. If the evil enters the interior and becomes bound in the region of the stomach, forming a repletion bind, then distention, fullness, and pain with bound stool will be present. In the pattern above, the absence of chest bind and presence of a soft abdomen indicate that the interior is not replete. The pulse is vacuous and not sunken or tight. The reversal in this pattern is not the result of a repletion evil in the interior obstructing the yáng qì; it is the result of blood vacuity. The blood and construction are insufficient to nourish the extremities; consequently, reversal occurs. This type of reversal cold should be clearly differentiated from that which occurs when obstruction and depression of yáng qì in the interior of the body gives rise to reversal and heat is also present.

For patterns of reversal that are caused by interior vacuity, one should attack with a precipitating formula. In these patterns the pulse is sunken, replete, and forceful; tidal heat effusion and abdominal fullness and pain are also present. In the blood vacuity reversal pattern above, the stool may be bound as a result of intestinal dryness caused by insufficiency of blood and construction, but the abdomen is not full, hard, and painful, and other signs of repletion bind, like tidal heat effusion, are absent. The pulse is vacuous and forceless, and the abdomen is soft; therefore precipitation is not the appropriate treatment. This pattern is also slightly different than reversal that is the result of faint yáng and exuberant yīn because in those patterns diarrhea is generally present; consequently, the treatment strategy is to return yáng and stem counterflow.

The signs present in the pattern above are the result of blood vacuity; therefore, one should nourish blood and supplement the center. This line is an example of the principle expressed in line 330, p. 554, that precipitation should not be used in reversal patterns with vacuity. If precipitation is used in this pattern, it constitutes the error of attacking vacuity, which will exacerbate vacuity and, in this case, cause death.

6 IDENTIFICATION OF DIARRHEA PATTERNS

Line 358

伤寒四五日，腹中痛，若转气下趣少腹者，此欲自利也。

Shāng hàn sì wǔ rì, fù zhōng tòng, ruò zhuǎn qì xià qù shào fù zhě, cǐ yù zì lì yě.

In cold damage [that has lasted] four or five days, if [there is] pain in the abdomen and shifting qì descending hastily* to the lesser abdomen, this [means there is] about to be spontaneous diarrhea.

Text Note

* Shifting qì descending hastily, 转气下趣 *zhuǎn qì xià qù*: A feeling of stirring in the intestines accompanied by frequent flatulence, which is called shifting qì. In this case, the moving qì is felt to be descending rapidly into the lesser abdomen.

Synopsis

Signs that spontaneous diarrhea is about to occur.

Commentary

In cold damage with abdominal pain it is likely that cold evil has congealed in the interior, inhibiting the qì dynamic. If the pain is accompanied by rapidly descending shifting qì, it can mean that yáng is vacuous and the qì is falling. Yáng vacuity and qì fall commonly manifests as diarrhea.

Abdominal pain and descending shifting qì is a sign of impending diarrhea. Many commentators interpret these signs as an indication of yáng vacuity and exuberant cold and this is supported by clinical experience, as this type of diarrhea is frequently seen. Nonetheless, one should not rule out the possibility of heat diarrhea, as Yóu Yí points out, noting that similar patterns in which a heat evil falls inward can produce heat diarrhea. One should, as in all cases, use this information as a guideline for the interpretation of the signs, and make a diagnosis after an analysis of the entire pattern.

Line 371

热利下重者，白头翁汤主之。

Rè lì xià zhòng zhě, bái tóu wēng tāng zhǔ zhī.

When [there is] heat diarrhea with rectal heaviness,* Pulsatilla Decoction (*bái tóu wēng tāng*) governs.

Text Notes

1. Heat diarrhea with rectal heaviness, 热利下重 *rè lì xià zhòng*: Loose stool which is accompanied by a feeling of heat and pressure in the anus. Rectal

heaviness, 下重 *xià zhòng*, is also read as pressure in the rectum, 后重 *hòu zhòng*.

FORMULA

Pulsatilla Decoction (*bái tóu wēng tāng*)

◦ Clear heat and dry dampness; cool the liver and resolve toxin.

白头翁二两　黄蘗三两　黄连三两　秦皮三两

(一) 右四味，以水七升，煮取二升，去滓，温服一升。(二) 不愈，更服一升。

Bái tóu wēng èr liǎng　huáng bǎi sān liǎng　huáng lián sān liǎng　qín pí sān liǎng.

(1) *Yòu sì wèi, yǐ shuǐ qī shēng, zhǔ qǔ èr shēng, qù zǐ, wēn fú yī shēng.* (2) *Bù yù, gèng fú yī shēng.*

pulsatilla (白头翁 *bái tóu wēng*, Pulsatillae Radix) 2 liǎng
phellodendron (黄蘗 *huáng bǎi*, Phellodendri Cortex) 3 liǎng
coptis (黄连 *huáng lián*, Coptidis Rhizoma) 3 liǎng
ash (秦皮 *qín pí*, Fraxini Cortex) 3 liǎng

(1) [For] the above four ingredients use seven shēng of water. Boil to get two shēng, remove the dregs, and take one shēng, warm. (2) [If there is] no recovery, take another shēng.

SYNOPSIS

The primary signs and treatment of reverting yīn heat diarrhea.

COMMENTARY

In the *Shāng Hán Lùn*, the term "diarrhea" includes simple diarrhea, as well as dysentery-type diarrhea. This line describes heat diarrhea. Liver heat descends into the large intestine and foul qì stagnates in the anus, causing heat diarrhea and a feeling of heaviness in the anus. Because of the terse text, this interpretation is based primarily on an analysis of Pulsatilla Decoction (*bái tóu wēng tāng*). This formula is appropriate for cases of heat-type diarrhea, particularly when rectal heaviness is present and the liver is involved.

Pulsatilla (*bái tóu wēng*) enters the liver channel and is the primary medicinal for the treatment of reverting yīn heat diarrhea. Ash (*qín pí*), which also enters the liver, clears heat and cools the liver. The combination of these two medicinals is particularly useful for heat diarrhea. The assistants phellodendron (*huáng bǎi*) and coptis (*huáng lián*) clear upper burner heat and drain lower burner heat. This bitter, cold formula not only clears heat, but also dries dampness, so it is effective for the treatment of liver channel damp-heat diarrhea. One must be certain that a repletion evil is present when using this formula. Its use in vacuity patterns is contraindicated.

Pulsatilla Decoction (*bái tóu wēng tāng*), Scutellaria Decoction (*huáng qín tāng*), and Pueraria, Scutellaria, and Coptis Decoction (*gé gēn huáng qín huáng lián tāng*) all clear heat and check diarrhea, but significant differences exist between the formulae. Scutellaria Decoction (*huáng qín tāng*), from line 172, p. 159, treats lesser yáng diseases with gallbladder heat in which diarrhea is accompanied by abdominal pain, bitter taste in the mouth, and a pulse that is stringlike. It clears heat and resolves the lesser yáng. Pueraria, Scutellaria, and Coptis Decoction (*gé gēn huáng qín huáng lián tāng*), from line 34, p. 158, clears heat and expels the evil to treat yáng brightness heat diarrhea. The diarrhea in these patterns is often accompanied by panting, sweating, thirst, and a pulse that is rapid. Pulsatilla Decoction (*bái tóu wēng tāng*) clears heat, dries dampness, cools the liver, and resolves toxins.

A final historical note with regard to the entering channels of pulsatilla (*bái tóu wēng*): throughout the materia medica of different historical periods, pulsatilla (*bái tóu wēng*) has been assigned different entering channels. Qián Huáng, after reviewing much of the literature, wrote that pulsatilla (*bái tóu wēng*) is a special medicinal for the reverting yīn channel. Furthermore, on the basis of years of clinical experience, we know that Pulsatilla Decoction (*bái tóu wēng tāng*) is particularly effective for the treatment of liver channel damp-heat with yīn mounting and sagging. Yīn mounting (a disease attributed to evils invading the liver channel) is characterized by acute pain of the testicles and genitals.

LINE 373

下利欲饮水者，以有热故也，白头翁汤主之。

Xià lì yù yǐn shuǐ zhě, yǐ yǒu rè gù yě, bái tóu wēng tāng zhǔ zhī.

When [there is] diarrhea with a desire to drink water, this means that [there is] heat; [therefore,] Pulsatilla Decoction (*bái tóu wēng tāng*) governs.

SYNOPSIS

A different identification of the signs of heat diarrhea.

COMMENTARY

In the previous line, Pulsatilla Decoction (*bái tóu wēng tāng*) is suggested for the treatment of heat-type diarrhea with rectal heaviness. The current line adds additional information to the pattern for which this formula is appropriate. Heat in the interior damages the fluids; therefore, in addition to diarrhea, thirst and a desire to drink are also present. These signs are important for the differentiation of this type of diarrhea.

In many patterns, thirst is an indication of heat; but it does not always indicate heat. Thirst may occur in patterns with lower burner fire debilitation in which the fluids cannot be steamed upward to the mouth. An example is lesser yīn disease with both diarrhea and thirst, as in line 282, p. 471. When thirst and desire for fluids are present, one must also consider the quantity of fluids consumed, if the fluids are hot or cold, and the status of urination.

Line 374

下利谵语者，有燥屎也，宜小承气汤。

Xià lì zhān yǔ zhě, yǒu zào shǐ yě, yí xiǎo chéng qì tāng.

When [there is] diarrhea with delirious speech, [there is] dry stool; [therefore,] Minor Qì-Coordinating Decoction (*xiǎo chéng qì tāng*) is appropriate.

Synopsis

The signs and treatment of heat bind circumfluence diarrhea.

Commentary

Delirious speech is generally considered an indication of repletion heat steaming in the interior and causing derangement of the spirit. If diarrhea occurs with delirious speech, the diarrhea is attributed not to vacuity cold, but to interior heat bind with circumfluence. Minor Qì-Coordinating Decoction (*xiǎo chéng qì tāng*) is used to precipitate this repletion evil.

The pattern in this line belongs to yáng brightness and the line should be considered in the context of the other yáng brightness patterns. This line appears in the reverting yīn section because it discusses a diarrhea pattern which must be differentiated from other patterns with diarrhea, not because it presents a reverting yīn disease.

Line 375

下利后，更烦，按之心下濡者，为虚烦也，宜栀子豉汤。

Xià lì hòu, gèng fán, àn zhī xīn xià rú zhě, wéi xū fán yě, yí zhī zǐ chǐ tāng.

When after diarrhea, [the person is] more vexed and [there is] sogginess below the heart* when pressed, this indicates vacuity vexation; [therefore,] Gardenia and Fermented Soybean Decoction (*zhī zǐ chǐ tāng*) is appropriate.

Text Note

* Sogginess below the heart, 心下濡 *xīn xià rú*: A soft and yielding quality in the area between the stomach and the heart.

Synopsis

Abdominal examination and treatment of a vacuity vexation pattern following diarrhea.

Commentary

If increased vexation follows diarrhea, one should consider, as in the previous line, that a repletion evil is bound in the interior. Nonetheless, here the area below the heart is soft and yielding; therefore, one knows that a substantial evil is not bound in the interior. A formless heat evil is depressed in the interior and it causes vacuity vexation. Gardenia and Fermented Soybean Decoction (*zhī zǐ chǐ tāng*) clears and diffuses depressed heat and treats vacuity vexation.

Previous lines in both the greater yáng and yáng brightness sections have described the signs of vacuity vexation in patterns for which Gardenia and Fermented Soybean Decoction (*zhī zǐ chǐ tāng*) is used. In addition to these signs (anguish in the heart and chest stuffiness), sogginess below the heart should also be considered a sign that can be used in the identification of vacuity vexation.

The differentiation of vacuity vexation patterns is important prior to determining an appropriate treatment. Gardenia and Fermented Soybean Decoction (*zhī zǐ chǐ tāng*) is contraindicated for use with any patient who has enduring diarrhea, because these patients generally have yáng insufficiency in the center burner. In this line, no evidence of enduring diarrhea or center burner yáng vacuity exists; therefore, this formula may be used.

LINE 366

㈠ 下利，脉沉而迟，其人面少赤，身有微热，下利清谷者，必郁冒汗出而解， 病人必微厥。 ㈡ 所以然者，其面戴阳，下虚故也。

(1) *Xià lì, mài chén ér chí, qí rén miàn shǎo chì, shēn yǒu wēi rè, xià lì qīng gǔ zhě, bì yù mào hàn chū ér jiě, bìng rén bì wēi jué.* (2) *Suǒ yǐ rán zhě, qí miàn dài yáng, xià xū gù yě.*

(1) When [there is] diarrhea, the pulse is sunken and slow, the person's face is slightly red and [there is] mild generalized heat and clear-food diarrhea, there will be depression veiling,[1] sweating, and resolution, and the person will have mild reversal. (2) Why [this is] so is because this facial [color means] upcast yáng[2] and [there is] lower body vacuity.

TEXT NOTES

1. Depression veiling, 郁冒 *yù mào*: A combined pattern of oppression from qì stagnation and dizziness. The *Shāng Hán Lùn Yán Jiū Dà Cí Diǎn* describes this pattern in more detail, writing that the patient may be in a daze and have periods in which their visual field goes black and they are unable to see anything. These signs are accompanied by a feeling of vexation and oppression.
2. This facial [color means] upcast yáng, 其面戴阳 *qí miàn dài yáng*: The facial color referred to is red, which is a yáng color. When cold is exuberant in the lower body and vacuous yáng qì floats upward, the complexion becomes red.

SYNOPSIS

In a pattern of yīn exuberance and yáng vacuity, although the vacuity is not yet severe, there can be depression veiling, sweating, and resolution.

Commentary

The combination of clear-food diarrhea with a pulse that is sunken and slow is a clear indication of vacuity cold. The pulse is not faint or fine, however, indicating that although yáng is vacuous, the vacuity is not yet severe. The complexion is red, the body is slightly hot, and mild reversal occurs. At this point, the disease could still resolve through sweating. Yáng is vacuous, though, and it floats upward. Contention between the right yáng and the evil, prior to the issuance of sweat, engenders depression veiling. This sign is a sign of the severe struggle between accumulated right qì and evil qì. When the right yáng prevails, sweat issues and the disease resolves.

Depression veiling does not only include dizziness and impaired vision, but also includes a feeling of vexation and oppression. This sign is differentiated from clouding (which occurs when vacuous yáng is about to desert prior to death) by the presence of agitation and oppression (which are absent in clouding patterns). The important point in this line is that yáng vacuity is not yet severe. If yáng vacuity was severe, the vacuous yáng would float upward and stray to the exterior. Sweating would then bring death as the yáng qì deserted; it would not bring resolution, as in the pattern described above.

Line 370

下利清谷，里寒外热，汗出而厥者，通脉四逆汤主之。

Xià lì qīng gǔ, lǐ hán wài rè, hàn chū ér jué zhě, tōng mài sì nì tāng zhǔ zhī.

When [there is] clear-food diarrhea, interior cold and external heat, sweating, and reversal, Vessel-Freeing Counterflow Cold Decoction (*tōng mài sì nì tāng*) governs.

Synopsis

The treatment of yáng qì collapsing to the exterior in a pattern of true cold and false heat.

Commentary

In this line, interior cold and exterior heat can be understood as true cold and false heat. This pattern, with clear-food diarrhea and reversal, is similar to the lesser yīn disease presented in line 317, p. 478. Just as in line 317, it is likely that the signs presented above are accompanied both by a pulse that is faint and verging on expiry and by absence of aversion to cold. This is a typical pattern of exuberant yīn repelling yáng. Sweating indicates that vacuous yáng is about to desert and suggests that this pattern is extremely dangerous. Vessel-Freeing Counterflow Cold Decoction (*tōng mài sì nì tāng*) causes the absorption of collapsing yáng.

Although, generally, sweating does not occur in lesser yīn disease, line 283, p. 473, reads, "When the person's yīn and yáng pulses are both tight, but [there is] sweating, it means yáng collapse, and belongs to the lesser yīn." The important sign in the line above is sweating. When sweat issues in patterns with exuberant yīn and vacuous yáng, it means that the yáng qì is collapsing to the exterior. At that point, a method to rescue yáng is urgently needed.

Line 372

下利腹胀满，身体疼痛者，先温其里，乃攻其表，温里宜四逆汤，攻表宜桂枝汤。

Xià lì fù zhàng mǎn, shēn tǐ téng tòng zhě, xiān wēn qí lǐ, nǎi gōng qí biǎo, wēn lǐ yí sì nì tāng, gōng biǎo yí guì zhī tāng.

When [there is] diarrhea with abdominal distention and pain, and generalized pain, first warm the interior, then attack the exterior. To warm the interior, Counterflow Cold Decoction (*sì nì tāng*) is appropriate. To attack the exterior, Cinnamon Twig Decoction (*guì zhī tāng*) is appropriate.

Synopsis

The treatment principle for an interior vacuity cold pattern with an exterior pattern.

Commentary

This line, in which yáng vacuity occurs simultaneously with an exterior pattern, is similar to line 91, p. 140. As in that line, it is likely that the diarrhea in this line is enduring clear-food diarrhea that has caused spleen-kidney yáng vacuity. Yáng is vacuous and cannot transform turbid yīn; consequently, distention and fullness are felt in the abdominal region. Diarrhea and abdominal fullness and distention are clear indications of yáng vacuity and exuberant cold. At the same time, generalized pain suggests an unresolved exterior pattern. Because the yáng vacuity is more severe than the exterior pattern, it is suggested that one first warm the interior with Counterflow Cold Decoction (*sì nì tāng*) and then resolve the exterior with Cinnamon Twig Decoction (*guì zhī tāng*).

Line 364

下利清谷，不可攻表，汗出必胀满。

Xià lì qīng gǔ, bù kě gōng biǎo, hàn chū bì zhàng mǎn.

[When there is] clear-food diarrhea, [one] cannot attack the exterior [because, if] sweat issues, there will be [abdominal] distention and fullness.

Synopsis

A transmuted pattern that occurs following the inappropriate promotion of sweating in a pattern of vacuity cold diarrhea with an exterior pattern.

Commentary

Clear-food diarrhea is an indication of yáng vacuity and exuberant cold. Even if it occurs simultaneously with an exterior pattern, one should not promote sweating. If sweating occurs, the yáng qì will stray outward and exacerbate the interior yáng vacuity. Vacuous yáng qì cannot transform turbid yīn, giving rise to abdominal distention and fullness. In this line, abdominal distention and fullness occurs following the inappropriate promotion of sweating, suggesting that it has caused or exacerbated yáng vacuity; in the previous line, it is a primary sign that reflects the patient's original condition.

7 IDENTIFICATION OF RETCHING AND HICCUP PATTERNS

7.1 Identification of Retching Patterns

Line 378

干呕，吐涎沫，头痛者，吴茱萸汤主之。

Gān ǒu, tù xián mò, tóu tòng zhě, wú zhū yú tāng zhǔ zhī.

When [there is] dry retching, ejection of drool and foam, and headache, Evodia Decoction (*wú zhū yú tāng*) governs.

Synopsis

The signs and treatment of turbid yīn ascending counterflow in a pattern of liver and stomach vacuity cold.

Commentary

Dry retching is a result of liver cold invading the stomach and causing stomach qì counterflow. When the stomach becomes cold, the spleen also becomes cold and the spleen yáng cannot retain and distribute fluids normally. Drool and foam follow the qì counterflow and are ejected from the mouth. The cold evil in the liver channel follows the channel pathway up to the head and causes a headache. Because the liver channel ascends to the vertex, most liver channel headaches are characterized by pain at the vertex. Evodia Decoction (*wú zhū yú tāng*) is suggested because it warms and downbears the liver and stomach, and discharges turbidity and frees yáng.

Line 377

呕而脉弱，小便复利，身有微热，见厥者难治，四逆汤主之。

Oǔ ér mài ruò, xiǎo biàn fù lì, shēn yǒu wēi rè, jiàn jué zhě nán zhì, sì nì tāng zhǔ zhī.

When [there is] retching and a pulse that is weak, then uninhibited urination and mild generalized heat, [if one] sees reversal, [this pattern] is difficult to treat. Counterflow Cold Decoction (*sì nì tāng*) governs.

Synopsis

The treatment of retching counterflow from yīn exuberance and yáng vacuity.

Commentary

When retching occurs with a pulse that is weak, it is an indication of vacuity of right qì and qì counterflow. Uninhibited urination is a sign of vacuous kidney qì and cold. The presence of generalized heat and reversal cold suggests that vacuous yáng is floating outward. This pattern is difficult to treat because cold counterflow is present in the upper body and yáng vacuity is present in the lower body; yīn is exuberant in the interior and yáng is floating to the exterior. Nonetheless, the basic pattern is one of exuberant yīn and vacuous yáng; therefore Counterflow Cold Decoction (*sì nì tāng*) is suggested.

If right qì is vacuous and qì ascends counterflow, one may wonder why Evodia Decoction (*wú zhū yú tāng*) is not used. It is because of the severity of the yáng vacuity. The primary action of Evodia Decoction (*wú zhū yú tāng*) is to warm and downbear. Its ability to restore the yáng is insufficient for this case. Counterflow Cold Decoction (*sì nì tāng*), although not generally useful for downbearing counterflow or checking retching, is used here because the retching is a result of exuberant yīn and vacuous yáng; once yáng is restored and yīn is eliminated, the retching will spontaneously cease. If one considers the additions made to Vessel-Freeing Counterflow Cold Decoction (*tōng mài sì nì tāng*) line 317, p. 478, it is likely that fresh ginger (*shēng jiāng*) would also be added here, to increase the formula's ability to check retching.

Line 379

呕而发热者，小柴胡汤主之。

Oǔ ér fā rè zhě, xiǎo chái hú tāng zhǔ zhī.

When [there is] retching and heat effusion, Minor Bupleurum Decoction (*xiǎo chái hú tāng*) governs.

Synopsis

The signs and treatment of reverting yīn disease shifting into the lesser yáng.

Commentary

Retching is one of the primary signs associated with lesser yáng diseases. When retching and heat effusion are observed together, they indicate a lesser yáng heat evil and are clearly different from a pattern of qì counterflow with exuberant yīn and vacuous yáng. Minor Bupleurum Decoction (*xiǎo chái hú tāng*) is used to check retching in lesser yáng diseases. The goal of placing this line in the reverting yīn section is to aid the reader in understanding the differences between these patterns.

Traditionally, this line is explained through the relationship between the reverting yīn and the lesser yáng. In a reverting yīn disease, when the yáng qì is restored, the disease may shift into the lesser yáng. In a reverting yīn disease, if retching and heat effusion signs appear, it indicates yīn is shifting to yáng, but this transmutation does not only occur in reverting yīn disease. For example, line 149, p. 234, presents almost the exact same content in a greater yáng pattern. "When cold damage [has lasted for] five or six days, [and is marked by] retching and heat effusion, and [Minor] Bupleurum Decoction ([*xiǎo*] *chái hú tāng*) signs are present, [if] other medicinals [are used] to precipitate, [and the] [Minor] Bupleurum [Decoction] ([*xiǎo*] *chái hú* [*tāng*]) signs are still present, one can still give [Minor] Bupleurum Decoction ([*xiǎo*] *chái hú tāng*)." Thus, generally, when retching and heat effusion appear together, one should consider the possibility of a lesser yáng disease, regardless of the previous diagnosis.

LINE 376

呕家有痈脓者，不可治呕，脓尽自愈。

Ǒu jiā yǒu yōng nóng zhě, bù kě zhì ǒu, nóng jìn zì yù.

When [treating] retching patients with suppurating welling-abscesses, one cannot treat the retching, and [when] the suppuration ceases, recovery will be spontaneous.

SYNOPSIS

Treatment contraindications for retching with a suppurating welling-abscess.

COMMENTARY

In this line, retching is the mechanism through which the body is trying to eliminate pus from abscesses; therefore, one should not attempt to check it. Once suppuration ceases and the pus is eliminated, retching will spontaneously cease, since it is only the tip of the disease. The root of the disease is the suppurating welling-abscess. The principle described in this line is that one must be aware of the momentum of the disease process, even if that means resisting the impulse to provide treatment. In the pattern described above, if one vigorously attempts to check retching, the treatment will go directly against the momentum of the body's own restorative process. Not only will retching persist, but the pus will have no way to escape the body. The combination of retching and suppurating abscesses is but one example of this general principle. Another example of this is in exterior patterns, where heat effusion indicates the struggle between the defensive qì and an evil fettering the exterior. Generally, one should not clear or drain heat, but should support the process of the body by giving medicinals that effuse the exterior and cause sweating, so that the evil can be expelled. Draining heat will result in the exterior evil falling inward and it is counter to the momentum of the body's own process.

7.2 Identification of Hiccup Patterns

Line 380

(一) 伤寒，大吐大下之，极虚，复极汗者，其人外气怫郁，复与之水，以发其汗，因得哕。(二) 所以然者，胃中寒冷故也。

(1) *Shāng hán, dà tù dà xià zhī, jí xū, fù jí hàn zhě, qí rén wài qì fú yù, fù yǔ zhī shuǐ, yǐ fā qí hàn, yīn dé yuē.* (2) *Suǒ yǐ rán zhě, wèi zhōng hán lěng gù yě.*

(1) When in cold damage, [after] great vomiting and great precipitation, [there is] extreme vacuity, and then extreme sweating [is promoted], the person has external qì depression.[1] Water is given to promote sweating,[2] and [this will] cause hiccup. (2) Why [this] is so is because of cold in the stomach.

Text Notes

1. External qì depression, 外气怫郁 *wài qì fú yù*: Exuberant heat depressed in the fleshy exterior, which impairs sweating.
2. Water is given to promote sweating, 复与之水，以发其汗 *fù yǔ zhī shuǐ, yǐ fā qí hàn*: Water is given to the patient to boost the fluids so that sweat will be able to issue.

Synopsis

Hiccup that is the result of vacuity cold in the stomach.

Commentary

In cold damage, precipitation and vomiting treatment is generally inappropriate and causes damage to right qì. In this pattern, a strong form of this treatment is used, resulting in extreme vacuity. The patient has external qì depression in which heat is depressed in the exterior and sweating cannot occur because the fluids of the body have been depleted by the inappropriate use of vomiting and precipitation. The physician mistakenly identifies this as a pattern of exterior repletion and strongly promotes sweating after giving the patient water. This inappropriate promotion of sweating exacerbates the existing yáng vacuity. Vacuous yáng is unable to warm the interior, and the stomach, which was damaged in the original mistreatment, becomes more cold. When yáng is vacuous, water collects in the interior and there is contention between the cold and water evils. The stomach qì ascends counterflow and gives rise to hiccups. Thus, Zhāng Jī explains that cold in the stomach is the cause of the hiccups.

Line 381

伤寒，哕而腹满，视其前后，知何部不利，利之即愈。
Shāng hán, yuē ér fù mǎn, shì qí qián hòu, zhī hé bù bù lì, lì zhī jí yù.

[For] cold damage with hiccup and abdominal fullness, observe the anterior and posterior* and know which region is inhibited. Disinhibiting [that region] [will bring] recovery.

Text Note

* Observe the anterior and posterior, 视其前后 *shì qí qián hòu*: "Anterior" and "posterior" refer to the orifices at the front and the rear of the body. One should investigate the status of the patient's urination and bowel movements.

Synopsis

The treatment principle for hiccups from a repletion evil.

Commentary

Hiccups indicate that the stomach qì is not downbearing properly and this sign occurs in many diseases, but it can mainly be divided into vacuity and repletion patterns. In vacuity patterns the sound of the hiccup will be low and faint and the episodes will be infrequent, indicating that the stomach qì has been vanquished. This pattern is similar to the hiccup pattern that occurs in the previous line. Line 194, p. 366, line 226, p. 386, and line 232, p. 398, all provide examples of hiccups occurring in vacuity patterns.

Repletion patterns occur when the qì of the stomach or lung is replete; consequently, the hiccup is high pitched and continuous. Examples of repletion patterns with hiccup can be found in line 231, p. 396, and line 98, p. 426. In the line above, the hiccups belong to a repletion pattern.

Hiccup can be the result of inhibited urine or stool. Line 111, p. 252, "[If this] endures, there will be delirious speech, and when severe, hiccuping, agitation of the extremities, and picking at bedclothes," provides an example of inhibited stool movement giving rise to hiccups. Line 231, p. 396, is an example of inhibited urination and hiccup. In the line above, the hiccup and abdominal fullness belong to repletion, and Zhāng Jī suggests that one should investigate the status of the urine and stool in order to choose the proper course of treatment. If urination is inhibited, then one must disinhibit urination. If the stool is blocked, then one must free the stool. Once the inhibited region is open, and urine and stool pass normally, the hiccups will cease.

8 PROGNOSIS

8.1 Identification of Signs of Recovery in Cold Patterns

Line 329

厥阴病，渴欲饮水者，少少与之愈。

Jué yīn bìng, kě yù yǐn shuǐ zhě, shǎo shǎo yǔ zhī yù.

When in reverting yīn disease, [there is] thirst with desire to drink water, give a small amount [of water] and [there will be] recovery.

Synopsis

The treatment of thirst from yáng return in reverting yīn disease.

Commentary

In reverting yīn disease with upper heat and lower cold, dispersion-thirst occurs. Yet in this line, the patient desires to drink water, and a small amount of water will resolve the disease. This appears to be a contradiction, but differences in the basic pathomechanisms producing thirst allow for differentiation on the basis of the degree of thirst.

Yáng qì return is a necessary condition for recovery, but if it is excessive, the heat will become exuberant and will engender great thirst. It is unlikely that great thirst will be relieved by consumption of a small amount of water. Likewise, when dispersion-thirst occurs in reverting yīn patterns with upper body heat, the degree of thirst is such that drinking a small amount of water is unlikely to resolve the thirst.

This line presents a reverting yīn disease in which the yīn evil is abating and the yáng qì is returning. Thirst with a desire to drink indicates that the fluids are insufficient. The thirst in this pattern is not as severe as in patterns of great thirst or dispersion-thirst. By giving the patient a small amount of water, one can differentiate these patterns. If the thirst is relieved, as it is here, one knows that the thirst was not severe, the prognosis is positive, and treatment is not necessary. Giving a small amount of water in mild disease patterns enriches the fluids, boosts yīn humor, and allows yīn and yáng to return to proper balance. It should be noted that the fluids should only be given a small amount at a time. Line 75, p. 271, and line 127, p. 200, present patterns in which the patient drinks copious amounts of water and as a result experiences a negative transmutation.

8.2 Identification of Signs of Impending Death in Vacuity Cold Patterns

Line 343

伤寒六七日，脉微，手足厥冷，烦躁，灸厥阴，厥不还者，死。

Shāng hán liù qī rì, mài wēi, shǒu zú jué lěng, fán zào, jiǔ jué yīn, jué bù huán zhě, sǐ.

When in cold damage [that has lasted] six or seven days, the pulse is faint, [there is] reversal cold of the extremities, and vexation and agitation, [use] moxibustion on reverting yīn,* [and if] the reversal is not restored [to normal], [the person will] die.

Text Note

* [Use] moxibustion on reverting yīn, 灸厥阴 *jiǔ jué yīn*: Moxibustion should be used on points on the reverting yīn channel. Cháng Qì-Zhī suggests Supreme Surge (*tài chōng,* LR-3). Zhāng Xī-Jū writes that the points should be Moving Between (*xíng jiān,* LR-2) and Camphorwood Gate (*zhāng mén,* LR-13).

Synopsis

In reversal cold, one can use moxibustion; if the reversal does not return, the patient will die.

Commentary

When cold damage has lasted for about a week and the pulse is faint and accompanied by reversal cold of the limbs, yīn is exuberant and yáng is debilitated. Vexation and agitation results from vacuous yáng being compelled to struggle with evil qì. This combination of signs indicates a severe pattern, and moxibustion is used on the liver channel to restore the yáng qì and dissipate cold. If the limbs become warm, yáng is returning and the patient will live, but if reversal cold persists, the prognosis is poor and it is likely that the patient will die.

Although no formula is suggested in the line, Evodia Decoction (*wú zhū yú tāng*) may be used if the vexation and agitation is severe. If the pulse is faint and verging on expiry, one may give Vessel-Freeing Counterflow Cold Decoction (*tōng mài sì nì tāng*). These formulae may be used simultaneously with the administration of moxibustion to improve the chances for recovery.

Line 344

伤寒发热，下利厥逆，躁不得卧者，死。

Shāng hán fā rè, xià lì jué nì, zào bù dé wò zhě, sǐ.

When in cold damage [there is] heat effusion, diarrhea, reverse-flow, agitation, and inability to sleep, [the person will] die.

Synopsis

When yīn cold is exuberant in the interior and vacuous yáng strays, the patient will die.

Commentary

In reverting yīn disease, heat effusion is often a sign of yáng qì return and recovery. Nonetheless, since it may also mean that vacuous yáng qì is floating outward, one must observe these patterns carefully. If heat effusion means that yáng qì is returning, the limbs should become warm and diarrhea should cease. In the pattern above, heat effusion occurs, but reversal cold and diarrhea persist, indicating that yīn is exuberant and vacuous yáng qì is floating outward. In addition, agitation and inability to sleep indicate that the yáng qì is about to expire and that death will follow.

In the pattern above and in line 298, p. 500, agitation occurs without vexation. In both these lines, the prognosis is death. Vexation is said to be the result of vacuous yáng struggling with evil qì, but when only agitation is present, it indicates pure yīn without yáng. This sign pattern occurs when yīn and yáng separate, prior to death.

Line 345

伤寒发热，下利至甚，厥不止者，死。

Shāng hán fā rè, xià lì zhì shèn, jué bù zhǐ zhě, sǐ.

When in cold damage [there is] heat effusion, severe diarrhea, and incessant reversal, [the person will] die.

Synopsis

In patterns of yīn exhaustion and yáng expiry, the patient will die.

Commentary

In this line, heat effusion is accompanied by severe diarrhea and incessant reversal. These signs should cease if heat effusion were an indication of yáng qì return. Because they do not, heat effusion is a sign that the yáng qì is floating outward. Furthermore, severe diarrhea exhausts yīn humor. Incessant reversal indicates that the yáng qì is not returning, but is expiring. Therefore, this is a critical pattern and the person will most likely die.

Line 346

伤寒六七日，不利，便发热而利，其人汗出不止者，死，有阴无阳故也。

Shāng hán liù qī rì, bù lì, biàn fā rè ér lì, qí rén hàn chū bù zhǐ zhě, sǐ, yǒu yīn wú yáng gù yě.

When in cold damage [that has lasted for] six or seven days, diarrhea is absent, and then [there is] heat effusion, diarrhea, and the person is sweating incessantly, [there will be] death because [there is] yīn without yáng.

SYNOPSIS

In patterns with yīn and without yáng, the patient will die.

COMMENTARY

Originally, a pattern of cold damage without diarrhea is observed, indicating that the disease is not severe. After a period of time, the pattern changes and heat effusion, diarrhea, and incessant sweating are observed. Zhāng Jī explains that the prognosis is death because yīn exists without yáng. Here, heat effusion, which can indicate yáng qì return when the accompanying signs resolve, suggests that this transmutation is negative. Heat effusion indicates the presence of exuberant yīn and vacuous yáng floating outward. Yáng is collapsing and the true yīn is being exhausted through the loss of fluids in the sweat and diarrhea. The only yīn that remains is the exuberant yīn evil, and yáng is absent; therefore, the prognosis is death.

LINE 362

㈠ 下利，手足厥冷，无脉者，灸之。㈡ 不温， 若脉不还，反微喘者，死。㈢ 少阴负趺阳者，为顺也。

(1) *Xià lì, shǒu zú jué lěng, wú mài zhě, jiǔ zhī.* (2) *Bù wēn, ruò mài bù huán, fǎn wēi chuǎn zhě, sǐ.* (3) *Shào yīn fù fū yáng zhě, wéi shùn yě.*

(1) When [there is] diarrhea, reversal cold of the extremities, and absent pulse, [use] moxibustion. (2) [In cases where the limbs are] not warm, if the pulse is not returning, but [there is] mild panting, [the person will] die. (3) If the lesser yīn [pulse],[1] is less than[2] the instep yáng [pulse][3] it means a favorable [outcome].

TEXT NOTES

1. Lesser yīn [pulse], 少阴 *shào yīn*: The pulse felt at Great Ravine (*tài xī,* KI-3).
2. Is less than, 负 *fù*: From its meaning of "negative" or "minus" comes the idea that one pulse is weaker than the other.
3. Instep yáng [pulse], 趺阳 *fū yáng*: The pulse felt at Surging Yáng (*chōng yáng,* ST-42).

SYNOPSIS

a) Critical signs in reverting yīn disease.

b) Two situations that may occur after moxibustion.

Commentary

The diarrhea, reversal, and pulse description in this line are reminiscent of the lesser yīn disease pattern described in line 315, p. 481, "incessant diarrhea, reverse-flow, absent pulse, dry retching and vexation." In that pattern, which also includes retching and vexation, the signs are the result of an exuberant yīn evil repelling the yáng medicinals. In this line, no treatment has been given, yet diarrhea and reversal are observed, and the pulse is absent, indicating that the pattern is a critical one. Moxibustion is used here as an emergency treatment. If reversal resolves and the limbs become warm, it is a positive transmutation. If reversal persists and the patient begins to experience slight panting, it indicates yáng qì exhaustion prior to desertion. These are negative transmutations and the patient will die.

If one can palpate the pulse in the feet, it means that the yáng qì has not expired and that the yáng qì may return. The instep yáng pulse is on the stomach channel and belongs to earth. The Great Ravine (*tài xī,* KI-3) pulse is on the kidney channel and belongs to water. The first governs the acquired constitution and the second the congenital constitution. When the Great Ravine (*tài xī,* KI-3) pulse is smaller than the instep yáng pulse, it indicates the presence of stomach qì. The source of transformation is still present, and "[when there is] stomach qì, then [there is] life." Thus, when the instep yáng pulse is greater than the Great Ravine (*tài xī,* KI-3) pulse, it is considered a favorable sign indicating that the patient will recover.

Over the years many commentators have written that this line does not belong in the reverting yīn section. Kē Qín suggests that this line should be expunged from the text. Many others suggest that it should be placed in another section of the text. For example, Fāng Yǒu-Zhí relates this line to the pattern for which Vessel-Freeing Counterflow Cold Decoction (*tōng mài sì nì tāng*) is used. Yù Chāng and Wāng Hǔ would place this line in the lesser yīn section on urgent precipitation. In any event, all these commentators agree that this line does not describe reverting yīn disease. In fact, the lines of the reverting yīn section do not only discuss reverting yīn disease. An absent pulse accompanied by reversal, diarrhea means that this line clearly has a relationship to the lesser yīn and in fact describes a lesser yīn disease. The reference to the lesser yīn is not only a reference to the pulse location, but also the pathomechanism of the disease.

Line 368

下利后脉绝，手足厥冷，晬时脉还，手足温者，生；脉不还者，死。

Xià lì hòu mài jué, shǒu zú jué lěng, zuì shí mài huán, shǒu zú wēn zhě, shēng; mài bù huán zhě, sǐ.

After diarrhea, the pulse expires and [there is] reversal cold of the extremities. In one day,* if the pulse returns and the extremities are warm, [the person will] live, [but] if the pulse does not return, [the person will] die.

TEXT NOTE

* In one day, 晬时 *zuì shí*: A period of twenty-four hours.

SYNOPSIS

After diarrhea, when the pulse expires and the limbs are cold, whether the patient will live or die can be decided after one day.

COMMENTARY

Following diarrhea, if the pulse expires and reversal cold occurs, it indicates fulminant desertion of the yáng qì. In this line, the changes are of a sudden nature and the disease is acute; hence Zhāng Jī does not present a treatment, but instead suggests that one should wait and observe the patient. Within 24 hours, one will know the prognosis. If the pulse returns and the limbs become warm, the prognosis is good and the patient should recover. If the pulse does not return, it means that the yáng qì is unable to return and the patient will die. This is considered to be an acute disease because in a protracted disease course, the right yáng would already be vacuous. If the pulse expired and reversal was observed, it would indicate exhaustion of the true yáng and imminent desertion. One would not be able to wait 24 hours, but would have to treat the patient immediately.

LINE 369

伤寒下利，日十余行，脉反实者，死。

Shāng hán xià lì, rì shí yú xíng, mài fǎn shí zhě, sǐ.

When in cold damage, [there is] diarrhea, more than ten times per day, but the pulse is replete, [the person will] die.

SYNOPSIS

When the pattern is vacuity, but the pulse is replete, the prognosis is poor.

COMMENTARY

When diarrhea occurs very frequently, as it does in this case, the pulse should be faint and weak because the yáng qì is vacuous. If the pulse is replete, it not only means that the evil is exuberant, but it also means that the stomach qì is about to expire. When the stomach qì expires, the patient will die.

LINE 360

下利，有微热而渴，脉弱者，今自愈。

Xià lì, yǒu wēi rè ér kě, mài ruò zhě, jīn zì yù.

When [there is] diarrhea with mild heat, thirst, and a pulse that is weak, [the person] [will] soon recover spontaneously.

SYNOPSIS

The pulse and signs of spontaneous recovery in a pattern of reverting yīn cold diarrhea.

Commentary

In this pattern the diarrhea belongs to vacuity cold. Mild heat and thirst indicate that the yáng qì is returning. A pulse that is weak indicates that the force of the evil is already debilitated; therefore, the disease in this line will resolve quickly. Here the diarrhea is not classified as heat-type diarrhea because if it were, mild heat and thirst would not be a sign of recovery, but simply a sign of internal heat.

The presence of mild heat is an important point to differentiate yáng qì return that leads to recovery from exuberant yáng qì that can cause further negative transmutations. When the heat is mild the thirst is also considered to be slight; if great heat and great thirst were observed, recovery would be unlikely. Furthermore, if yáng were exuberant, the pulse would not be weak, but instead would be rapid and large. This illustrates the principle of "a small [pulse] indicates the disease [is] abating," 小则病退 *xiǎo zé bìng tuì*, from the *Sù Wèn*.

Line 361

㈠ 下利脉数，有微热汗出，今自愈。㈡ 设复紧，为未解。

(1) Xià lì mài shuò, yǒu wēi rè hàn chū, jīn zì yù. (2) Shè fù jǐn, wéi wèi jiě.

(1) [When there is] diarrhea, a pulse that is rapid, mild heat and sweating, [the person] [will] soon recover spontaneously. (2) If [the pulse] is again tight, it means that [the disease has] not yet resolved.

Synopsis

a) The pulse and signs indicating that recovery is about to occur in a cold diarrhea pattern.

b) The pulse that means this pattern has not yet resolved.

Commentary

In the previous line a pulse that is weak indicated that the evil is debilitated. In this line, a pulse that is rapid indicates the return of the yáng qì. In the previous line mild heat and thirst occured, whereas in this line mild heat and sweating occur. Although these presentations are slightly different, they are both manifestations of yáng qì return and recovery. If the pulse becomes tight again, the yáng qì has not returned sufficiently, the yīn cold is prevailing, and the disease has not yet resolved. Because the pulse is described as being tight "again," one knows that originally the pulse was tight. This presentation of different pulse descriptions should serve as a guide to the meaning of different pulses and their interpretations, not as pulse definitions.

8.3 Identification of Scenarios in Vacuity Cold Diarrhea Patterns

Line 363

下利，寸脉反浮数，尺中自濇者，必清脓血。

Xià lì, cùn mài fǎn fú shuò, chǐ zhōng zì sè zhě, bì qīng nóng xuè.

When [there is] diarrhea but the inch pulse is floating and rapid and the cubit [pulse] is spontaneously rough, there will be pus and blood in the stool.*

Text Note

* Pus and blood in the stool, 清脓血 *qīng nóng xuè*: In this phrase, 清 *qīng* is read as 圊 *qīng*, 'toilet', used here in the extended sense of defecation.

Synopsis

A transmuted pattern that can occur when yáng returns excessively.

Commentary

On account of the pulse descsription, the diarrhea in this pattern is considered to belong to reverting yīn vacuity cold. The pulse, described as floating and rapid, is considered contrary to expectations, 反 *fǎn*. In vacuity cold diarrhea, the pulse should be weak and slow or tight, not floating and rapid. A pulse that is floating and rapid indicates that the cold evil has transformed to heat and the yáng qì has returned. The cubit pulse is rough, indicating that the lower burner blood aspect has been damaged. The movement of blood is inhibited and heat steams the blood and construction-yīn, forcing pus and blood into the stool. It is possible that if early in the disease process this patient was given a formula to clear heat from the construction and cool the blood, this transmutation might have been avoided.

Line 367

㈠ 下利，脉数而渴者，今自愈。㈡ 设不差，必清脓血，以有热故也。

(1) *Xià lì, mài shuò ér kě zhě, jīn zì yù.* (2) *Shè bù chài, bì qīng nóng xuè, yǐ yǒu rè gù yě.*

(1) When [there is] diarrhea with a pulse that is rapid, and thirst, [the person is] about to recover spontaneously. (2) If [the person is] not cured, pus and blood [will appear] in the stool because of heat.

Synopsis

a) When yáng returns, diarrhea ceases.

b) When yáng returns excessively, there is pus and blood in the stool.

Commentary

In vacuity cold reverting yīn disease, when the yáng qì returns, the patient recovers. Nonetheless, if the yáng qì returns too strongly, it can cause negative transmutations instead of recovery. Thirst and a pulse that is rapid are indications of yáng qì return and recovery, but if recovery does not occur, it means that the yáng qì returned excessively. Heat damages the blood network vessels in the lower burner and, as a result, pus and blood appear in the stool. As in the previous line, it is important to investigate the degree of thirst and the rapidity of the pulse carefully. If the thirst is mild and the pulse is only slightly rapid, it is likely that the yáng qì is returning normally and the patient will recover. If great thirst is observed and the pulse is very rapid and large, the yáng qì is likely excessive and may cause a negative transmutation.

Line 365

下利，脉沉弦者，下重也；脉大者，为未止；脉微弱数者，为欲自止，虽发热，不死。

Xià lì, mài chén xián zhě, xià zhòng yě; mài dà zhě, wéi wèi zhǐ; mài wēi ruò shuò zhě, wéi yù zì zhǐ, suī fā rè, bù sǐ.

When [there is] diarrhea and a pulse that is sunken and stringlike, [it indicates] rectal heaviness. A pulse that is large indicates that it has not yet ceased, [but] a pulse that is faint, weak, and rapid indicates that it is about to cease and although [there is] heat effusion, [the person] will not die.

Synopsis

Combining the pulse and signs to determine the scenario and prognosis when there is diarrhea because yáng returned excessively.

Commentary

Here, diarrhea is characterized by abdominal urgency and rectal heaviness. In simple diarrhea, the stool pours out and is accompanied by intestinal rumbling and abdominal pain. After evacuation the rectum feels loose or slack and not heavy. This line emphasizes the the importance of the pulse in differentiating diarrhea patterns, signs, and prognoses.

A pulse that is sunken indicates an interior pattern. A pulse that is stringlike indicates pain and stagnation of the qì mechanism. In this pattern, diarrhea occurs and the pulse is sunken and stringlike. That the pulse is sunken reflects the interior pattern and the stringlike quality indicates stagnation of the qì dynamic, which is also reflected in rectal heaviness.

Two possible transmutations are presented. In the first, the pulse becomes large, indicating that the disease is not resolving. The evil continues to progress and is not abating. This description illustrates the principle, "a large [pulse] means the disease [is] advancing (大则病进 *dà zé bìng jìn*)," from the *Sù Wèn*. If the pulse is weak and rapid, it means that the yáng qì is returning and the evil is abating.

The weak quality of the pulse does not mean right qì is weak, but that evil qì is debilitated. The rapid quality of the pulse indicates the return of the yáng qì. When the yáng qì returns, heat effusion will occur and the diarrhea will spontaneously cease.

9 CHAPTER APPENDIX

Line 327

厥阴中风，脉微浮，为欲愈，不浮，为未愈。

Jué yīn zhòng fēng, mài wēi fú, wéi yù yù, bù fú, wéi wèi yù.

In reverting yīn wind strike, a pulse that is slightly floating* indicates [the person is] about to recover. [If the pulse] is not floating, it means [the person will] not yet recover.

Text Note

* A pulse that is slightly floating, 脉微浮 *mài wēi fú*: It should be noted that the character 微 *wēi* in this phrase can be translated as "faint" instead of "slightly," in which case this line reads, "the pulse is faint [and] floating." The commentary in *Yī Zōng Jīn Jiàn* supports this interpretation. "A pulse that is faint is the pulse of the reverting yīn. [A pulse that is] floating is an exterior yáng pulse. When in reverting yīn disease one obtains a yáng floating pulse, [it means that] the evil is already in the exterior; therefore, [the person is] about to recover. [If the pulse] is not floating, then [it is] sunken. A sunken [pulse] is an interior yīn pulse, and [means that] the evil is still in the interior; therefore, [the person will] not yet recover."

Synopsis

Whether or not the pulse is floating is used to determine the prognosis.

Commentary

In this pattern, the reverting yīn directly contracts an exterior evil. This line presents no signs other than the pulse for pattern identification. When the pulse is floating, it can indicate an exterior pattern, but it can also be a sign that the disease is moving outwards prior to recovery. When the pulse is not floating, the evil remains in the interior; consequently, recovery is not imminent. This line is included in the Appendix because the signs presented are insufficient to enable one to assess the pattern reliably. The commentary of Kē Qín is provided for reference.

> [When] reverting yīn contracts disease, then the bar and cubit pulses are slightly moderate and not floating. Now, [the pulse is] slightly floating indicating that yáng is issuing from yīn. This is a yīn disease with a yáng pulse.... [There is] a pulse for reverting yīn wind strike [in which the patient] is about to recover, so there should be a pattern [in which the patient] has not yet recovered. If the patient is struck by wind during the time when the viscus of wood and wind [i.e., the liver] happens to be governing qì [i.e., the

spring], the [associated] transmutations will be more severe than [if] other channels [were affected].

Line 348

发热而厥，七日，下利者，为难治。

Fā rè ér jué, qī rì, xià lì zhě, wéi nán zhì.

When [there is] heat effusion and reversal for seven days with diarrhea, this is difficult to treat.

Synopsis

Exuberant evil and interior vacuity is difficult to treat.

Commentary

This line is placed in the Chapter Appendix because the information is insufficient to decide if it is a pattern of heat reversal or cold reversal. Both interpretations can be substantiated. Two commentaries are included below to illustrate these two interpretations.

Gāo Xué-Shān writes:

> From seven days of interior heat and reversal [one can] already see that this is yīn and yáng repulsion, with each [acting] separately. At seven days, this is the period when disease springing from yáng should recover. The reversal should cease and [the patient should] recover; [that is] good fortune. [If] diarrhea occurs instead, yáng is defeated and the yīn cold will prevail. Although [this pattern] is not at the point of sudden death, [one must] contend with [a pattern] in which yáng is faint and yīn is exuberant and [this is] difficult.

Yóu Yí writes:

> Heat effusion and reversal means generalized heat effusion and reversal of the limbs. The disease belongs to yáng, and the interior, it follows, is vacuous. At seven days the right [qì] is gradually returning and the evil is about to abate. Then, [it] should [be that] first the reversal ceases and afterward the heat is eliminated. [With] reversal heat as before, and in addition (contrary to expectations) [there is] diarrhea, [it means] the right is not returning and the interior is increasingly vacuous. [This] disease is not yīn cold, so [one] cannot [treat] the interior with acrid, sweet, and warm [medicinals]. [There is] interior vacuity and insufficiency, [so one] cannot [treat] this diarrhea with bitter, cold [medicinals that] consolidate [yīn in] the lower body. Therefore, this [pattern] is difficult to treat.

Chapter Seven

Sudden Turmoil

Pulses and Signs; Treatment

辨霍乱脉证并治

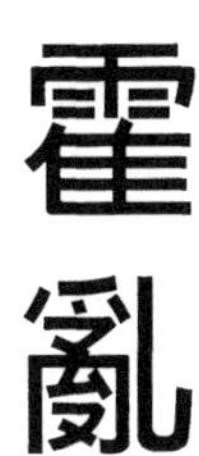

Sudden turmoil is a disease characterized by the sudden appearance of alternating vomiting and diarrhea. Heat effusion, aversion to cold, headache, and generalized pain may also be observed.

The treatment of sudden turmoil can be arranged in six main sections according to the formula used to treat each.

1. When there is a concurrent exterior pattern, a water-dampness evil is present, and urination is inhibited, the appropriate formula is Poria (Hoelen) Five Powder (*wǔ líng sǎn*).
2. If exuberant interior cold dampness gives rise to a pattern of vacuity cold in the center, the appropriate formula is Center-Rectifying Pill (*lǐ zhōng wán*).
3. When in a pattern of yáng vacuity and yīn exuberance, vomiting and diarrhea is accompanied by sweating, heat effusion and aversion to cold, hypertonicity of the limbs, reverse-flow, and a pulse that is faint and verging on expiry, the appropriate formula is Counterflow Cold Decoction (*sì nì tāng*).
4. If damage to yáng and humor desertion give rise to signs such as aversion to cold, a pulse that is faint, and diarrhea that ceases, the appropriate formula is Counterflow Cold Decoction Plus Ginseng (*sì nì jiā rén shēn tāng*).
5. When yáng collapses and yīn is exhausted, giving rise to signs such as vomiting that ceases, sweating, reversal, hypertonicity of the limbs, and a pulse that is faint and verging on expiry, the appropriate formula is Vessel-Freeing Counterflow Cold Decoction Plus Pig's Bile (*tōng mài sì nì jiā zhū dǎn (zhī) tāng*).
6. In sudden turmoil, if vomiting and diarrhea cease, but the exterior has not yet resolved, the appropriate formula is Cinnamon Twig Decoction (*guì zhī tāng*).

In modern Western medicine, 霍乱 *huò luàn* is the term used for the equivalent of the English cholera, which now refers to a specific disease caused by *Vibrio cholerae*. In Chinese medicine, 霍乱 *huò luàn*, as indeed the English term cholera prior to the modern era, has the traditional meaning of any condition characterized by simultaneous vomiting and diarrhea. To avoid confusion, the Chinese term is literally translated here as "sudden turmoil."

LINE 382

㈠ 问曰：病有霍乱者何？ ㈡ 答曰：呕吐而利，此名霍乱。

(1) *Wèn yuē: bìng yǒu huò luàn zhě hé?* (2) *Dá yuē: ǒu tù ér lì, cǐ míng huò luàn.*

(1) Question: What of the disease sudden turmoil? (2) Answer: Retching and vomiting and diarrhea is called sudden turmoil.

SYNOPSIS

The primary signs of sudden turmoil.

COMMENTARY

Sudden turmoil is characterized by alternating vomiting and diarrhea. It begins suddenly and changes rapidly and is an acute and severe disease pattern. The dynamic in these patterns is sudden and uncontrolled, 霍 *huò*, and chaotic, 乱 *luàn*. It is described as sudden and uncontrolled because of the degree of vomiting and diarrhea, and as chaotic because of the feeling of disquiet, and distention and pain in the heart and abdomen. Sudden turmoil is due to the following mechanism: "clear qì is in yīn, turbid qì is in yáng, the clear and turbid mutually offend, and chaos [arises] in the stomach and intestines." In this pattern the functions of the spleen and stomach become chaotic. The spleen cannot upbear the clear qì and diarrhea occurs. The stomach cannot downbear the turbid qì and vomiting occurs.

LINE 383

㈠ 问曰：病发热，头痛，身疼，恶寒，吐利者，此属何病？ ㈡ 答曰：此名霍乱。 ㈢ 霍乱自吐下，又利止，复更发热也。

(1) *Wèn yuē: bìng fā rè, tóu tòng, shēn téng, wù hán, tù lì zhě, cǐ shǔ hé bìng?* (2) *Dá yuē: cǐ míng huò luàn.* (3) *Huò luàn zì tù xià, yòu lì zhǐ, fù gèng fā rè yě.*

(1) Question: When [there is] illness with heat effusion, headache, generalized pain, aversion to cold, and vomiting and diarrhea, what disease is this? (2) Answer: This [disease] is called sudden turmoil. (3) [When in] sudden turmoil, [there is] spontaneous vomiting and diarrhea, and the diarrhea ceases, there will be even more heat effusion.

SYNOPSIS

a) The signs of sudden turmoil interior and exterior patterns.

b) Differentiation of sudden turmoil from cold damage.

Commentary

This line presents a pattern of sudden turmoil in which an exterior evil is present. Heat effusion, aversion to cold, headache, and generalized pain indicate a cold damage exterior pattern. If these signs are accompanied by severe diarrhea and vomiting, the pattern is called "sudden turmoil."

Spontaneous diarrhea and vomiting spring from the interior and are not the result of an exterior evil. Disease is present in the interior and the exterior; disharmony exists between the interior and exterior. This disharmony is reflected in the simultaneous appearance of a) diarrhea and vomiting, and b) heat effusion and aversion to cold. If the vomiting and diarrhea cease and the heat effusion continues, it means that although the interior has harmonized, the exterior has still not resolved.

Line 384

㈠ 伤寒，其脉微濇者，本是霍乱，今是伤寒， 却四五日，至阴经上，转入阴必利，本呕下利者，不可治也。 ㈡ 欲似大便，而反失气，仍不利者，此属阳明也，便必硬，十三日愈。 ㈢ 所以然者，经尽故也。 ㈣ 下利后，当便硬，硬则能食者愈。 ㈤ 今反不能食，到后经中，颇能食，复过一经能食，过之一日当愈。 ㈥ 不愈者，不属阳明也。

(1) *Shāng hán, qí mài wēi sè zhě, běn shì huò luàn, jīn shì shāng hán, què sì wǔ rì, zhì yīn jīng shàng, zhuǎn rù yīn bì lì, běn ǒu xià lì zhě, bù kě zhì yě.* (2) *Yù sì dà biàn, ér fǎn shī qì, réng bù lì zhě, cǐ shǔ yáng míng yě, biàn bì yìng, shí sān rì yù.* (3) *Suǒ yǐ rán zhě, jīng jìn gù yě.* (4) *Xià lì hòu, dāng biàn yìng, yìng zé néng shí zhě yù.* (5) *Jīn fǎn bù néng shí, dào hòu jīng zhōng, pǒ néng shí, fù guò yì jīng néng shí, guò zhī yí rì dāng yù.* (6) *Bù yù zhě, bù shǔ yáng míng yě.*

(1) When in cold damage, the pulse is faint and rough, originally [there] was sudden turmoil and now [there] is cold damage. However at four or five days, [the evil] is proceeding to the yīn channels and [when it] shifts into the yīn [channels] there will be diarrhea. The original [pattern with] retching and diarrhea cannot be treated. (2) When it seems [there is] about to be defecation but instead [there is] fecal qì and still no diarrhea, this belongs to yáng brightness. The stool will be hard and [there will be] recovery in thirteen days. (3) Why [this] is so is because [the evil] has gone through the channel. (4) After diarrhea, there should be hard stool. [When the patient has] hard [stool], and is able to eat, [he/she

will] recover. (5) But in the present [case], [the person] is unable to eat. After reaching the next channel, [the person] is to some extent able to eat. Passing through one more channel, [the person is] able to eat. The day of passage there should be recovery. (6) If [there is] no recovery, [the pattern] did not belong to yáng brightness.

SYNOPSIS

Differentiation of the pathomechanism, transmutations, and scenarios in sudden turmoil and cold damage.

COMMENTARY

In this pattern sudden turmoil changes to cold damage. In sudden turmoil, vomiting and diarrhea damage right qì and the fluids. Afterward, the patient contracts an exterior evil, which gives rise to signs such as heat effusion, aversion to cold, and headache. The pulse is weak and rough, not floating and tight, because right qì has already been damaged; hence the pulse is forceless. After four or five days, the evil enters the yīn channels and causes diarrhea. Previously, diarrhea occurred and, after the evil enters the yīn, it occurs again; consequently, right qì is extremely vacuous. Diarrhea can occur in both cold damage and sudden turmoil, but the timing of its occurrence is different. In cold damage, the patient contracts an evil and, generally, it is only after the passage of a number of days that diarrhea may begin. In sudden turmoil, at the onset of the disease severe diarrhea and vomiting are already present.

If the evil does not enter the yīn, diarrhea will not occur. The patient desires to defecate but is unable to do so and instead only expels gas. This means that the stomach qì is returning and right qì is overcoming evil qì. After the original diarrhea and vomiting, the fluids are damaged and the stomach and intestines are not moistened; the stool becomes hard and this pattern belongs to the yáng brightness. Thirteen days means the period of time for the complete passage of the channel qì; hence at the end of this time, the patient may spontaneously recover.

The final section of the line, from "After diarrhea" to the end of the line, discusses the prognosis. The designation of this pattern as belonging to the yáng brightness is not the same as "stomach domain repletion." The stool should be hard because of fluid damage, but this is not a pattern in which the stomach domain is replete because the bowel qì is still free and the stomach is in harmony. In this case, if the patient is able to eat, he/she will recover. If the patient is unable to eat, it means that the stomach qì has not yet returned. After a few days, if the patient's appetite is slightly improved, it means that the stomach qì is gradually returning and the patient should slowly recover. If following a short period of time he/she does not recover, it means that this pattern was not the result of fluid damage affecting the yáng brightness, and another pathomechanism must be sought.

LINE 385

恶寒脉微而复利，利止亡血也，四逆加人参汤主之。

Wù hán mài wēi ér fù lì, lì zhǐ wáng xuè yě, sì nì jiā rén shēn tāng zhǔ zhī.

When [there is] aversion to cold and a pulse that is faint, then diarrhea, and the diarrhea stops and [there is] blood collapse,* Counterflow Cold Decoction Plus Ginseng (*sì nì jiā rén shēn tāng*) governs.

TEXT NOTE

* Blood collapse, 血亡 *xuè wáng*: Interpreted as fluid collapse in this context. Chéng Wǔ-Jí writes, "Aversion to cold, a pulse that is weak, and diarrhea indicate yáng vacuity and prevailing yīn. [When] the diarrhea ceases, the interior fluids are exhausted; hence [it] says 'blood collapse.'"

FORMULA

Counterflow Cold Decoction Plus Ginseng (*sì nì jiā rén shēn tāng*)

○ Return yáng and stem counterflow; boost qì and engender liquid.

甘草二两（炙） 附子一枚（生，去皮，破八片） 干姜一两半 人参一两

右四味，以水三升，煮取一升二合，去滓，分温再服。

Gān cǎo èr liǎng (zhì) fù zǐ yī méi (shēng, qù pí, pò bā piàn) gān jiāng yī liǎng bàn rén shēn yī liǎng

Yòu sì wèi, yǐ shuǐ sān shēng, zhǔ qǔ yī shēng èr gě, qù zǐ, fēn wēn zài fú.

mix-fried licorice (甘草 *gān cǎo*, Glycyrrhizae Radix) 2 liǎng

aconite (附子 *fù zǐ*, Aconiti Tuber Laterale) 1 piece (raw, remove skin, break into eight pieces)

dried ginger (干姜 *gān jiāng*, Zingiberis Rhizoma Exsiccatum) 1.5 liǎng

ginseng (人参 *rén shēn*, Ginseng Radix) 1 liǎng

[For] the above four ingredients use three shēng of water. Boil to get one shēng two gě and remove the dregs. Divide [into two parts], and take warm twice a day.

SYNOPSIS

The signs and treatment of yáng collapse and fluid desertion from sudden turmoil with vomiting and diarrhea.

COMMENTARY

In this line, following the vomiting and diarrhea of sudden turmoil, the yáng qì is debilitated and yīn humor are exhausted. Aversion to cold, a pulse that is weak, and diarrhea indicate that the yáng qì is vacuous and the yīn evil is exuberant. This line presents a critical pattern of yáng debilitation. Diarrhea ceases because the yáng qì is vacuous, yīn humor are exhausted, and no stool remains in the body to be expelled.

When diarrhea ceases, the aversion to cold persists and the pulse is still weak. It is likely that these signs would be accompanied by counterflow cold of the extremities and other signs of yáng collapse and fluid desertion. This pattern should be differentiated from those in which diarrhea ceases because yáng is returning. When yáng returns, not only will the diarrhea cease, but the pulse should improve and the limbs should be warm.

Counterflow Cold Decoction Plus Ginseng (*sì nì jiā rén shēn tāng*) returns yáng and stems counterflow. It also boosts the qì and engenders fluids. This formula is Counterflow Cold Decoction (*sì nì tāng*) plus ginseng (*rén shēn*). Counterflow Cold Decoction (*sì nì tāng*) warms and supplements the spleen and stomach, and returns yáng and stems counterflow. The addition of ginseng (*rén shēn*) greatly supplements the original qì, secures desertion, engenders fluids, and helps to avoid further damage to yīn from the warm yáng medicinals. This formula may be used in patterns of yáng collapse and vacuity desertion in which both yīn and yáng are damaged, or it can be used in patterns of blood collapse and fluid exhaustion, as above.

LINE 386

霍乱，头痛发热，身疼痛，热多欲饮水者，五苓散主之；寒多不用水者，理中丸主之。

Huò luàn, tóu tòng fā rè, shēn téng tòng, rè duō yù yǐn shuǐ zhě, wǔ líng sǎn zhǔ zhī; hán duō bù yòng shuǐ zhě, lǐ zhōng wán zhǔ zhī.

When in sudden turmoil, [there is] headache, heat effusion, and generalized pain, [if there is] more heat and [the patient] desires to drink water, Poria (Hoelen) Five Powder (*wǔ líng sǎn*) governs; [but if there is] more cold and [the patient] does not drink water, Center-Rectifying Pill (*lǐ zhōng wán*) governs.

FORMULA
Poria (Hoelen) Five Powder (*wǔ líng sǎn*)

◦ Course the exterior and disinhibit the interior.

(See line 71, p. 195, for a complete discussion of the formula.)

FORMULA
Center-Rectifying Pill (*lǐ zhōng wán*)

◦ Warm the center and dissipate cold.

人参　干姜　甘草（炙）　白术各三两

㈠ 右四味，捣筛，蜜和为丸如鸡子黄许大，以沸汤数合和一丸，研碎，温服之，日三四、夜二服。㈡ 腹中未热，益至三四丸，然不及汤。㈢ 汤法：以四物依两数切，用水八升，煮取三升，去滓，温服一升，日三服。㈣ 若脐上筑者，肾气动也，去术加桂四两。㈤ 吐多者，去术加生姜三两。(六)下多者，还用术。(七)悸者，加茯苓二两。(八)渴欲得水者，加术，足前成四两半。(九)腹中痛者，加人参，足前成四两半。(十)寒者加干姜，足前成四两半。(十一)腹满者，去术加附子一枚。(十二)服汤后，如食顷，饮热粥一升许，微自温，勿发揭衣被。

Rén shēn gān jiāng gān cǎo (zhì) bái zhú gè sān liǎng

(1) *Yòu sì wèi, dǎo shāi, mì huò wéi wán rú jī zǐ huáng xǔ dà, yǐ fèi tāng shù gě huò yī wán, yán suì, wēn fú zhī, rì sān sì、 yè èr fú.* (2) *Fù zhōng wèi rè, yì zhì sān sì wán, rán bù jí tāng.* (3) *Tāng fǎ: yǐ sì wù yī liǎng shù qiē, yòng shuǐ bā shēng, zhǔ qǔ sān shēng, qù zǐ, wēn fú yī shēng, rì sān fú.* (4) *Ruò qí shàng zhú zhě, shèn qì dòng yě, qù zhú jiā guì sì liǎng.* (5) *Tù duō zhě, qù zhú jiā shēng jiāng sān liǎng.* (6) *Xià duō zhě, huán yòng zhú.* (7) *Jì zhě, jiā fú qín èr liǎng.* (8) *Kě yù dé shuǐ zhě, jiā zhú, zú qián chéng sì liǎng bàn.* (9) *Fù zhōng tòng zhě, jiā rén shēn, zú qián chéng sì liǎng bàn.* (10) *Hán zhě jiā gān jiāng, zú qián chéng sì liǎng bàn.* (11) *Fù mǎn zhě, qù zhú jiā fù zǐ yī méi.* (12) *Fú tāng hòu, rú shí qǐng, yǐn rè zhōu yī shēng xǔ, wēi zì wēn, wù fā jiē yī bèi.*

ginseng (人参 *rén shēn*, Ginseng Radix)
dried ginger (干姜 *gān jiāng*, Zingiberis Rhizoma Exsiccatum)
mix-fried licorice (甘草 *gān cǎo*, Glycyrrhizae Radix)
ovate atractylodes (白术 *bái zhú*, Atractylodis Ovatae Rhizoma)
each 3 liǎng

(1) [For] the above four ingredients, pound and sieve, [then] mix with honey to make pills about the size of a chicken's egg yolk. Use several gě of boiling water, mix in one pill, crush and take warm. [Take] three or four [times] a day, and twice at night. (2) If [there is] still no heat in the abdomen, [take] up to three or four more pills. However, [the preceeding method] is not as good as a decoction. (3) For the decoction method: take the four ingredients in the amounts suggested above and cut. Use eight shēng of water and boil to get three shēng. Remove the dregs and take one shēng warm, three times a day. (4) If [there is] pounding above the umbilicus, the kidney qì has been stirred and [one should] remove ovate atractylodes ([*bái*] *zhú*) and add 4 liǎng of cinnamon twig (*guì* [*zhī*]). (5) [For] excessive vomiting, remove ovate atractylodes ([*bái*] *zhú*) and add 3 liǎng of fresh ginger (*shēng jiāng*). (6) [For] excessive diarrhea, still use ovate atractylodes ([*bái*] *zhú*). (7) [For] palpitations, add 2 liǎng of poria (*fú líng*). (8) [For] thirst with a desire to drink water, add ovate atractylodes ([*bái*] *zhú*) to the previous [amount] to make 4.5 liǎng. (9) [For] pain in the abdomen, add ginseng (*rén shēn*) to the previous [amount] to make 4.5 liǎng. (10) [For] cold, add dried ginger (*gān jiāng*) to the previous [amount] to make 4.5 liǎng. (11) [For] abdominal fullness, remove ovate atractylodes ([*bái*] *zhú*) and add one piece of aconite (*fù zǐ*). (12) After taking the decoction, [wait] about the time it takes to eat a meal, [then] drink about one shēng of hot gruel to warm oneself slightly. Do not remove the clothes and bedclothes.

SYNOPSIS

Differentiation of the signs and treatment of sudden turmoil disease with exterior and interior cold and heat.

COMMENTARY

Sudden turmoil is characterized by alternating vomiting and diarrhea. If these signs are accompanied by headache, heat effusion, and generalized pain, it indicates the presence of an unresolved exterior evil. This line presents a pattern of simultaneous disease of the exterior and interior. One must analyze the disease pattern and determine what method should be used to address these two conditions.

If heat is predominant, as suggested by a desire to drink water, it means that the exterior evil is unresolved and disharmony exists in the interior. Because Poria (Hoelen) Five Powder (*wǔ líng sǎn*) is used to treat this pattern, one knows that a water evil is present in the interior, causing an inhibition of the qì dynamic; consequently, the clear and the turbid are not moving properly. Poria (Hoelen) Five Powder (*wǔ líng sǎn*) courses the exterior and disinhibits the interior. It treats the exterior and interior simultaneously.

If the cold is predominant and the patient has no desire to drink, it means that the evil has entered the yīn portion. The suggestion of Center-Rectifying Pill (*lǐ zhōng wán*) suggests the presence of yáng vacuity cold affecting the center burner, giving rise to exuberant cold and dampness in the interior, and disturbing transformation and movement.

Center-Rectifying Pill (*lǐ zhōng wán*) warms the center, dissipates cold, and rectifies yīn and yáng in order to restore normal upbearing and downbearing. Ginseng (*rén shēn*) and mix-fried licorice (*gān cǎo*) supplement the spleen and boost the qì. Dried ginger (*gān jiāng*) and ovate atractylodes (*bái zhú*) warm and transform cold-damp. Once the spleen yáng is roused, the cold and dampness will be eliminated. Normal upbearing of the clear and downbearing of the turbid will then be restored and vomiting and diarrhea will cease. Center-Rectifying Pill (*lǐ zhōng wán*) is the primary formula for treating greater yīn vacuity cold patterns. It may be used as a decoction or in pill form. The decoction is appropriate for severe and acute patterns; the pills are better for long-term use.

After taking Center-Rectifying Pill (*lǐ zhōng wán*), cold sensations in the abdomen should be replaced by a feeling of warmth. This change substantiates that the formula is appropriate and its use can be continued. If no feeling of warmth occurs, it may be a sign that the formula is not strong enough for the severity of the pattern. The dosage may then be increased or the decoction may be used instead.

In order to increase the effect of the medicinals for warming and nourishing the center burner, about an hour after taking the pills the patient should eat a bowl of hot gruel.

For stirring in the abdomen, which indicates kidney vacuity cold with water qì, ovate atractylodes (*bái zhú*) is removed to prevent it from causing stagnation, and cinnamon twig (*guì zhī*) is added to warm yáng and control water. Excessive vomiting indicates rheum evil is harassing the stomach. Ovate atractylodes (*bái zhú*) is removed because of its upbearing and supplementing actions, and fresh ginger (*shēng jiāng*) is added to harmonize the stomach, downbear counterflow, and dissipate rheum. Excessive diarrhea indicates that spleen yáng is unable to upbear and dampness is pouring downward. Ovate atractylodes (*bái zhú*) is kept in the formula in order to fortify the spleen and dry dampness. For palpitations below the heart in which water qì intimidates the heart, poria (*fú líng*), which quells water, is added. Thirst and a desire to drink, in this case, indicate that spleen movement is impaired and fluids are not being distributed properly. Ovate atractylodes (*bái zhú*), which fortifies the spleen and transforms dampness, is added to restore fluid distribution. Abdominal pain that improves when pressure is applied indicates vacuity in the center burner; hence a large dose of ginseng (*rén shēn*) is used to supplement vacuity and relieve pain. Cold pain in the abdomen indicates spleen vacuity and more severe interior cold; hence dried ginger (*gān jiāng*) is added to warm the center and dissipate cold. For abdominal fullness, which indicates yáng vacuity and congealed cold with stagnant qì, ovate atractylodes (*bái zhú*) is removed because of its stagnating qualities; aconite (*fù zǐ*) is added to free yáng and expel cold.

Line 387

吐利止而身痛不休者，当消息和解其外，宜桂枝汤小和之。

Tù lì zhǐ ér shēn tòng bù xiū zhě, dāng xiāo xī hé jiě qí wài, yí guì zhī tāng xiǎo hě zhī.

When vomiting and diarrhea cease and [there is] persistent generalized pain, after considering* [the patient's condition], resolve the exterior [accordingly]. Cinnamon Twig Decoction (*guì zhī tāng*) is appropriate for mildly resolving.

Text Note

* After considering, 消息 *xiāo xī*: One should stop and consider the appropriate action.

Synopsis

The signs and treatment of sudden turmoil in which the interior is harmonized and the exterior has not resolved.

Commentary

In this pattern the interior is in harmony and the exterior is still unresolved. Vomiting and diarrhea cease, indicating that upbearing and downbearing have returned to normal. The sudden turmoil pattern has already ceased and the disease progression is towards recovery. Nonetheless, the presence of generalized pain suggests disharmony between the construction and defense and an unresolved exterior pattern. At this point, Zhāng Jī suggests that one should pause in the treatment and consider the next step carefully. Then, if one is convinced of the diagnosis, Cinnamon Twig Decoction (*guì zhī tāng*) can be used to resolve the exterior pattern.

Cinnamon Twig Decoction (*guì zhī tāng*) is used in this pattern for several reasons. The first is that vomiting and diarrhea have already damaged right qì and weakened the spleen and stomach. Ephedra Decoction (*má huáng tāng*) is too harsh to be used with this degree of vacuity. Furthermore, the evil is already moving outward and strong sweating is not required. This pattern requires the use of a moderate formula to resolve the exterior without further damaging the qì.

LINE 388

吐利汗出，发热恶寒，四肢拘急，手足厥冷者，四逆汤主之。

Tù lì hàn chū, fā rè wù hán, sì zhī jū jí, shǒu zú jué lěng zhě, sì nì tāng zhǔ zhī.

When [there is] vomiting and diarrhea, sweating, heat effusion and aversion to cold, hypertonicity of the limbs, and reversal cold of the extremities, Counterflow Cold Decoction (*sì nì tāng*) governs.

SYNOPSIS

The signs and treatment of vomiting and diarrhea in yáng collapse.

COMMENTARY

In this pattern, the vomiting and diarrhea of sudden turmoil damage the yáng qì, and result in exuberant yīn cold in the interior with vacuous yáng collapsing outward. Yīn humor is also damaged as a result of the vomiting and diarrhea and the result is a pattern of yáng collapse and fluid desertion.

In patterns of yáng vacuity and exuberant yīn cold, sweating may occur because the yáng qì is insecure. Furthermore, vacuous yáng floats outward and causes heat effusion. Counterflow cold of the limbs is a result of the inability of vacuous yáng qì to warm the limbs. In this pattern, vomiting, diarrhea, and sweating not only damages yáng qì, but also the yīn humor. The sinews and the vessels lose normal moistening and the limbs become hypertonic. In the *Líng Shū* it is written, "In liquid desertion, the interstices are open and great sweat discharges. In humor desertion, extension of the bones is inhibited."

Although in this pattern both yīn and yáng are damaged, the yáng vacuity is considered to be more severe; therefore, Counterflow Cold Decoction (*sì nì tāng*) is used to rescue yáng because once yáng qì is secure, yīn humor will be constrained.

LINE 389

既吐且利，小便复利，而大汗出，下利清谷，内寒外热，脉微欲绝者，四逆汤主之。

Jì tù qiě lì, xiǎo biàn fù lì, ér dà hàn chū, xià lì qīng gǔ, nèi hán wài rè, mài wēi yù jué zhě, sì nì tāng zhǔ zhī.

When [there is] vomiting as well as diarrhea, then uninhibited urination, and great sweating, clear-food diarrhea, internal cold and external heat, and the pulse is faint and verging on expiry, Counterflow Cold Decoction (*sì nì tāng*) governs.

SYNOPSIS

The signs and treatment of interior cold and exterior heat after vomiting.

Commentary

This line presents a pattern of exuberant yīn cold in the interior and vacuous yáng straying to the exterior. When the spleen and kidney yáng are debilitated, movement and transformation are impaired. Yīn cold causes qì counterflow and alternating vomiting and clear-food diarrhea. Yáng qì is severely damaged and the fleshy exterior is insecure, which gives rise to great sweating. Damage to both yáng and yīn causes the pulse to become weak to the point that it is about to expire. "Internal cold" refers to exuberant yīn in the interior, and this evil forces vacuous yáng to the exterior. Vacuous yáng is referred to here as "external heat."

One of the unique characteristics of this pattern is that urination is uninhibited. Following damage to the fluids from vomiting and diarrhea, it is expected that urination would be short, scant, and inhibited. The fact that it is not indicates yáng collapse. When kidney yáng is vacuous, it cannot perform its office of securing and containing; consequently, urination is uninhibited. Counterflow Cold Decoction (*sì nì tāng*), which stems counterflow and returns yáng, is used to constrain the fluids.

Line 390

吐已下断，汗出而厥，四肢拘急不解，脉微欲绝者，通脉四逆加猪胆汤主之。

Tù yǐ xià duàn, hàn chū ér jué, sì zhī jū jí bù jiě, mài wēi yù jué zhě, tōng mài sì nì jiā zhū dǎn tāng zhǔ zhī.

When the vomiting has ceased and the diarrhea has stopped, [but there is] sweating and reversal, unresolved hypertonicity of the limbs, and a pulse that is faint and verging on expiry, Vessel-Freeing Counterflow Cold Decoction Plus Pig's Bile (*tōng mài sì nì jiā zhū dǎn (zhī) tāng*) governs.

Formula

Vessel-Freeing Counterflow Cold Decoction Plus Pig's Bile (*tōng mài sì nì jiā zhū dǎn (zhī) tāng*)

◦ Return yáng and stem counterflow; boost yīn and harmonize yáng.

甘草二两（炙） 干姜三两（强人可四两） 附子大者一枚（生，去皮，破八片） 猪胆汁半合

右四味，以水三升，煮取一升二合，去滓，内猪胆汁，分温再服，其脉即来，无猪胆，以羊胆代之。

Gān cǎo èr liǎng (zhì) gān jiāng sān liǎng (qiáng rén kě sì liǎng) fù zǐ dà zhě yī méi (shēng, qù pí, pò bā piàn) zhū dǎn zhī bàn gě

Yòu sì wèi, yǐ shuǐ sān shēng, zhǔ qǔ yī shēng èr gě, qù zǐ, nà zhū dǎn zhī, fēn wēn zài fú, qí mài jí lái, wú zhū dǎn, yǐ yáng dǎn dài zhī.

mix-fried licorice (甘草 *gān cǎo*, Glycyrrhizae Radix) 2 liǎng

dried ginger (干姜 *gān jiāng*, Zingiberis Rhizoma Exsiccatum) 3 liǎng (strong people can [be given] 4 liǎng)

aconite (附子 *fù zǐ*, Aconiti Tuber Laterale) 1 large piece (raw, remove skin, break into eight pieces)

pig's bile (猪胆汁 *zhū dǎn zhī*, Suis Bilis) half gě

[For] the four ingredients above, use three shēng of water. Boil [the first three ingredients] to get one shēng two gě and remove the dregs. Add pig's bile (*zhū dǎn zhī*). Divide [into two parts], and take warm twice a day. The pulse will then return. [If there is] no pig's gallbladder (*zhū dǎn*), goat's gallbladder (*yáng dǎn*) [can be] substituted.

SYNOPSIS

The signs and treatment of sudden turmoil vomiting and diarrhea with yáng collapse and yīn exhaustion.

COMMENTARY

In this pattern, as a result of vomiting and diarrhea yáng qì is debilitated and yīn humor is exhausted. After the vomiting and diarrhea have ceased, if the extremities become warm and the pulse is harmonious, it means that the yáng qì is returning, the yīn evil is dissipating, and recovery will soon occur. In the text above, the vomiting and diarrhea have ceased, but reverse-flow of the extremities, hypertonicity of the limbs, sweating, and a pulse that is about to expire are observed. These signs do not indicate the return of yáng, but instead indicate that the qì and blood are vacuous and yīn humor is exhausted.

In this pattern, signs of yáng and yīn expiry already exist. If one does not use an acrid, warm formula, it will be insufficient to return yáng, but this type of formula may stir the floating yáng and damage the remaining yīn humor. Therefore, Vessel-Freeing Counterflow Cold Decoction Plus Pig's Bile (*tōng mài sì nì jiā zhū dǎn (zhī) tāng*) is used to return the yáng qì and break the yīn evil, while also boosting yīn.

This pattern is similar to the one for which Counterflow Cold Decoction Plus Ginseng (*sì nì jiā rén shēn tāng*) is used. Both patterns belong to yáng collapse and yīn exhaustion, but differ in severity. In the pattern associated with Counterflow Cold Decoction Plus Ginseng (*sì nì jiā rén shēn tāng*), aversion to cold, reverse flow, and a pulse that is weak begin after the diarrhea ceases. The pattern above is considered more severe given that after the diarrhea and vomiting cease, sweating, reverse-flow, hypertonicity of the limbs, and a pulse that is about to expire are observed. This is a more severe pattern of yáng collapse and yīn exhaustion with mutual repelling of yīn and yáng.

Vessel-Freeing Counterflow Cold Decoction (*tōng mài sì nì tāng*) breaks yīn cold evil and returns deserting yáng. The addition of pig's bile (*zhū dǎn zhī*) has several actions. It boosts yīn and enriches the fluids, in order to supplement yīn damaged by vomiting and diarrhea. At the same time, it assists in preventing damage to yīn from the acrid, hot medicinals used to return yáng. Furthermore, pig's bile (*zhū dǎn zhī*) has a cold nature and is able to conduct the hot yáng medicinals into yīn. This helps prevent the repulsion of the hot medicinals by the exuberant yīn cold.

LINE 391

吐利发汗，脉平，小烦者，以新虚不胜谷气故也。

Tù lì fā hàn, mài píng, xiǎo fán zhě, yǐ xīn xū bù shèng gǔ qì gù yě.

When [there is] vomiting and diarrhea and sweating is promoted, the pulse is calm, and [there is] mild vexation because of the new vacuity, [the body] cannot overcome grain qì.

SYNOPSIS

Following sudden turmoil, one must pay attention to regulation of dietary intake.

COMMENTARY

The vomiting and diarrhea in this line represent a pattern of sudden turmoil. After this type of illness, when the pulse becomes harmonious, it means that the evil has been eliminated and both the interior and exterior are in harmony. Normal downbearing and upbearing has been restored and recovery should follow. Following sudden turmoil, "new vacuity" means that the spleen and stomach are still weak and unable to transform food. Vexation reflects the struggle of the weak center burner to move and transform grain qì. In this pattern one must carefully regulate the diet and should not treat the vexation as if it were the result of residual or bound evil qì.

Chapter Eight

Yīn-Yáng Exchange and Taxation Relapse

Pulses and Signs; Treatment

辨阴阳易差後劳复病脉证并治

1 OVERVIEW

This chapter discusses lifestyle during recuperation, prevention of relapse, and consolidation of treatment effect. After a major illness, when yīn and yáng are not yet balanced, qì and blood have not fully returned, and residual evil qì has not yet been eliminated, incautious activities can result in taxation relapse.

The first line of this chapter concerns sexual transmission of disease, what in the text is called "yīn-yáng exchange." Following a major illness, when the patient has not fully recovered, sexual intercourse can lead to a pattern of generalized heaviness, shortage of qì, lesser abdominal urgency, genital spasms, heat ascending and insulting the chest, heaviness of the head, flowery vision, and hypertonicity of the knee and lower leg. This pattern is treated with Burnt Pants Decoction (*shāo kūn sǎn*).

Taxation relapse patterns occur when, following a major illness, the patient does not properly attend to regulating activities and food intake in order to consolidate the treatment effect. If there is relapse with signs such as heat vexation, glomus, and fullness, the appropriate formula is Unripe Bitter Orange, Gardenia, and Fermented Soybean Decoction (*zhǐ shí zhī zǐ chǐ tāng*). In this pattern, if abdominal fullness is accompanied by inability to defecate, one can add rhubarb (*dà huáng*).

After recovery from an illness, if heat effusion recurs, the evil is in the exterior and one can promote sweating in order to resolve the exterior. If there is repletion heat, precipitation can be employed. If exterior and interior signs are absent, harmonization can be employed using Minor Bupleurum Decoction (*xiǎo chái hú tāng*). If one observes water qì below the lumbus, the appropriate formula is Oyster Shell and Alisma Powder (*mǔ lì zé xiè sǎn*), which disinhibits urination and expels water evil. For cold above the chest with frequent spitting, use Center-Rectifying Pill (*lǐ zhōng wán*) to warm. Vacuity and marked emaciation, shortage of qì, and qì counterflow with a desire to vomit is treated with Bamboo Leaf and Gypsum Decoction (*zhú yè shí gāo tāng*), which clears vacuity heat, and boosts qì and engenders liquid.

2 YĪN-YÁNG EXCHANGE

Line 392

伤寒阴［阳］易之为病，其人身体重，少气，少腹里急，或引阴中拘挛，热上冲胸，头重不欲举，眼中生花，膝胫拘急者，烧裈散主之。

Shāng hán yīn [yáng] yì zhī wéi bìng, qí rén shēn tǐ zhòng, shǎo qì, shào fù lǐ jí, huò yǐn yīn zhōng jū luán, rè shàng chōng xiōng, tóu zhòng bù yù jǔ, yǎn zhōng shēng huā, xī jìng jū jí zhě, shāo kūn sǎn zhǔ zhī.

When in the disease [pattern] of cold damage with yīn[-yáng] exchange,[1] the person has generalized heaviness, shortage of qì, lesser abdominal urgency, or it causes hypertonicity of the yīn,[2] heat ascending and insulting the chest, heaviness of the head with no desire to lift it, flowery vision,[3] and hypertonicity of the knee and lower leg, Burnt Pants Powder (*shāo kūn sǎn*) governs.

Text Notes

1. Yīn-[yáng] exchange, 阴［阳］易 *yīn [yáng] yì*: Interaction between yīn-female and yáng-male, as in sexual intercourse. The word "yáng" is missing from the Sòng version.
2. Hypertonicity of the yīn, 阴中拘挛 *yīn zhōng jū luán*: Spasms in the genitals.
3. Flowery vision, 眼中生花 *yǎn zhōng shēng huā*: This is a general term embracing various kinds of visual disturbances such as blurring, distortion, floaters, and nearsightedness. It is the same as 眼花 *yǎn huā*.

Formula

Burnt Pants Powder (*shāo kūn sǎn*)

○ Abduct the evil outward.

妇人中裈，近隐处，取烧作灰。

(一) 右一味，水服方寸匕，日三服，小便即利，阴头微肿，此为愈矣。(二) 妇人病，取男子裈烧服。

Fù rén zhōng kūn, jìn yǐn chù, qǔ shāo zuò huī

(1) *Yòu yī wèi, shuǐ fú fāng cùn bǐ, rì sān fú, xiǎo biàn jí lì, yīn tóu wēi zhǒng, cǐ wéi yù yǐ.* (2) *Fù rén bìng, qǔ nán zǐ kūn shāo fú.*

The part of a woman's pants close to the hidden part,[1] charred

(1) [For] the above one ingredient take a square-inch-spoonful with water, three times a day. [When] urination is uninhibited and the yīn head[2] [becomes] slightly swollen, this indicates recovery. (2) [For a] woman [with this] disease, use charred men's pants..

FORMULA NOTE

1. Close to the hidden part, 隐处 *yǐn chù*: The crotch.
2. Yīn head, 阴头 *yīn tóu*: The glans penis.

SYNOPSIS

The signs and treatment of yīn-yáng exchange.

COMMENTARY

This line provides further commentary on patterns that may follow recovery from illness. After recovery, because of the general state of vacuity, one must be cautious in daily life and eat properly to avoid a relapse. These suggestions also include prudence in sexual relations. In this pattern, disease may be passed from yīn-female to yáng-male or from yáng-male to yīn-female.

Sexual activity most easily damages the essential qì and the signs of generalized heaviness and shortage of qì reflect insufficiency of essential qì. Abdominal urgency, hypertonicity of the yīn, and hypertonicity of the knee and lower leg reflect damage to the yīn aspect and loss of normal nourishment to the sinews and vessels. Residual heat from cold damage enters the yīn and toxic heat from the lower burner attacks upward, causing a feeling of heat ascending and insulting the chest, heaviness of the head with no desire to lift it, and flowery vision.

Xiāo Kāng-Bǎi (肖康伯) provides another perspective on the meaning of this line.

> With regard to "yīn-yáng exchange" disease in the *Shāng Hán Lùn*, most commentators have suggested that a newly recovered patient transmits the disease to a person without disease during sexual intercourse. Thus, this disease is referred to as yīn-yáng exchange. Careful inspection of the original text, however, reveals that it does not say following recovery, nor does it say that the disease has already resolved; therefore, why should we explain this as following recent recovery? If [the patient] has already recovered from the disease, how can it then be transmitted to another person? Why should transmission of the disease occur through sexual intercourse and not via some other route? There are contradictions between the original text and the explanations. Recently, I read an explanation of this problem written by Chén Bǎi-Tán (陈伯坛, style 山农 Shān-Nóng). He writes, "speaking of cold damage, generally we are referring to the early [stages] of greater yáng disease. Early in greater yáng disease, the disease dynamic has not yet fully broken out. If at this time one has sexual relations, the lesser yīn first [becomes] vacuous. The greater yáng evil exploits this vacuity and invades the lesser yīn. Therefore, the signs that appear in yīn-yáng exchange are primarily those of lesser yīn vacuity. What is called 'yīn-yáng exchange' is greater yáng disease shifting into the lesser yīn. This is also to say that in this case of greater yáng disease transmuting into yīn-yáng exchange disease, the problem of mode of transmission does not exist. Yīn-yáng exchange is a disease name.... In this case, yīn and yáng refer to yīn channels and yáng channels, not to male and female.'

Burnt Pants Powder (*shāo kūn sǎn*) abducts the evil outwards. Charred pants do not appear in the traditional materia medica, but information about their use has been passed down through the generations. This ingredient is reported to have the ability to vanquish turbidity.

3 TAXATION RELAPSE

Line 393

大病差后，劳复者，枳实栀子豉汤主之。

Dà bìng chài hòu, láo fù zhě, zhǐ shí zhī zǐ chǐ tāng zhǔ zhī.

When after a major illness is cured, [there is] taxation relapse,* Unripe Bitter Orange, Gardenia, and Fermented Soybean Decoction (*zhǐ shí zhī zǐ chǐ tāng*) governs.

Text Note

* Taxation relapse, 劳复 *láo fù*: Recurrence of a disease due to fatigue. Before qì and blood have returned to normal or when residual heat is still present, physical exertion, or dietary or sexual intemperance, can damage right qì and cause a relapse of the disease.

Formula

Unripe Bitter Orange, Gardenia, and Fermented Soybean Decoction (*zhǐ shí zhī zǐ chǐ tāng*)

∘ Clear heat and eliminate vexation; loosen the center and move qì.

枳实三枚（炙） 栀子十四个（擘） 豉一升（绵裹）

(一) 右三味，以清浆水七升，空煮取四升，内枳实、栀子，煮取二升，下豉，更煮五六沸，去滓，温分再服。(二) 覆令微似汗。(三) 若有宿食者，内大黄如博棋子五六枚，服之愈。

Zhǐ shí sān méi (zhì) zhī zǐ shí sì ge (bò) chǐ yī shēng (mián guǒ)

(1) *Yòu sān wèi, yǐ qīng jiāng shuǐ qī shēng, kōng zhǔ qǔ sì shēng, nà zhǐ shí、zhī zǐ, zhǔ qǔ èr shēng, xià chǐ, gèng zhǔ wǔ liù fèi, qù zǐ, wēn fēn zài fú.* (2) *Fù lìng wēi sì hàn.* (3) *Ruò yǒu sù shí zhě, nà dà huáng rú bó qí zǐ wǔ liù méi, fú zhī yù.*

unripe bitter orange (枳实 *zhǐ shí*, Aurantii Fructus Immaturus) 3 pieces (mix-fried)
gardenia (栀子 *zhī zǐ*, Gardeniae Fructus) 14 pieces (broken)
fermented soybean (香豉 *xiāng chǐ*, Glycines Semen Fermentatum) 1 shēng (cotton-wrapped)

(1) [For] the above three ingredients use seven shēng of clear starch water.* Boil without [any ingredients] to get four shēng. Add unripe bitter orange (*zhǐ shí*) and gardenia (*zhī zǐ*) and boil to get two shēng. Add fermented soybean (*xiāng chǐ*) and boil five or six more times. Remove the dregs. Divide [into two parts], and take warm twice a day. (2) Cover [with bedclothes] to obtain slight sweating. (3) If [there is]

abiding food add five or six pieces of rhubarb (*dà huáng*) about the size of a go stone. [See line 107, p. 439, for this measurement.] [After] taking [there will be] recovery.

FORMULA NOTE

* Clear starch water, 清浆水 *qīng jiāng shuǐ*: Wú Yí-Luò writes, "Another name is 'sour starch water.' Cook millet [until] thoroughly cooked. Put into cold water and steep for five or six days [until] the odor is sour and it engenders "flowers" and the color is starchy; hence [it gets its] name." Xú Dà Chūn writes, "'Starch water' means the sieved water from washing rice [which is] stored for a period [until] the odor is sour, [then] [it is] ready."

SYNOPSIS

The treatment of taxation relapse.

COMMENTARY

After recovery from an illness, when right qì is still vacuous, yīn and yáng are not yet harmonized, the blood and qì have not yet returned, the residual heat has not yet been cleared, and the stomach and spleen are not yet in harmony, one must be cautious in everyday life and regulate the diet to avoid relapse of the disease. If one exerts oneself to the point of fatigue, the disease may relapse and heat effusion may recur, in a pattern called "taxation relapse." The signs of this pattern are not elaborated in the text, but from analyzing the formula, we can imagine that some of the following signs would be seen: heart vexation, anguish in the heart, heat effusion, glomus below the heart, and abdominal distention and fullness. This is a pattern of depressed heat in the chest and diaphragm, and congestion of the qì dynamic. Unripe Bitter Orange, Gardenia, and Fermented Soybean Decoction (*zhǐ shí zhī zǐ chǐ tāng*) is used to clear heat and eliminate vexation, move qì and disperse glomus.

Unripe Bitter Orange, Gardenia, and Fermented Soybean Decoction (*zhǐ shí zhī zǐ chǐ tāng*) is based on Gardenia and Fermented Soybean Decoction (*zhī zǐ chǐ tāng*) with the addition of unripe bitter orange (*zhǐ shí*) and an increase in the amount of fermented soybean (*xiāng chǐ*). Gardenia (*zhī zǐ*) drains heat and eliminates vexation. A large amount of fermented soybean (*xiāng chǐ*) diffuses and outthrusts the evil. These two ingredients diffuse evil heat, resolve depression, and eliminate vexation. Unripe bitter orange (*zhǐ shí*) loosens the center, moves the qì, and disperses glomus. Clear starch water is cool and penetrating; it clears heat and eliminates vexation, rectifies the qì, loosens the center, opens the stomach and transforms stagnation, and assists in dispersing the glomus. If abiding food is present, rhubarb (*dà huáng*) can be added to flush the stomach and intestines.

This pattern is similar to the pattern for which Gardenia and Magnolia Bark Decoction (*zhī zǐ hòu pò tāng*) is given. Both patterns involve depressed heat in the chest and diaphragm, and qì bind, but in the Gardenia and Magnolia Bark Decoction (*zhī zǐ hòu pò tāng*) pattern, qì stagnation in the abdomen gives rise to heart vexation, abdominal fullness, and disquiet sitting and lying. In the pattern above, the qì stagnation is more in the chest and less in the abdomen. These two formulae are very similar, only differing by one ingredient. In Gardenia and Magnolia Bark Decoction (*zhī zǐ hòu pò tāng*), the diffusing action of fermented soybean (*xiāng chǐ*) is not considered necessary, and magnolia bark (*hòu pò*) and unripe bitter orange (*zhǐ shí*) are combined to move qì, loosen the center, and dissipate fullness and eliminate distention. Unripe Bitter Orange, Gardenia, and Fermented Soybean Decoction (*zhǐ shí zhī zǐ chǐ tāng*) contains a large amount of fermented soybean (*xiāng chǐ*) to clear and diffuse depressed heat in the chest and diaphragm. It is combined with unripe bitter orange (*zhǐ shí*), which discharges fullness, and clear starch water, which regulates the center and harmonizes the stomach.

Line 394

㈠ 伤寒差以后，更发热，小柴胡汤主之。㈡ 脉浮者，以汗解之，脉沉实者，以下解之。

(1) *Shāng hán chài yǐ hòu, gèng fā rè, xiǎo chái hú tāng zhǔ zhī.*
(2) *Mài fú zhě, yǐ hàn jiě zhī, mài chén shí zhě, yǐ xià jiě zhī.*

(1) [When] after cold damage is cured, [there is] heat effusion again, Minor Bupleurum Decoction (*xiǎo chái hú tāng*) governs. (2) If the pulse is floating, [the promotion of] sweating [will] resolve [the disease and] if the pulse is sunken and replete, precipitation [will] resolve [the disease].

Synopsis

An example of the treatment of heat effusion that again occurs after an illness has been cured.

Commentary

Following recovery from a cold damage disease, if heat effusion occurs again one must carefully analyze the situation. It may be that a residual heat evil has not been completely eliminated or it may be a pattern of taxation relapse due to lifestyle or dietary irregularities. Because different pathomechanisms can produce heat effusion following recovery, one must investigate the pulse in order to decide on the appropriate treatment.

Following recovery, if interior and exterior signs are absent, and only heat effusion from residual heat is present, one may use Minor Bupleurum Decoction (*xiǎo chái hú tāng*) to harmonize the pivot mechanism. It courses and harmonizes, supports the right, and eliminates the evil. If the pulse is floating, it indicates an unresolved exterior evil, and the promotion of sweating is appropriate. If the pulse is sunken and replete, it indicates stagnation in the interior; hence precipitation should be used.

This line presents three methods that may be used to treat heat effusion after recovery from an illness. These methods are harmonizing, promoting sweating, and precipitating. This line cannot be considered to cover all transmuted patterns that may occur following recovery from an illness, but the spirit of the line is in pattern identification and treatment determination, not the specific methods that are indicated.

Line 395

大病差后，从腰以下有水气者，牡蛎泽泻散主之。

Dà bìng chài hòu, cóng yāo yǐ xià yǒu shuǐ qì zhě, mǔ lì zé xiè sǎn zhǔ zhī.

When after a major illness has been cured, [there is] water qì from the lumbus down, Oyster Shell and Alisma Powder (*mǔ lì zé xiè sǎn*) governs.

Formula

Oyster Shell and Alisma Powder (*mǔ lì zé xiè sǎn*)

∘ Clear heat and expel water.

牡蛎（熬） 泽泻 蜀漆（暖水洗去腥） 葶苈子（熬） 商陆根（熬） 海藻（洗去咸） 栝楼根各等分

(一)右七味，异捣，下筛为散，更于臼中治之，白饮和，服方寸匕，日三服。(二)小便利，止后服。

Mǔ lì (áo) zé xiè shǔ qī (nuǎn shuǐ xǐ qù xīng) tíng lì zǐ (áo) shāng lù gēn (áo) hǎi zǎo (xǐ qù xián) guā lóu gēn gè děng fēn

(1) *Yòu qī wèi, yì dǎo, xià shāi wéi sǎn, gèng yú jiù zhōng zhì zhī, bái yǐn huò, fú fāng cùn bǐ, rì sān fú.* (2) *Xiǎo biàn lì, zhǐ hòu fú.*

oyster shell (牡蛎 *mǔ lì*, Ostreae Concha) (dry-fry)
alisma (泽泻 *zé xiè*, Alismatis Rhizoma)
dichroa leaf (蜀漆 *shǔ qī*, Dichroae Folium) (wash with warm water to eliminate fishy smell)
tingli (葶苈子 *tíng lì zǐ*, Descurainiae seu Lepidii Semen) (dry-fry)
phytolacca (商陆根 *shāng lù gēn*, Phytolaccae Radix) (dry-fry)
sargassum (海藻 *hǎi zǎo*, Sargassi Herba) (wash to eliminate salt)
trichosanthes root (栝楼根 *guā lóu gēn*, Trichosanthis Radix)

[Use] equal parts [of each ingredient].

(1) [For] the above seven ingredients pound separately and sieve into a powder. Work [the powder] in a mortar to blend with a white [rice] cool decoction. Take a square-inch-spoonful three times a day. (2) [If] urination is uninhibited cease taking [the decoction].

Synopsis

The treatment of water qì from the lumbus down after an illness has been cured.

Commentary

Following recovery from an illness, the appearance of water qì can be a sign of vacuity or repletion. Using the information from an analysis of the formula and the information provided in the text, we can infer that this line presents a pattern involving repletion. Water-swelling from the lumbus down indicates damp-heat congestion and a loss of normal qì transformation in the lower burner. Consequently, water qì collects in the lower part of the body and water-swelling is observed from the lumbus downward. Qì vacuity water qì often causes swelling in the head and face. If the spleen is vacuous, these signs may be accompanied by abdominal distention and fullness.

The treatment of this disease follows the principle described in *Jīn Guì Yào Lüè*, "[For] all [diseases] with water and swelling from the lumbus down, [one] should disinhibit the urine." Oyster Shell and Alisma Powder (*mǔ lì zé xiè sǎn*) clears heat and expels water. Alisma (*zé xiè*) and phytolacca (*shāng lù gēn*) drain water and disinhibit the urine in order to treat water swelling. Dichroa leaf (*shǔ qī*) and tingli (*tíng lì zǐ*) dispel congelation and expel water, and break binds caused by water and heat. Oyster shell (*mǔ lì*) and sargassum (*hǎi zǎo*) soften hardness in order to disperse glomus. Trichosanthes root (*guā lóu gēn*) enriches fluids and disinhibits stagnant blood vessels. The formula is taken as a powder, not as a decoction, in order to moderate the effect of the medicinals. This is an example of using harsh medicinals in a moderate way. By not using a decoction, the possibility that the water in the decoction will assist the water qì is also avoided. The formula is taken with a rice decoction to protect the stomach fluids and support the spleen qì. In the directions for the formula are the instructions that once the urine is disinhibited, one should stop taking the formula because Oyster Shell and Alisma Powder (*mǔ lì zé xiè sǎn*) is a harsh formula for expelling water and its continued use would damage yīn humor and right qì.

LINE 396

大病差后，喜唾，久不了了，胸上有寒，当以丸药温之，宜理中丸。

Dà bìng chài hòu, xǐ tuò, jiǔ bù liǎo liǎo, xiōng shàng yǒu hán, dāng yǐ wán yào wēn zhī, yí lǐ zhōng wán.

After a major illness is cured, frequent spitting[1] [that] endures without clearly [resolving][2] [indicates] cold above the chest, so one should warm with a pill medicine;[3] [therefore,] Center-Rectifying Pill (*lǐ zhōng wán*) is appropriate.

TEXT NOTES

1. Frequent spitting, 喜唾 *xǐ tuò*: Recurrent ejection of spittle and foam from the mouth.
2. Endures without clearly [resolving], 久不了了 *jiǔ bù liǎo liǎo*: 久 *jiǔ* means that the disease course is protracted. 不了了 *bù liǎo liǎo* means that the disease may have begun to resolve, but the progression is not definite.
3. Pill medicine, 丸药 *wán yào*: Previously this term was used in reference to a harsh precipitant in pill form, but in this case it refers to Center-Rectifying Pill (*lǐ zhōng wán*).

SYNOPSIS

The signs and treatment of vacuity cold and frequent spitting after an illness has been cured.

COMMENTARY

Following recovery from a severe disease, the right yáng is weakened. This weakness may affect multiple areas of the body. An analysis of the suggested formula shows that in this case, the yáng of the spleen and lung is vacuous. Vacuous spleen yáng causes abnormal movement and transformation; consequently, fluids are not properly distributed. When lung vacuity exists, diffusion and downbearing become abnormal. The fluids, which are already not being distributed properly, become further congealed. In this case the congealed fluids transform into cold-rheum, which gathers in the chest and diaphragm. The spleen is the source of phlegm formation and the lung is the receptacle that holds phlegm. One must trace back to the source and treat the root. Center-Rectifying Pill (*lǐ zhōng wán*) warms the center and supplements the spleen. The formula also contains medicinals, such as dried ginger (*gān jiāng*), which warm the lung and transform rheum. Once the spleen and lung are warmed, the fluids will be properly distributed and the cold-rheum will be eliminated.

In this pattern, cold-rheum gathers in the chest, producing frequent spitting. Nonetheless, it has not yet caused lung qì counterflow; therefore, coughing and panting are absent. When cold-rheum in the chest invades the lung and causes qì counterflow, Minor Green-Blue Dragon Decoction (*xiǎo qīng lóng tāng*) is appropriate.

LINE 397

伤寒解后，虚羸少气，气逆欲吐，竹叶石膏汤主之。

Shāng hán jiě hòu, xū léi shǎo qì, qì nì yù tù, zhú yè shí gāo tāng zhǔ zhī.

After resolution of cold damage, [when there is] vacuity and marked emaciation, shortage of qì, and qì counterflow with a desire to vomit, Bamboo Leaf and Gypsum Decoction (*zhú yè shí gāo tāng*) governs.

FORMULA

Bamboo Leaf and Gypsum Decoction (*zhú yè shí gāo tāng*)

∘ Clear and abate vacuity heat; boost qì and engender liquid.

竹叶二把　石膏一斤　半夏半升（洗）　麦门冬一升（去心）　人参二两　甘草二两（炙）粳米半升

右七味，以水一斗，煮取六升，去滓，内粳米，煮米熟，汤成去米，温服一升，日三服。

Zhú yè èr bǎ　shí gāo yī jīn　bàn xià bàn shēng (xǐ)　mài mén dōng yī shēng (qù xīn)　rén shēn èr liǎng　gān cǎo èr liǎng (zhì)　gēng mǐ bàn shēng

Yòu qī wèi, yǐ shuǐ yī dǒu, zhǔ qǔ liù shēng, qù zǐ, nà gēng mǐ, zhǔ mǐ shú, tāng chéng qù mǐ, wēn fú yī shēng, rì sān fú.

bamboo leaf (竹叶 *zhú yè*, Lophatheri Folium) 2 bunches*
gypsum (石膏 *shí gāo*, Gypsum) 1 jīn
pinellia (半夏 *bàn xià*, Pinelliae Tuber) half shēng (washed)
ophiopogon (麦门冬 *mài mén dōng*, Ophiopogonis Tuber) 1 shēng (remove hearts)
ginseng (人参 *rén shēn*, Ginseng Radix) 2 liǎng
mix-fried licorice (甘草 *gān cǎo*, Glycyrrhizae Radix) 2 liǎng
rice (粳米 *gēng mǐ*, Oryzae Semen) half shēng

[For] the above seven ingredients use one dǒu of water. Boil [the first six ingredients] to get six shēng. Remove the dregs and add rice (*gēng mǐ*). Boil [until] the rice is cooked and it becomes a soup. Remove the rice and take one shēng warm, three times a day.

Formula Note

* bamboo leaf (*zhú yè*) 2 bunches: According to the authors of *Shāng Hán Lùn Tāng Zhèng Lùn Zhì* (伤寒论汤证论治 "*Shāng Hán Lùn* Formulae, Patterns, and Treatment Differentiation"), the amount is 10 grams.

Synopsis

The signs and treatment of the pattern in which, after an illness, there is residual heat that has not been cleared and damage to the qì and humor.

Commentary

Following recovery from a severe disease, the qì and fluids may still be damaged. When the qì and fluids are insufficient, they cannot adequately enrich and nourish the body; consequently, vacuity and marked emaciation may be observed. Damage to the qì can result in shortage of qì (since the qì is insufficient to support the breath) and difficulty breathing. In addition to these signs of vacuity, residual heat in the interior may harass the stomach and disturb normal downbearing. As a result, qì ascends counterflow and the patient desires to vomit. The description of this pattern is terse and it can be supplemented through an analysis of the formula. It is likely that the signs above would be accompanied by heat effusion, heart vexation, thirst, reduced sleep, a red tongue with scant fur, and a pulse that is vacuous and rapid.

Bamboo Leaf and Gypsum Decoction (*zhú yè shí gāo tāng*) clears and discharges residual heat, and boosts the qì and nourishes the fluids. Sweet and cold, bamboo leaf (*dàn zhú yè*) clears vexation heat. Gypsum (*shí gāo*), which is very cold, clears yáng brightness heat. These two medicinals, used together, clear heat and eliminate vexation. Ginseng (*rén shēn*) boosts the qì, engenders fluids, and supports vacuity. Ophiopogon (*mài mén dōng*) enriches fluids, moistens dryness, and clears heat. Mix-fried licorice (*gān cǎo*) and rice (*gēng mǐ*) supplement the center, boost the qì, and nourish the stomach. Acrid and dissipating, pinellia (*bàn xià*) harmonizes the stomach and downbears counterflow in order to check retching. It also balances the medicinals, such as ophiopogon (*mài mén dōng*), that may cause stagnation.

Line 398

病人脉已解，而日暮微烦，以病新差，人强与谷，脾胃气尚弱，不能消谷，故令微烦，损谷则愈。

Bìng rén mài yǐ jiě, ér rì mù wēi fán, yǐ bìng xīn chài, rén qiáng yǔ gǔ, pí wèi qì shàng ruò, bù néng xiāo gǔ, gù lìng wēi fán, sǔn gǔ zé yù.

The person's pulse has already resolved and in the evening [there is] mild vexation. Because the disease is newly cured, the person is forced to eat food,* [but] the spleen and stomach qì is still weak, [so] food cannot be swiftly digested; hence [there is] mild vexation. Decrease food [intake] [and] then [there will be] recovery.

Text Note

* Food, 谷 *gǔ*, This word, which means "grain," refers to food in general, not only grains.

Synopsis

After an illness is cured, one should pay attention to regulation of dietary intake.

Commentary

After recovery from disease, the pulse no longer reflects the disease pattern, but reflects the fact that the spleen and stomach may not yet have returned to normal strength. If those around the patient force him/her to eat food, in order to speed recovery, it may cause a negative transmutation. This patient's spleen and stomach are still weak; when food is given, the weak stomach and spleen have difficulty digesting the food, causing mild vexation. Vexation occurs primarily in the evening because this is the time when the yáng qì is beginning to abate. Yáng qì of the center is already weakened, and in the evening it becomes even more weak. Food is not digested properly, the stomach qì becomes depressed, and food accumulates, engendering mild heat, which gives rise to mild vexation. This pattern is caused by giving the patient too much food too early in the process of recovery. It does not involve abiding food or severe stagnation; therefore, the only treatment necessary is to reduce the food intake. Once the spleen and stomach qì returns, digestion will occur naturally and vexation will cease.

Appendix I
Text in Sòng Version Order

The present appendix presents the original text of the *Shāng Hán Lùn* in complex characters, with the lines arranged in the order in which they appear in the Sòng version (see Introduction), though with formulas attached to lines under which they appear in the modern order.

太陽病脈證并治

1. 太陽之爲病，脈浮，頭項強痛而惡寒。
2. 太陽病，發熱汗出，惡風，脈緩者， 名爲中風。
3. 太陽病，或已發熱，或未發熱，必惡寒，體痛，嘔逆，脈陰陽俱緊者，名爲傷寒。
4. 傷寒一日，太陽受之，脈若靜者，爲不傳； 頗欲吐，若躁煩，脈數急者，爲傳也。
5. 傷寒二三日，陽明、少陽證不見者， 爲不傳也。
6. 太陽病，發熱而渴，不惡寒者，爲溫病。 若發汗已，身灼熱者，名風溫。 風溫爲病，脈陰陽俱浮，自汗出，身重，多眠睡，鼻息必鼾，語言難出。 若被下者，小便不利，直視失溲；若被火者，微發黃色，劇則如驚癇，時瘛瘲， 若火熏之；一逆尚引日，再逆促命期。
7. 病有發熱惡寒者，發於陽也； 無熱惡寒者，發於陰也。 發於陽，七日愈。 發於陰，六日愈。 以陽數七、陰數六故也。
8. 太陽病，頭痛至七日以上自愈者，以行其經盡故也。 若欲作再經者，針足陽明，使經不傳則愈。
9. 太陽病，欲解時，從巳至未上。
10. 風家，表解而不了了者，十二日愈。
11. 病人身大熱，反欲得衣者，熱在皮膚，寒在骨髓也； 身大寒，反不欲近衣者，寒在皮膚，熱在骨髓也。
12. 太陽中風，陽浮而陰弱，陽浮者，熱自發，陰弱者，汗自出。 嗇嗇惡寒，淅淅惡風，翕翕發熱，鼻鳴乾嘔者，桂枝湯主之。

    桂枝三兩（去皮） 芍藥三兩 甘草二兩（炙） 生薑三兩（切） 大棗十二枚（擘） 右五味， 㕮咀三味，以水七升，微火煮取三升，去滓，適寒溫，服一升。 服已須臾，歠熱稀粥一升餘，以助藥力。 溫覆令一時許，遍身漐漐微似有汗者益佳，不可令如水流漓，病必不除。 若一服汗病差，停後服，不必盡劑。 若不汗，更服依前法。 又不汗， 後服小促其間，半日許令三服盡。 若病重者，一日一夜服，週時觀之。 服一劑盡，病證猶在者，更作服。 若汗不出，乃服至二、三劑。 禁生冷、粘滑、肉麵、五辛、酒酪，臭惡等物。

13. 太陽病，頭痛，發熱，汗出，惡風，桂枝湯主之。
14. 太陽病，項背強几几，反汗出惡風者，桂枝加葛根湯主之。

葛根四兩　麻黃三兩（去節）　桂枝二兩（去皮）　芍藥二兩　生薑三兩（切）　甘草二兩（炙）　大棗十二枚（擘）　右七味，以水一斗，先煮麻黃、葛根，減二升，去上沫，內諸藥，煮取三升，去滓，溫服一升，覆取微似汗，不須歠粥，餘如桂枝法將息及禁忌。

15. 太陽病，下之後，其氣上衝者，可與桂枝湯，方用前法。若不上衝者，不得與之。

16A. 太陽病三日，已發汗，若吐、若下、若溫針，仍不解者，此爲壞病，桂枝不中與之也。觀其脈證，知犯何逆，隨證治之。...

16B. ...桂枝本爲解肌，若其人脈浮緊，發熱汗不出者，不可與之也。常須識此，勿令誤也。

17. 若酒客病，不可與桂枝湯，得之則嘔，以酒客不喜甘故也。

18. 喘家作桂枝湯，加厚朴、杏子佳。

桂枝三兩（去皮）　甘草二兩（炙）　生薑三兩（切）　芍藥三兩　大棗十二枚（擘）　厚朴二兩（炙，去皮）　杏仁五十枚（去皮尖）　右七味，以水七升，微火煮取三升，去滓，溫服一升，覆取微似汗。

19. 凡服桂枝湯吐者，其後必吐膿血也。

20. 太陽病，發汗，遂漏不止，其人惡風，小便難，四肢微急，難以屈伸者，桂枝加附子湯主之。

桂枝三兩（去皮）　芍藥三兩　甘草三兩（炙）　生薑三兩（切）　大棗十二枚（擘）　附子一枚（炮，去皮，破八片）　右六味，以水七升，煮取三升，去滓，溫服一升。本云，桂枝湯，今加附子。將息如前法。

21. 太陽病，下之後，脈促，胸滿者，桂枝去芍藥湯主之。

桂枝三兩（去皮）　甘草二兩（炙）　生薑三兩（切）　大棗十二枚（擘）　右四味，以水七升，煮取三升，去滓，溫服一升。本云，桂枝湯，今去芍藥。將息如前法。

22. 若微寒者，桂枝去芍藥加附子湯主之。

桂枝三兩（去皮）　甘草二兩（炙）　生薑三兩（切）　大棗十二枚（擘）　附子一枚（炮，去皮，破八片）　右五味，以水七升，煮取三升，去滓，溫服一升。本云，桂枝湯，今去芍藥加附子。將息如前法。

23. 太陽病，得之八九日，如瘧狀，發熱惡寒，熱多寒少，其人不嘔，清便欲自可，一日二三度發。脈微緩者，爲欲愈也；脈微而惡寒者，此陰陽俱虛，不可更發汗、更下、更吐也；面色反有熱色者，未欲解也，以其不能得小汗出，身必癢，宜桂枝麻黃各半湯。

桂枝一兩十六銖（去皮）　芍藥　生薑（切）　甘草（炙）　麻黃（去節）各一兩　大棗四枚（擘）　杏仁二十四枚（湯浸，去皮尖及兩仁者）　右七味，以水五升，先煮麻黃一二沸，去上沫，內諸藥，煮取一升八合，去滓，溫服六合。本云，桂枝湯三合，麻黃湯三合，并爲六合，頓服。將息如上法。

24. 太陽病，初服桂枝湯，反煩不解者，先刺風池、風府，却與桂枝湯則愈。

25. 服桂枝湯，大汗出，脈洪大者，與桂枝湯，如前法。若形似瘧，一日再發者，汗出必解，宜桂枝二麻黃一湯。

桂枝一兩十七銖（去皮）　芍藥一兩六銖　麻黃十六銖（去節）　生薑一兩六銖（切）　杏仁十六箇（去皮尖）　甘草一兩二銖（炙）　大棗五枚（擘）　右七味，以水五升，先煮麻黃一二沸，去上沫，內諸藥，煮取二升，去滓，溫服一升，日再服。本云，桂枝湯二分，麻黃湯一分，合爲二升，分再服。今合爲一方，將息如前法。

26. 服桂枝湯，大汗出後，大煩渴不解，脈洪大者，白虎加人參湯主之。

知母六兩　石膏一斤（碎，綿裹）　甘草二兩（炙）　粳米六合　人參三兩　右五味，以水一斗，煮米熟，湯成，去滓，溫服一升，日三服。

27. 太陽病，發熱惡寒，熱多寒少，脈微弱者，此無陽也，不可發汗，宜桂枝二越婢一湯。

桂枝（去皮）　芍藥　麻黃　甘草（炙）各十八銖　大棗四枚（擘）　生薑一兩二銖（切）　石膏二十四銖（碎，綿裹）　右七味，以水五升，煮麻黃一二沸，去上沫，內諸藥，煮取二升，去滓，溫服一升。本云，當裁爲越婢湯、桂枝湯合之，飲一升。今合爲一方，桂枝湯二分，越婢湯一分。

28. 服桂枝湯，或下之，仍頭項強痛，翕翕發熱，無汗，心下滿微痛，小便不利者，桂枝去桂加茯苓白朮湯主之。

芍藥三兩　甘草二兩（炙）　生薑（切）、白朮、茯苓各三兩　大棗十二枚（擘）　右六味，以水八升，煮取三升，去滓，溫服一升。小便利則愈。本云，桂枝湯，今去桂枝加茯苓、白朮。

29. 傷寒脈浮，自汗出，小便數，心煩，微惡寒，脚攣急，反與桂枝欲攻其表，此誤也。得之便厥，咽中乾，煩躁吐逆者，作甘草乾薑湯與之，以復其陽；若厥愈足溫者，更作芍藥甘草湯與之，其脚即伸；若胃氣不和，讝語者，少與調胃承氣湯；若重發汗，復加燒針者，四逆湯主之。

甘草四兩（炙）　乾薑二兩　右二味，以水三升，煮取一升五合，去滓，分溫再服。

白芍藥、甘草（炙）各四兩　右二味，以水三升，煮取一升五合，去滓，分溫再服。

30. 問曰：證象陽旦，按法治之而增劇，厥逆，咽中乾，兩脛拘急而讝語。師曰：言夜半手足當溫，兩脚當伸，後如師言。何以知此？答曰：寸口脈浮而大，浮爲風，大爲虛，風則生微熱，虛則兩脛攣，病形象桂枝，因加附子參其間，增桂令汗出，附子溫經，亡陽故也。厥逆，咽中乾，煩躁，陽明內結，讝語煩亂，更飲甘草乾薑湯。夜半陽氣還，兩足當熱，脛尙微拘急，重與芍藥甘草湯，爾乃脛伸。以承氣湯微溏，則止其讝語，故知病可愈。

31. 太陽病，項背強几几，無汗惡風，葛根湯主之。

葛根四兩　麻黃三兩（去節）　桂枝二兩（去皮）　生薑三兩（切）　甘草二兩（炙）　芍藥二兩　大棗十二枚（擘）　右七味，以水一斗，先煮麻黃、葛根，減二升，去白沫，內諸藥，煮取三升，去滓，溫服一升。覆取微似汗。餘如桂枝法將息及禁忌。諸湯皆仿此。

32. 太陽與陽明合病者，必自下利，葛根湯主之。

33. 太陽與陽明合病，不下利，但嘔者，葛根加半夏湯主之。

葛根四兩　麻黃三兩（去節）　甘草二兩（炙）　芍藥二兩　桂枝二兩（去皮）　生薑二兩（切）　半夏半升（洗）　大棗十二枚（擘）　右八味，以水一斗，先煮葛根、麻黃，減二升，去白沫，內諸藥，煮取三升，去滓，溫服一升。覆取微似汗。

34. 太陽病，桂枝證，醫反下之，利遂不止，脈促者，表未解也；喘而汗出者，葛根黃芩黃連湯主之。

葛根半斤　甘草二兩（炙）　黃芩三兩　黃連三兩　右四味，以水八升，先煮葛根，減二升，內諸藥，煮取二升，去滓，分溫再服。

35. 太陽病，頭痛發熱，身疼腰痛，骨節疼痛，惡風，無汗而喘者，麻黃湯主之。

麻黃三兩（去節）　桂枝二兩（去皮）　甘草一兩（炙）　杏仁七十箇（去皮尖）　右四味，以水九升，先煮麻黃，減二升，去上沫，內諸藥，煮取二升半，去滓，溫服八合。覆取微似汗，不須歠粥。餘如桂枝法將息。

36. 太陽與陽明合病，喘而胸滿者，不可下，宜麻黃湯。

37. 太陽病，十日以去，脈浮細而嗜臥者，外已解也。設胸滿脅痛者，與小柴胡湯；脈但浮者，與麻黃湯。

柴胡半斤　黃芩、人參、甘草（炙）、生薑（切）各三兩　大棗十二枚（擘）　半夏半升（洗）　右七味，以水一斗二升，煮取六升，去滓，再煎取三升，溫服一升，日三服。

38. 太陽中風，脈浮緊，發熱惡寒，身疼痛，不汗出而煩躁者，大青龍湯主之。若脈微弱，汗出惡風者，不可服之。服之則厥逆，筋惕肉瞤，此爲逆也。

麻黃六兩（去節）　桂枝二兩（去皮）　甘草二兩（炙）　杏仁四十枚（去皮尖）　生薑三兩（切）　大棗十枚（擘）　石膏如雞子大（碎）　右七味，以水九升，先煮麻黃，減二升，去上沫，內諸藥，煮取三升，去滓，溫服一升。取微似汗。汗出多者，溫粉粉之。一服汗者，停後服。若復服，汗多亡陽遂虛，惡風，煩躁，不得眠也。

39. 傷寒脈浮緩，身不疼，但重，乍有輕時，無少陰證者，大青龍湯發之。

40. 傷寒表不解，心下有水氣，乾嘔發熱而咳，或渴，或利，或噎，或小便不利，少腹滿，或喘者，小青龍湯主之。

麻黃（去節）　芍藥　細辛　乾薑　甘草（炙）　桂枝（去皮）各三兩　五味子半升　半夏（洗）半升　右八味，以水一斗，先煮麻黃，減二升，去上沫，內諸藥，煮取三升，去滓，溫服一升。若渴，去半夏，加栝樓根三兩。若微利，去麻黃，加蕘花，如一雞子，熬令赤色。若噎者，去麻黃，加附子一枚，炮。若小便不利，少腹滿者，去麻黃，加茯苓四兩。若喘，去麻黃，加杏仁半升，去皮尖。且蕘花不治利，麻黃主喘，今此語反之，疑非仲景意。

41. 傷寒心下有水氣，咳而微喘，發熱不渴；服湯已，渴者，此寒去欲解也；小青龍湯主之。

42. 太陽病，外證未解，脈浮弱者，當以汗解，宜桂枝湯。

桂枝（去皮）　芍藥　生薑（切）各三兩　甘草二兩（炙）　大棗十二枚（擘）　右五味，以水七升，煮取三升，去滓，溫服一升。須臾歠熱稀粥一升，助藥力，取微汗。

43. 太陽病，下之微喘者，表未解故也，桂枝加厚朴杏子湯主之。

44. 太陽病，外證未解，不可下也，下之爲逆，欲解外者，宜桂枝湯。

45. 太陽病，先發汗不解，而復下之，脈浮者不愈。浮爲在外，而反下之，故令不愈，今脈浮，故在外，當須解外則愈，宜桂枝湯。

46. 太陽病，脈浮緊，無汗發熱，身疼痛，八九日不解，表證仍在，此當發其汗。服藥已，微除，其人發煩目瞑，劇者必衄，衄乃解。所以然者，陽氣重故也。麻黃湯主之。

47. 太陽病，脈浮緊，發熱，身無汗，自衄者愈。

48. 二陽併病，太陽初得病時，發其汗，汗先出不徹，因轉屬陽明，續自微汗出，不惡寒。若太陽病證不罷者，不可下，下之爲逆，如此可小發汗。設面色緣緣正赤者，陽氣怫鬱在表，當解之、熏之。若發汗不徹，不足言，陽氣怫鬱不得越，當汗不汗，其人躁煩，不知痛處，乍在腹中，乍在四肢，按之不可得，其人短氣但坐，以汗出不徹故也，更發汗則愈。何以知汗出不徹，以脈濇故知也。

49. 脈浮數者，法當汗出而愈。若下之，身重心悸者，不可發汗，當自汗出乃解。所以然者，尺中脈微，此裏虛，須表裏實，津液自和，便自汗出愈。

50. 脈浮緊者，法當身疼痛，宜以汗解之。假令尺中遲者，不可發汗。何以知然？以榮氣不足，血少故也。

51. 脈浮者，病在表，可發汗，宜麻黃湯。

52. 脈浮而數者，可發汗，宜麻黃湯。

53. 病常自汗出者，此爲榮氣和，榮氣和者，外不諧，以衛氣不共榮氣諧和故爾。以榮行脈中，衛行脈外，復發其汗，榮衛和則愈，宜桂枝湯。

54. 病人藏無他病，時發熱自汗出而不愈者，此衛氣不和也，先其時發汗則愈，宜桂枝湯。

55. 傷寒脈浮緊，不發汗，因致衄者，麻黃湯主之。

56. 傷寒不大便六七日，頭痛有熱者，與承氣湯。其小便清者，知不在裏，仍在表也，當須發汗；若頭痛者，必衄，宜桂枝湯。

57. 傷寒發汗已解，半日許復煩，脈浮數者，可更發汗，宜桂枝湯。

58. 凡病，若發汗、若吐、若下、若亡血、亡津液，陰陽自和者，必自愈。

59. 大下之後，復發汗，小便不利者，亡津液故也。勿治之，得小便利，必自愈。

60. 下之後，復發汗，必振寒，脈微細。所以然者，以內外俱虛故也。

61. 下之後，復發汗，晝日煩躁不得眠，夜而安靜，不嘔不渴，無表證，脈沉微，身無大熱者，乾薑附子湯主之。

乾薑一兩　附子一枚（生用，去皮，切八片）　右二味，以水三升，煮取一升，去滓，頓服。

62. 發汗後，身疼痛，脈沉遲者，桂枝加芍藥生薑各一兩人參三兩新加湯主之。

桂枝三兩（去皮）　芍藥四兩　甘草二兩（炙）　人參三兩　大棗十二枚（擘）　生薑四兩　右六味，以水一斗二升，煮取三升，去滓，溫服一升。本云，桂枝湯，今加芍藥、生薑、人參。

63. 發汗後，不可更行桂枝湯，汗出而喘，無大熱者，可與麻黃杏仁甘草石膏湯。

麻黃四兩（去節）　杏仁五十箇（去皮尖）　甘草二兩（炙）　石膏十斤（碎，綿裹）　右四味，以水七升，煮麻黃，減二升，去上沫，內諸藥，煮取二升，去滓，溫服一升。本云，黃耳杯。

64. 發汗過多，其人叉手自冒心，心下悸，欲得按者，桂枝甘草湯主之。

桂枝四兩（去皮）　甘草二兩（炙）　右二味，以水三升，煮取一升，去滓，頓服。

65. 發汗後，其人臍下悸者，欲作奔豚，茯苓桂枝甘草大棗湯主之。

茯苓半斤　桂枝四兩（去皮）　甘草二兩（炙）　大棗十五枚（擘）。右四味，以甘瀾水一斗，先煮茯苓，減二升，內諸藥，煮取三升，去滓，溫服一升，日三服。作甘瀾水法：取水二斗，置大盆內，以杓揚之，水上有珠子五六千顆相逐，取用之。

66. 發汗後，腹脹滿者，厚朴生薑半夏甘草人參湯主之。

厚朴半斤（炙，去皮）　生薑十斤（切）　半夏半升（洗）　甘草二兩　人參一兩　右五味，以水一斗，煮取三升，去滓，溫服一升，日三服。

67. 傷寒，若吐若下後，心下逆滿，氣上衝胸，起則頭眩，脈沉緊，發汗則動經，身爲振振搖者，茯苓桂枝白朮甘草湯主之。

茯苓四兩　桂枝三兩（去皮）　白朮　甘草各二兩（炙）　右四味，以水六升，煮取三升，去滓，分溫三服。

68. 發汗，病不解，反惡寒者，虛故也，芍藥甘草附子湯主之。

芍藥　甘草（炙）各三兩　附子一枚（炮，去皮，破八片）　右三味，以水五升，煮取一升五合，去滓，分溫三服。疑非仲景方。

69. 發汗，若下之，病仍不解，煩躁者，茯苓四逆湯主之。

茯苓四兩　人參一兩　附子一枚（生用，去皮，破八片）　甘草二兩（炙）　乾薑一兩半　右五味，以水五升，煮取三升，去滓，溫服七合，日二服。

70. 發汗後惡寒者，虛故也。不惡寒，但熱者，實也。當和胃氣，與調胃承氣湯。

芒消半升　甘草二兩（炙）　大黃四兩（去皮，清酒洗）　右三味，以水三升，煮取一升，去滓，內芒消，更煮兩沸，頓服。

71. 太陽病，發汗後，大汗出，胃中乾，煩躁不得眠，欲得飲水者，少少與飲之，令胃氣和則愈。若脈浮，小便不利，微熱消渴者，五苓散主之。

豬苓十八銖（去皮）　澤瀉一兩六銖　白朮十八銖　茯苓十八銖　桂枝半兩（去皮）　右五味，擣爲散，以白飲和服方寸匕，日三服。多飲煖水，汗出愈。如法將息。

72. 發汗已，脈浮數，煩渴者，五苓散主之。

73. 傷寒汗出而渴者，五苓散主之；不渴者，茯苓甘草湯主之。

茯苓二兩　桂枝二兩（去皮）　甘草一兩（炙）　生薑三兩（切）　右四味，以水四升，煮取二升，去滓，分溫三服。

74. 中風發熱，六七日不解而煩，有表裏證，渴欲飲水，水入則吐者，名曰水逆，五苓散主之。

75. 未持脈時，病人手叉自冒心，師因教試令咳，而不咳者，此必兩耳聾無聞也，所以然者，以重發汗虛故如此。發汗後，飲水多必喘，以水灌之亦喘。

76A. 發汗後，水藥不得入口，爲逆；若更發汗，必吐下不止。

76B. 發汗吐下後，虛煩不得眠，若劇者，必反覆顛倒，心中懊憹，梔子豉湯主之；若少氣者，梔子甘草豉湯主之；若嘔者，梔子生薑豉湯主之。

梔子十四箇（擘）　香豉四合（綿裹）　右二味，以水四升，先煮梔子，得二升半，內豉，煮取一升半，去滓，分爲二服，溫進一服，得吐者，止後服。

梔子十四箇（擘）　甘草二兩（炙）　香豉四合（綿裹）　右三味，以水四升，先煮梔子、甘草取二升半，內豉，煮取一升半，去滓，分二服，溫進一服，得吐者，止後服。

梔子十四箇（擘）　生薑五兩　香豉四合（綿裹）　右三味，以水四升，先煮梔子、生薑，取二升半，內豉，煮取一升半，去滓，分二服，溫進一服，得吐者，止後服。

77. 發汗，若下之，而煩熱，胸中窒者，梔子豉湯主之。

78. 傷寒五六日，大下之後，身熱不去，心中結痛者，未欲解也，梔子豉湯主之。

79. 傷寒下後，心煩腹滿，臥起不安者，梔子厚朴湯主之。

梔子十四箇（擘）　厚朴四兩（炙，去皮）　枳實四枚（水浸，炙令黃）　右三味，以水三升半，煮取一升半，去滓，分二服，溫進一服，得吐者，止後服。

80. 傷寒，醫以丸藥大下之，身熱不去，微煩者，梔子乾薑湯主之。

梔子十四箇（擘）　乾薑二兩　右二味，以水三升半，煮取一升半，去滓，分二服，溫進一服，得吐者，止後服。

81. 凡用梔子湯，病人舊微溏者，不可與服之。

82. 太陽病發汗，汗出不解，其人仍發熱，心下悸，頭眩，身瞤動，振振欲擗地者，眞武湯主之。

茯苓　芍藥　生薑各三兩（切）　白朮二兩　附子一枚（炮，去皮，破八片）　右五味，以水八升，煮取三升，去滓，溫服七合，日三服。

83. 咽喉乾燥者，不可發汗。

84. 淋家，不可發汗，發汗必便血。

85. 瘡家，雖身疼痛， 不可發汗，汗出則痓。

86. 衄家，不可發汗， 汗出必額上陷脈急緊，直視不能眴，不得眠。

87. 亡血家，不可發汗，發汗則寒慄而振。

88. 汗家，重發汗， 必恍惚心亂，小便已陰疼，與禹餘糧丸。
方本闕。

89. 病人有寒，復發汗，胃中冷，必吐蚘。

90. 本發汗，而復下之，此爲逆也； 若先發汗，治不爲逆。 本先下之，而反汗之，爲逆； 若先下之，治不爲逆。

91. 傷寒，醫下之，續得下利，清穀不止，身疼痛者，急當救裏。 後身疼痛，清便自調者，急當救表。 救裏宜四逆湯，救表宜桂枝湯。

92. 病發熱頭痛，脈反沉，若不差，身體疼痛，當救其裏。 四逆湯方。
甘草二兩（炙） 乾薑一兩半 附子一枚（生用，去皮，破八片）。 右三味，以水三升，煮取一升二合，去滓，分溫再服，強人可大附子一枚， 乾薑三兩。

93. 太陽病，先下而不愈，因復發汗，以此表裏俱虛，其人因致冒。 冒家汗出自愈。所以然者，汗出表和故也。 裏未和，然後復下之。

94. 太陽病未解，脈陰陽俱停，必先振慄汗出而解。 但陽脈微者，先汗出而解；但陰脈微者，下之而解。 若欲下之，宜調胃承氣湯。

95. 太陽病，發熱汗出者，此爲榮弱衛強，故使汗出，欲救邪風者，宜桂枝湯。

96. 傷寒五六日，中風，往來寒熱，胸脅苦滿，嘿嘿不欲飲食，心煩喜嘔，或胸中煩而不嘔，或渴，或腹中痛，或脅下痞硬，或心下悸、小便不利，或不渴、身有微熱，或咳者，小柴胡湯主之。
柴胡半斤 黃芩三兩 人參三兩 半夏半升（洗） 甘草（炙） 生薑（切）各三兩 大棗十二枚（擘） 右七味，以水一斗二升，煮取六升，去滓，再煎取三升，溫服一升，日三服。 若胸中煩而不嘔者，去半夏、人參，加栝樓實一枚。 若渴，去半夏，加人參合前成四兩半，栝樓根四兩。 若腹中痛者，去黃芩，加芍藥三兩。 若脅下痞硬，去大棗，加牡蠣四兩。 若心下悸，小便不利者，去黃芩，加茯苓四兩。 若不渴、外有微熱者，去人參，加桂枝三兩，溫覆微汗愈。 若咳者，去人參、大棗、生薑，加五味子半升， 乾薑二兩。

97. 血弱氣盡，腠理開，邪氣因入，與正氣相摶，結於脅下。 正邪分爭，往來寒熱，休作有時，嘿嘿不欲飲食。 藏府相連，其痛必下，邪高痛下，故使嘔也，小柴胡湯主之。 服柴胡湯已，渴者屬陽明，以法治之。

98. 得病六七日，脈遲浮弱，惡風寒，手足溫，醫二三下之，不能食，而脅下滿痛，面目及身黃，頸項強，小便難者，與柴胡湯， 後必下重。 本渴飲水而嘔者，柴胡湯不中與也，食穀者噦。

99. 傷寒四五日，身熱惡風，頸項強，脅下滿，手足溫而渴者，小柴胡湯主之。

100. 傷寒，陽脈濇，陰脈弦，法當腹中急痛，先與小建中湯，不差者，小柴胡湯主之。
桂枝三兩（去皮） 甘草二兩（炙） 大棗十二枚（擘） 芍藥六兩 生薑三兩（切） 膠飴一升 右六味，以水七升，煮取三升，去滓，內飴，更上微火消解。 溫服一升，日三服。 嘔家不可用建中湯，以甜故也。

101. 傷寒中風，有柴胡證，但見一證便是，不必悉具。 凡柴胡湯病證而下之，若柴胡證不罷者，復與柴胡湯，必蒸蒸而振， 却復發熱汗出而解。

102. 傷寒二三日，心中悸而煩者，小建中湯主之。

桂枝三兩（去皮） 芍藥六兩 生薑三兩（切） 甘草二兩（炙） 大棗十二枚（擘） 膠飴一升 右六味，以水七升，煮取三升，去滓，溫服一升，日三服。嘔家不可用小建中湯，以甜故也。

103. 太陽病，過經十餘日，反二三下之，後四五日，柴胡證仍在者，先與小柴胡。嘔不止，心下急，鬱鬱微煩者，爲未解也，與大柴胡湯下之則愈。

柴胡半斤 黃芩三兩 芍藥三兩 半夏半升（洗） 生薑五兩（切） 枳實四枚（炙） 大棗十二枚（擘） 右七味，以水一斗二升，煮取六升，去滓，再煎，溫服一升，日三服。一方，加大黃二兩。若不加，恐不爲大柴胡湯。

104. 傷寒十三日不解，胸脅滿而嘔，日晡所發潮熱，已而微利。此本柴胡證，下之以不得利，今反利者，知醫以丸藥下之，此非其治也。潮熱者，實也。先宜服小柴胡湯以解外，後以柴胡加芒消湯主之。

柴胡二兩十六銖 黃芩一兩 人參一兩 甘草一兩（炙） 生薑一兩（切） 半夏二十銖（本云五枚，洗） 大棗四枚（擘） 芒消二兩 右八味，以水四升，煮取二升，去滓，內芒消，更煮微沸，分溫再服。不解，更作。

105. 傷寒十三日，過經譫語者，以有熱也，當以湯下之。若小便利者，大便當硬，而反下利，脈調和者，知醫以丸藥下之，非其治也。若自下利者，脈當微厥，今反和者，此爲內實也，調胃承氣湯主之。

106. 太陽病不解，熱結膀胱，其人如狂，血自下，下者愈。其外不解者，尙未可攻，當先解其外。外解已，但少腹急結者，乃可攻之，宜桃核承氣湯。

桃仁五十箇（去皮尖） 大黃四兩 桂枝二兩（去皮） 甘草二兩（炙） 芒消二兩 右五味，以水七升，煮取二升半，去滓，內芒消，更上火微沸，下火，先食溫服五合，日三服。當微利。

107. 傷寒八九日，下之，胸滿煩驚，小便不利，譫語，一身盡重，不可轉側者，柴胡加龍骨牡蠣湯主之。

柴胡四兩 龍骨 黃芩 生薑（切） 鉛丹 人參 桂枝（去皮） 茯苓各一兩半 半夏二合半（洗） 大黃二兩 牡蠣一兩半（熬） 大棗六枚（擘） 右十二味，以水八升，煮取四升，內大黃，切如碁子，更煮一兩沸，去滓，溫服一升。本云，柴胡湯，今加龍骨等。

108. 傷寒腹滿譫語，寸口脈浮而緊，此肝乘脾也，名曰縱，刺期門。

109. 傷寒發熱，嗇嗇惡寒，大渴欲飲水，其腹必滿，自汗出，小便利，其病欲解，此肝乘肺也，名曰橫，刺期門。

110. 太陽病二日，反躁，凡熨其背而大汗出，大熱入胃，胃中水竭，躁煩，必發譫語。十餘日，振慄，自下利者，此爲欲解也。故其汗從腰以下不得汗，欲小便不得，反嘔，欲失溲，足下惡風，大便硬，小便當數而反不數及不多；大便已，頭卓然而痛，其人足心必熱，穀氣下流故也。

111. 太陽病中風，以火劫發汗，邪風被火熱，血氣流溢，失其常度，兩陽相熏灼，其身發黃。陽盛則欲衄，陰虛小便難。陰陽皆虛竭，身體則枯燥，但頭汗出，劑頸而還，腹滿微喘，口乾咽爛，或不大便，久則譫語，甚者至噦，手足躁擾，捻衣摸床，小便利者，其人可治。

112. 傷寒脈浮，醫以火迫劫之，亡陽，必驚狂，臥起不安者，桂枝去芍藥加蜀漆牡蠣龍骨救逆湯主之。

桂枝三兩（去皮） 甘草二兩（炙） 生薑三兩（切） 大棗十二枚（擘） 牡蠣五兩（熬） 蜀漆三兩（洗去腥） 龍骨四兩 右七味，以水一斗二升，先煮蜀漆，減二升，內諸藥，煮取三升，去滓，溫服一升。本云，桂枝湯，今去芍藥，加蜀漆、牡蠣、龍骨。

113. 形作傷寒，其脈不弦緊而弱，弱者必渴，被火必讝語，弱者發熱脈浮，解之當汗出愈。

114. 太陽病，以火熏之，不得汗，其人必躁，到經不解，必清血，名爲火邪。

115. 脈浮熱甚，而反灸之，此爲實，實以虛治，因火而動，必咽燥吐血。

116. 微數之脈，愼不可灸。 因火爲邪，則爲煩逆，追虛逐實，血散脈中，火氣雖微，內攻有力，焦骨傷筋，血難復也。 脈浮，宜以汗解。 用火灸之，邪無從出，因火而盛，病從腰以下，必重而痹，名火逆也。 欲自解者，必當先煩，煩乃有汗而解。 何以知之？脈浮，故知汗出解。

117. 燒針令其汗，針處被寒，核起而赤者，必發奔豚。 氣從少腹上衝心者，灸其核上各一壯，與桂枝加桂湯，更加桂二兩也。

桂枝五兩（去皮） 芍藥三兩 生薑三兩（切） 甘草二兩（炙） 大棗十二枚（擘） 右五味，以水七升，煮取三升，去滓，溫服一升。 本云，桂枝湯，今加桂滿五兩，所以加桂者，以能泄奔豚氣也。

118. 火逆下之，因燒針煩躁者，桂枝甘草龍骨牡蠣湯主之。

桂枝一兩（去皮） 甘草二兩（炙） 牡蠣二兩（熬） 龍骨二兩 右四味，以水五升，煮取二升半，去滓，溫服八合，日三服。

119. 太陽傷寒者，加溫針，必驚也。

120. 太陽病，當惡寒發熱，今汗自出，反不惡寒發熱，關上脈細數者，以醫吐之過也。 一、二日吐之者，腹中飢，口不能食；三、四日吐之者，不喜糜粥，欲食冷食，朝食暮吐，以醫吐之所致也，此爲小逆。

121. 太陽病吐之，但太陽病當惡寒，今反不惡寒，不欲近衣，此爲吐之內煩也。

122. 病人脈數，數爲熱，當消穀引食，而反吐者，此以發汗，令陽氣微，膈氣虛，脈乃數也。 數爲客熱，不能消穀， 以胃中虛冷，故吐也。

123. 太陽病，過經十餘日，心下溫溫欲吐，而胸中痛，大便反溏，腹微滿，鬱鬱微煩，先此時自極吐下者，與調胃承氣湯。 若不爾者，不可與。 但欲嘔，胸中痛，微溏者，此非柴胡湯證，以嘔，故知極吐下也。

124. 太陽病六七日，表證仍在，脈微而沉，反不結胸，其人發狂者，以熱在下焦，少腹當硬滿， 小便自利者，下血乃愈。 所以然者，以太陽隨經，瘀熱在裏故也，抵當湯主之。

水蛭（熬） 虻蟲各三十箇（去翅足，熬） 桃仁二十箇（去皮尖） 大黃三兩（酒洗） 右四味，以水五升，煮取三升，去滓，溫服一升。 不下，更服。

125. 太陽病，身黃，脈沉結，少腹硬，小便不利者，爲無血也；小便自利，其人如狂者，血證諦也，抵當湯主之。

126. 傷寒有熱，少腹滿，應小便不利，今反利者，爲有血也，當下之，不可餘藥，宜抵當丸。

水蛭二十箇（熬） 虻蟲二十箇（去翅足，熬） 桃仁二十五箇（去皮尖） 大黃三兩 右四味，擣分四丸。 以水一升，煮一丸，取七合服之。 晬時當下血，若不下者，更服。

127. 太陽病，小便利者，以飲水多，必心下悸； 小便少者，必苦裏急也。

128. 問曰：病有結胸，有藏結，其狀何如？ 答曰：按之痛，寸脈浮，關脈沉，名曰結胸也。

129. 何謂藏結？ 答曰：如結胸狀，飲食如故，時時下利，寸脈浮，關脈小細沉緊，名曰藏結。 舌上白胎滑者，難治。

130. 藏結無陽證，不往來寒熱，其人反靜，舌上胎滑者，不可攻也。

131. 病發於陽，而反下之，熱入因作結胸，病發於陰，而反下之，因作痞也。 所以成結胸者，以下之太早故也。 結胸者，項亦強，如柔痓狀，下之則和，宜大陷胸丸。

大黃半斤　葶藶子半升（熬）　芒消半升　杏仁半升（去皮尖，熬黑）　右四味，擣篩二味，內杏仁、芒消合研如脂，和散。 取如彈丸一枚，別擣甘遂末一錢匕，白蜜二合，水二升，煮取一升；溫頓服之，一宿乃下；如不下，更服，取下爲效。 禁如藥法。

132. 結胸證，其脈浮大者，不可下，下之則死。

133. 結胸證悉具，煩躁者亦死。

134. 太陽病，脈浮而動數，浮則爲風，數則爲熱，動則爲痛，數則爲虛， 頭痛發熱，微盜汗出，而反惡寒者，表未解也。 醫反下之，動數變遲，膈內拒痛，胃中空虛， 客氣動膈，短氣躁煩，心中懊憹，陽氣內陷，心下因硬，則爲結胸，大陷胸湯主之。 若不結胸，但頭汗出， 餘處無汗，劑頸而還，小便不利，身必發黃。

大黃六兩（去皮）　芒消一升　甘遂一錢匕　右三味，以水六升，先煮大黃取二升，去滓，內芒消，煮一兩沸，內甘遂末，溫服一升。 得快利，止後服。

135. 傷寒六七日，結胸熱實，脈沉而緊，心下痛，按之石硬者，大陷胸湯主之。

136. 傷寒十餘日，熱結在裏，復往來寒熱者，與大柴胡湯；但結胸，無大熱者，此爲水結在胸脅也，但頭微汗出者，大陷胸湯主之。

柴胡半斤　枳實四枚（炙）　生薑五兩（切）　黃芩三兩　芍藥三兩　半夏半升（洗）　大棗十二枚（擘）　右七味，以水一斗二升，煮取六升，去滓，再煎，溫服一升，日三服。 一方，加大黃二兩。 若不加，恐不名大柴胡湯。

137. 太陽病，重發汗而復下之，不大便五六日，舌上燥而渴，日晡所小有潮熱，從心下至少腹硬滿而痛不可近者，大陷胸湯主之。

138. 小結胸病，正在心下，按之則痛，脈浮滑者，小陷胸湯主之。

黃連一兩　半夏半升（洗）　栝樓實大者一枚　右三味，以水六升，先煮栝樓，取三升，去滓，內諸藥，煮取二升，去滓，分溫三服。

139. 太陽病，二三日，不能臥，但欲起，心下必結，脈微弱者，此本有寒分也。 反下之，若利止，必作結胸，未止者，四日復下之，此作協熱利也。

140. 太陽病，下之，其脈促，不結胸者，此爲欲解也；脈浮者，必結胸；脈緊者，必咽痛；脈弦者，必兩脅拘急；脈細數者，頭痛未止；脈沉緊者，必欲嘔；脈沉滑者，協熱利；脈浮滑者，必下血。

141A. 病在陽，應以汗解之，反以冷水潠之，若灌之，其熱被劫不得去，彌更益煩，肉上粟起，意欲飲水，反不渴者，服文蛤散；若不差者，與五苓散。. . .

141B. . . .寒實結胸，無熱證者，與三物小陷胸湯，白散亦可服。

文蛤五兩　右一味，爲散。 以沸湯和一方寸匕服，湯用五合。

豬苓十八銖（去黑皮）　白朮十八銖　澤瀉一兩六錢　茯苓十八銖　桂枝半兩（去皮）　右五味，爲散，更於臼中杵之，白飲和方寸匕服之，日三服。 多飲煖水。 汗出愈。

桔梗三分　巴豆一分（去皮心，熬黑，研如脂）　貝母三分　右三味，爲散，內巴豆，更於臼中杵之，以白飲和服，強人半錢匕，羸者減之。 病在膈上必吐，在膈下必利。 不利，進熱粥一杯；利過不止，進冷粥一杯。

142. 太陽與少陽併病，頭項強痛，或眩冒，時如結胸，心下痞硬者，當刺大椎第一間、肺俞、肝俞，愼不可發汗，發汗則譫語，脈弦。 五日譫語不止，當刺期門。

143. 婦人中風，發熱惡寒，經水適來，得之七八日，熱除而脈遲身涼，胸脅下滿，如結胸狀， 譫語者，此爲熱入血室也，當刺期門，隨其實而取之。

144. 婦人中風，七八日續得寒熱，發作有時，經水適斷者，此爲熱入血室，其血必結，故使如瘧狀，發作有時，小柴胡湯主之。

柴胡半斤　黃芩三兩　人參三兩　半夏半升（洗）　甘草三兩　生薑三兩（切）　大棗十二枚（擘）　右七味，以水一斗二升，煮取六升，去滓，再煎取三升，溫服一升，日三服。

145. 婦人傷寒發熱，經水適來，晝日明瞭，暮則譫語，如見鬼狀者，此爲熱入血室，無犯胃氣及上二焦，必自愈。

146. 傷寒六七日，發熱，微惡寒，肢節煩疼，微嘔，心下支結，外證未去者，柴胡桂枝湯主之。

桂枝（去皮）　黃芩一兩半　人參一兩半　甘草一兩（炙）　半夏二合半（洗）　芍藥一兩半　大棗六枚（擘）　生薑一兩半（切）　柴胡四兩　右九味，以水七升，煮取三升，去滓，溫服一升。

147. 傷寒五六日，已發汗而復下之，胸脅滿微結，小便不利，渴而不嘔，但頭汗出，往來寒熱，心煩者，此爲未解也，柴胡桂枝乾薑湯主之。

柴胡半斤　桂枝三兩（去皮）　乾薑二兩　栝樓根四兩　黃芩三兩　牡蠣二兩（熬）　甘草二兩（炙）　右七味，以水一斗二升，煮取六升。去滓，再煎取三升，溫服一升，日三服。初服微煩，復服，汗出便愈。

148. 傷寒五六日，頭汗出，微惡寒，手足冷，心下滿，口不欲食，大便硬，脈細者，此爲陽微結，必有表，復有裏也。脈沉，亦在裏也。汗出爲陽微。假令純陰結，不得復有外證，悉入在裏；此爲半在裏半在外也。脈雖沉緊，不得爲少陰病。所以然者，陰不得有汗，今頭汗出，故知非少陰也。可與小柴胡湯，設不了了者，得屎而解。

149. 傷寒五六日，嘔而發熱者，柴胡湯證具，而以他藥下之，柴胡證仍在者，復與柴胡湯。此雖已下之，不爲逆，必蒸蒸而振，却發熱汗出而解。若心下滿而硬痛者，此爲結胸也，大陷胸湯主之。但滿而不痛者，此爲痞，柴胡不中與之，宜半夏瀉心湯。

半夏半升（洗）　黃芩　乾薑　人參　甘草（炙）各三兩　黃連一兩　大棗十二枚（擘）　右七味，以水一斗，煮取六升，去滓，再煎取三升，溫服一升，日三服。須大陷胸湯者，方用前第二法。

150. 太陽少陽併病，而反下之，成結胸，心下硬，下利不止，水漿不下，其人心煩。

151. 脈浮而緊，而復下之，緊反入裏，則作痞，按之自濡，但氣痞耳。

152. 太陽中風，下利，嘔逆，表解者，乃可攻之。其人漐漐汗出，發作有時，頭痛，心下痞硬滿，引脅下痛，乾嘔短氣，汗出不惡寒者，此表解裏未和也，十棗湯主之。

芫花（熬）　甘遂　大戟　右三味，等分，各別擣爲散。以水一升半，先煮大棗肥者十枚，取八合，去滓，內藥末。強人服一錢匕，羸人服半錢，溫服之，平旦服。若下少，病不除者，明日更服加半錢，得快下利後，糜粥自養。

153. 太陽病，醫發汗，遂發熱惡寒。因復下之，心下痞，表裏俱虛，陰陽氣並竭，無陽則陰獨。復加燒針，因胸煩。面色青黃，膚瞤者，難治；今色微黃，手足溫者，易愈。

154. 心下痞，按之濡，其脈關上浮者，大黃黃連瀉心湯主之。

大黃二兩　黃連一兩　上二味以麻沸湯二升漬之須臾，絞去滓，分溫再服。

155. 心下痞，而復惡寒汗出者，附子瀉心湯主之。

大黃二兩　黃連一兩　黃芩一兩　附子一枚（炮，去皮，破，別煮取汁）右四味，切三味，以麻沸湯二升漬之，須臾，絞去滓，內附子汁，分溫再服。

156. 本以下之，故心下痞，與瀉心湯。 痞不解，其人渴而口燥煩，小便不利者，五苓散主之。

一方云：忍之一日乃愈。

157. 傷寒汗出，解之後，胃中不和，心下痞硬， 乾噫食臭，脅下有水氣，腹中雷鳴，下利者，生薑瀉心湯主之。

生薑四兩（切） 甘草三兩（炙） 人參三兩 乾薑一兩 黃芩三兩 半夏半升（洗） 黃連一兩 大棗十二枚（擘） 右八味，以水一斗，煮取六升，去滓，再煎取三升，溫服一升，日三服。

158. 傷寒中風，醫反下之，其人下利日數十行， 穀不化，腹中雷鳴，心下痞硬而滿，乾嘔，心煩不得安。 醫見心下痞，謂病不盡，復下之，其痞益甚，此非結熱，但以胃中虛，客氣上逆，故使硬也，甘草瀉心湯主之。

甘草四兩（炙） 黃芩三兩 乾薑三兩 半夏半升（洗） 大棗十二枚（擘） 黃連一兩 右六味，以水一斗，煮取六升，去滓，再煎取三升，溫服一升，日三服。

159. 傷寒服湯藥，下利不止，心下痞硬。 服瀉心湯已，復以他藥下之，利不止。 醫以理中與之，利益甚。 理中者，理中焦，此利在下焦，赤石脂禹餘糧湯主之。復不止者，當利其小便。

赤石脂一斤（碎） 太一禹餘糧一斤（碎） 右二味，以水六升，煮取二升，去滓，分溫三服。

159. 傷寒吐下後，發汗，虛煩，脈甚微，八九日心下痞硬，脅下痛，氣上衝咽喉，眩冒，經脈動惕者，久而成痿。

161. 傷寒發汗，若吐若下，解後，心下痞硬，噫氣不除者，旋覆代赭湯主之。

旋覆花三兩 人參二兩 生薑五兩 代赭一兩 甘草三兩（炙） 半夏半升（洗） 大棗十二枚（擘） 右七味，以水一斗，煮取六升，去滓，再煎取三升，溫服一升，日三服。

162. 下後，不可更行桂枝湯，若汗出而喘，無大熱者，可與麻黃杏子甘草石膏湯。

麻黃四兩（去節） 杏仁五十箇（去皮尖） 甘草二兩（炙） 石膏半斤（碎、綿裹） 右四味，以水七升，先煮麻黃，減二升，去上沫，內諸藥，煮取二升，去滓，溫服一升。 本云，黃耳杯。

163. 太陽病，外證未除，而數下之，遂協熱而利，利下不止，心下痞硬，表裏不解者，桂枝人參湯主之。

桂枝四兩（別切） 甘草四兩（炙） 白朮三兩 人參三兩 乾薑三兩 右五味，以水九升，右煮四味，取五升，內桂，更煮取三升，去滓，溫服一升，日再、夜一服。

164. 傷寒大下後，復發汗，心下痞，惡寒者，表未解也。 不可攻痞，當先解表，表解乃可攻痞。 解表宜桂枝湯，攻痞宜大黃黃連瀉心湯。

165. 傷寒發熱，汗出不解，心中痞硬，嘔吐而下利者，大柴胡主之。

166. 病如桂枝證，頭不痛，項不強，寸脈微浮，胸中痞硬，氣上衝喉咽不得息者，此為胸有寒也，當吐之，宜瓜蒂散。

瓜蒂一分（熬黃） 赤小豆一分 右二味，各別擣篩，為散已，合治之， 取一錢匕，以香豉一合，用熱湯七合，煮作稀糜，去滓。 取汁和散，溫，頓服之。不吐者，少少加， 得快吐乃止。 諸亡血虛家， 不可與瓜蒂散。

167. 病脅下素有痞，連在臍傍，痛引少腹，入陰筋者，此名藏結，死。

168. 傷寒若吐若下後，七八日不解，熱結在裏，表裏俱熱，時時惡風，大渴，舌上乾燥而煩，欲飲水數升者，白虎加人參湯主之。

知母六兩　石膏一斤（碎）　甘草二兩（炙）　人參二兩　粳米六合　右五味，以水一斗，煮米熟湯成，去滓，溫服一升，日三服。此方立夏後立秋前，乃可服，立秋後不可服，正月、二月、三月尙凜冷，亦不可與服之，與之則嘔利而腹痛，諸亡血、虛家，亦不可與，得之則腹痛利者，但可溫之，當愈。

169. 傷寒無大熱，口燥渴，心煩，背微惡寒者，白虎加人參湯主之。

170. 傷寒，脈浮，發熱無汗，其表不解，不可與白虎湯；渴欲飲水，無表證者，白虎加人參湯主之。

171. 太陽少陽併病，心下硬，頸項強而眩者，當刺大椎、肺俞、肝俞，愼勿下之。

172. 太陽與少陽合病，自下利者，與黃芩湯；若嘔者，黃芩加半夏生薑湯主之。

黃芩三兩　芍藥二兩　甘草二兩（炙）　大棗十二枚（擘）　右四味，以水一斗，煮取三升，去滓，溫服一升，日再、夜一服。

黃芩三兩　芍藥二兩　甘草二兩（炙）　大棗十二枚（擘）　半夏半升（洗）　生薑一兩半（一方三兩，切）　右六味，以水一斗，煮取三升，去滓，溫服一升，日再、夜一服。

173. 傷寒胸中有熱，胃中有邪氣，腹中痛，欲嘔吐者，黃連湯主之。

黃連三兩　甘草三兩（炙）　乾薑三兩　桂枝三兩（去皮）　人參二兩　半夏半升（洗）　大棗十二枚（擘）　右七味，以水一斗，煮取六升，去滓，溫服，晝三、夜二。疑非仲景方。

174. 傷寒八九日，風濕相搏，身體疼煩，不能自轉側，不嘔不渴，脈浮虛而濇者，桂枝附子湯主之。若其人大便硬，小便自利者，去桂加白朮湯主之。

桂枝四兩（去皮）　附子三枚（炮，去皮，破）　生薑三兩（切）　大棗十二枚（擘）　甘草二兩（炙）　右五味，以水六升，煮取二升，去滓，分溫三服。

附子三枚（炮，去皮，破）　白朮四兩　生薑三兩（切）　甘草二兩（炙）　大棗十二枚（擘）　右五味，以水六升，煮取二升，去滓，分溫三服。初一服，其人身如痹，半日許復服之，三服都盡，其人如冒狀，勿怪，此以附子、朮併走皮內，逐水氣未得除，故使之耳，法當加桂四兩。此本一方二法：以大便硬、小便自利，去桂也；以大便不硬、小便不利，當加桂。附子三枚，恐多也。虛弱家及產婦，宜減服之。

175. 風濕相搏，骨節疼煩，掣痛不得屈伸，近之則痛劇，汗出短氣，小便不利，惡風不欲去衣，或身微腫者，甘草附子湯主之。

甘草二兩（炙）　附子二枚（炮，去皮，破）　白朮二兩　桂枝四兩（去皮）　右四味，以水六升，煮取三升，去滓，溫服一升，日三服。初服得微汗則解。能食汗止復煩者，將服五合，恐一升多者，宜服六七合爲始。

176. 傷寒，脈浮滑，此表有熱，裏有寒，白虎湯主之。

知母六兩　石膏一斤（碎）　甘草二兩（炙）　粳米六合　右四味，以水一斗，煮米熟，湯成去滓，溫服一升，日三服。

177. 傷寒脈結代，心動悸，炙甘草湯主之。

甘草四兩（炙）　生薑三兩（切）　人參二兩　生地黃一斤　桂枝三兩（去皮）　阿膠二兩　麥門冬半升（去心）　麻仁半升　大棗三十枚（擘）　右九味，以清酒七升，水八升，右煮八味，取三升，去滓，內膠烊消盡，溫服一升，日三服。一名復脈湯。

178. 脈按之來緩，時一止復來者，名曰結。又脈來動而中止，更來小數，中有還者反動，名曰結，陰也。脈來動而中止，不能自還，因而復動者，名曰代，陰也。得此脈者，必難治。

179. 問曰：病有太陽陽明，有正陽陽明，有少陽陽明，何謂也？ 答曰：太陽陽明者，脾約是也；正陽陽明者，胃家實是也；少陽陽明者，發汗利小便已，胃中燥煩實，大便難是也。

陽明病脈證并治

180. 陽明之爲病，胃家實是也。

181. 問曰： 何緣得陽明病？ 答曰：太陽病，若發汗，若下，若利小便，此亡津液，胃中乾燥，因轉屬陽明。 不更衣，內實，大便難者，此名陽明也。

182. 問曰：陽明病外證云何？ 答口：身熱，汗自出，不惡寒，反惡熱也。

183. 問曰： 病有得之一日，不發熱而惡寒者，何也？ 答曰：雖得之一日，惡寒將自罷，即自汗出而惡熱也。

184. 問曰：惡寒何故自罷？ 答曰：陽明居中，主土也，萬物所歸，無所復傳，始雖惡寒，二日自止，此爲陽明病也。

185. 本太陽初得病時，發其汗，汗先出不徹，因轉屬陽明也。 傷寒發熱無汗，嘔不能食，而反汗出濈濈然者，是轉屬陽明也。

186. 傷寒三日，陽明脈大。

187. 傷寒脈浮而緩，手足自溫者，是爲繫在太陰。 太陰者，身當發黃，若小便自利者，不能發黃。 至七八日，大便硬者，爲陽明病也。

188. 傷寒轉繫陽明者，其人濈然微汗出也。

189. 陽明中風，口苦咽乾，腹滿微喘，發熱惡寒，脈浮而緊，若下之，則腹滿，小便難也。

190. 陽明病，若能食，名中風；不能食，名中寒。

191. 陽明病，若中寒者，不能食，小便不利，手足濈然汗出，此欲作固瘕，必大便初硬後溏。 所以然者，以胃中冷，水穀不別故也。

192. 陽明病，初欲食，小便反不利，大便自調，其人骨節疼，翕翕如有熱狀，奄然發狂，濈然汗出而解者，此水不勝穀氣，與汗共并，脈緊則愈。

193. 陽明病，欲解時，從申至戌上。

194. 陽明病，不能食，攻其熱必噦，所以然者，胃中虛冷故也。 以其人本虛，攻其熱必噦。

195. 陽明病，脈遲，食難用飽，飽則微煩頭眩，必小便難，此欲作穀癉。 雖下之，腹滿如故，所以然者，脈遲故也。

196. 陽明病，法多汗，反無汗，其身如蟲行皮中狀者，此以久虛故也。

197. 陽明病，反無汗而小便利，二三日嘔而咳，手足厥者，必苦頭痛；若不咳，不嘔，手足不厥者，頭不痛。

198. 陽明病，但頭眩，不惡寒，故能食而咳，其人咽必痛；若不咳者，咽不痛。

199. 陽明病，無汗，小便不利，心中懊憹者，身必發黃。

200. 陽明病，被火，額上微汗出，而小便不利者，必發黃。

201. 陽明病，脈浮而緊者， 必潮熱，發作有時。 但浮者，必盜汗出。

202. 陽明病，口燥，但欲漱水，不欲嚥者，此必衄。

203. 陽明病，本自汗出，醫更重發汗，病已差，尚微煩不了了者，此必大便硬故也。以亡津液，胃中乾燥，故令大便硬。 當問其小便，日幾行。 若本小便日三四行，今日再行，故知大便不久出，今爲小便數少，以津液當還入胃中，故知不久必大便也。

204. 傷寒嘔多，雖有陽明證，不可攻之。

205. 陽明病，心下硬滿者，不可攻之，攻之利遂不止者死，利止者愈。

206. 陽明病，面合色赤，不可攻之，必發熱，色黃者，小便不利也。

207. 陽明病，不吐不下，心煩者，可與調胃承氣湯。

甘草二兩（炙） 芒消半斤 大黃四兩（清酒洗） 右三味，切，以水三升，煮二物至一升，去滓，內芒消，更上微火一二沸，溫頓服之，以調胃氣。

208. 陽明病，脈遲，雖汗出不惡寒者，其身必重，短氣，腹滿而喘，有潮熱者，此外欲解，可攻裏也。手足濈然汗出者，此大便已硬也，大承氣湯主之；若汗多，微發熱惡寒者，外未解也，其熱不潮，未可與承氣湯；若腹大滿不通者，可與小承氣湯，微和胃氣，勿令至大泄下。

209. 陽明病，潮熱，大便微硬者，可與大承氣湯，不硬者，不可與之。若不大便六七日，恐有燥屎，欲知之法，少與小承氣湯，湯入腹中，轉失氣者，此有燥屎也，乃可攻之；若不轉失氣者，此但初頭硬，後必溏，不可攻之，攻之必脹滿不能食也。欲飲水者，與水則噦。其後發熱者，必大便復硬而少也，以小承氣湯和之。不轉失氣者，慎不可攻也。

210. 夫實則譫語，虛則鄭聲。鄭聲者，重語也。直視譫語，喘滿者死，下利者亦死。

211. 發汗多，若重發汗者，亡其陽，譫語，脈短者死，脈自和者不死。

212. 傷寒，若吐若下後，不解，不大便五六日，上至十餘日，日晡所發潮熱，不惡寒，獨語如見鬼狀，若劇者，發則不識人，循衣摸床，惕而不安，微喘直視，脈弦者生，濇者死；微者，但發熱譫語者，大承氣湯主之。若一服利，則止後服。

213. 陽明病，其人多汗，以津液外出，胃中燥，大便必硬，硬則譫語，小承氣湯主之。若一服譫語止者，更莫復服。

大黃四兩（酒洗） 厚朴二兩（炙，去皮） 枳實三枚（大者，炙） 右三味，以水四升，煮取一升二合，去滓，分溫二服。初服湯當更衣，不爾者盡飲之，若更衣者，勿服之。

214. 陽明病，譫語，發潮熱，脈滑而疾者，小承氣湯主之。因與承氣湯一升，腹中轉氣者，更服一升，若不轉氣者，勿更與之，明日又不大便，脈反微濇者，裏虛也，爲難治，不可更與承氣湯也。

215. 陽明病，譫語，有潮熱，反不能食者，胃中必有燥屎五六枚也。若能食者，但硬耳，宜大承氣湯下之。

216. 陽明病，下血譫語者，此爲熱入血室，但頭汗出者，刺期門，隨其實而寫之，濈然汗出則愈。

217. 汗出譫語者，以有燥屎在胃中，此爲風也，須下者，過經乃可下之。下之若早，語言必亂，以表虛裏實故也。下之愈，宜大承氣湯。

218. 傷寒四五日，脈沉而喘滿，沉爲在裏，而反發其汗，津液越出，大便爲難，表虛裏實，久則譫語。

219. 三陽合病，腹滿身重，難以轉側，口不仁面垢，譫語遺尿，發汗則譫語，下之則額上生汗，手足厥冷。若自汗出者，白虎湯主之。

知母二兩 石膏一斤（碎） 甘草二兩（炙） 粳米六合 右四味，以水一斗，煮米熟湯成，去滓，溫服一升，日三服。

220. 二陽併病，太陽證罷，但發潮熱，手足漐漐汗出，大便難而譫語者，下之則愈，宜大承氣湯。

大黃四兩（酒洗） 厚朴半斤（炙，去皮） 枳實五枚（炙） 芒消三合 右四味，以水一斗，先煮二物，取五升，去滓，內大黃，更煮取二升，去滓，內芒消，更上微火一兩沸，分溫再服。得下，餘勿服。

221. 陽明病，脈浮而緊，咽燥口苦，腹滿而喘，發熱汗出，不惡寒，反惡熱，身重。若發汗則躁，心憒憒，反譫語； 若加溫針，必怵惕，煩躁不得眠； 若下之，則胃中空虛，客氣動膈，心中懊憹，舌上胎者，梔子豉湯主之。

肥梔子十四枚（擘） 香豉四合（綿裹） 右二味，以水四升，煮梔子取二升半，去滓，內豉，更煮取一升半，去滓，分二服，溫進一服，得快吐者，止後服。

222. 若渴欲飲水，口乾舌燥者，白虎加人參湯主之。

知母六兩 石膏一斤（碎） 甘草二兩（炙） 粳米六合 人參三兩 右五味，以水一斗，煮米熟，湯成去滓，溫服一升，日三服。

223. 若脈浮發熱，渴欲飲水，小便不利者，豬苓湯主之。

豬苓（去皮） 茯苓 澤瀉 阿膠 滑石（碎）各一兩 右五味，以水四升，先煮四味取二升，去滓，內阿膠烊消，溫服七合，日三服。

224. 陽明病，汗出多而渴者，不可與豬苓湯，以汗多胃中燥，豬苓湯復利其小便故也。

225. 脈浮而遲，表熱裏寒，下利清穀者，四逆湯主之。

甘草二兩（炙） 乾薑一兩半 附子一枚（生用，去皮，破八片） 右三味，以水三升，煮取一升二合，去滓，分溫二服，強人可大附子一枚， 乾薑三兩。

226. 若胃中虛冷，不能食者，飲水則噦。

227. 脈浮發熱，口乾鼻燥，能食者則衄。

228. 陽明病，下之，其外有熱，手足溫，不結胸，心中懊憹，飢不能食，但頭汗出者，梔子豉湯主之。

229. 陽明病，發潮熱，大便溏，小便自可，胸脅滿不去者，與小柴胡湯。

柴胡半斤 黃芩三兩 人參三兩 半夏半升（洗） 甘草三兩（炙） 生薑三兩（切） 大棗十二枚（擘） 右七味，以水一斗二升，煮取六升，去滓，再煎取三升，溫服一升，日三服。

230. 陽明病，脅下硬滿，不大便，而嘔，舌上白胎者，可與小柴胡湯，上焦得通，津液得下，胃氣因和，身濈然汗出而解。

231. 陽明中風，脈弦浮大，而短氣，腹都滿，脅下及心痛，久按之，氣不通，鼻乾，不得汗，嗜臥，一身及目悉黃，小便難，有潮熱，時時噦，耳前後腫。 刺之小差，外不解，病過十日，脈續浮者，與小柴胡湯。

232. 脈但浮，無餘證者，與麻黃湯。 若不尿，腹滿加噦者，不治。

麻黃三兩（去節） 桂枝二兩（去皮） 甘草一兩（炙） 杏仁七十箇（去皮尖） 右四味，以水九升，煮麻黃，減二升，去白沫，內諸藥，煮取二升半，去滓，溫服八合，覆取微似汗。

233. 陽明病，自汗出，若發汗，小便自利者，此為津液內竭，雖硬不可攻之，當須自欲大便，宜蜜煎導而通之。 若土瓜根及大豬膽汁，皆可為導。

食蜜七合 右一味， 於銅器內，微火煎，當須凝如飴狀，攪之勿令焦著。欲可丸，併手捻作挺，令頭銳，大如指，長二寸許，當熱時急作，冷則硬。 以內穀道中，以手急抱，欲大便時乃去之。 疑非仲景意， 已試甚良。

又大豬膽一枚，瀉汁，和少許法醋，以灌穀道內，如一食頃，當大便出宿食惡物，甚效。

234. 陽明病，脈遲，汗出多，微惡寒者，表未解也，可發汗，宜桂枝湯。

桂枝三兩（去皮） 芍藥三兩 生薑三兩 甘草二兩（炙） 大棗十二枚（擘） 右五味，以水七升，煮取三升，去滓，溫服一升，須臾歠熱稀粥一升，以助藥力取汗。

235. 陽明病，脈浮，無汗而喘者，發汗則愈，宜麻黃湯。

236. 陽明病，發熱汗出者，此爲熱越，不能發黃也；但頭汗出，身無汗，劑頸而還，小便不利，渴引水漿者，此爲瘀熱在裏，身必發黃，茵陳蒿湯主之。

茵陳蒿六兩　梔子十四枚（擘）　大黃二兩（去皮）　右三味，以水一斗二升，先煮茵陳，減六升，右二味，煮取三升，去滓，分三服。小便當利，尿如皂莢汁狀，色正赤。一宿腹減，黃從小便去也。

237. 陽明證，其人喜忘者，必有蓄血。所以然者，本有久瘀血，故令喜忘，屎雖硬，大便反易，其色必黑者，宜抵當湯下之。

水蛭（熬）　虻蟲（去翅足，熬）各三十箇　大黃三兩（酒洗）　桃仁二十箇（去皮尖及兩人者）　右四味，以水五升，煮取三升，去滓，溫服一升，不下更服。

238. 陽明病，下之，心中懊憹而煩，胃中有燥屎者，可攻，腹微滿，初頭硬，後必溏，不可攻之，若有燥屎者，宜大承氣湯。

239. 病人不大便五六日，繞臍痛，煩躁，發作有時者，此有燥屎，故使不大便也。

240. 病人煩熱，汗出則解，又如瘧狀，日晡所發熱者，屬陽明也。脈實者，宜下之；脈浮虛者，宜發汗。下之與大承氣湯；發汗宜桂枝湯。

241. 大下後，六七日不大便，煩不解，腹滿痛者，此有燥屎也。所以然者，本有宿食故也，宜大承氣湯。

242. 病人小便不利，大便乍難乍易，時有微熱，喘冒不能臥者，有燥屎也，宜大承氣湯。

243. 食穀欲嘔，屬陽明也，吳茱萸湯主之；得湯反劇者，屬上焦也。

吳茱萸一升（洗）　人參三兩　生薑六兩（切）　大棗十二枚（擘）　右四味，以水七升，煮取二升，去滓，溫服七合，日三服。

244. 太陽病，寸緩、關浮、尺弱，其人發熱汗出，復惡寒，不嘔，但心下痞者，此以醫下之也，如其不下者，病人不惡寒而渴者，此轉屬陽明也，小便數者，大便必硬，不更衣十日無所苦也，渴欲飲水，少少與之，但以法救之，渴者，宜五苓散。

豬苓（去皮）　白朮　茯苓各十八銖　澤瀉一兩六銖　桂枝半兩（去皮）　右五味，爲散，白飲和，服方寸匕，日三服。

245. 脈陽微而汗出少者，爲自和也；汗出多者，爲太過。陽脈實，因發其汗，出多者，亦爲太過。太過者，爲陽絕於裏，亡津液，大便因硬也。

246. 脈浮而芤，浮爲陽，芤爲陰，浮芤相搏，胃氣生熱，其陽則絕。

247. 趺陽脈浮而濇，浮則胃氣強，濇則小便數，浮濇相搏，大便則硬，其脾爲約，麻子仁丸主之。

麻子仁二升　芍藥半斤　枳實半斤（炙）　大黃一斤（去皮）　厚朴一尺（炙，去皮）　杏仁一升（去皮尖，熬，別作脂）　右六味，蜜和丸，如梧桐子大，飲服十丸，日三服。漸加，以知爲度。

248. 太陽病三日，發汗不解，蒸蒸發熱者，屬胃也，調胃承氣湯主之。

大黃四兩（去皮，清酒洗）　甘草二兩（炙）　芒消半升　右三味，切，以水三升，煮二物至一升，去滓，內芒消，更上火一二沸，溫頓服之以調胃氣。

249. 傷寒吐後，腹脹滿者，與調胃承氣湯。

250. 太陽病，若吐、若下、若發汗後，微煩，小便數，大便因硬者，與小承氣湯和之愈。

251. 得病二三日，脈弱，無太陽、柴胡證，煩躁，心下硬，至四五日，雖能食，以小承氣湯少少與，微和之，令小安，至六日，與承氣湯一升。若不大便六七日，小便少者，雖不受食，但初頭硬，後必溏，未定成硬，攻之必溏。須小便利，屎定硬，乃可攻之，宜大承氣湯。

252. 傷寒六七日，目中不了了，睛不和，無表裏證，大便難，身微熱者，此爲實也，急下之，宜大承氣湯。

253. 陽明病，發熱汗多者，急下之，宜大承氣湯。

254. 發汗不解，腹滿痛者，急下之，宜大承氣湯。

255. 腹滿不減，減不足言，當下之，宜大承氣湯。

256. 陽明少陽合病，必下利，其脈不負者，爲順也。負者，失也，互相剋賊，名爲負也，脈滑而數者，有宿食也。當下之，宜大承氣湯。

257. 病人無表裏證，發熱七八日，雖脈浮數者，可下之。假令已下，脈數不解，合熱則消穀善飢，至六七日，不大便者，有瘀血，宜抵當湯。

258. 若脈數不解，而下不止，必協熱便膿血也。

259. 傷寒發汗已，身目爲黃，所以然者，以寒濕在裏不解故也。以爲不可下也，於寒濕中求之。

260. 傷寒七八日，身黃如橘子色，小便不利，腹微滿者，茵陳蒿湯主之。

261. 傷寒身黃，發熱，梔子蘗皮湯主之。

肥梔子十五箇（擘） 甘草一兩（炙） 黃蘗二兩。 右三味，以水四升，煮取一升半，去滓，分溫再服。

262. 傷寒瘀熱在裏，身必黃，麻黃連軺赤小豆湯主之。

麻黃二兩（去節） 連軺二兩（連翹根是） 杏仁四十箇（去皮尖） 赤小豆一升 大棗十二枚（擘） 生梓白皮（切）一升 生薑二兩（切） 甘草二兩（炙）。 右八味，以潦水一斗，先煮麻黃再沸，去上沫，內諸藥，煮取三升，去滓，分溫三服，半日服盡。

辨少陽病脈證并治

263. 少陽之爲病，口苦，咽乾，目眩也。

264. 少陽中風，兩耳無所聞，目赤，胸中滿而煩者，不可吐下，吐下則悸而驚。

265. 傷寒，脈弦細，頭痛發熱者，屬少陽。少陽不可發汗，發汗則譫語，此屬胃，胃和則愈，胃不和，煩而悸。

266. 本太陽病，不解，轉入少陽者，脅下硬滿，乾嘔不能食，往來寒熱，尚未吐下，脈沉緊者，與小柴胡湯。

柴胡八兩 人參三兩 黃芩三兩 甘草三兩（炙） 半夏半升（洗） 生薑三兩（切） 大棗十二枚（擘）。 右七味，以水一斗二升，煮取六升，去滓，再煎取三升，溫服一升，日三服。

267. 若已吐、下、發汗、溫針，譫語，柴胡證罷，此爲壞病，知犯何逆，以法治之。

268. 三陽合病，脈浮大，上關上，但欲眠睡，目合則汗。

269. 傷寒六七日，無大熱，其人躁煩者，此爲陽去入陰故也。

270. 傷寒三日，三陽爲盡，三陰當受邪，其人反能食而不嘔，此爲三陰不受邪也。

271. 傷寒三日，少陽脈小者，欲已也。

272. 少陽病，欲解時，從寅至辰上。

辨太陰病脈證并治

273. 太陰之爲病，腹滿而吐，食不下，自利益甚，時腹自痛，若下之，必胸下結硬。

274. 太陰中風，四肢煩疼，陽微陰濇而長者，爲欲愈。

275. 太陰病，欲解時，從亥至丑上。

276. 太陰病，脈浮者，可發汗，宜桂枝湯。

桂枝三兩（去皮）　芍藥三兩　甘草二兩（炙）　生薑三兩（切）　大棗十二枝（擘）。 右五味，以水七升，煮取三升，去滓，溫服一升，須臾歠熱稀粥一升，以助藥力，溫覆取汗。

277. 自利不渴者，屬太陰，以其藏有寒故也，當溫之，宜服四逆輩。

278. 傷寒脈浮而緩，手足自溫者，繫在太陰；太陰當發身黃，若小便自利者，不能發黃；至七八日，雖暴煩下利，日十餘行，必自止，以脾家實，腐穢當去故也。

279. 本太陽病，醫反下之，因爾腹滿時痛者，屬太陰也，桂枝加芍藥湯主之；大實痛者，桂枝加大黃湯主之。

桂枝三兩（去皮）　芍藥六兩　甘草二兩（炙）　大棗十二枚（擘）　生薑三兩（切）　右五味，以水七升，煮取三升，去滓，溫分三服。 本云，桂枝湯，今加芍藥。

桂枝三兩（去皮）　大黃二兩　芍藥六兩　生薑三兩（切）　甘草二兩（炙）　大棗十二枚（擘）　右六味，以水七升，煮取三升，去滓，溫服一升，日三服。

280. 太陰爲病，脈弱，其人續自便利，設當行大黃、芍藥者，宜減之，以其人胃氣弱，易動故也。

辨少陰病脈證并治

281. 少陰之爲病，脈微細，但欲寐也。

282. 少陰病，欲吐不吐，心煩但欲寐，五六日，自利而渴者，屬少陰也，虛故引水自救；若小便色白者，少陰病形悉具，小便白者，以下焦虛有寒，不能制水，故令色白也。

283. 病人脈陰陽俱緊，反汗出者，亡陽也，此屬少陰，法當咽痛而復吐利。

284. 少陰病，咳而下利， 譫語者，被火氣劫故也，小便必難，以強責少陰汗也。

285. 少陰病，脈細沉數，病爲在裏，不可發汗。

286. 少陰病，脈微，不可發汗，亡陽故也；陽已虛，尺脈弱濇者，復不可下之。

287. 少陰病，脈緊，至七八日，自下利，脈暴微，手足反溫，脈緊反去者，爲欲解也，雖煩下利，必自愈。

288. 少陰病，下利，若利自止，惡寒而踡臥，手足溫者，可治。

289. 少陰病，惡寒而踡，時自煩，欲去衣被者，可治。

290. 少陰中風，脈陽微陰浮者，爲欲愈。

291. 少陰病，欲解時，從子至寅上。

292. 少陰病，吐利，手足不逆冷，反發熱者，不死，脈不至者，灸少陰七壯。

293. 少陰病，八九日，一身手足盡熱者，以熱在膀胱，必便血也。

294. 少陰病，但厥無汗，而強發之，必動其血，未知從何道出，或從口鼻，或從目出者，是名下厥上竭，爲難治。

295. 少陰病，惡寒身踡而利，手足逆冷者，不治。

296. 少陰病，吐利躁煩，四逆者，死。

297. 少陰病，下利止而頭眩，時時自冒者，死。

298. 少陰病，四逆惡寒而身踡，脈不至，不煩而躁者死。

299. 少陰病，六七日，息高者死。

300. 少陰病，脈微細沉，但欲臥，汗出不煩，自欲吐，至五六日，自利，復煩躁不得臥寐者死。

301. 少陰病，始得之，反發熱，脈沉者，麻黃細辛附子湯主之。

麻黃二兩（去節）　細辛二兩　附子一枚（炮，去皮，破八片）　右三味，以水一斗，先煮麻黃，減二升，去上沫，內諸藥，煮取三升，去滓，溫服一升，日三服。

302. 少陰病，得之二三日，麻黃附子甘草湯微發汗，以二三日無證，故微發汗也。

麻黃二兩（去節）　甘草二兩（炙）　附子一枚（炮，去皮，破八片）　右三味，以水七升，先煮麻黃一兩沸，去上沫，內諸藥，煮取三升，去滓，溫服一升，日三服。

303. 少陰病，得之二三日以上，心中煩，不得臥，黃連阿膠湯主之。

黃連四兩　黃芩二兩　芍藥二兩　雞子黃二枚　阿膠三兩　右五味，以水六升，先煮三物，取二升，去滓，內膠烊盡，小冷，內雞子黃，攪令相得，溫服七合，日三服。

304. 少陰病，得之一二日，口中和，其背惡寒者，當灸之，附子湯主之。

305. 少陰病，身體痛，手足寒，骨節痛，脈沉者，附子湯主之。

附子二枚（炮，去皮，破八片）　茯苓三兩　人參二兩　白朮四兩　芍藥三兩　右五味，以水八升，煮取三升，去滓，溫服一升，日三服。

306. 少陰病，下利便膿血者，桃花湯主之。

赤石脂一斤（一半全用，一半篩末）　乾薑一兩　粳米一升　右三味，以水七升，煮米令熟，去滓，溫服七合，內赤石脂末方寸匕，日三服。若一服愈，餘勿服。

307. 少陰病，二三日至四五日，腹痛，小便不利，下利不止，便膿血者，桃花湯主之。

308. 少陰病，下利便膿血者，可刺。

309. 少陰病，吐利，手足逆冷，煩躁欲死者，吳茱萸湯主之。

吳茱萸一升　人參二兩　生薑六兩（切）　大棗十二枚（擘）　右四味，以水七升，煮取二升，去滓，溫服七合，日三服。

310. 少陰病，下利，咽痛，胸滿，心煩，豬膚湯主之。

豬膚一斤。　右一味，以水一斗，煮取五升，去滓，加白蜜一升，白粉五合，熬香，和令相得，溫分六服。

311. 少陰病，二三日，咽痛者，可與甘草湯；不差，與桔梗湯。

甘草二兩　右一味，以水三升，煮取一升半，去滓，溫服七合，日二服。

桔梗一兩　甘草二兩　右二味，以水三升，煮取一升，去滓，溫分再服。

312. 少陰病，咽中傷，生瘡，不能語言，聲不出者，苦酒湯主之。

半夏十四枚（洗，破如棗核）　雞子一枚（去黃，內上苦酒，著雞子殼中）。　右二味，內半夏，著苦酒中，以雞子殼置刀環中，安火上，令三沸，去滓，少少含嚥之。不差，更作三劑。

313. 少陰病，咽中痛，半夏散及湯主之。

半夏（洗）　桂枝（去皮）　甘草（炙）　右三味，等分，各別擣篩已，合治之。白飲和，服方寸匕，日三服。若不能散服者，以水一升，煎七沸，內散兩方寸匕，更煮三沸，下火令小冷，少少咽之。半夏有毒，不當散服。

314. 少陰病，下利，白通湯主之。

蔥白四莖　乾薑一兩　附子一枚（生，去皮，破八片）。　右三味，以水三升，煮取一升，去滓，分溫再服。

315. 少陰病，下利，脈微者，與白通湯。利不止，厥逆無脈，乾嘔煩者，白通加豬膽汁湯主之。服湯脈暴出者死，微續者生。

蔥白四莖　乾薑一兩　附子一枚（生，去皮，破八片）　人尿五合　豬膽汁一合。　右五味，以水三升，煮取一升，去滓，內膽汁、人尿，和令相得，分溫再服。若無膽，亦可用。

316. 少陰病，二三日不已，至四五日，腹痛，小便不利，四肢沉重疼痛，自下利者，此爲有水氣，其人或咳，或小便利，或下利，或嘔者，眞武湯主之。

茯苓三兩　芍藥三兩　白朮二兩　生薑三兩（切）　附子一枚（炮，去皮，破八片）　右五味，以水八升，煮取三升，去滓，溫服七合，日三服。若咳者，加五味子半升，細辛一兩，乾薑一兩。若小便利者，去茯苓。若下利者，去芍藥加乾薑二兩。若嘔者，去附子加生薑，足前爲半斤。

317. 少陰病，下利清穀，裏寒外熱，手足厥逆，脈微欲絕，身反不惡寒。其人面色赤，或腹痛，或乾嘔，或咽痛，或利止脈不出者，通脈四逆湯主之。

甘草二兩（炙）　附子大者一枚（生用，去皮，破八片）　乾薑三兩（強人可四兩）　右三味，以水三升，煮取一升二合，去滓，分溫再服，其脈即出者愈。面色赤者，加蔥九莖。腹中痛者，去蔥加芍藥二兩。嘔者，加生薑二兩。咽痛者，去芍藥加桔梗一兩。利止脈不出者，去桔梗加人參二兩，病皆與方相應者，乃服之。

318. 少陰病，四逆，其人或咳，或悸，或小便不利，或腹中痛，或泄利下重者，四逆散主之。

甘草（炙）　枳實（破，水漬，炙乾）　柴胡　芍藥　右四味，各十分，擣篩，白飲和，服方寸匕，日三服。咳者，加五味子、乾薑各五分，并主下利。悸者，加桂枝五分。小便不利者，加茯苓五分。腹中痛者，加附子一枚，炮令坼。泄利下重者，先以水五升，煮薤白三升，煮取三升，去滓，以散三方寸匕，內湯中，煮取一升半，分溫再服。

319. 少陰病，下利，六七日，咳而嘔渴，心煩不得眠者，豬苓湯主之。

320. 少陰病，得之二三日，口燥咽乾者，急下之，宜大承氣湯。

枳實五枚（炙）　厚朴半斤（去皮，炙）　大黃四兩（酒洗）　芒消三合　右四味，以水一斗，先煮二味，取五升，去滓，內大黃，更煮取二升，去滓，內芒消，更上火，令一兩沸，分溫再服。一服得利，止後服。

321. 少陰病，自利清水，色純青，心下必痛，口乾燥者，可下之，宜大承氣湯。

322. 少陰病，六七日，腹脹，不大便者，急下之，宜大承氣湯。

323. 少陰病，脈沉者，急溫之，宜四逆湯。

甘草二兩（炙）　乾薑一兩半　附子一枚（生用，去皮，破八片）　右三味，以水三升，煮取一升二合，去滓，分溫再服。強人可大附子一枚，乾薑三兩。

324. 少陰病，飲食入口則吐，心中溫溫欲吐，復不能吐，始得之，手足寒，脈弦遲者，此胸中實，不可下也，當吐之。若膈上有寒飲，乾嘔者，不可吐也，當溫之，宜四逆湯。

325. 少陰病，下利，脈微濇，嘔而汗出，必數更衣，反少者，當溫其上，灸之。

辨厥陰病脈證并治

326. 厥陰之爲病，消渴，氣上撞心，心中疼熱，飢而不欲食，食則吐蚘，下之利不止。

327. 厥陰中風，脈微浮，爲欲愈，不浮，爲未愈。

328. 厥陰病，欲解時，從丑至卯上。

329. 厥陰病，渴欲飲水者，少少與之愈。

330. 諸四逆厥者，不可下之，虛家亦然。

331. 傷寒先厥，後發熱而利者，必自止；見厥復利。

332. 傷寒始發熱六日，厥反九日而利。凡厥利者，當不能食，今反能食者，恐爲除中。食以索餅，不發熱者，知胃氣尚在，必愈。恐暴熱來出而復去也。後日脈之，其熱續在者，期之旦日夜半愈。所以然者，本發熱六日，厥反九日，復發熱三日，并前六日，亦爲九日，與厥相應，故期之旦日夜半愈。後三日脈之而脈數，其熱不罷者，此爲熱氣有餘，必發癰膿也。

333. 傷寒脈遲，六七日，而反與黃芩湯徹其熱，脈遲爲寒，今與黃芩湯復除其熱，腹中應冷，當不能食，今反能食，此名除中，必死。

334. 傷寒，先厥後發熱，下利必自止。而反汗出，咽中痛者，其喉爲痹。發熱無汗，而利必自止，若不止，必便膿血。便膿血者，其喉不痹。

335. 傷寒一二日，至四五日，厥者，必發熱，前熱者，後必厥。厥深者熱亦深，厥微者，熱亦微。厥應下之，而反發汗者，必口傷爛赤。

336. 傷寒病，厥五日，熱亦五日，設六日，當復厥，不厥者自愈。厥終不過五日，以熱五日，故知自愈。

337. 凡厥者，陰陽氣不相順接，便爲厥。厥者，手足逆冷者是也。

338. 傷寒，脈微而厥，至七八日，膚冷，其人躁無暫安時者，此爲藏厥，非蚘厥也。蚘厥者，其人當吐蚘。令病者靜，而復時煩者，此爲藏寒。蚘上入其膈，故煩，須臾復止，得食而嘔，又煩者，蚘聞食臭出，其人常自吐蚘。蚘厥者，烏梅丸主之。又主久利。

　　烏梅三百枚　細辛六兩　乾薑十兩　黃連十六兩　當歸四兩　附子六兩（炮，去皮）　蜀椒四兩（出汗）　桂枝六兩（去皮）　人參六兩　黃蘗六兩　右十味，異擣篩，合治之。以苦酒漬烏梅一宿，去核，蒸之五斗米下，飯熟擣成泥，和藥令相得，內臼中，與蜜杵二千下，丸如梧桐子大，先食飲服十丸，日三服，稍加至二十丸。禁生冷、滑物、臭食等。

339. 傷寒，熱少微厥，指頭寒，嘿嘿不欲食，煩躁。數日，小便利，色白者，此熱除也，欲得食，其病爲愈。若厥而嘔，胸脅煩滿者，其後必便血。

340. 病者手足厥冷，言我不結胸，小腹滿，按之痛者，此冷結在膀胱關元也。

341. 傷寒發熱四日，厥反三日，復熱四日，厥少熱多者，其病當愈。四日至七日，熱不除者，必便膿血。

342. 傷寒，厥四日，熱反三日，復厥五日，其病爲進。寒多熱少，陽氣退，故爲進也。

343. 傷寒六七日，脈微，手足厥冷，煩躁，灸厥陰，厥不還者，死。

344. 傷寒發熱，下利厥逆，躁不得臥者，死。

345. 傷寒發熱，下利至甚，厥不止者，死。

346. 傷寒六七日，不利，便發熱而利，其人汗出不止者，死，有陰無陽故也。

347. 傷寒五六日，不結胸，腹濡，脈虛復厥者，不可下，此亡血，下之死。

348. 發熱而厥，七日，下利者，爲難治。

349. 傷寒脈促，手足厥逆，可灸之。

350. 傷寒，脈滑而厥者，裏有熱，白虎湯主之。

知母六兩　石膏一斤（碎，綿裹）　甘草二兩（炙）　粳米六八　右四味，以水一斗，煮米熟，湯成去滓，溫服一升，日三服。

351. 手足厥寒，脈細欲絕者，當歸四逆湯主之。

當歸三兩　桂枝三兩（去皮）　芍藥三兩　細辛三兩　甘草二兩（炙）　通草二兩　大棗二十五枚（擘，一法，十二枚）　右七味，以水八升，煮取三升，去滓，溫服一升，日三服。

352. 若其人內有久寒者，宜當歸四逆加吳茱萸生薑湯。

當歸三兩　芍藥三兩　甘草二兩（炙）　通草二兩　桂枝三兩（去皮）　細辛三兩　生薑半斤（切）　吳茱萸二升　大棗二十五枚（擘）　右九味，以水六升，清酒六升和，煮取五升，去滓，溫分五服。

353. 大汗出，熱不去，內拘急，四肢疼，又下利，厥逆而惡寒者，四逆湯主之。

甘草二兩（炙）　乾薑一兩半　附子一枚（生用，去皮，破八片）　右三味，以水三升，煮取一升二合，去滓，分溫再服。若強人可用大附子一枚，乾薑三兩。

354. 大汗，若大下利而厥冷者，四逆湯主之。

355. 病人手足厥冷，脈乍緊者，邪結在胸中，心下滿而煩，飢不能食者，病在胸中，當須吐之，宜瓜蒂散。

瓜蒂　赤小豆　右二味，各等分，異擣篩，合內臼中，更治之。別以香豉一合，用熱湯七合，煮作稀糜，去滓，取汁和散一錢匕，溫頓服之。不吐者，少少加，得快吐乃止。諸亡血虛家，不可與瓜蒂散。 356. 傷寒，厥而心下悸，宜先治水，當服茯苓甘草湯，却治其厥。不爾，水漬入胃，必作利也。

茯苓二兩　甘草一兩（炙）　生薑三兩（切）　桂枝二兩（去皮）　右四味，以水四升，煮取二升，去滓，分溫三服。

357. 傷寒六七日，大下後，寸脈沉而遲，手足厥逆，下部脈不至，喉咽不利，唾膿血，泄利不止者，爲難治，麻黃升麻湯主之。

麻黃二兩半（去節）　升麻一兩一分　當歸一兩一分　知母十八銖　黃芩十八銖　萎蕤十八銖　芍藥六銖　天門冬六銖（去心）　桂枝六銖（去皮）　茯苓六銖　甘草六銖（炙）　石膏六銖（碎，綿裹）　白朮六銖　乾薑六銖　右十四味，以水一斗，先煮麻黃一兩沸，去上沫，內諸藥，煮取三升，去滓，分溫三服。相去如炊三斗米頃，令盡，汗出愈。

358. 傷寒四五日，腹中痛，若轉氣下趣少腹者，此欲自利也。

359. 傷寒本自寒下，醫復吐下之，寒格更逆吐下，若食入口即吐，乾薑黃芩黃連人參湯主之。

乾薑　黃芩　黃連　人參各三兩　右四味，以水六升，煮取二升，去滓，分溫再服。

360. 下利，有微熱而渴，脈弱者，今自愈。

361. 下利脈數，有微熱汗出，今自愈。設復緊，爲未解。

362. 下利，手足厥冷，無脈者，灸之。不溫，若脈不還，反微喘者，死。少陰負趺陽者，爲順也。

363. 下利，寸脈反浮數，尺中自濇者，必清膿血。

364. 下利清穀，不可攻表，汗出必脹滿。

365. 下利，脈沉弦者，下重也；脈大者，爲未止；脈微弱數者，爲欲自止，雖發熱，不死。

366. 下利，脈沉而遲，其人面少赤，身有微熱，下利清穀者，必鬱冒汗出而解，病人必微厥。所以然者，其面戴陽，下虛故也。

367. 下利，脈數而渴者，今自愈。設不差，必清膿血，以有熱故也。

368. 下利後脈絕，手足厥冷，晬時脈還，手足溫者，生；脈不還者，死。

369. 傷寒下利，日十餘行，脈反實者，死。

370. 下利清穀，裏寒外熱，汗出而厥者，通脈四逆湯主之。

甘草二兩（炙） 附子大者一枚（生，去皮，破八片） 乾薑三兩（強人可四兩） 右三味，以水三升，煮取一升二合，去滓，分溫再服。其脈即出者愈。

371. 熱利下重者，白頭翁湯主之。

白頭翁二兩 黃蘗三兩 黃連三兩 秦皮三兩 右四味，以水七升，煮取二升，去滓，溫服一升。不愈，更服一升。

372. 下利腹脹滿，身體疼痛者，先溫其裏，乃攻其表，溫裏宜四逆湯，攻表宜桂枝湯。

桂枝三兩（去皮） 芍藥三兩 甘草二兩（炙） 生薑三兩（切） 大棗十二枚（擘） 右五味，以水七升，煮取三升，去滓，溫服一升，須臾歠熱稀粥一升，以助藥力。

373. 下利欲飲水者，以有熱故也，白頭翁湯主之。

374. 下利讝語者，有燥屎也，宜小承氣湯。

大黃四兩（酒洗） 枳實三枚（炙） 厚朴二兩（去皮，炙） 右三味，以水四升，煮取一升二合，去滓，分二服。初一服讝語止，若更衣者，停後服。不爾，盡服之。

375. 下利後，更煩，按之心下濡者，為虛煩也，宜梔子豉湯。

肥梔子十四箇（擘） 香豉四合（綿裹） 右二味，以水四升，先煮梔子，取二升半，內豉，更煮取一升半，去滓，分再服。一服得吐，止後服。

376. 嘔家有癰膿者，不可治嘔，膿盡自愈。

377. 嘔而脈弱，小便復利，身有微熱，見厥者難治；四逆湯主之。

378. 乾嘔，吐涎沫，頭痛者，吳茱萸湯主之。

吳茱萸一升（湯洗七遍） 人參三兩 大棗十二枚（擘） 生薑六兩（切） 右四味，以水七升，煮取二升，去滓，溫服七合，日三服。

379. 嘔而發熱者，小柴胡湯主之。

柴胡八兩 黃芩三兩 人參三兩 甘草三兩（炙） 生薑三兩（切） 半夏半升（洗） 大棗十二枚（擘） 右七味，以水一斗二升，煮取六升，去滓，更煎取三升，溫服一升，日三服。

380. 傷寒，大吐大下之，極虛，復極汗者，其人外氣怫鬱，復與之水，以發其汗，因得噦。所以然者，胃中寒冷故也。

381. 傷寒，噦而腹滿，視其前後，知何部不利，利之即愈。

辨霍亂病脈證并治

382. 問曰：病有霍亂者何？答曰：嘔吐而利，此名霍亂。

383. 問曰：病發熱，頭痛，身疼，惡寒，吐利者，此屬何病？答曰：此名霍亂。霍亂自吐下，又利止，復更發熱也。

384. 傷寒，其脈微濇者，本是霍亂，今是傷寒，却四五日，至陰經上，轉入陰必利，本嘔下利者，不可治也。欲似大便，而反失氣，仍不利者，此屬陽明也，便必硬，十三日愈。所以然者，經盡故也。下利後，當便硬，硬則能食者愈。今反不能食，到後經中，頗能食，復過一經能食，過之一日當愈。不愈者，不屬陽明也。

385. 惡寒脈微而復利，利止亡血也，四逆加人參湯主之。

甘草二兩（炙） 附子一枚（生，去皮，破八片） 乾薑一兩半 人參一兩 右四味，以水三升，煮取一升二合，去滓，分溫再服。

386. 霍亂，頭痛發熱，身疼痛，熱多欲飲水者，五苓散主之；寒多不用水者，理中丸主之。

人參 乾薑 甘草（炙） 白朮各三兩 右四味，擣篩，蜜和爲丸如雞子黃許大，以沸湯數合和一丸，研碎，溫服之，日三四、夜二服。腹中未熱，益至三四丸，然不及湯。湯法：以四物依兩數切，用水八升，煮取三升，去滓，溫服一升，日三服。若臍上築者，腎氣動也，去朮加桂四兩。吐多者，去朮加生薑三兩。下多者，還用朮。悸者，加茯苓二兩。渴欲得水者，加朮，足前成四兩半。腹中痛者，加人參，足前成四兩半。寒者加乾薑，足前成四兩半。腹滿者，去朮加附子一枚。服湯後，如食頃，飲熱粥一升許，微自溫，勿發揭衣被。

387. 吐利止而身痛不休者，當消息和解其外，宜桂枝湯小和之。

桂枝三兩（去皮） 芍藥三兩 生薑三兩 甘草二兩（炙） 大棗十二枚（擘） 右五味，以水七升，煮取三升，去滓，溫服一升。

388. 吐利汗出，發熱惡寒，四肢拘急，手足厥冷者，四逆湯主之。

甘草二兩（炙） 乾薑一兩半 附子一枚（生，去皮，破八片） 右三味，以水三升，煮取一升二合，去滓，分溫再服。強人可大附子一枚，乾薑三兩。

389. 既吐且利，小便復利，而大汗出，下利清穀，內寒外熱，脈微欲絕者，四逆湯主之。

390. 吐已下斷，汗出而厥，四肢拘急不解，脈微欲絕者，通脈四逆加豬膽湯主之。

甘草二兩（炙） 乾薑三兩（強人可四兩） 附子大者一枚（生，去皮，破八片） 豬膽汁半合 右四味，以水三升，煮取一升二合，去滓，內豬膽汁，分溫再服，其脈即來，無豬膽，以羊膽代之。

391. 吐利發汗，脈平，小煩者，以新虛不勝穀氣故也。

392. 傷寒陰〔陽〕易之爲病，其人身體重，少氣，少腹裏急，或引陰中拘攣，熱上衝胸，頭重不欲舉，眼中生花，膝脛拘急者，燒褌散主之。

婦人中褌，近隱處，取燒作灰。 右一味，水服方寸匕，日三服，小便即利，陰頭微腫，此爲愈矣。婦人病，取男子褌燒服。

393. 大病差後，勞復者，枳實梔子豉湯主之。

枳實三枚（炙） 梔子十四箇（擘） 豉一升（綿裹） 右三味，以清漿水七升，空煮取四升，內枳實、梔子，煮取二升，下豉，更煮五六沸，去滓，溫分再服。覆令微似汗。若有宿食者，內大黃如博碁子五六枚，服之愈。

394. 傷寒差以後，更發熱，小柴胡湯主之。脈浮者，以汗解之，脈沉實者，以下解之。

柴胡八兩 人參二兩 黃芩二兩 甘草二兩（炙） 生薑二兩 半夏半升（洗） 大棗十二枚（擘） 右七味，以水一斗二升，煮取六升，去滓，再煎取三升，溫服一升，日三服。

395. 大病差後，從腰以下有水氣者，牡蠣澤瀉散主之。

牡蠣（熬） 澤瀉 蜀漆（煖水洗去腥） 葶藶子（熬） 商陸根（熬） 海藻（洗去鹹） 栝樓根各等分 右七味，異擣，下篩爲散，更於臼中治之，白飲和，服方寸匕，日三服。小便利，止後服。

396. 大病差後，喜唾，久不了了，胸上有寒，當以丸藥溫之，宜理中丸。

人參　白朮　甘草（炙）　乾薑各三兩　右四味，擣篩，蜜和爲丸，如雞子黃許大，以沸湯數合，和一丸，研碎，溫服之，日三服。

397. 傷寒解後，虛羸少氣，氣逆欲吐，竹葉石膏湯主之。

竹葉二把　石膏一斤　半夏半升（洗）　麥門冬一升（去心）　人參二兩　甘草二兩（炙）　粳米半升　右七味，以水一斗，煮取六升，去滓，內粳米，煮米熟，湯成去米，溫服一升，日三服。

398. 病人脈已解，而日暮微煩，以病新差，人強與穀，脾胃氣尚弱，不能消穀，故令微煩，損穀則愈。

Appendix II
Shāng Hán Lùn Language Study

We hope that students who have already acquired notions of the Chinese language will apply their developing skills to reading the Chinese text of the *Shāng Hán Lùn* as well as the translation. The *Shāng Hán Lùn* is an ideal text for learners of classical Chinese because of the relative simplicity of its grammatical structures and smallness of its vocabulary. To help beginning students, we offer a concise description of the language of the *Shāng Hán Lùn*, presenting the basic grammatical patterns and vocabulary it uses.

The *Shāng Hán Lùn*, as the earlier classics of Chinese medicine, is written in classical Chinese, the language of the philosophical writings of Confucius, Mencius, and Laozi. Classical Chinese is the traditional name given to the written form of Old Chinese, the language of the period from the end of the Spring and Autumn period down to the end of the Hàn Dynasty (5th century B.C.E. to 3rd century C.E.). Old Chinese differs from modern Chinese in certain grammatical patterns, vocabulary, and use of words. One of the most striking changes that has taken place in the spoken language is the increase in compounds; thus while the equivalent of an English word in classical Chinese is usually a single syllable (in writing, a single character), in the modern language it is often a compound. Despite these changes, a great continuity exists between classical Chinese and modern Chinese, so much so that the former is accessible to modern Chinese people in a way that Latin, say, is not accessible to modern Italian people. A major reason for this continuity is that in spite of the huge changes in pronunciation that have occurred, the written form of words has retained a continuous identity.

For those wishing to learn Chinese to gain access to medical knowledge, familiarity with the classical language is just as important as familiarity with the modern written and spoken language. Despite the changes that took place in the spoken language over the centuries, the written language for centuries remained relatively conservative, continuing to take classical Chinese as its model. New literary forms of writing developed, partly under the influence of changes in the spoken language, yet also partly independently of them. In the early twentieth century, the standard written language was remodeled on the cultivated speech of northern China (Mandarin, now called Pǔtōnghuà in the PRC), thus bringing the written language up-to-date with the times. All modern writing—newspapers, scientific and technical literature, creative literature—is expressed in the modern vernacular form of writing, 白话文 *bái huà wén* ("plain-speech writing"), even though it is often liberally peppered with classical expressions and turns of phrase. In Chinese medicine, which is still strongly rooted in classical medical literature, the switch to modern vernacular writing was not so easily made. Though the general expression of modern Chinese medical texts has been vernacularized, Chinese medical terminology is still largely classical. Although, for example, in vernacular writing the classical 目 *mù*, eye, has now been replaced by 眼睛 and 足 *zú*, foot, by 脚 *jiǎo*, the classical terms are still very much in use in modern Chinese medical literature.

The study of Chinese usually begins with the script. This is the greatest hurdle in learning Chinese, but the effort it takes rewards the assiduous student with access not only to modern, but also to classical writing. As regards sentence patterns and word usage, classical Chinese can be learned in tandem with the modern language without much difficulty. Those studying Chinese specifically for medical purposes will find in some ways that they make swifter headway in gaining the passive knowledge needed to read classical texts than they make in gaining the active knowledge required to communicate verbally in modern Chinese. The *Shāng Hán Lùn* provides an excellent introduction to the language of Chinese medicine since it is expressed in a limited gamut of sentence patterns, and uses a vocabulary of a little over 900 characters, probably considerably fewer than the number used in modern Chinese medical books. Most of the characters appearing in the *Shāng Hán Lùn* are among the most commonly used in the everyday modern language. Given the prominent place of the *Shāng Hán Lùn* in the history of medicine in China, much of the terminology it contains is still used in modern literature. Students who have mastered the basic rules of character composition (signific, phonetics) and know how to look up words in a Chinese dictionary will find that by studying the material contained in this appendix they will be able to approach the text without too many difficulties.

Our sketch of the language of the *Shāng Hán Lùn* falls into two parts: basic grammatical structures and vocabulary.

Grammar

The vocabulary of the Chinese language can, as in all languages, be classified according to word-classes (or parts of speech). Chinese, just as English, has nouns representing objects, phenomena, and concepts; it has verbs denoting action, and adjectives describing states. It also has pronouns, which stand for nouns, and adverbs, which qualify verbs, as well as prepositions and conjunctions, which provide various links. Words of these classes interact in a sentence according to certain grammatical patterns.

The chief feature of classical Chinese is that words retain the same form no matter what function they perform in a sentence.[1] Words in general show no word-class marking (as English "-ize," "-ation," "-ly"). Verbs have no personal or tense inflection ("give," "gives," "gave" are represented by a single form). Nouns have no singular/plural distinction, and do not require any article ("a patient," "patients," "the patient" are represented by a single form). Furthermore, although most words can be basically classified according to word-classes, many words can be used with different word-class functions (e.g., the noun 篩 *shāi*, "sieve," can also be used as a verb to mean to "sift").

In the absence of complex variations in word forms, grammatical relationships are largely by word order. Since Chinese, like English, follows a "subject-verb-object" order (e.g., "the physician cures the patient"), English-speaking students find the grammar of classical Chinese relatively easy. Difficulties for foreign learners lie mainly in certain specific constructions (e.g., those involving 者 *zhě* and 所

[1] This may not have always been so. A distinction between subject and object pronouns may constitute the vestiges of a case system. A difference in pronunciation of certain verbs according to whether they are used intransitively or causatively may be evidence of a former inflectional system.

suǒ), in the multiple meanings of words, and in overall interpretation of sentences comprising loosely strung clauses. Apart from these difficulties, the grammatical structures appearing in the *Shāng Hán Lùn* can be learned quite quickly.

Subject-verb-object

One of the recurrent needs of any language is to express the action of a subject, and very often, the action of a subject on an object. Sentences involving subjects, verbs, and objects are therefore of particularly high frequency.

As we have said, basic Chinese sentences follow a subject-verb-object pattern, that is, subject-verb-object is the basic order of a sentence that has a subject, verb, and object. Since English also follows the same subject-verb-object order, many Chinese sentences follow a pattern familiar to English speakers. The following Chinese sentence is identically structured in English:

1. 医发汗 *yī fā hàn*, [the] physician promotes sweating[2]

Simple sentences with intransitive verbs or adjectives have no objects. In the following examples, the order of the English sentence is again identical to that of the Chinese. English requires more words than Chinese to make sense and the words appearing in the English sentences that do not appear in Chinese are written in brackets.

2. 头痛 *tóu tòng*, [the] head aches/[is] painful
3. 脉沉迟 *mài chén chí*, [the] pulse [is] sunken [and] slow

The last example shows two further features of Chinese. One is that adjectives can follow their subjects without any equivalent of the English verb "to be," so that "subject + adjective" constructions are formally indistinguishable from "subject + verb" constructions. For this reason, adjectives and verbs in Chinese are often referred to as "stative verbs" and "active verbs," respectively. The other feature is that two stative verbs can succeed one another without being separated by any word equivalent to "and," which in English is mandatory.

In English, a verb invariably has a subject (there are exceptions, such as imperatives), but in Chinese (classical and modern) a subject is not necessary. When the subject can be deduced from context, it is often redundant. Thus in a medical text such as the *Shāng Hán Lùn*, descriptions of pathological states, for instance, do not require a subject, since the we know that "the patient" is the subject. Thus the following two examples can be said to be complete Chinese sentences, whereas complete sentences in English require the addition of a subject.

4. 吐血 *tù xuè*, [the patient] vomits blood
5. 发热 *fā rè*, [the patient] effuses heat, [i.e., is running a fever]

In Chinese (modern as well as classical), a verb-object construction is used to express the idea that something exists, which we express in English by "there" with the verb "to be." In Chinese, the verb 有 *yǒu* is followed by an object.

6. 有热 *yǒu rè*, there is heat
7. 有燥屎 *yǒu zào shǐ*, there is dry stool

The same verb when preceded by a subject is equivalent to the English "have."

[2]The Chinese 发汗 *fā hàn* means literally "to effuse (put forth) sweat." In the *Shāng Hán Lùn*, this expression generally means "to cause (the patient) to sweat"; in modern Chinese, the same expression usually means "to sweat" or "perspire."

8. 病人有寒 *bìng rén yǒu hán*, the patient (lit. "sick person") has cold

The verb 有 *yǒu* has a special negative form, 无 *wú*, which will be discussed ahead.

9. 无寒 *wú hán*, there is no cold, [the patient] has no cold

Equational sentences

Besides subject-verb-object sentences, there are sentences—in Chinese and English alike—that equate one thing with another (e.g., "the patient is a child"). These are called equational or copulative sentences. In English, equation is expressed by the verb "to be," in the form "X is Y." In Old Chinese, there was originally no verb equivalent to the English verb "to be" that coupled two nominal expressions. The two items were placed one in front of the other, usually followed by a final particle 也 *yě* at the end of the sentence, expressing the notion that the second item was a definition or explanation of the first item: "X Y 也." In the *Shāng Hán Lùn*, we find the following example:

10. 此误也 *cǐ wù yě*, this [is a] mistake PARTICLE

The subject of the sentence can also be marked as such with the particle 者 *zhě*: "X 者， Y 也." In the *Shāng Hán Lùn*, this construction is more common than the one previously described.

11. 郑声者，重语也 *zhèng shēng zhě, chóng yǔ yě*, muttering is repetitious speech PARTICLE
12. 但热者，实也 *dàn rè zhě, shí yě*, heat alone [is] repletion PARTICLE

Note that although it is modern typographical convention to place a comma after 者 *zhě*, the comma, as all other punctuation marks, was originally absent in classical Chinese.

The "X Y 也" equational sentence is called a "nominal sentence" because it consists of nouns (or words that stand in for nouns) without a verb. Alongside the nominal copulative sentence, there developed a verbal copulative sentence, in which the verb 为 *wéi*, "to act," was used very much as the verb "to be" in English. This kind of verbal sentence, like the nominal sentence, usually terminates with 也 *yě*: "X 为 Y 也."

13. 此为逆也 *cǐ wéi nì yě*, this is adverse [treatment] PARTICLE

Note that 为 *wéi* has a number of other meanings including "to make" and "to cause."

A more complex version of the nominal sentence uses the demonstrative pronoun 是 *shì*, "this": "X （者） Y （者）是也."

14. 阳明之为病，胃家实是也 *yáng míng zhī wéi bìng, wéi jiā shí shì yě*, disease of yáng brightness is stomach domain repletion
15. 厥者，手足逆冷者是也 *jué zhě, shǒu zú nì lěng shì yě*, lit. "reversal: counterflow cold of the extremities [is what] this [is]," i.e., reversal is counterflow cold of the extremities

Another nominal sentence pattern using 是 is "X 是 Y 也," where 是 *shì*, "this," recapitulates the subject. Probably because of a structural analogy with the "X 为 Y 也," the 是 in such sentences gradually came to be reinterpreted as an equational verb like 为 *wéi*, "to be." In modern Chinese, 是 *shì* is the standard equational verb, and its use as a demonstrative pronoun is obsolete. A couple of examples of 是 *shì* as an equational verb are found in the *Shāng Hán Lùn*:[3]

16. 本是霍乱，今是伤寒 *bǔ shì huò luàn, jīn shì shāng hán*, originally, [it] was cholera; now [it] is cold damage

Finally, Chinese has yet one further verb that is equivalent to our verb "to be." The word 属 *shǔ*, which in some contexts means "to belong," is often used to express the notion of one thing being a subset of another.

17. 此属胃 *cǐ shǔ wèi*, this is [a] stomach [problem]

Copulative sentences in Chinese, whether nominal or verbal, are used to express a wider range of meanings than mere equation. In translation, it is often clearer to express the intended meaning with "to mean" or "to indicate," rather than "to be."

18. 潮热者，实也 *cháo rè zhě, shí yě*, tidal heat [effusion] is/means/indicates repletion.
19. 浮为风 *fú wéi fēng*, floating (of the pulse) means wind

The verbs 似 *sì*, 象 *xiàng*, and 如 *rú*, all meaning "to resemble," can also be considered to be copulative verbs. In the *Shāng Hán Lùn*, the last one is more commonly used as a preposition equivalent to the English "like."

20. 形似疟 *xíng sì nüè*, the form (appearance) [of the disease] resembles malaria
21. 证象阳旦 *zhèng xiàng yáng dàn*, the signs resemble [those of] yáng dawn
22. 如惊痫 *rú jīng xián*, like fright epilepsy
23. 饮食如故 *yǐn shí rú gù*, eating and drinking as before [the illness] (i.e., as normal)
24. 丸如梧桐子大 *wán rú wú tóng zǐ dà*, [make into] pills like firmiana seeds large, [i.e., make into pills the size of firmiana seeds]

Finally, we should introduce the verb 然 *rán*, "to be so," which is believed to be a fusion of 如 *rú* and a no longer identifiable pronoun ending in the sound [n]. The expression 如此 *rú cǐ*, "to be like this," "to be so," is the same in meaning, although it can also be used adverbially ("like this," "in this way").

Expressing location

Location, which is yet another idea that English expresses with the verb "to be," is expressed in classical Chinese, as indeed still in modern Chinese, by a special verb, 在 *zài*. While English expresses location with the verb "to be" followed by a preposition (in, on, at, etc.), Chinese does not necessarily require a preposition. Thus, in its simplest form, the Chinese construction is "X 在 Y," corresponding to the English "X is/are at/in/on... Y."

25. 病在表 *bìng zài biǎo*, [the] disease is [in the] exterior
26. 热在下焦 *rè zài xià jiāo*, heat is [in the] lower burner

The verb 在 *zài* not followed by a word indicating location simply implies presence.

27. 表证仍在 *biǎo zhèng réng zài*, [the] exterior signs [are] still present

[3] A mark of the reinterpretation of 是 as a verb is seen in its ability to be negated by 不 *bù*, which can (with few exceptions) precede only a verb. Nevertheless, there is no example of 不是 *bù shì* in the *Shāng Hán Lùn*.

For location at a point, no word corresponding to the English prepositions "in," "at," "on," etc., is necessarily required. Only when a specific location is indicated within or outside the object in question is any additional word required. Locative words appearing in the *Shāng Hán Lùn* include: 内 *nèi*, "in," "within;" 外 *wài*, "outside;" 中 *zhōng*, "in," "within;" 上 *shàng*, "on," "on top of," or "above;" and 下 *xià*, "below." A feature of these words is that they *follow* the nouns they refer to; hence they are "postpositions" rather than "prepositions" as the corresponding words are in English.

28. 盆内 *pén nèi*, lit. "pot inside," i.e., in [a] pot
29. 脉外 *mài wài*, lit. "vessels outside," i.e., outside the vessels
30. 胸中 *xiōng zhōng*, in the chest
31. 胃中 *wèi zhōng*, in the stomach
32. 胁下 *xié xià*, under the rib-side
33. 舌上 *shé shàng*, on the tongue
34. 额上 *é shàng*, on the forehead

These locative phrases may follow 在 *zài*:

35. 病在膈上 *bìng zài gé shàng*, the disease is above the diaphragm

They can be used adverbially before a verb:

36. 胸中有热 *xiōng zhōng yǒu rè*, lit. "in the chest there is heat," i.e., there is heat in the chest
37. 膈上有寒饮 *gé shàng yǒu hán yǐn*, there is cold rheum above (or on) the diaphragm
38. 心下有水气 *xīn xià yǒu shuǐ qì*, there is water-qì below the heart

The words 前 *qián*, "in front of," and 后 *hòu*, "behind," are two more important locatives. These are encountered in the *Shāng Hán Lùn*, but only in their extended senses of "before" and "after."

39. 秋前 *qiū qián*, before autumn
40. 大汗出后 *dà hàn chū hòu*, after great sweat [has] issued

In addition to locative words placed after the noun they refer to, Chinese possesses a number of prepositions that are placed before the noun. The most important one is 于 *yú*, "at" or "to" (in some cases even "from").

41. 阳绝于里 *yáng jué yú lǐ*, yáng cut off in the interior
42. 邪气结于胁下 *xié qì jié yú xié xià*, evil qì binds below the rib-side

Expressing movement

The generic notion of "to move," "to go," in classical Chinese is expressed as 行 *xíng*.

43. 行其经 *xíng qí jīng*, move [through] the channels
44. 卫行脉外 *wèi xíng mài wài*, defense [qì] moves outside the vessels
45. 荣行脉外 *róng xíng mài wài*, construction [qì] moves inside the vessels

The words 上 *shāng* and 下 *xià*, in addition to indicating location ("on" and "under"), also act as verbs, "to ascend" and "to descend." The words 出 *chū* and 入 *rù* mean "to exit" or "to issue" (to come out or go out) and "to enter," respectively.

46. 谷气下流 *gǔ qì xià liú*, grain qì flows down
47. 客气上逆 *kè qì shàng nì*, visiting qì ascends counterflow

The locatives 内 *nèi*, "in(side)," and 外 *wài*, "out(side)," may also be combined with verbs in the sense of "toward the inside" and "toward the outside."

48. 阳气内陷 *yáng qì nèi xiàn*, lit. "yáng qì inward(ly) falls," i.e., yáng qì falls inward

Sometimes a destination is added to a verb of movement:

49. 气上冲咽喉 *qì shàng chōng yān hóu*, qì surges up [into] the throat
50. 蚘上入其膈 *huí shàng rù qí gé*, [the] roundworms rise [and] enter the diaphragm

We have already introduced the preposition 于 *yú*. Two other prepositions should be mentioned, both originally verbs. The term 从 *cóng*, "to follow," is also used prepositionally in the sense of "via" or "from"; 至 *zhì*, "to arrive," is used in the sense of "to" (equivalent of the modern 到 *dào*).

51. 从心下至少腹 *cóng xīn xià zhì shào fù*, from [the region] below the heart to the lesser abdomen
52. 气从少腹上冲心 *qì cóng shào fù shàng chōng xīn*, lit. "qì from the lesser abdomen upwardly surges [into the] heart," i.e., qì surges up from the lesser abdomen into the heart
53. 从目出 *cóng mù chū*, lit. "issues via (or from) the eyes," i.e., comes out of the eyes

Note the idiomatic nature of the following construction:

54. 邪无从出 *xié wú cóng chū*, lit. "evil has no [way] via [which to] issue," i.e., evil has no way out

至 *zhì* is often used in the sense of "up to" with numbers:

55. 至七八日 *zhì qī bā rì*, up to seven or eight days

Auxiliary verbs

A number of auxiliary verbs appear in the *Shāng Hán Lùn*. These include modal auxiliaries, which are verbs used to modify the sense of the main verb to express possibility, ability, desire, obligation, etc. In addition, there are two causative verbs.

可 *kě*, may, can	宜 *yí*, to be appropriate to
能 *néng*, can, able to	欲 *yù*, desire to, want to, about to
得 *dé*, may, can, able to	须 *xū*, need to; to wait
当 *dāng*, should, ought to	使 *shǐ*, cause to
必 *bì*, will be, bound to be; must be	令 *lìng*, cause to

The use of most auxiliary verbs is relatively straightforward, as the following examples show:

56. 可与桂枝汤 *kě yǔ guì zhī tāng*, [one] can give Cinnamon Twig Decoction
57. 不能食 *bù néng shí*, cannot/is unable to eat
58. 大便当硬 *dà biàn dāng yìng*, [the] stool should be hard
59. 必渴 *bì kě*, will be (bound to be) thirsty
60. 欲吐 *yù tù*, wants to vomit
61. 欲解 *yù jiě*, about to resolve
62. 不得眠 *bù dé mián*, cannot/is unable to sleep
63. 宜服小柴胡汤 *yí fú xiǎo chái hú tāng*, [one] can/should (it is appropriate for one to) take Minor Bupleurum Decoction

The word 宜 *yí* has the sense of "appropriate," but when it is used as an auxiliary verb, it can be translated as "can" or "should." In the *Shāng Hán Lùn*, 宜 *yí* is usually not an auxiliary but a full verb, meaning "to be appropriate to use."

64. 宜麻黄汤 *yí má huáng tāng*, it is appropriate to use Ephedra Decoction; Ephedra Decoction is appropriate

The causative verbs 使 *shǐ* and 令 *lìng* are both used in similar fashion.

65. 使不大便 *shǐ bù dà biàn*, causes [the patient] not [to] defecate
66. 增桂令汗出 *zēng guì lìng hàn chū*, increase [the] cinnamon to make sweat issue

Negatives

We have already seen 无 *wú*, the negative form of 有 *yǒu*.

67. 无汗 *wú hàn*, there is no sweat
68. 病人无他病 *bìng rén wú tā bìng*, the patient has no other illness

Chinese (classical and modern) has a number of other negatives. Those appearing in the *Shāng Hán Lùn* are the following:

非 *fēi*, negative in nominal sentences
不 *bù*, not
未 *wèi*, not yet
勿 *wù*, negative in the imperative
莫 *mò*, not at all; negative in the imperative

非 *fēi* is the negative used in nominal sentences, that is, in copulative sentences in which there is no verb.

69. 此非结热 *cǐ fēi jié rè*, this [is] not heat bind

In verbal sentences, 不 *bù* is the general negative for all verbs except 有 *yǒu*, "there is/are," "have."

70. 不可发汗 *bù kě fā hàn*, lit. "[you, the physician] not can promote sweating," [one] cannot promote sweating

Sometimes 不 *bù* is used in a more loaded sense:

71. 不治 *bù zhì*, [can, will] not cure
72. 不去 *bù qù*, won't go away

The negative 未 *wèi* is used to negate an action or event that fails to occur as expected. It is often translated as "not yet," although the expression 尚未 *shàng wèi*, which corresponds more literally to the English "not yet," is used when an action or event has not occurred at the expected time.

73. 未发汗 *wèi fā hàn*, [has] not promote[d] sweating
74. 表未解 *biǎo wèi jiě*, [the] exterior [has] not resolve[d]
75. 面色反有热色者，未欲解也 *miàn sè fǎn yǒu rè sè zhě, wèi yù jiě yě*, but facial complexion with the color of heat indicates [the disease] is not about to resolve
76. 尚未可攻 *shàng wèi kě gōng*, [one] cannot attack yet

The negative 勿 *wù* is used with imperatives.

77. 勿治之 *wù zhī zhī*, do not treat it

无 *wú* is sometimes used as an imperative negative:

78. 无犯胃气及上二焦 *wú fàn wèi qì jí shàng èr jiāo*, do not assail the stomach qì and the upper two burners

莫 *mò* has certain specialized usages in classical Chinese. In its single occurrence in the *Shāng Hán Lùn*, however, it is used like 勿 *wù*.

79. 更莫复服 *gèng mò fù fú*, don't take any more

Adverbs

Adverbs include adverbs proper, and adverbs derived from other word-classes. The adverbs proper that occur in the *Shāng Hán Lùn* are the following:

乃 *nǎi*, in fact, precisely; then, thereupon, consequently (equivalent to the modern 就 *jiù*)
则 *zé*, then
即 *jí*, then immediately
亦 *yì*, also
又 *yòu*, again, further
再 *zài*, again, then, twice
却 *què*, then
仍 *réng*, still
初 *chū*, at the beginning
今 *jīn*, now
先 *xiān*, first
后 *hòu*, afterwards
久 *jiǔ*, for a long time
常 *cháng*, often, constantly
都 *dōu*, all, both
皆 *jiē*, all, both
俱 *jù*, all, both
悉 *xī*, all, entirely
全 *quán*, all, entirely
乍 *zhà*, suddenly
互 *hù*, mutually, reciprocally, each other
相 *xiāng*, mutually, reciprocally, each other
因 *yīn*, so, accordingly, thereby, as a result
尚 *shàng*, still
但 *dàn*, only

Other adverbs are most commonly derived from verbs (stative and active), nouns, and, in one case, a pronoun. Those given in the preceding list are the main ones encountered in the *Shāng Hán Lùn*, but there are many others.

将 *jiāng* (intend to), about to
复 *fù* (return, restore), again, then
更 *gèng* (change), again, then
反 *fǎn* (turn over), but, instead
益 *yì* (increase), even (more)
已 *yǐ* (finish), already
适 *shì* (appropriate, right, just), just, coincidentally (happen to)
甚 *shèn*, (very, marked, pronounced, very), markedly
微 *wēi* (faint, slight), slightly
太 *tài* (supreme, great), too
少 *shǎo* (little, few), in little amounts, to a small extent
小 *xǎo* (small), in small amounts, to a small extent
稍 *shāo* (little), in little amounts, to a small extent
过 *guò* (cross, pass, exceed), excessively
暴 *bào* (fulminant), fulminantly (suddenly and violently)
本 *běn* (stem-root), originally
自 *zì* (self), spontaneously ([of] itself)

Many of the adverbs listed above are self-explanatory, so we will limit the discussion here to the ones that are most troublesome to students.

Like negatives, simple adverbs such as those listed above are also placed in front of the verb. In the following examples, the adverbs 仍 *réng*, "still," and 已 *yǐ*, "already," are interposed between the subject and verb.

80. 表证仍在 *biǎo zhèng réng zài*, the exterior signs are still present

81. 外已解 *wài yǐ jiě*, [the] outer [body] [has] already resolve[d]
82. 复发汗 *fù fā hàn*, again promote sweating

The classical 乃 *nǎi* is used in nominal sentences with a mild sense of "in fact" ("X 乃 Y 也," "X is in fact Y"). It is also used in a second clause indicating that the action or event is chronological or the logical consequence of the action or event described in the first clause.

83. 先温其里，乃攻其表 *xiān wēn qí lǐ, nǎi gōng qí biǎo*, first warm the interior, then attack the exterior

When translating into English, "action/event X, 乃 action/event Y" is sometimes best rendered as "When X, (then) Y":

84. 表解乃可攻痞 *biǎo jiě nǎi kě gōng pǐ*, lit. "exterior resolves, then [one] can attack the glomus," i.e., when the exterior resolves, (then) one can attack the glomus.

则 *zé* functions like 乃 *nǎi* in the sense of "then" or "consequently," but is not used in nominal sentences. Since it may introduce a full clause, a preceding subject and verb, it is also considered as a conjunction (see below).

即 *jí*, "then," "immediately," is used like 乃 *nǎi* and 则 *zé*, usually implying that the one action follows straight after the other.

85. 若食入口即吐 *ruò shí rù kǒu jí tù*, if food enters the mouth, [the patient] immediately vomits

皆 *jiē*, 都 *dōu*, 俱 *jù*, and 悉 *xī* are all adverbs meaning "all" or "both." Nevertheless, they are often best translated by the corresponding adjectives in English:

86. 结胸证悉具 *jié xiōng zhèng xī jù*, "chest bind signs [are] all present" or "all chest bind signs [are] present"

Two words meaning "again" appear in the *Shāng Hán Lùn*, 复 *fù* and 更 *gèng*.

87. 复服 *fù fú*, take [the medicine] again
88. 不可更发汗 *bù kě gèng fā hàn*, cannot promote sweating again

Rather confusingly for the learner, 更 *gèng* and 复 *fù* are also both used adverbially in the sense of "then" or "further," as the examples below show. Note that the same ambiguity attaches to the modern 再 *zài*.

89. 大下之后，复发汗 *dà xià zhī hòu, fù fā hàn*, [when] after great precipitation, sweating is then promoted
90. 其人发热汗出，复恶寒 *qí rén fā rè hàn chū, fù wù hán*, the person effuses heat, sweats, and then [has] aversion to cold

Both these words are also used as verbs: 复 *fù* means "to restore" (as in 复脉汤 *fù mài tāng*, Pulse-Restorative Decoction), while 更 *gēng* (here in the first rather than the fourth tone) means "to change" (as in 更衣 *gēng yī*, to change [one's] clothes).

互 *hù* and 相 *xiāng* are both adverbs meaning reciprocally or mutually, and often translate into English as "each other." They appear singly or paired.

91. 互相克贼 *hù xiàng kè zéi*, restraining and robbing
92. 风湿相搏 *fēng shī xiāng bó*, wind and dampness contending with each other

Although all the adverbs listed above have survived into modern Chinese, a good number are now used differently. For example, 亦 *yì*, in the *Shāng Hán Lùn* and in classical Chinese in general, is the standard expression for "also"; in modern standard Chinese, it has been replaced by 也 *yě*, which in classical Chinese serves only as a final particle. In the *Shāng Hán Lùn*, 益 *yì*, whose primary meaning is "to increase," is used in the sense of "even (more)," although it no longer has the latter meaning in the modern spoken language. 但 *dàn* usually means "only" in the *Shāng Hán Lùn*, while in the modern language it retains this meaning only in 不但... 也 *bú dàn... yě*, "not only... but also." The word 但 *dàn* means "but" in the modern language, yet it is rarely used in this sense in the *Shāng Hán Lùn*.[4] 更 *gèng* in the *Shāng Hán Lùn* means "again," while nowadays it means "even (more)." 复 *fù*, also meaning "again," is now no longer a free-standing word and only appears in bound verb compounds.[5] Both 更 *gèng* and 复 *fù* in the sense of "then" or "further" have been replaced in the modern language with 再 *zài*.

Pronouns

The pronouns most commonly occurring in the *Shāng Hán Lùn* are the third-person pronouns, namely the subject pronoun 其 *qí*, "he," "she," "it," "they," or (more commonly) "his," "her," "its," "their," and the object pronoun 之 *zhī*.

Two of several first-person pronouns appear in the *Shāng Hán Lùn*: 余 *yú* and 我 *wǒ*. The former is the word by which Zhāng Jī refers to himself in his preface; and 我 *wǒ* is the word by which a patient refers to himself in a quotation.

Both 其 *qí* and 之 *zhī* are somewhat idiomatic in their usage. Since Chinese requires no subject in a sentence, subject pronouns are essentially redundant. The word 其 *qí* is used rarely as the subject pronoun in the *Shāng Hán Lùn*, and its most common usage is as a possessive equivalent to the English "his," "her," or "its." Nevertheless, in most contexts where it appears, 其 *qí* is often best translated into English simply as "the." Consider the following typical examples:

93. 观其脉证 *guān qí mài zhèng*, look at the pulse [and] signs
94. 攻其表 *gōng qí biǎo*, attack the exterior
95. 熨其背 *yùn qí bèi*, apply a hot pack to his back

The word 之 *zhī* has the idiomatic usage of marking a verb as transitive. In classical Chinese, transitive verbs need not be followed by an object when the object is clearly understood. Nevertheless, 之 *zhī* tends to be added when the verb phrase is only one character. Thus, while 不可下 *bù kě xià*, "cannot precipitate" is acceptable, 下 *xià* would tend to be followed by 之 *zhī* rather than appearing alone, as the example below shows. Of course, it can be argued that here 之 *zhī* stands for "the patient," but this would not be the intuition of the native speaker.[6]

96. 若下之，身重心悸 *ruò xià zhī, shēn zhòng xīn jì*, if [one] precipitates, [there will be] heavy body and heart palpitations
97. 太阳受之 *tài yáng shòu zhī*, the greater yáng contracts it (the disease)

Of the two reflexive pronouns 自 *zì* and 己 *jǐ*, only the former appears in the *Shāng Hán Lùn*.

---

[4]The sense of "but" developed from the sense of "only." Note also that in colloquial English "only" has undergone a parallel development (e.g., "I would go, only I don't have the money").

[5]E.g., 复建 *fù jiàn*, rehabilitate; 复审 *fù shěn*, reassess.

[6]The transitivizing function of "it" in the English expression "go it alone" is comparable to this.

98. 病人手叉自冒心 *bìng rén shǒu chā zì mào xīn*, lit. "the patient [with] hands crossed self covers heart" —the patient has his/her hands crossed over his/her heart

自 *zì* is also used in the sense of "of itself" (or "spontaneously"), for which reason we included it in the list of adverbs above.

Interrogatives

Although classical Chinese has quite a variety of question words, the only one that appears in the *Shāng Hán Lùn* is 何 *hé*. Used alone, it means "what." With 以 *yǐ*, "by" or "for," it forms the combination 何以 *hé yǐ*, meaning "how" or "why." With 如 *rú*, "like," it can be combined either as 如何 *rú hé* or 何如 *hé rú*, meaning "what like" or "how."

99. 何以知此？ *hé yǐ zhī cǐ?*, how [does one] know this?
100. 其状何如？ *qí zhuàng hé rú?*, what does it look like?
101. 此属何病？ *cǐ shǔ hé bìng?*, what disease is this?
102. 何谓藏结？ *hé wèi zàng jié?*, what [does] "storehouse bind" mean?

We should note the use of 何谓 *hé wèi* in the last example above. The verb 谓 *wèi* means "to say," "to be called" or "to mean." The above example 何谓藏结？ *hé wèi zàng jié* is equivalent to the modern Chinese 什么叫藏结？ *shén me jiào zàng jié*, "what [is the thing that] is called 'storehouse bind'?"

Topics

We have said that Chinese is basically a subject-verb-object language. Nevertheless, the notion of "subject" is different in Chinese than in English. Very often it is more loosely tied to the rest of the sentence, and for this reason it is often referred to as a "topic" rather than a subject.

103. 病人身大热 *bìng rén shēn dà rè*, patient: body greatly hot

Simple English sentences can be divided into two main parts, the subject and the predicate, the latter being composed of a verb and possibly other elements, such as an object. In classical Chinese, the two main parts are the topic and comment. The comment may be structured like an English predicate, but it also may consist of "subject + predicate" phrases. In the example above, the topic of the sentence is 病人 *bìng rén*, "the patient," and the comment is a kernel sentence consisting of the subject 身 *shēn*, "the body," and predicate 大热 *dà rè*, "[is] greatly hot." To render this sentence in English, the "topic + comment" pattern has to be changed to "subject + predicate" pattern, e.g., "the patient's body is greatly hot" or "the patient has a body that is greatly hot" (and, of course, more changes would be necessary to achieve idiomatic English).

104. 其人脉浮紧 *qí rén mài fú jǐn*, lit. "the person (patient), pulse [is] floating [and] tight," i.e., the person has a pulse that is floating and tight

The Chinese topic further differs from the English subject in that it may be the object of a verb. The object of a transitive verb, that is, one that normally takes an object, can be made into the topic of the sentence, so that the sentence takes on a passive sense.

105. 阳明少阳证不见 *yáng míng shào yáng zhèng bù jiàn*, yáng brightness and lesser yáng signs [are] not see[n] (i.e., are not present)

In this example, 见 *jiàn*, "to see," is the verb, and its grammatical object (yáng brightness and lesser yáng signs) is here brought up in front of it to form the topic. The real subject (the human observer) is not mentioned.

Building word groups

In most of the examples we have seen so far, the components of sentences (subjects, verbs, objects, etc.) have largely been represented by single characters. Nevertheless, we have seen examples of stative verbs being placed together in an additive sense, that is, in a way that, for English speakers, the insertion of the English word "and" is required to complete the sense.

106. 脉沉迟 *mài chén chí*, [the] pulse [is] sunken [and] slow

Active verbs are also juxtaposed in an additive sense:

107. 捣筛 *dǎo shāi*, pound and sift

And nouns too:

108. 头项 *tóu xiàng*, head and nape
109. 项背 *xiàng bèi*, nape and back
110. 颈项 *jǐng xiàng*, neck and nape
111. 手足 *shǒu zú*, hands and feet
112. 阴阳 *yīn yáng*, yīn and yáng

Despite this kind of additive juxtaposition, classical Chinese does have words equivalent to the English "and," notably 与 *yǔ*. Nonetheless, 与 *yǔ* tends to be used only when an interaction or a relationship between two things is being discussed. In the above examples, no word equivalent to "and" appears.

Numerals may be combined in an alternative sense: 二三 *èr sān*, two or three; 八九 *bā jiǔ*, eight or nine. If the first of the numbers is 十 *shí*, ten, 百 *bǎi*, hundred, or 千 *qiān*, thousand, the sense is additive, e.g., 十二 *shí èr*, twelve (ten plus two). If, on the other hand, the second of the numbers is 十 *shí*, 百 *bǎi*, or 千 *qiān*, then the number preceding it is a multiple, 二十 *èr shí*, twenty (two times ten).

The word 之 *zhī* has already been encountered in its use as a third-person pronoun. In addition to this use, it is also the main "word joiner" of classical Chinese, equivalent to the modern 的 *de*, to which it is thought to be etymologically related. In this role, 之 *zhī* can join noun to noun or qualifier (stative or active verb) to noun. When joining one noun to another, it can be most simply thought of as the equivalent to the English *'s*. Thus, for example, 肝经之病 *gān jīng zhī bìng*, translates word for word "liver channel's disease." Note that in more idiomatic English, "disease of the liver channel," the word order is the opposite of the Chinese.

When linking a qualifying phrase (or qualifier) to a noun, 之 *zhī* is likewise placed between the two. Normally, this construction is only used when the qualifying phrase consists of more than one character. A single stative verb placed before a noun does not require this formal link.

113. 微数之脉 *wēi shuò zhī mài*, a faint, rapid pulse

As explained above, the time words 前 *qián*, "before," and 后 *hòu*, "after," follow the nouns they qualify. Sometimes 之 *zhī* is interposed, as the following examples show:

114. 下之后 *xià zhī hòu*, after precipitation
115. 解之后 *jiě zhī hòu*, after resolution

The addition of 之 *zhī* in these phrases helps to clarify why words like "before" and "after" follow the nouns in Chinese. If we think of the time words as nouns indicating points in time, the phrases can be seen to follow the "noun + 之 + noun" pattern.

A further use of 之 *zhī* is to turn a simple sentence into a noun phrase:

116. 太阳之为病，脉浮，头项强痛而恶寒 *tài yáng zhī wéi bìng, mài fú, tóu xiàng qiáng tòng ér wù hán*, in greater yáng disease, the pulse is floating, the head and nape are stiff and painful, and [the patient] is averse to cold.

The opening phrase 太阳之为病 *tài yáng zhī wéi bìng* literally means "greater yáng's being ill/diseased." Without 之 *zhī*, 太阳为病 *tài yáng wéi bìng* might, if considered in isolation, be interpreted as a full sentence, "greater yáng is ill/diseased."

In most cases, the addition of the word joiner 之 *zhī* is optional. In some cases, it cannot be inserted, notably after a single-character stative verb (adjective) placed directly before the noun.

117. 燥屎 *zào shǐ*, dry stool
118. 邪气 *xié qì*, evil qì
119. 他病 *tā bìng*, other disease
120. 清水 *qīng shuǐ*, clear water

Locative words can be used as qualifiers in the same way as qualifiers, and again 之 *zhī* cannot be interposed.

121. 上焦 *shàng jiāo*, upper burner
122. 中焦 *zhōng jiāo*, center burner
123. 下焦 *xì jiāo*, lower burner

Above we saw how two nouns could be juxtaposed in an additive sense. Nouns may also be juxtaposed in a subordinative relationship, without 之 *zhī*.

124. 淋家 *lín jiā*, strangury patients
125. 桂枝 *guì zhī*, cinnamon twig[s]
126. 谷气 *gǔ qì*, grain qì

Combinations taking the form of a "single stative verb + noun" and "noun + noun" are used not only as a way of qualifying nouns descriptively; very often they are set compounds for the purposes of denotation. Thus, 病人 *bìng rén*, lit. "sick person" (a person who is sick), is used to mean "sickperson," i.e., "patient." In the examples below, the first seven are "stative verb + noun" combinations, while the rest are "noun + noun" combinations.

127. 太阳 *tài yáng*, greater yáng
128. 大椎 *dà zhuī*, Great Hammer, GV-14
129. 少阳 *shào yáng*, lesser yáng
130. 小便 *xiǎo biàn*, lit. "smaller convenience," i.e., urine, urination
131. 大便 *dà biàn*, lit. "greater convenience," i.e., stool
132. 短气 *duǎn qì*, lit. "short breath," i.e., shortness of breath
133. 少腹 *shào fù*, lesser abdomen
134. 腠理 *còu lǐ*, interstices
135. 气海 *qì hǎi*, Sea of Qì, CV-6
136. 风池 *fēng chí*, Wind Pool, GB-20
137. 期门 *qī mén*, Cycle Gate, LR-14
138. 芍药 *sháo yào*, peony medicine (i.e., peony)
139. 石膏 *shí gāo*, lit. "stone paste," gypsum

140. 人参 *rén shēn*, lit. "man wort," ginseng

141. 半夏 *bàn xià*, lit. "half summer," pinellia

Note that the ability of "noun + noun" constructions to express both additive and subordinating relationships can lead to confusion. The expression 骨髓 *gǔ suǐ*, for example, could be interpreted as "bone and marrow" or as "bone marrow." In fact, in Chinese medicine, it means "bone and marrow," while in modern Western medical terminology it means bone marrow.

As regards "stative verb + noun" collocations, it is useful to contrast the fixed naming compounds above with the descriptive terminology of symptomatology in the *Shāng Hán Lùn*. Many discomforts associated with parts of the body are expressed in "subject + verb" form, e.g., 目眩 *mù xuàn*, "eyes [are] dizzy"; 腹痛 *fù tòng*, "abdomen [is] painful." The pulse descriptions also follow the same pattern, e.g., 脉浮 *mài fú*, "pulse [is] floating"; 脉紧 *mài jǐn*, "pulse [is] tight." It is interesting to note that in development of sphygmology after the *Shāng Hán Lùn*, Wáng Shū-Hé (王叔和) introduced set definitions of pulses, and with them the practice of referring to individual pulses as, for example, 浮脉 *fú mài*, "floating pulse" and 紧脉 *jǐn mài*, "tight pulse." Wáng Shū-Hé's definitions were largely accepted by physicians after him, but the "stative verb + noun" expression is reserved for single pulse types in the context of pulse discussions, while the single or multiple pulse types in the context of descriptions of pathological states have always followed the "noun + stative verb" pattern. As a result, a term composed of a double stative verb preceding 脉 *mài* is rare in Chinese medical literature, and the only example of this construction found in the *Shāng Hán Lùn* is 微数之脉 *wēi shuò zhī mài*, "a faint, rapid pulse."

Compounds of the form of a "single stative verb + noun" and "noun + noun" were used to name new items and concepts. Although we often characterize classical Chinese (Old Chinese) as being fundamentally monosyllabic, compounding has always been one of its features. Among the early types of compound are reduplications in which the whole syllable is reduplicated (we will see examples of this further ahead), or where part of the syllable is reduplicated (膀胱 *páng guāng*, bladder, may be an example of this).

A tendency toward compounding appears to have been further fostered by a reduction in the number of sounds in the language. Although the *Shāng Hán Lùn* was written largely in classical style, it nevertheless reflects the tendency toward compounding in the spoken language. One method of compounding increasingly used with nouns was the addition of suffixes such as 子 *zi*, originally meaning "offspring" and 头 *tou*, originally meaning "head." When used as suffixes, however, these words lost their original meanings (and in the modern language, both are pronounced in the neutral tone), and provided a distinguishing mark to a noun that might have been confused with others now pronounced in the same way. A couple of examples of nouns with suffixes appear in the *Shāng Hán Lùn*:

142. 橘子 *jú zi*, tangerine

143. 指头 *zhǐ tou*, finger

Few languages share the same degree of monosyllabism as Chinese, and not surprisingly therefore, many loans from other languages take the form of compounds (e.g., 莱菔 *lái fú*, radish, akin to the Latin *raphanus*), but the *Shāng Hán Lùn* contains none that we can be sure of. The Chinese 霍乱 *huò luàn* may, like the

English cholera, have come from the Greek, but the evidence rests only on the similarity of sound.

A method of compounding that was increasingly used in the spoken language, apparently to cope with phonetic attrition, was that of combining two synonyms. This practice is an essential feature of the modern language by contrast to Old Chinese. An example of synonym compounding is the word for "body," 身体 *shēn tǐ*, which is composed of two characters of almost identical meaning. This tendency was already well established in the Hàn Dynasty. In the *Shāng Hán Lùn*, the body is usually referred to simply as 身 *shēn*, although in five of its more than 60 occurrences, it appears in the collocation 身体 *shēn tǐ*.

144. 身体重 *shēn tǐ zhòng*, [the] body-body [is] heavy

145. 身体痛 *shēn tǐ tòng*, [the] body-body aches, [is] painful

146. 热在皮肤 *rè zài pí fú*, the heat is in the skin (lit. skin-skin)

The borderline between additive compounds denoting like entities and synonym compounds is poorly drawn. Whether 咽喉 *yān hóu* is to be interpreted as "pharynx [and] larynx" in an additive sense or whether the two component characters are to be taken as near-synonyms in the looser meaning of "throat" is debatable.

Generally speaking in the *Shāng Hán Lùn*, "noun + noun" collocations express synonymy much less than they do addition or subordination. Among verbs, both stative and active, synonym collocations are much more common, as the following examples show:

147. 疼痛 *téng tòng*, hurts-hurts, [is] painful-painful

148. 枯燥 *kū zào*, withered [and] dry

149. 干燥 *gān zào*, "dry-dry"

150. 眠睡 *mián shuì*, "sleep-sleep"

151. 空虚 *kōng xū*, "empty-vacuous"

152. 谐和 *xié hé*, "concordant-harmonious"

153. 安静 *ān jìng*, "quiet-still"

154. 发作 *fā zuò*, "happen-act," to occur (as of an episode of a disease)

Many synonym collocations such as these gradually became fixed compounds in the spoken language. They came to appear more frequently in literature of the post-classical period, but in the written language, where homophones continued to be represented by distinct characters, collocations were essentially redundant, and hence remained optional.

Reduplications

Reduplication and semi-reduplication of sounds is one method of compounding. It was used in the naming of certain animals, particularly insects (two examples not appearing the *Shāng Hán Lùn* are 螟蛉 *míng líng*, corn moth, and 螳螂 *táng láng*, praying mantis). As we have said, 膀胱 *páng guāng*, "bladder," may be a compound of this type.

Another common use of reduplication was that of expressing intensification. 时 *shí*, "time," can be doubled to express the notion of "many times" or "frequently." In the modern language, this usage of reduplication is still seen in set expressions, but it has virtually ceased to be an active principle. In the *Shāng Hán Lùn*, there are over ten examples of intensifying reduplication.

155. 时时恶风 *shí shí è fēng*, frequent aversion to wind

156. 少少与之 *shǎo shǎo yǔ zhī*, lit. "little-little give it," i.e., give just a little of it
157. 蒸蒸发热 *zhēng zhēng fà rè*, lit. "steamingly-steaming(ly) effusing heat," steaming heat effusion
158. 项背强几几 *xiàng bèi qiáng shū shū*, lit. "nape and back stiff stretch-stretched," stretched stiff nape and back
159. 漐漐汗出 *zhé zhé hàn chū*, lit. " drizzly-drizzly sweat issues"
160. 啬啬恶寒 *sè sè wù hán*, lit. "huddlingly-huddlingly averse to cold"
161. 淅淅恶风 *xī xī wù fēng*, lit. "wettedly-wettedly averse to wind"
162. 翕翕发热 *xì xì fā rè*, lit. "warm-featheredly warm-featheredly effusing heat"
163. 汗出濈濈然 *hàn chū jí jí rán*, lit. "sweat issuing streamingly-streamingly"
164. 振振摇 *zhèn zhèn yáo*, lit. "vibrantly-vibrantly shaking"
165. 蒸蒸而振 *zhēng zhēng ér zhèn*, lit. "steamingly-steamingly shaking"
166. 嘿嘿不欲饮食 *mò mò bù yù yǐn shí*, taciturn-taciturn [and] not wanting to eat or drink
167. 振振欲擗地 *zhèn zhèn yù pì dì*, lit. "quivering-quivering, about to fall to the ground"
168. 郁郁微烦 *yù yù wēi fán*, lit. "depression-depression mildly vexed,"
169. 不了了 *bù liǎo liǎo*, lit. "not definitively-definitively," not clearly, not definitively
170. 心愦愦 *xīn kuì kuì*, restiveness in the heart

Conjunctions

Conjunctions are words used to connect words, phrases, clauses, and sentences. The following appear commonly in the *Shāng Hán Lùn*:

与 *yǔ*, and (joining nouns)
而 *ér*, and (joining verbs and clauses), but
及 *jí*, to, and
或 *huò*, or, possibly
虽 *suī*, although
若 *ruò*, if
设 *shè*, if, supposing
假令 *jiǎ lìng*, if, supposing
以 *yǐ*, because, in order to
因 *yīn*, because (in the *Shāng Hán Lùn*, also 因尔 *yīn ěr*)
故 *gù*, therefore, hence (it also means "formerly")
则 *zé*, then
即 *jí*, then immediately
既 *jì*, both (... and)
且 *qiě*, and

Two nouns may be joined by 与 *yǔ* in an additive sense expressed in English by the word "and."

171. 太阳与阳明 *tài yáng yǔ yáng míng*, greater yáng and yáng brightness

The word 及 *jí* is also used in the sense of "and":

172. 胃气及上二焦 *wèi qì jí shàng èr jiāo*, stomach qì and the two upper burners

Two verbs can be juxtaposed without any link (e.g., 强痛 *qiáng tòng*, [is] stiff and painful). Nevertheless, they may also be joined with the conjunction 而 *ér*, which means "and," very often in a resultative sense ("and as a result")

173. 无汗而喘 *wú hàn ér chuǎn*, [the patient] has no sweat, and pants
174. 发热而渴 *fā rè ér kě*, [the patient] effuses heat and [(as a result) is] thirsty

而 *ér* also has the meaning of "but."

175. 表解而不了了 *biǎo jiě ér bù liǎo liǎo*, the exterior has resolved, but not clearly

When used in the sense of "but" in the *Shāng Hán Lùn*, 而 *ér* is usually followed by 反 *fǎn*, "instead."

176. 小便当数而反不数 *xiǎo biàn dāng shuò ér fǎn bù shuò*, urine should be frequent, but instead is not frequent

The word 虽 *suī* matches the English "although," "even though," or "even if." It often appears after the subject rather than before it, as can be seen in the second example below:

177. 虽身疼痛，不可发汗 *suī shēn téng tòng, bù kě fā hàn*, although the body is painful, [one] cannot promote sweating

178. 屎虽硬，大便反易 *shǐ suī yìng, dà biàn fǎn yì*, although the stool is hard, defecation is nevertheless easy

故 *gù*, "therefore," is a conjunction that links two clauses. The 故 *gù* clause is often terminated by 也 *yě*.

179. 脉浮，故知汗出解 *mài fú, gù zhī hàn chū jiě*, the pulse is floating; hence one knows the effusion of sweat will resolve [the disease]

180. 邪高痛下，故使呕也 *xié gāo tòng xià, gù shǐ ǒu yě*, the evil is high [up] and pain is [low] down, therefore [this] causes vomiting

181. 以重发汗虚故如此 *yǐ chóng fā hàn xū gù rú cǐ*, lit. "because of repeated promotion of sweating [which caused] vacuity, therefore it is like this," i.e., this is because of the repeated promotion of sweating, which [caused] vacuity.

The last of the above examples represents a typically Chinese way of expressing causal connections, which, when literally translated, strikes an English speaker as odd. In this pattern of expression, the final 如此 *rú cǐ* is commonly omitted, so that in such cases 故 *gù*, followed by the particle 也 *yě*, takes on the sense of "that's why," rounding off a causal explanation.

182. ... 以酒客不喜甘故也 ... *yǐ jiǔ kè bù xǐ gān gù yě*, lit. "... because drinkers do not like sweet [things], that's why," i.e., ... this is because drinkers do not like sweet [things]

We have already met 则 *zé* as an adverb. As a conjunction, it establishes a logical link between the actions/events described in separate clauses. Such a link in English is often best expressed using "when," "if," or "since."

183. 无阳则阴独 *wú yáng zé yīn dú*, lit. "there is no yáng, then yīn is solitary," i.e., when (if, since) there is no yáng, yīn is solitary

184. 按之则痛 *àn zhī zé tòng*, lit."press it [and it] is painful," i.e., painful when pressed, painful under pressure

Note that 则 *zé* is often omitted. Thus 按之痛 *àn zhī tòng* is identical in meaning to the latter example above.

Prepositions

于 *yú*, at, to, from
从 *cóng*, from
至 *zhì*, to, up to
以 *yǐ*, by, according to
依 *yī*, according to
随 *suí*, following, according to
按 *àn*, according to

The first three of the prepositions listed above, 于 *yú*, 从 *cóng*, and 至 *zhì* have already been discussed.

The preposition 以 *yǐ* has the primary sense of "using" or "by (means of)," but it also has other senses such as "according to." Furthermore, 以 *yǐ* also serves as a conjunction in the sense of "because of" and "in order to," being able to express reason or cause on the one hand and intention on the other. This word survives in the modern language, although its primary meaning of "using" has largely been supplanted in the modern language by 用 *yòng*, a prepositional usage of the verb "to use."

As a preposition, 以 *yǐ* introduces an adverbial phrase that in older classical texts usually followed the verb. In the *Shāng Hán Lùn*, we see it preceding the verb:

185. 当以汗解 *dāng yǐ hàn jiě*, lit. "should by sweating resolve," i.e., should resolve by sweating
186. 以小承气汤和之 *yǐ xiǎo chéng qì tāng hé zhī*, harmonize [the patient] by means of (or with) Minor Qì-Coordinating Decoction

Sometimes 以 *yǐ* is omitted:

187. 清酒洗 *qīng jiǔ xǐ*, wash with clear liquor
188. 微火煮 *wéi huǒ zhǔ*, boil over a mild flame

We have 以 *yǐ* in the sense of "because" and "by." Readers will now see that 何以 *hé yǐ*, "how," "why," literally means "because of what," "by what" (or "what for").

以 *yǐ* also corresponds to the English "to" that precedes infinitive verbs. It can be used to join two verbs together.

189. 难以屈伸 *nán yǐ shēn qū*, difficult to bend and stretch

It can also be used to introduce a subordinate clause explaining the purpose of the action in the preceding main clause:

190. 以助药力 *yǐ zhù yào lì*, (in order) to help the medicinal strength

Another meaning is "according to" or "as":

191. 实以虚治 *shí yǐ xū zhì*, to treat repletion as vacuity

以 *yǐ* may precede time and location words. 以后 *yǐ hòu*, "after," has exactly the same meaning as 之后 *zhī hòu*.

192. 伤寒差以后 *shāng hán chài yǐ hòu*, after cold damage has [been] recovered [from]

Both 上 *shàng*, "on," "up," and 下 *xià*, "below," "down" may be preceded by 以 *yǐ*. Look at the following examples:

193. 从腰以下 *cóng yāo yǐ xià*, from the waist downward

194. 七日以上 *qī rì yǐ shàng*, over (i.e., more than) seven days

In the *Shāng Hán Lùn*, 以 *yǐ* is regularly used in the sense of "because" (this usage is obsolete in the modern language).

195. 以有热也 *yǐ yǒu rè yě*, because there is heat

196. 以酒客不喜甘故也 *yǐ jiǔ kè bù xǐ gān gù yě*, "because drinkers do not like sweet [things], that's why," i.e., this is because drinkers do not like sweet things

The verbs 依 *yī*, "to rely on," 按 *àn*, "to press," and 随 *suí*, "to follow" are all used prepositionally in the sense of "according to."

197. 更服依前法 *gèng fú yī qián fǎ*, take again according to the previous method

198. 按法治之 *àn fǎ zhì zhī*, treat according to [the proper] method

199. 随证治之 *suí*, treat according to pattern

Note that in the first of the three examples above, the phrase introduced by 依 *yī* follows the verb.

Initial and final particles

Traditional Chinese grammarians recognized that many words in their language did not represent concrete objects, actions, or states, although they helped to make sentences meaningful. They called these 虚字 *xū zì*, "empty words." Words listed under the headings of adverbs and prepositions above were all traditionally considered "empty words." In addition to these, there are a number of "empty words" that occur at the beginning or end of a sentence that we here call initial and final particles ("particles," even though they are not necessarily shorter than other words). The initial and final particles that appear in the *Shāng Hán Lùn* are as follows:

夫 *fū*, initial particle implying obviousness

也 *yě*, final particle implying explanation or judgment

矣 *yǐ*, final particle implying affirmation or exclamation

尔 *ěr*, final particle implying affirmation or sureness

耳 *ěr*, final particle implying limitation or finality

已 *yǐ*, final particle indicating perfective

The only initial particle occurring in the *Shāng Hán Lùn* is 夫 *fū*, which expresses certainty or obviousness. In some cases, it can be translated as "now," "well," or "of course."

200. 夫实则谵语，虚则郑声 *fū shí zé zhān yǔ, xū zé zhēng shēng*, (Now, as we know,) when there is repletion there is delirious speech, and when there is vacuity, there is muttering

Of the final particles, 也 *yě* we have already seen in equational sentences. The same particle is used more widely to end sentences expressing firm statements, explanations, or judgments.

201. 脉微缓者，为欲愈也 *mài wēi huǎn zhě, wéi yù yù yě*, a pulse that is slightly moderate is (i.e., means) [the patient] is about to recover

202. 表未解故也 *biǎo wèi jiě gù yě*, lit. "the exterior has not resolved, that's why," i.e., this is because the exterior has not resolved

The particle 矣 *yǐ* indicates affirmation or exclamation.

203. 此为愈矣 *cǐ wéi yù yǐ*, this means [the patient] is recovering!

The word 尔 *ĕr* is a final particle implying affirmation or sureness.

204. 以卫气不共荣气谐和故尔 *yǐ wèi qì bù gòng róng qì xiē hé gù ĕr*, because defense is not in concordant harmony with construction, that's why

We have already encountered 已 *yǐ* in the adverbial sense of "already." Originally, this word was a verb meaning "to finish." It came to serve as an adverb placed before the verb, and also as a particle indicating perfectiveness placed at the end of a sentence.

205. 发汗已 *fā hàn yǐ*, [one has] promoted sweating

Three other important particles have already been discussed above, under the categories of adverbs and conjunctions, the word-classes in which modern grammarians place them. These are as follows:

者 *zhě*, nominalizing particle
以 *yǐ*, because of, in order to
所 *suǒ*, particle

The particle 者 *zhě* has already been discussed in the context of nominal sentences. Nevertheless, its use as a topic marker is by no means confined to a nominal sentence, as the following examples show:

206. 风家，表解而不了了者，十二日愈 *fēng jiā, biǎo jiě ér bù liǎo liǎo zhě, shí èr rì yù*, lit. "wind patients, exterior resolves but not clearly, recover in 12 days," i.e., wind patients in whom the exterior has resolved but not clearly, will recover in 12 days

In the *Shāng Hán Lùn*, 者 *zhě* often ends a clause beginning with 虽 *suī*, "although," "even if."

207. 虽汗出不恶寒者，其身必重 *suī hàn chū bù wù hán zhě, qí shēn bì zhòng*, although there is sweating and no aversion to cold, there will be generalized heaviness

者 *zhě* is also used as a nominalizing particle for stative or active verbs. Thus, 病者 *bìng zhě* means patient, and is identical in meaning to (the more common) 病人 *bìng rén*. Nouns formed in this way may be used in subject or object position.

208. 令病者静 *lìng bìng zhě jìng*, make the patient tranquil

The particle 所 *suǒ* means "a place," and this seems to have been the original meaning of the word. Followed by a verb, it can mean "place where."

209. 万物所归 *wàn wù suǒ guī*, lit. "the myriad things place where [to] return," i.e., the place to which the myriad things return

It is from "place where" that all extensions of the 所 *suǒ* flow: "thing which" ("that which," "what"), "person who," "reason why."

Thus 所见 *suǒ jiàn* means "that [which] [one] sees," "what [one] sees." The *Shāng Hán Lùn* offers no example of this otherwise common construction, except in the negative 无所 *wú suǒ*. Chinese has no single word corresponding to the English "nothing." In some cases, 无所 *wú suǒ* fills the need.

210. 两耳无所闻 *liǎng ĕr wú suǒ wén*, lit. "[the] two ears have no[thing] that [they] hear," i.e., both ears hear nothing, or no hearing in either ear

211. 无所苦 *wú suǒ kǔ*, lit. "[the patient] has no[thing] from which [he/she] suffers," i.e., the patient suffers from nothing

The phrase 所以 *suǒ yǐ*, in modern Chinese, is commonly used in the sense of "so," "for that reason" or "therefore." In the *Shāng Hán Lùn*, it does not appear in this sense, but it does appear in the sense of "the reason why." We have already met 以 *yǐ* in the sense of "by means of" and "because." Here, 所以 *suǒ yǐ* means "that because of which."

212. 所以加桂者，以能泄奔豚气也 *suǒ yǐ jiā guì zhě, yǐ néng xiè bēn tún qì yě*, the reason why [we add] cinnamon is to be able to discharge the running piglet qì

The phrase 所以然 *suǒ yǐ rán*, often followed by 者 *zhě*, lit. "that by [which it] is thus," means "the reason why [it] is so," or "the reason for this."

213. 所以然者，以内外俱虚故也 *suǒ yǐ rán zhě, yǐ nèi wài jù xū gù yě*, lit. "the reason it is so [is] because the inner [body] and outer [body] are both vacuous, that's why," i.e., the reason for this is that the inner [body] and outer [body] are both vacuous

The preceding example is typical of recapitulative causal explanations in classical Chinese. The word 故 *gù* means "therefore" when it introduces a clause, but here it has the sense of "that's why," and merely rounds off the explanation.

In some constructions, 所 has the function of simply marking the passive. Thus X 所致 *suǒ zhì*, "caused by X." In the following, we see this usage combined with the somewhat redundant use of the 以 *yǐ*, "because":

214. 以医吐之所致也 *yǐ yī tù zhī suǒ zhì yě*, [this is] caused because the physician's [inducing] vomiting

Passive constructions

As we have already explained, although the object of a transitive verb is normally placed after the verb, it can also form the topic of the sentence. This is often equivalent to the passive construction of English. The agent could be stated after the verb with the interposition of 于 *yú*: "object topic + verb + 于 + agent." No such constructions are found in the *Shāng Hán Lùn*. Nevertheless, the terms 伤寒 *shāng hán*, translated in this text as "cold damage," and 中风 *zhòng fēng*, "wind strike," are actually passive constructions with the 于 *yú* dropped: "damaged by cold" and "struck by wind." These phrases also serve as nouns, and indeed we render them as nouns ("cold damage" and "wind strike") in this text.

Another passive construction involving the use of 所 *suǒ* has already been described.

Measure words

Classical Chinese, like English, qualifies the amount of something by a series of words for weights and measures. In English, a "number + measure" expression precedes the noun (e.g., five *bottles* of milk). Classical Chinese differs by placing the "number + measure" expression after the noun:

215. 水一斗 *shuǐ yī dǒu*, a dǒu of water

216. 桂枝二两 *guì zhī èr liǎng*, two liǎng of cinnamon twig

Most measure words were originally nouns, but verbs also came to be used as measure words. In the *Shāng Hán Lùn*, we find the following expressions:

217. 杵千下 *chǔ qiān xià*, lit. "pestle a thousand downs," i.e., pound a thousand times with a pestle

218. 小便日三四行 *xiǎo biàn rì sān sì xíng*, lit. "urinate a day three four goes," i.e., "urinate three or four times a day"

Note that after the classical period two changes occurred in the use of measure words. First, they tended to be placed, as in English, before the noun, although the older order has been preserved to this day in formal lists of items, such as the ingredients of medicinal formulae. Second, their use was extended to all nouns, even those whose referents occur in a naturally defined units, whenever used with numbers. Thus the classical 三牛 *sān niú*, "three oxen," became 三头牛 *sān tóu niú*, "three *head* of oxen." Measure words are virtually obligatory in the modern language except in certain expressions that preserve the classical pattern.

Expressions of time

Time expressions may either precede or follow the verb or verb + object. Although students may find the following explanation somewhat complex, the meaning is always clear from the context.

A word or phrase expressing the point in time when an action or event occurs precedes the verb.

219. 下之后，脉促 *xià zhī hòu, mài cù*, after precipitation, the pulse is skipping

Expressions of duration of time follow the verb or verb + object.

220. 伤寒发热四日 *shāng hán fā rè sì rì*, lit. "cold damage effuse heat four days," i.e., in cold damage, when there has been heat effusion for four days...

221. 头痛至七日以上 *tóu tòng zhì qī rì yǐ shàng*, lit. "head aches up to seven days or over," i.e., when the headache has lasted for up to seven days or more...

222. 太阳病，得之八九日 *tài yáng bìng, dé zhī bā jiǔ rè*, lit. "greater yáng disease, got it for eight nine days," i.e., when in greater yáng disease that [the patient] has had for eight or nine days...

Expressions of length of time in which an action does not take place precede the verb.

223. 八九日不解 *bā jiǔ rì bù jiě*, lit. "eight nine days not resolve," i.e., when there is no resolution for eight or nine days...

Phrases expressing the time that elapses before an action or event takes place are placed before the verb.

224. 十二日愈 *shí rì yù*, lit. "12 days recover," i.e., recover in 12 days

Phrases expressing the number of times an action takes place follow the verb or verb + object.

225. 杵千下 *chǔ qiān xià*, lit. "pestle a thousand downs," i.e., pound a thousand times with a pestle

There are different ways of expressing the number of times an action or event takes place within a given length of time. In the *Shāng Hán Lùn*, we find two patterns: "verb + length of time + number of times" and "length of time + number of times + verb."

226. 下利日数十行 *xià lì rì shù shí xíng*, lit. "have diarrhea day several tens [of] times," i.e., have diarrhea several tens of times a day

227. 日三服 *rì sān fú*, take three times a day

Multiple meanings

Two features of classical Chinese is the wide variety of senses in which a single word can be used, and the freedom words have to serve different grammatical functions. We have already seen a number of examples of words used in different senses. 上 *shàng*, for example, means "on," "over" ("above" physically or "more than" numerically), "upper," "rise," and "above-mentioned." 下 *xià* is similarly used in the senses of "under," "down," "below," "lower," "fall." In the medical context, 下 *xià* also has the specific meaning of "to cause the contents of the digestive tract to descend." Here, we see not only words being used in different senses, but also in different grammatical categories.

Not all Chinese words have the same number of uses as those given as examples above. Yet there are some general tendencies. Intransitive verbs can be used transitively in a causative sense. Thus 吐 *tù*, "to vomit," can be used transitively to mean "to cause someone to vomit" (in the *Shāng Hán Lùn*, we find 吐之 *tù zhī*, "to cause [him] to vomit"). The word 厚 *hòu*, "thick," is also used in the sense of "thicken."

Nouns can be used as verbs: 杵 *chǔ*, a pestle, is also used to mean "to pound with a pestle." The word 筛 *shāi*, a sieve, is also used in the sense of "to sift." The word 丸 *wán*, a pill, could mean "to form into pill." In the context of the pulse, 芤 *kōu*, scallion-stalk, and 弦 *xián*, string, are both used as stative verbs. The word for pulse itself, 脉 *mài* in the phrase 脉之 *mài zhī*, means to "take the pulse."

Less commonly, nouns can be used adverbially. In the following example 雷 *léi*, "thunder," is used as an adverb:

228. 雷鸣 *léi míng*, rumble thunderously

Much more commonly, verbs (stative or active) and verb phrases can serve as nouns. The word 甘 *gān* means "sweet" but also "sweetness." Also very commonly, verb phrases (verbs with subjects or objects) can serve as nouns.

229. 恶寒 *wù hán*, "averse to cold" or "aversion to cold"
230. 头痛 *tóu tòng*, "head aches" or "headache"

Depending on the grammatical function, the negative form can vary: 头不痛 *tóu bú tòng*, "the head does not ache"; 无头痛 *wú tóu tòng*, "no headache."

Complex sentences

Most of the lines of the *Shāng Hán Lùn* describe a pathological condition and the appropriate treatment for it. Some lines offer explanations for the condition; some offer a rationale for the choice of treatment. Most of the lines thus follow a narrow format.

Let us the look at the first line of the *Shāng Hán Lùn*.

230. 太阳之为病，脉浮，头项强痛而恶寒。
Tài yáng zhī wéi bìng, mài fú, tóu xiàng jiàng tòng ér wù hán.
[In] greater yáng's being sick, [the] pulse [is] floating, [the] head and nape [are] stiff and painful, and [the patient is] averse [to] cold

The opening phrase is 太阳为病 *tài yáng wéi bìng*, "greater yáng is sick," with 之 *zhī* added to turn a full sentence into a noun phrase, "greater yáng's being sick," which forms the topic of the sentence. The rest of the line is composed of general statements about greater yáng disease. These statements include "subject + verb" phrases (脉浮 *mài fú*; 头项强痛 *tóu xiàng jiàng tòng*) and a "verb + object" phrase (恶寒 *wù hán*), but they all form part of a complex comment on the topic "greater yáng's being sick."

We can adjust the literal translation somewhat to make the ideas clearer:

> In disease of greater yáng, the pulse is floating, the head and nape are stiff and painful, and there is aversion to cold.

This less literal translation dispenses with the idiomatic "greater yáng's being sick" in preference for "disease of greater yáng." Furthermore, the Chinese topic phrase becomes an adverbial phrase in English ("*in* disease of greater yáng"). Finally, "[the patient] is averse to cold" is changed to "aversion to cold" in accordance with the English tendency to express signs in terms of noun phrases.

Let us now move on to line 2 of the *Shāng Hán Lùn*.

230. 太阳病，发热汗出，恶风脉缓者，名为中风。
Tài yáng bìng, fā rè hàn chū, wù fēng mài huǎn zhě, míng wéi zhòng fēng.
Greater yáng [is] sick, [the patient] effuses heat, sweat issues, [the patient] is averse to cold, the pulse is moderate, name is wind strike.

In this case the opening phrase is 太阳病 *tài yáng bìng*. This can be read as a full sentence ("greater yáng is sick"). Nevertheless, the reader's interpretation is naturally colored by his reading of the first line, in which 之 *zhī* was added to mark the opening phrase clearly as a noun topic. The 之 *zhī* is optional, and is here omitted. (In actual fact, only the first lines of each channel contain the 之 *zhī*).

Line 2 is more complex than line 1. The opening phrase is followed by four signs marked off by the particle 者 *zhě*, which is followed by the complex comment in which the name of the condition is stated (wind strike). The four signs describe a restricted form of greater yáng disease, which is called "wind strike." The majority of lines in the *Shāng Hán Lùn* follow this format of stating a channel disease and then narrowing its scope. A more idiomatic translation of the line reads as follows:

> Greater yáng disease, with heat effusion, sweating, aversion to wind, and a pulse that is moderate, is called "wind strike."

Let us move on to line 11.

230. 太阳病，头痛，发热，汗出，恶风，桂枝汤主之。
Tài yáng bìng, tóu tòng, fā rè, hàn chū, wù fēng, guì zhī tāng zhǔ zhī.
Greater yáng [is] sick, [the] head ache[s], [the patient] effuses heat, sweat issue[s], [the patient] is averse to wind, Cinnamon Twig Decoction govern[s] it.

This line, like the previous two, opens with "greater yáng." The disease is again narrowed down, and in the comment a treatment is suggested.

> Greater yáng disease with headache, heat effusion, sweating, and aversion to wind is governed by Cinnamon Twig Decoction.

Vocabulary

In this section, we present under various headings most of the characters appearing in the *Shāng Hán Lùn*, together, in most cases, with examples of character combinations.

Immediately apparent from the lists of single characters is the smallness and simplicity of the vocabulary. The lists contain less than 900 characters—only a fraction of the number of characters literate people today know. As can be seen from the literal translations we give them here, most of the words used in the *Shāng Hán Lùn* are ordinary, everyday words such as body parts, discomforts, plant names, food items, etc. Some of the words are a little old-fashioned in flavor, but most are in fact still used in the senses in which they were used when the *Shāng Hán Lùn* was written.

The simplicity of the vocabulary makes the *Shāng Hán Lùn* a good text for language learners. In fact, knowledge of very much less than 900 characters carries the beginning student a long way: quite astoundingly, the 50 characters most commonly appearing in the text account for nearly 50% of the total text; the 100 most commonly appearing characters account for nearly 70% of the text; and the 150 most commonly used characters account for almost 80% of the text. Once students have learned the fundamentals of character composition, they should be able to master the 150 characters listed below in a very short time. This initial study is grueling and time-consuming. Nevertheless, for students wishing to read Chinese for the purposes of reading the *Shāng Hán Lùn* and Chinese medical texts in general, this initial investment will be highly rewarding because it will facilitate the crossing of a very much exaggerated language barrier. In order to read the remaining 20% of the *Shāng Hán Lùn* text, one admittedly has to acquire a further 700 or more characters; however, after the initial study of the Chinese characters, the learning process speeds up dramatically.

In the list of 150 most commonly used characters below, and the complete lists that follow it in this section, simplified characters are followed by their signific in brackets, and these are followed by the complex characters with their signific in brackets.

The 150 most frequent characters in the *Shāng Hán Lùn*

1–50

者 [耂]; 者 [老] *zhě*, nominalizing particle
两 [一]; 兩 [入] *liǎng*, two; liǎng (unit of weight)
不 [不]; 不 [一] *bù*, not
升 [丿]; 升 [十] *shēng*, shēng (unit of volume)
之 [丶]; 之 [丿] *zhī*, subordinating particle
三 [一]; 三 [一] *sān*, three
一 [一]; 一 [一] *yī*, one
二 [二]; 二 [一] *èr*, two
去 [去]; 去 [厶] *qù*, go away; remove
汤 [氵]; 湯 [水] *tāng*, decoction
服 [月]; 服 [肉] *fú*, take (medicines)
下 [卜]; 下 [一] *xià*, below, down; precipitate
以 [人]; 以 [人] *yǐ*, because; objectifying particle
汗 [氵]; 汗 [氵] *hàn*, sweat
病 [疒]; 病 [疒] *bìng*, disease, illness
大 [大]; 大 [大] *dà*, large, great
脉 [月]; 脈 [肉] *mài*, vessel; pulse

阳 [阝]; 陽 [阜] *yáng*, yáng
热 [灬]; 熱 [火] *rè*, heat
发 [又]; 發 [癶] *fā*, effuse
日 [日]; 日 [日] *rì*, sun, day
也 [乛]; 也 [乙] *yě*, final particle indicating equation or judgment
寒 [宀]; 寒 [宀] *hán*, cold
水 [氵]; 水 [水] *shuǐ*, water
而 [而]; 而 [而] *ér*, and, but
利 [禾]; 利 [刀] *lì*, uninhibited; disinhibit
四 [口]; 四 [口] *sì*, four
煮 [灬]; 煮 [火] *zhě*, boil
黄 [廿]; 黃 [黃] *huáng*, yellow
温 [氵]; 溫 [水] *wēn*, warm
取 [耳]; 取 [又] *qǔ*, take
味 [口]; 味 [口] *wèi*, flavor; ingredient
右 [𠂇]; 右 [口] *yòu*, right (opposite of left)
半 [丨]; 半 [十] *bàn*, half
便 [亻]; 便 [人] *biàn*, convenience (stool, urine)
桂 [木]; 桂 [木] *guì*, cinnamon
主 [王]; 主 [丶] *zhǔ*, govern
若 [艹]; 若 [艸] *ruò*, if
为 [丶]; 爲 [火] *wéi*, be; make
滓 [氵]; 滓 [水] *zǐ*, dregs
人 [人]; 人 [人] *rén*, person
中 [中]; 中 [丨] *zhōng*, center; in
小 [小]; 小 [小] *xiǎo*, small
枝 [木]; 枝 [木] *zhī*, twig, branch
其 [八]; 其 [八] *qí*, his, hers, its; the
甘 [甘]; 甘 [甘] *gān*, sweet
六 [亠]; 六 [八] *liù*, six
出 [屮]; 出 [凵] *chū*, go/come out, issue, exit
微 [彳]; 微 [彳] *wēi*, slight; mild

51–100

草 [艹]; 草 [艸] *cǎo*, herb, grass
气 [气]; 氣 [气] *qì*, qì
十 [十]; 十 [十] *shí*, ten
五 [二]; 五 [二] *wǔ*, five
少 [小]; 少 [小] *shào*, lesser
皮 [皮]; 皮 [皮] *pí*, skin
子 [子]; 子 [子] *zǐ*, offspring; noun suffix
必 [丶]; 必 [心] *bì*, must, will
姜 [羊]; 薑 [艸] *jiāng*, ginger
枚 [木]; 枚 [木] *méi*, piece (disk-like objects)
阴 [阝]; 陰 [阜] *yīn*, yīn
炙 [火]; 炙 [火] *zhì*, mix-fry
可 [口]; 可 [口] *kě*, can
七 [一]; 七 [一] *qī*, seven
解 [角]; 解 [角] *jiě*, resolve
伤 [亻]; 傷 [人] *shāng*, damage
此 [止]; 此 [止] *cǐ*, this
药 [艹]; 藥 [艸] *yào*, medicinal
加 [力]; 加 [力] *jiā*, add
生 [丿]; 生 [生] *shēng*, engender; arise
太 [大]; 太 [大] *tài*, supreme; greater
痛 [疒]; 痛 [疒] *tòng*, pain
欲 [谷]; 欲 [欠] *yù*, desire
烦 [火]; 煩 [火] *fán*, vexation
心 [心]; 心 [心] *xīn*, heart
自 [自]; 自 [自] *zì*, self; spontaneously
当 [⺌]; 當 [田] *dāng*, ought to
与 [一]; 與 [臼] *yǔ*, give
有 [𠂇]; 有 [月] *yǒu*, there is/are; have
合 [人]; 合 [口] *hé*, combine; *gě*, gě (unit of volume)
吐 [口]; 吐 [口] *tù*, vomit
得 [彳]; 得 [彳] *dé*, get; be able
内 [冂]; 內 [入] *nèi*, inward, inner (body); *nà*, put in
愈 [心]; 愈 [心] *yù*, recover
浮 [氵]; 浮 [水] *fú*, float
则 [贝]; 則 [刀] *zé*, then
明 [日]; 明 [日] *míng*, bright
厥 [厂]; 厥 [厂] *jué*, reserve, revert
反 [厂]; 反 [又] *fǎn*, but, instead
故 [攵]; 故 [攴] *gù*, therefore, that's why
八 [八]; 八 [八] *bā*, eight
恶 [亚]; 惡 [心] *wù*, aversion to
分 [八]; 分 [刀] *fēn*, fēn (unit of weight)
上 [⺊]; 上 [一] *shàng*, on, up, rise
宜 [宀]; 宜 [宀] *yí*, to be appropriate
逆 [辶]; 逆 [辵] *nì*, (move) counterflow; adverse [treatment]
腹 [月]; 腹 [肉] *fù*, abdomen
复 [𠂉]; 復 [彳] *fù*, again
身 [身]; 身 [身] *shēn*, body
麻 [麻]; 麻 [麻] *má*, hemp
胸 [月]; 胸 [肉] *xiōng*, chest

101–150

白 [白]; 白 [白] *bái*, white
擘 [手]; 擘 [手] *bò*, break
满 [氵]; 滿 [水] *mǎn*, full
食 [食]; 食 [食] *shí*, eat, food
更 [一]; 更 [日] *gēng*, change; *gèng*, again, further
止 [止]; 止 [止] *zhǐ*, stop
枣 [朿]; 棗 [木] *zǎo*, jujube
柴 [木]; 柴 [木] *chái*, brushwood; 柴胡 bupleurum
胡 [月]; 胡 [肉] *hú*, foreign
硬 [石]; 硬 [石] *yìng*, hard
附 [阝]; 附 [阜] *fù*, appendage; 附子, aconite
芍 [艹]; 芍 [艸] *sháo*, peony
如 [女]; 如 [女] *rú*, like, resemble
证 [讠]; 證 [言] *zhèng*, pattern, sign
呕 [口]; 嘔 [口] *ǒu*, retching
方 [方]; 方 [方] *fāng*, formula
参 [厶]; 參 [厶] *shēn*, ginseng
切 [刀]; 切 [刀] *qiē*, cut
先 [儿]; 先 [儿] *xiān*, first of all
结 [纟]; 結 [糸] *jié*, bind
和 [禾]; 和 [口] *hé*, harmonious
胃 [月]; 胃 [肉] *wèi*, stomach
足 [足]; 足 [足] *zú*, foot, leg
苓 [艹]; 苓 [艸] *líng*, poria
无 [尢]; 無 [火] *wú*, there is/are not; have not
治 [氵]; 治 [水] *zhì*, treat
再 [一]; 再 [冂] *zài*, again, as a further step
虚 [虍]; 虛 [虍] *xū*, vacuity
承 [乛]; 承 [丿] *chéng*, inherit, carry on
在 [𠂇]; 在 [土] *zài*, to be (located)
风 [风]; 風 [風] *fēng*, wind
血 [血]; 血 [血] *xuè*, blood
头 [大]; 頭 [頁] *tóu*, head
数 [攵]; 數 [攴] *shù*, number, several
渴 [氵]; 渴 [水] *kě*, thirst(y)
能 [厶]; 能 [肉] *néng*, can
时 [日]; 時 [日] *shí*, time, hour; at times
斗 [斗]; 斗 [斗] *dǒu*, dǒu (unit of volume)
里 [里]; 裏 [衣] *lǐ*, interior
语 [讠]; 語 [言] *yǔ*, speak, speech
实 [宀]; 實 [宀] *shí*, repletion
饮 [饣]; 飲 [食] *yǐn*, drink
洗 [氵]; 洗 [水] *xiǎn*, wash
表 [龶]; 表 [衣] *biǎo*, exterior
但 [亻]; 但 [人] *dàn*, only
夏 [夊]; 夏 [夊] *xià*, summer
本 [木]; 本 [木] *běn*, root
令 [人]; 令 [人] *lìng*, cause to
手 [手]; 手 [手] *shǒu*, hand
散 [攵]; 散 [攴] *sàn*, dissipate; *sǎn*, powder

The characters are divided into four major categories: grammatical vocabulary, nouns, active verbs, and stative verbs. Each category is divided into subcategories based on similarity of meaning of the characters included in them. The categorization aims only to provide an overall impression of the nature of *Shāng Hán Lùn* vocabulary; it is in no way definitive, since many words listed under one category could also be listed under others. Characters are categorized according to the relevant meanings in the ordinary language at the time the *Shāng Hán Lùn* was written. Thus under "internal organs" are listed characters denoting internal organs, whereas the characters composing the term 中焦 *zhōng jiāo*, "center burner," are listed under other categories since in neither case is the primary meaning of the character an internal organ. A number of words fall into categories that have now changed. For example, 坏 *huài* is characterized as an active verb meaning to deteriorate, whereas its dominant meaning now is that of a stative verb ("bad"). 椎 *zhuī*, a mallet, hammer (as in the term 大椎 *dà zhuī*, Great Hammer, CV-14) was probably still a live metaphor in the Hàn Dynasty; hence it is placed under "artifacts." Nowadays, the same character is used almost exclusively in the sense of "vertebra" (bones that stick out like mallets), and hence would be placed under body parts.

Classified list of characters appearing in the *Shāng Hán Lùn*

Grammatical vocabulary

Basic verbs

有 [ナ]; 有 [月] *yǒu*, there is/are; have
为 [丶]; 爲 [火] *wéi*, act, be
属 [尸]; 屬 [尸] *shǔ*, belong to, be
在 [ナ]; 在 [土] *zài*, be [located] in, on, at, etc.
似 [亻]; 似 [人] *sì*, to resemble, to be like
如 [女]; 如 [女] *rú*, to be like, to be as if
象 [刀]; 象 [豕] *xiàng*, resemble, like
然 [灬]; 然 [火] *rán*, to be so
具 [八]; 具 [八] *jù*, to be present

Auxillary verbs

可 [口]; 可 [口] *kě*, may, can
能 [厶]; 能 [肉] *néng*, can, able to
得 [彳]; 得 [彳] *dé*, may, can, able to
当 [小]; 當 [田] *dāng*, should, ought to
应 [广]; 應 [心] *yīng*, ought
必 [丶]; 必 [心] *bì*, will be, bound to be
宜 [宀]; 宜 [宀] *yí*, to be appropriate
欲 [谷]; 欲 [欠] *yù*, desire to, want to, about to
须 [彡]; 須 [頁] *xū*, need to; to wait
使 [亻]; 使 [人] *shǐ*, cause to
令 [人]; 令 [人] *lìng*, cause to;
致 [至]; 致 [至] *zhì*, cause to: 以医吐之所致 *yǐ yī tù zhī suǒ zhì*, caused by the doctor making him vomit

Adverbs

乃 [丿]; 乃 [丿] *nǎi*, in fact, precisely; then, thereupon, consequently (equivalent to the modern 就 *jiù*)
则 [贝]; 則 [刀] *zé*, then
亦 [亦]; 亦 [亠] *yì*, also
又 [又]; 又 [又] *yòu*, again, further
再 [一]; 再 [冂] *zài*, again, then, twice
郑 [阝]; 鄭 [邑] *zhèng*, again, repeatedly
却 [去]; 卻 [卩] *què*, then
即 [艮]; 即 [卩] *jí*, then immediately
仍 [亻]; 仍 [人] *réng*, still
犹 [犭]; 猶 [犬] *yóu*, still
都 [阝]; 都 [邑] *dōu*, all, both
皆 [比]; 皆 [白] *jiē*, all, both
俱 [亻]; 俱 [人] *jù*, all, both
悉 [釆]; 悉 [心] *jù*, all, entirely
全 [入]; 全 [入] *quán*, all, entirely
遍 [辶]; 遍 [辵] *piàn*, whole, entirely
乍 [𠂉]; 乍 [丿] *zhà*, suddenly
奄 [大]; 奄 [大] *yān*, suddenly
卓 [⺊]; 卓 [十] *zhuó*, suddenly
霍 [雨]; 霍 [雨] *zhà*, rapidly, suddenly
趣 [走]; 趣 [走] *qù*, rapidly
渐 [氵]; 漸 [水] *jiàn*, gradually, little by little
互 [一]; 互 [二] *hù*, mutually, reciprocally, each other
相 [木]; 相 [目] *xiāng*, mutually, reciprocally, each other
因 [囗]; 因 [囗] *yīn*, so, accordingly, thereby, as a result
尚 [小]; 尙 [小] *shàng*, still
但 [亻]; 但 [人] *dàn*, only
颇 [皮]; 頗 [頁] *pǒ*, very
暂 [日]; 暫 [日] *zàn*, for a short time; for the time being
谛 [讠]; 諦 [言] *dì*, truly: 血证谛也 *xuè zhèng dì yě*, truly a blood pattern
初 [衤]; 初 [刀] *chū*, at the beginning
今 [人]; 今 [人] *jīn*, now
先 [儿]; 先 [儿] *xiān*, first of all
后 [厂]; 後 [彳] *hòu*, afterwards
久 [丿]; 久 [丿] *jiǔ*, for a long time
常 [⺍]; 常 [巾] *cháng*, often, constantly

Adverbs derived from other word-classes

将 [丬]; 將 [寸] *jiāng* (intend to), about to

复 [𠂉]; 復 [彳] *fù* (return, restore), again, then
更 [一]; 更 [日] *gèng (gēng)* again, then (change)
反 [厂]; 反 [又] *fǎn* (turn over), but, instead
益 [皿]; 益 [皿] *yì* (increase), more
弥 [弓]; 彌 [弓] *mí* (fill), more
已 [己]; 已 [己] *yǐ* (finish), already
甚 [一]; 甚 [甘] *shèn* (very, marked, prounounced, very), markedly
极 [木]; 極 [木] *jí* (ridgepole) extreme(ly)
微 [彳]; 微 [彳] *wēi* (faint, slight), slightly
太 [大]; 太 [大] *tài* (supreme, great), too
少 [小]; 少 [小] *shǎo* (little, few), in little amounts, to a small extent
小 [小]; 小 [小] *xǎo* (small), in small amounts, to a small extent
适 [辶]; 適 [辵] *shì* (appropriate, right, just), just, coincidentially (happen to)
过 [辶]; 過 [辵] *guò* (cross, pass, exceed), excessively
遂 [辶]; 遂 [辵] *suì* (pursue), then
稍 [禾]; 稍 [禾] *shāo* (little), in little amounts, to a small extent
暴 [日]; 暴 [日] *bào* (fulminant), fulminantly (suddenly and violently)
本 [木]; 本 [木] *běn* (stem-root), originally
自 [自]; 自 [自] *zì* (self), spontaneously ([of] itself)
素 [龶]; 素 [糸] *sù* (plain), usually
并 [丷]; 並 [丨] *bìng* (side by side), together

Negatives

非 [非]; 非 [非] *fēi*, not (in nominal sentences)
无 [尢]; 無 [火] *wú*, negative of 有 *yǒu*: there is/are not; have not
不 [不]; 不 [一] *bù*, not
未 [木]; 未 [木] *wèi*, not yet
勿 [勹]; 勿 [勹] *wù*, negative in the imperative
莫 [艹]; 莫 [艸] *mò*, not at all; negative in the imperative

Prepositions

于 [二]; 於 [方] *yú*, to, at
从 [人]; 從 [彳] *cóng*, from
至 [至]; 至 [至] *zhì*, to (equivalent of the modern 到 *dào*)
如 [女]; 如 [女] *rú*, like, as
共 [龷]; 共 [八] *gòng*, with: 卫气不共荣气谐和 *wèi qì bù gòng róng qì xié hé*, because defense qì is not in harmony with construction qì

Locatives

中 [中]; 中 [丨] *zhōng*, in, within
内 [冂]; 內 [入] *nèi*, in, within
外 [夕]; 外 [夕] *wài*, outside
上 [⺊]; 上 [一] *shàng*, above,
下 [⺊]; 下 [一] *xià*, below
前 [丷]; 前 [刀] *qián*, in front of, before
后 [厂]; 後 [彳] *hòu*, behind, after

Pronouns

我 [戈]; 我 [戈] *wǒ*, I
其 [八]; 其 [八] *qí*, his, her, its, their
之 [丶]; 之 [丿] *zhī*, him, her, it; them, their
自 [自]; 自 [自] *zì*, self

Demonstrative pronouns

是 [是]; 是 [日] *shì*, this
此 [止]; 此 [止] *cǐ*, this

Conjunctions

而 [而]; 而 [而] *ér*, and, but
或 [戈]; 或 [戈] *huò*, or
虽 [口]; 雖 [隹] *suī*, although, even though
若 [艹]; 若 [艸] *ruò*, if
设 [讠]; 設 [言] *shè*, if, supposing
假 [亻]; 假 [人] *jiǎ*, if, supposing (combined with next)
令 [人]; 令 [人] *lìng*, if, supposing
以 [人]; 以 [人] *yǐ*, because; in order to
因 [口]; 因 [口] *yīn*, because
故 [攵]; 故 [攴] *gù*, therefore, that's why
则 [贝]; 則 [刂] *zé*, then
即 [艮]; 即 [卩] *jí*, then immediately
既 [艮]; 既 [旡] *jì*, both (... and)
且 [一]; 且 [一] *qiě*, and

并 [丷]; 并 [干] *bìng*, and: 脉证并治 *mài, zhèng bìng zhì*, pulse, patterns, and treatment

及 [丿]; 及 [又] *jí*, and: 虚弱家及产妇 *xū ruò jiā jí chǎn fù*, weak patients and women who have just given birth

Particles

何 [亻]; 何 [人] *hé*, what

者 [耂]; 者 [老] *zhě*, nominalizing particle

也 [乛]; 也 [乙] *yě*, final particle implying a statement of fact

尔 [小]; 爾 [爻] *ěr*, final particle implying affirmation or sureness

耳 [耳]; 耳 [耳] *ěr*, final particle implying limitation or finality

矣 [厶]; 矣 [矢] *yǐ*, final particle implying affirmation or exclamation

已 [己]; 已 [己] *yǐ*, final particle indicating perfective

以 [人]; 以 [人] *yǐ*, multiple uses

所 [斤]; 所 [戶] *suǒ*, subordinating particle

夫 [大]; 夫 [大] *fū*, initial particle introducing a statement of commonly known fact

Nouns

Words for people

人 [人]; 人 [人] *rén*, human being, person: 病人 *bìng rèn*, patient

妇 [女]; 婦 [女] *fù*, woman: 妇人 *fù rén*, woman

母 [一]; 母 [毋] *mǔ*, mother: 知母 *zhī mǔ*, lit. "knowledge mother," anemarrhena

翁 [八]; 翁 [羽] *wēng*, old man: 白头翁 *bái tóu wēng*, lit. "white-headed old man," pulsatilla

医 [匚]; 醫 [酉] *yī*, physician, doctor, healer

家 [宀]; 家 [宀] *jiā*, person (with a particular problem): 淋家 *lín jiā*, strangury patient

客 [宀]; 客 [宀] *kè*, person (with some vice): 酒客 *jiǔ kè*, drinker

婢 [女]; 婢 [女] *bì*, maiden: 越婢汤 *yuè bì tāng*, Spleen-Effusing Decoction (婢 representing 脾 *pí* spleen)

男 [田]; 男 [田] *nán*, male, man: 男子 *nán zǐ*, male

子 [子]; 子 [子] *zǐ*, child, person; *zi*, noun suffix: 男子 *nán zǐ*, male; 橘子 *jú zi*, tangerine

师 [丨]; 師 [巾] *shī*, teacher, master

盗 [皿]; 盜 [皿] *dào*, thief: 盗汗 *dào hàn*, night sweating, lit. "thief" sweating

贼 [贝]; 賊 [貝] *zéi*, robber, robbery: 互相克贼 *hù xiàng kèi zéi*, mutual restraint and robbing

鬼 [鬼]; 鬼 [鬼] *guǐ*, ghost, demon: 如见鬼状 *rú jiàn guǐ zhuàng*, as if seeing ghosts

Internal organs[7]

肝 [月]; 肝 [肉] *gān*, liver

心 [心]; 心 [心] *xīn*, heart

脾 [月]; 脾 [肉] *pí*, spleen

肺 [月]; 肺 [肉] *fèi*, lung

肾 [月]; 腎 [肉] *shèn*, kidney

膀 [月]; 膀 [肉] *páng*, bladder (compounded with following as 膀胱 *páng guāng*)

胱 [月]; 胱 [肉] *guāng*, bladder

胃 [月]; 胃 [肉] *wèi*, stomach

[7]In the original text of the *Shāng Hán Lùn*, no mention is to be found of 胆 *dǎn*, gallbladder, except denoting animal gallbladders used as medicinals. The terms 三焦 *sān jiāo*, triple burner, 心包络 *xīn bāo luò*, pericardiac network, 大肠 *dà cháng*, large intestine, 小肠 *xiǎo cháng*, small intestine, do not appear in the text.

Body parts

身 [身]; 身 [身] *shēn*, body: 身重 *shēn zhòng*, heavy body

体 [亻]; 體 [骨] *tǐ*, body: 身体 *shēn tǐ*, body

头 [大]; 頭 [頁] *tóu*, head: 头痛 *tóu tòng*, headache

额 [页]; 額 [頁] *é*, forehead: 额上微汗出 *é shàng wēi hàn chū*, slight sweating on the forehead

目 [目]; 目 [目] *mù*, eye: 目眩 *mù xuàn*, dizzy eyes, dizzy vision

眼 [目]; 眼 [目] *yǎn*, eye: 眼中生花 *yǎn zhōng shēng huā*, flowery vision

睛 [目]; 睛 [目] *jīng*, eye: 睛不和 *jīng bù hé*, the eyes are in disharmony (unclear vision)

耳 [耳]; 耳 [耳] *ěr*, ear: 两耳无所闻 *liǎng ěr wú suǒ wén*, no hearing in either ear

口 [口]; 口 [口] *kǒu*, mouth: 口苦 *kǒu kǔ*, bitter taste in the mouth

舌 [舌]; 舌 [舌] *shé*, tongue: 舌燥 *shé zào*, dry tongue

胎 [月]; 胎 [肉] *tāi*, [tongue] fur: 胎滑 *tái huá*, glossy tongue fur

鼻 [鼻]; 鼻 [鼻] *bí*, nose: 鼻燥 *bí zào*, dry nose

颈 [页]; 頸 [頁] *jǐng*, neck: 颈项强 *jǐng xiàng qiáng*, stiff nape and neck

项 [工]; 項 [頁] *xiàng*, nape

咽 [口]; 咽 [口] *yān*, pharynx, throat: 咽喉干燥 *yān hóu gān zào*, dry throat

喉 [口]; 喉 [口] *hóu*, larynx

背 [月]; 背 [肉] *bèi*, back: 背恶寒 *bèi wù hán*, aversion to cold in the back

胸 [月]; 胸 [肉] *xiōng*, chest: 胸满 *xiōng mǎn*, fullness in the chest

胁 [月]; 脅 [肉] *xié*, rib-side: 胁痛 *xié tòng*, rib-side pain

腰 [月]; 腰 [肉] *yāo*, lumbus: 腰痛 *yāo tòng*, lumbar pain

腹 [月]; 腹 [肉] *fù*, abdomen: 少腹满 *shào fù mǎn*, lesser abdominal fullness

脐 [月]; 臍 [肉] *qí*, umbilicus: 脐下悸 *qí xià jì*, palpitations below the umbilicus

肢 [月]; 肢 [肉] *zhī*, limb: 肢节烦疼 *zhī jié fán téng*, vexing pain in the limb joints

手 [手]; 手 [手] *shǒu*, hand, arm: 手足温 *shǒu zú wēn*, warm hands and feet

寸 [寸]; 寸 [寸] *cùn*, thumb, inch: 方寸匕 *fāng cùn bǐ*, square-inch-spoon; 寸口 *cùn kǒu*, inch opening

尺 [尺]; 尺 [尸] *chǐ*, cubit, chǐ: 一尺 *yī chǐ*, one chǐ; 尺弱 *chǐ ruò*, the cubit [pulse] is weak

足 [足]; 足 [足] *zú*, foot, leg; sufficient: 針足陽明 *zhēn zú yáng míng*, needle the foot yáng brightness; 去翅足 *qù chì zú*, remove the wings and legs; 榮氣不足 *róng qì bù zú*, construction qi is insufficient

指 [扌]; 指 [手] *zhǐ*, finger: 指头寒 *zhǐ tóu hán*, the fingers are cold

脚 [月]; 腳 [肉] *jiǎo*, foot, leg: 脚挛急 *jiǎo luán jí*, hypertonicity of the legs

膝 [月]; 膝 [肉] *xī*, knee: 膝胫拘急 *xī jìng jù jí*, hypertonicity of the knee and lower leg

胫 [月]; 脛 [肉] *jìng*, lower leg: 膝胫拘急 *xī jìng jù jí*, hypertonicity of the knee and lower leg

趺 [足]; 趺 [足] *fū*, instep: 趺阳脉 *fū yáng mài*, instep yáng pulse

筋 [竹]; 筋 [竹] *jīn*, sinew: 筋惕肉瞤 *jīn tì ròu rùn*, jerking sinews and twitching flesh

皮 [皮]; 皮 [皮] *pí*, skin: 皮肤 *pí fū*, skin

肤 [月]; 膚 [肉] *fū*, skin

肉 [冂]; 肉 [肉] *ròu*, flesh: 筋惕肉瞤 *jīn tì ròu rùn*, jerking sinews and twitching flesh

肌 [月]; 肌 [肉] *jī*, flesh: 解肌 *jiě jī*, resolve the flesh

骨 [骨]; 骨 [骨] *gǔ*, bone: 骨节疼痛 *gǔ jié téng tòng*, pain in the bones and joints

髓 [骨]; 髓 [骨] *suǐ*, marrow: 骨髓 *gǔ suǐ*, bone and marrow

膈 [月]; 膈 [肉] *gé*, diaphragm: 膈上有寒饮 *gé shàng yǒu hán yǐn*, cold rheum above the diaphragm

俞 [入或人]; 兪 [入或人] *shū*, acupuncture point, transport hole: 肺俞 *fèi shū*, BL-13 (Lung Transport)

腠 [月]; 腠 [肉] *còu*, interstices: 腠理 *còu lǐ*, interstices

脉 [月]; 脈 [肉] *mài*, vessel; pulse: 衛行脈外 *wèi xíng mài wài*, defense moves outside the vessels; 脈浮 *mài fú*, the pulse is floating

Bodily substances[8]

气 [气]; 氣 [气] *qì*, qì: 卫气 *wèi qì*, defense qi

血 [血]; 血 [血] *xuè*, blood: 吐脓血 *tù nóng xuè*, vomit pus and blood

汗 [氵]; 汗 [水] *hàn*, sweat: 汗出 *hàn chū*, to sweat

津 [氵]; 津 [水] *jīn*, liquid: 津液 *jīn yè*, liquid and humor

液 [氵]; 液 [水] *yè*, humor

尿 [尸]; 尿 [尸] *niào*, urine: 遗尿 *yí niào*, enuresis

屎 [尸]; 屎 [尸] *shǐ*, stool: 燥屎 *zào shǐ*, dry stool

溲 [氵]; 溲 [水] *sōu*, urine: 失溲 *shī sōu*, urinary incontinence

涎 [氵]; 涎 [水] *xián*, drool: 涎沫 *xián mò*, drool and foam

便 [亻]; 便 [人] *biàn*, excretions (stool, urine): 便血 *biàn xuè*, bloody excretions; 大便 *dà biàn*, stool; 小便 *xiǎo biàn*, urine

脓 [月]; 膿 [肉] *nóng*, pus: 便脓血 *biàn nóng xuè*, pus and blood in the stool

Diseases

病 [疒]; 病 [疒] *bìng*, disease, illness

衄 [血]; 衄 [血] *nǜe*, spontaneous external bleeding

瘀 [疒]; 瘀 [疒] *yū*, stasis, static: 瘀热 *yū rè*, heat stasis

疟 [疒]; 瘧 [疒] *nüè*, malaria

痹 [疒]; 痹 [疒] *bì*, impediment

痿 [疒]; 痿 [疒] *wěi*, wilting

痉 [疒]; 痙 [疒] *jìng*, tetany

痓 [疒]; 痓 [疒] *cì*, tetany: 柔痓 *róu cì*, soft tetany

痫 [疒]; 癇 [疒] *xián*, epilepsy

痈 [疒]; 癰 [疒] *yōng*, welling-abscess

瘅 [疒]; 癉 [疒] *dǎn*, jaundice

疭 [疒]; 瘲 [疒] *zòng*, slackening

瘛 [疒]; 瘛 [疒] *qì*, tugging

瘕 [疒]; 瘕 [疒] *jiǎ*, conglomeration

Food

谷 [谷]; 穀 [禾] *gǔ*, grain, food: 谷道 *gǔ dào*, grain tract (alimentary tract)

粳 [米]; 粳 [米] *gēng*, non-glutinous rice: 粳米 *gēng mǐ*, rice

米 [米]; 米 [米] *mǐ*, rice (uncooked)

饭 [饣]; 飯 [食] *fàn*, rice (cooked)

面 [一]; 麵 [麥] *miàn*, noodles: 肉面 *ròu miàn*, meat and noodles

粉 [米]; 粉 [米] *fěn*, flour, powder: 白粉 *bái fěn*, rice flour

饼 [饣]; 餠 [食] *bǐng*, noodles; flat unleavened cake: 索饼 *suǒ bǐng*, string noodles

粥 [弓]; 粥 [米] *zhōu*, gruel (thick): 饮热粥 *yǐn rè zhōu*, eat hot gruel

糜 [广]; 糜 [米] *mí*, gruel (thin): 稀糜 *xī mí*, thin gruel

蜜 [宀]; 蜜 [虫] *mì*, honey: 食蜜 *shí mì*, eating honey

脂 [月]; 脂 [肉] *zhī*, fat: 研如脂 *yán rú zhī*, grind until like fat

酪 [酉]; 酪 [酉] *luò*, kumiss, cheese

膏 [高]; 膏 [肉] *gāo*, paste, unctuous substance: 石膏 *shí gāo*, lit. "stone paste," gypsum

浆 [水]; 漿 [水] *jiāng*, (thick) beverages: 水浆 *shuǐ jiāng*, fluids

酒 [氵]; 酒 [水] *jiǔ*, liquor: 清酒 *qīng jiǔ*, clear liquor

饴 [饣]; 飴 [食] *yí*, malt sugar

---

[8]The word 痰 *tán* does not occur in the *Shāng Hán Lùn*, nor does the word 唾 *tuò*, "spittle" (except as a verb, "to spit").

汤 [氵]; 湯 [水] *tāng*, hot water, soup, decoction

醋 [酉]; 醋 [酉] *cù*, vinegar

Clothing

衣 [衣]; 衣 [衣] *yī*, clothes, clothing: 去衣 *qù yī*, take off one's clothes

被 [衤]; 被 [衣] *bèi*, bedclothes: 衣被 *yī bèi*, clothes and bedclothes

褌 [衤]; 褌 [衣] *kūn*, pants: 烧褌散 *shāo kūn sǎn*, Burnt Pants Powder

Buildings, artifacts, and other man-made things

室 [宀]; 室 [宀] *shì*, chamber, room: 血室 *xuè shì*, blood chamber

藏 [艹]; 藏 [艸] *zàng*, storehouse, viscus: 藏结 *zàng jié*, storehouse bind

府 [广]; 府 [广] *fǔ*, mansion, bowel: 藏府 *zàng fǔ*, storehouses and mansions; viscera and bowels

门 [门]; 門 [門] *mén*, gate, door: 期门 *qí mén*, Cycle Gate, LR-14

杓 [木]; 杓 [木] *sháo*, spoon, ladle: 以杓扬之 *yǐ sháo yáng zhī*, lift it with a spoon

匕 [匕]; 匕 [匕] *bǐ*, spoon: 方寸匕 *fāng cùn bǐ*, square-inch-spoon

针 [钅]; 針 [金] *zhēn*, needle: 针足阳明 *zhēn zú yáng míng*, needle the foot yáng brightness

弦 [弓]; 弦 [弓] *xián*, string (of bow or musical instrument), stringlike: 脉弦 *mài xián*, stringlike pulse

索 [十]; 索 [糸] *suǒ*, rope: 索饼 *suǒ bǐng*, string noodle

杯 [木]; 杯 [木] *bēi*, cup: 热粥一杯 *rè zhōu yī bēi*, a cup of hot gruel

柸 [木]; 柸 [木] *pēi*, cup

杵 [木]; 杵 [木] *chǔ*, pestle, to pound: 杵二千下 *chū sān qiān xià*, pound two thousand times

臼 [臼]; 臼 [臼] *jiù*, mortar: 于臼中杵之 *yú jiù zhōng chǔ zhī*, pound it in a mortar

刀 [刀]; 刀 [刀] *dāo*, knife: 以鸡子壳置刀环中 *yǐ jī zǐ ké zhì dāo huán zhōng*, place the egg shell in the ring of a knife

盆 [八]; 盆 [皿] *pén*, basin: 置大盆内 *zhì dà pén nèi*, place in a large basin

筛 [竹]; 篩 [竹] *shāi*, sieve, to sift: 捣筛 *dǎo shāi*, pound and sift

器 [口]; 器 [口] *qì*, vessel, container, pot (and now also machine): 铜器 *tóng qì*, copper pot

漆 [氵]; 漆 [水] *qī*: 蜀漆 *shǔ qī*, dichroa leaf

棋 [木]; 棋 [木] *qí*: 棋子 *qí zǐ*, go stone (chess piece)

椎 [木]; 椎 [木] *zhuī*, mallet, hammer: 大椎 *dà zhuī*, Great Hammer (GV-14)

极 [木]; 極 [木] *jí*, ridgepole, by extension extreme(ly): 极虚 *jí xū*, extremely vacuous

床 [广]; 床 [广] *chuáng*, bed

道 [辶]; 道 [辵] *dào*, road, path, tract: 谷道 *gǔ dào*, grain tract

戟 [卓]; 戟 [戈] *jǐ*: spear: 大戟 *dà jǐ*, lit. "big spear," euphorbia/knoxia

药 [艹]; 藥 [艸] *yào*, medicinal: 药力 *yào lì*, strenth of the medicine

丸 [丸]; 丸 [丶] *wán*, pill: 大陷胸丸 *dà xiàn xiōng wán*, Major Chest Bind Pill

末 [木]; 末 [木] *mò*, powder (original meaning: tip of a branch): 甘遂末 *gān suì mò*, gansui powder

散 [攵]; 散 [攴] *sǎn*, powder (preparation): 五苓散 *wǔ líng sǎn*, Poria Five Powder

剂 [刂]; 劑 [刀] *jì*, pack (of medicine): 三剂 *sān jì*, three packs

文 [文]; 文 [文] *wén*, markings, writing: 文蛤 *wēn gé*, clam (lit. "marked clam")

环 [王]; 環 [玉] *huán*, ring: 刀环 *dāo huán*, ring of a knife

弹 [弓]; 彈 [弓] *tán*, pellet (hurled by a catapult): 弹丸 *dàn wán*, pellet

Natural things and phenomena

天 [天]; 天 [大] *tiān*, Heaven: 天门冬 *tiān mén dōng*, lit. "heaven gate winter," asparagus

地 [土]; 地 [土] *dì*, Earth: 地黄 *dì huáng*, lit. "earth yellow," rehmannia

陆 [阝]; 陸 [阜] *lù*, land (as opposed to water): 商陆 *shāng lù*, phytolacca

土 [土]; 土 [土] *shuǐ*, earth

水 [水]; 水 [水] *shuǐ*, water

日 [日]; 日 [日] *rì*, sun; day

月 [月]; 月 [月] *yuè*, moon; month

阴 [阝]; 陰 [阜] *yīn*, dark side of a mountain, yīn; private parts: 阴虚 *yīn xū*, yīn vacuity; 小便已阴疼 *xiǎo biàn yǐ yīn téng*, yīn pain after urination

阳 [阝]; 陽 [阜] *yáng*, sunny side of a mountain, yáng: 复其阳 *fù qí yáng*, restore the yáng

阿 [阝]; 阿 [阜] *ē*, large mound: 阿胶 *ē jiāo*, ass-hide glue (lit. ē glue, ē standing for Dōngē, East-Mound, a production area in Shāngdōng)

海 [氵]; 海 [水] *hǎi*, sea: 海藻 *hǎi zǎo*, lit. "seaweed," sargassum

潮 [氵]; 潮 [水] *cháo*, tide: 潮热 *cháo rè*, tidal heat

泥 [氵]; 泥 [水] *ní*, mud, by extension anything of mudlike consistency: 捣成泥 *dǎo chéng ní*, pound to a paste

泽 [氵]; 澤 [水] *zé*, marsh: 泽泻 *zé xiè*, lit. "marsh drain," alisma

池 [氵]; 池 [水] *chí*, pool: 风池 *fēng chí*, Wind Pool, GB-20

潦 [氵]; 潦 [水] *liáo*, rain water: 潦水一斗 *liáo shuǐ yī dǒu*, one dǒu of rainwater

澜 [氵]; 瀾 [水] *lán*, wave; swash, ruffle, agitate: 甘澜水 *gān lán shuǐ*, worked water

风 [风]; 風 [風] *fēng*, wind: 风湿相搏 *fēng shī xiāng bó*, wind and dampness contending with each other

寒 [宀]; 寒 [宀] *hán*, cold: 恶风寒 *wù fēng hán*, aversion to wind or cold

湿 [氵]; 濕 [水] *shī*, dampness: 寒湿 *hán shī*, cold-damp

雷 [雨]; 雷 [雨] *léi*, thunder: 腹中雷鸣 *fù zhōng léi míng*, thunderous rumbling in the abdomen

火 [火]; 火 [火] *huǒ*, fire; a cause of disease: 火邪 *huǒ xié*, fire evil

灰 [𠂇]; 灰 [火] *huī*, ash, cinders: 烧作灰 *shāo zuò huī*, burn to ashes

胶 [月]; 膠 [肉] *jiāo*, glue

绵 [纟]; 綿 [糸] *mián*, 绵裹 *mián guǒ*, cotton-wrapped

滓 [氵]; 滓 [水] *zǐ*, dregs

Minerals and metals

石 [石]; 石 [石] *shí*, stone

硝 [石]; 硝 [石] *xiāo*, niter

铜 [钅]; 銅 [金] *tóng*, copper, brass, bronze

铅 [钅]; 鉛 [金] *qiān*, lead

Plant types and parts

草 [艹]; 草 [艸] *cǎo*, grass, herb: 甘草 *gān cǎo*, licorice

木 [木]; 木 [木] *mù*, tree, wood

粮 [米]; 糧 [米] *liáng*, grain (as stored for human consumption): 禹余粮 *yǔ yú liáng*limonite,

根 [木]; 根 [木] *gēn*, root: 葛根 *gé gēn*, pueraria

枝 [木]; 枝 [木] *zhī*, branch, twig: 桂枝 *guì zhī*, cinnamon twig

支 [十]; 支 [支] *zhī*, branch; prop: 心下支结 *xīn xià zhī jié*, propping bind below the heart

实 [宀]; 實 [宀] *shí*, fruit: 枳实 *zhǐ shí*, bitter orange

子 [子]; 子 [子] *zǐ*, seed: 五味子 *wǔ wèi zǐ*, schisandra

花 [艹]; 花 [艸] *huā*, flower: 旋覆花 *xuán fù huā*, inula flower

仁 [亻]; 仁 [人] *rén*, kernel: 杏仁 *xìng rén*, apricot kernel; 桃仁 *táo rén*, peach pit

核 [木]; 核 [木] *hé*, kernel, pit: 桃核 *táo hé*, peach pit

叶 [口]; 葉 [艸] *yè*, leaf: 竹叶 *zhú yè*, bamboo leaf

汁 [氵]; 汁 [水] *zhī*, juice, sap: 皂荚汁 *zào jiá zhī*, gleditsia juice; 胆汁 *dǎn zhī*, gall, bile (lit. gallbladder juice)

蒂 [艹]; 蒂 [艸] *guā*, stalk, pedicel: 瓜蒂 *guā dì*, melon stalk

茎 [艹]; 莖 [艸] *jīng*, stem; a measure word 葱白四茎 *cōng bái sì jīng*, four scallion-whites

梗 [木]; 梗 [木] *gěng*, stem: 桔梗 *jié gěng*,

荚 [艹]; 莢 [艸] *jiá*, pod fruit: 皂荚 *zào jiá*, gleditsia [fruit]

节 [艹]; 節 [竹] *jié*, node, joint: 麻黄三两去节 *má huáng sān liǎng qù jié*, ephedra 3 liǎng (remove nodes)

芤 [艹]; 芤 [艸] *kōu*, scallion-stalk; (like a) scallion-stalk: 脉芤 *mài kōu*, the pulse is scallion-stalk

瓜 [瓜]; 瓜 [瓜] *guā*, melon, gourd: 瓜蒂 *guā dì*, melon stalk

Plants

麦 [麦]; 麥 [麥] *mài*, grain crops other than rice: 麦门冬 *mài mén dōng*, ophiopogon

粟 [西]; 粟 [米] *mài*, millet: 肉上粟起 *ròu shàng sù qǐ*, millet [papules] on the skin

桂 [木]; 桂 [木] *guì*, cinnamon: 桂枝 *guì zhī*, cinnamon twig

枳 [木]; 枳 [木] *zhǐ*, bitter orange: 枳实 *zhǐ shí*, bitter orange

梅 [木]; 梅 [木] *méi*, plum: 乌梅 *wū méi*, mume

竹 [竹]; 竹 [竹] *zhú*, bamboo: 竹叶 *zhú yè*, bamboo leaf

枣 [朿]; 棗 [木] *zǎo*, jujube: 大枣 *dà zǎo*, jujube

参 [厶]; 參 [厶] *shēn*, a root herb, ginseng: 人参 *rén shēn*, ginseng

杏 [木]; 杏 [木] *xìng*, apricot: 杏仁 *xìng rén*, apricot kernel

芍 [艹]; 芍 [艸] *sháo*, peony: 芍药 *sháo yào*, peony

豆 [豆]; 豆 [豆] *dòu*, bean: 巴豆 *bā dòu*, croton

豉 [豆]; 豉 [豆] *chǐ*: 香豉 *xiāng chǐ*, fermented soybean

麻 [麻]; 麻 [麻] *má*, hemp: 麻黄 *má huáng*, ephedra

葛 [艹]; 葛 [艸] *gé*, a trailing plant: 葛根 *gé gēn*, pueraria

姜 [⺶]; 薑 [艸] *jiāng*, ginger

芒 [艹]; 芒 [艸] *máng*: 芒消 *máng xiāo*, mirabilite

芩 [艹]; 芩 [艸] *qín*: 黄芩 *huáng qín*, scutellaria

苓 [艹]; 苓 [艸] *líng*: 茯苓 *fú líng*, poria

芍 [艹]; 芍 [艸] *sháo*: 芍药 *sháo yào*, peony

茯 [艹]; 茯 [艸] *fú*: 茯苓 *fú líng*, poria

芫 [艹]; 芫 [艸] *yuán*: 芫花 *yuán huā*,

蒂 [艹]; 蒂 [艸] *dì*: 瓜蒂 *guā dì*, melon stalk

茵 [艹]; 茵 [艸] *yīn*: 茵陈蒿 *yīn chén hāo*, capillaris

蒿 [艹]; 蒿 [艸] *hāo*: 茵陈蒿 *yīn chén hāo*, capillaris

葱 [艹]; 蔥 [艸] *cōng*: 葱白 *cōng bái*, scallion white

薤 [艹]; 薤 [艸] *xiè*: 薤白 *xiè bái*, Chinese chive

萎 [艹]; 萎 [艸] *wěi*: 萎蕤 *wēi ruí*, Solomon's seal

蕤 [艹]; 蕤 [艸] *ruí*:

葶 [艹]; 葶 [艸] *tíng*: 葶苈子 *tíng lì zǐ*, tingli seed

苈 [艹]; 藶 [艸] *lì*

茱 [艹]; 茱 [艸] *zhū*: 吴茱萸 *wú zhū yú*, evodia

萸 [艹]; 萸 [艸] *yú*

藻 [艹]; 藻 [艸] *zǎo*: 海藻 *hǎi zǎo*, sargassum

荛 [艹]; 蕘 [艸] *ráo*, gray wikstroemia: 荛花 *ráo huā*, gray wikstroemia flowers

桃 [木]; 桃 [木] *táo*, peach: 桃仁 *táo rén*, peach pit

橘 [木]; 橘 [木] *jú*, orange: 橘子 *jú zi*

栝 [木]; 栝 [木] *guā*: 栝楼 *guā lóu*, trichosanthes

楼 [木]; 樓 [木] *lóu*

术 [木]; 朮 [木] *zhú*: 白术 *bái zhú*, ovate atractylodes

桔 [木]; 桔 [木] *jié*: 桔梗 *jié gěng*, platycodon

梧 [木]; 梧 [木] *wú*: 梧桐 *wú tóng*, firmiana

桐 [木]; 桐 [木] *tóng*

梓 [木]; 梓 [木] *zǐ*: 梓白皮 *zǐ bái pí*, catalpa bark

柴 [木]; 柴 [木] *chái* firewood: 柴胡 *chái hú*, bupleurum

栀 [木]; 梔 [木] *zhī*: 栀子 *zhī zǐ*, gardenia

蘖 [艹]; 蘖 [艸] *bó*, biota, same as 柏 *bó*, *bǎi*: 黄蘖 *huáng bó*, biota

朴 [木]; 朴 [木] *pò*: 后朴 *hòu pò*, magnolia bark

椒 [木]; 椒 [木] *jiāo*: 蜀椒 *shǔ jiāo*, zanthoxylum [husk]

皂 [白]; 皀 [白] *zào*, gleditsia: 皂荚 *zào jiá*, gleditsia [fruit]

Animals and animal parts

羊 [羊]; 羊 [羊] *yáng*, goat, sheep: 羊胆 *yáng dǎn*, goat's bile

猪 [犭]; 豬 [豕] *zhū*, pig: 猪胆 *zhū dǎn*, pig's bile

豚 [月]; 豚 [肉] *tún*, piglet: 奔豚 *bēn tún*, running piglet

鸡 [又]; 雞 [隹] *jī*, chicken: 鸡子黄 *jī zǐ huáng*, chicken egg yolk

龙 [龙]; 龍 [龍] *lóng*, dragon: 小青龙汤 *xiǎo qīng lóng tāng*, Minor Green-Blue Dragon Decoction

虎 [虍]; 虎 [虍] *hǔ*, tiger: 白虎汤 *bái hǔ tāng*, White Tiger Decoction

虫 [虫]; 蟲 [虫] *chóng*, bug, insect, grub: 虻虫 *méng chóng*, tabanus

蛤 [虫]; 蛤 [虫] *gé*: 文蛤 *wén gé*, (meretrix) clam shell

蛎 [虫]; 蠣 [虫] *lì*: 牡蛎 *mǔ lì*, oyster shell

蛭 [虫]; 蛭 [虫] *zhì*: 水蛭 *shuǐ zhì*, leech

虻 [虫]; 虻 [虫] *méng*: 虻虫 *méng chóng*, tabanus

牡 [牛]; 牡 [牛] *mǔ*: 牡蛎 *mǔ lì*, oyster shell

蚘 [虫]; 蚘 [虫] *huí*, now written as 蛔, roundworm: 吐蚘 *tù huí*, vomit roundworm

翅 [羽]; 翅 [羽] *chì*: wing 去翅 *qù chì*, remove the wings

贝 [贝]; 貝 [貝] *bèi*, cowerie 贝母 *bèi mǔ*, fritilliaria

珠 [王]; 珠 [玉] *zhū*, pearl; bead: 珠子 *zhū zi*, bead

壳 [士]; 殼 [殳] *ké* (*qiáo*), shell: 鸡子壳 *jī zǐ ké*, chicken eggshell

Proper nouns

秦 [𡗗]; 秦 [禾] *qín*, Qín (Dynasty): 秦皮 *qín pí*, ash bark

巴 [乛]; 巴 [己] *bā*, Bā: name of an ancient state occupying what is now eastern Sìchuān: 巴豆 *bā dòu*, croton seed

吴 [口]; 吳 [口] *wú*, Wú, name of a state: 吴茱萸 *wú zhū yú*, evodia

禹 [丿]; 禹 [内] *yǔ*, Yǔ, a legendary ruler: 禹馀粮 *yǔ yú liáng*, limonite

胡 [月]; 胡 [肉] *hú*, Hú, people living to the north and west of China in ancient times; from the north or west: 柴胡 *chái hú*, bupleurum

蜀 [罒]; 蜀 [虫] *shǔ*, Shǔ, the name of a state: 蜀漆 *shǔ qī*, dichroa leaf

商 [亠]; 商 [口] *shāng*, Shāng, commerce: 商陆 *shāng lù*, phytolacca

Parts of objects

表 [丰]; 表 [衣] *biǎo*, exterior: 表未解 *biǎo wèi jiě*, the exterior has not resolved

里 [里]; 裏 [衣] *lǐ*, interior: 表里俱虚 *biǎo lǐ jù xū*, exterior and interior are both vacuous

侧 [亻]; 側 [人] *cè*, side: 不可转侧 *bù kě zhuǎn cè*, unable to turn sides

Properties of objects

形 [彡]; 形 [彡] *xíng*, form, body: 形似疟 *xíng sì nüè*, the form of the disease resembles malaria

状 [丬]; 狀 [犬] *zhuàng*, appearance, shape, form: 凝如饴状 *níng rú yí zhuàng*, congeal to form like malt sugar

味 [口]; 味 [口] *wèi*: flavor; in *Shāng Hán Lùn* mostly used as a measure word for medicinals, 右三味 *yòu sān wèi*, the above three (medicinals)

色 [刀]; 色 [色] *sè*, color, complexion: 面色青黄 *miàn sè qīng huáng*, green-yellow complexion

Miscellaneous

始 [女]; 始 [女] *shǐ*, start, beginning: 宜服六七合为始 *yí fú liù qī gě wéi shí*, it is appropriate to take six or seven gě to start with (lit. "as a start"); 始虽恶寒 *shǐ suī wù hán*, although at the beginning there is aversion to cold

元 [二]; 元 [儿] *yuán*, origin, starting point, head: 关元 *guān yuán*, Pass Head

终 [纟]; 終 [糸] *zhōng*, end; to end; from beginning to end: 厥终不过五日 *jué zhōng bù guò wǔ rè*, the entire [phase of] reversal will not surpass five days

命 [人或入]; 命 [口] *mìng*, life: 命期 *mìng qí*, term of life

关 [ ]; 關 [門] *guān*, bar: 关上脉细数 *guān shàng mài xì shuò*, a pulse that is fine and rapid at the bar

证 [讠]; 證 [言] *zhèng*, testimony; sign, pattern: 表证 *biǎo zhèng*, exterior pattern

法 [氵]; 法 [水] *fǎ*, method: 作甘澜水法 *zuò gān lán shuǐ fǎ*, the method to make worked water

度 [广]; 度 [广] *dù*, standard; degree: 常度 *cháng dù*, normalcy

处 [夂]; 處 [虍] *chù*, place: 不知痛处 *bù zhī tòng chù*, does not know where the pain is located

间 [门]; 間 [門] *jiān*, space; amidst: 其间 *qí jiān*, amongst them

荣 [艹]; 榮 [火] *yíng*, luxuriance; used for 营 *yíng*, military camp; construction: 荣气不足 *róng qì bù zú*, construction qi is insufficient

卫 [卩]; 衛 [行] *wèi*, defense: 荣卫和 *róng wèi hé*, construction and defense are in harmony

经 [纟]; 經 [糸] *jīng*, warp; any main line; channel; menses: 经脉 *jīng mài*, channel vessels; 经水 *jīng shuǐ*, menses

毒 [丰]; 毒 [毋] *dú*, poison, toxin

沫 [氵]; 沫 [水] *mò*, foam, scum: 去白沫 *qù bái mò*, remove the white foam

景 [日]; 景 [日] *jǐng*: 仲景 *zhòng jǐng*, Zhāng Jī's style

辈 [非]; 輩 [車] *bèi*, generation; class, type: 四逆辈 *sì nì bèi*, Counterflow Cold [Decoction] type [of formula]

部 [阝]; 部 [邑] *bù*, part, region: 知何部不利 *zhī hé bù bù lì*, know which region is inhibited

方 [方]; 方 [方] *fāng*, formula: 合为一方 *hé wéi yī fāng*, combined into one formula

力 [力]; 力 [力] *lì*, force, strength: 药力 *yào lì*, strength of the medicine

Numbers

半 [丨]; 半 [十] *bàn*, half

一 [一]; 一 [一] *yī*, one, first

二 [二]; 二 [二] *er*, two, second

三 [一]; 三 [一] *sān*, three, third

四 [口]; 四 [口] *sì*, four, fourth

五 [二]; 五 [二] *wǔ*, five, fifth

六 [亠]; 六 [八] *liù*, six, sixth

七 [一]; 七 [一] *qī*, seven, seventh

八 [八]; 八 [八] *bā*, eight, eighth

九 [乙]; 九 [乙] *jiǔ*, nine, ninth

十 [十]; 十 [十] *shí* ten, tenth

百 [白]; 百 [白] *bǎi*, hundred

千 [十]; 千 [十] *qiān*, thousand

万 [一]; 萬 [艸] *wàn*, ten thousand, myriad

Measures

斤 [斤]; 斤 [斤] *jīn*, jīn (catty), 250 grams

两 [一]; 兩 [入] *liǎng*, liǎng (tael), 15.625 grams

钱 [钅]; 錢 [金] *qián*, qián (mace)

分 [八]; 分 [刀] *fēn*, fēn

合 [人]; 合 [口] *gě*, gě

升 [丿]; 升 [十] *shēng*, shēng, 200 milliliters

铢 [钅]; 銖 [金] *zhū*, zhū, 1/24th of a liǎng

斗 [斗]; 斗 [斗] *dǒu*, dǒu (dipper): 水一斗 *shuǐ yī dǒu*, 1 dǒu of water

枚 [木]; 枚 [木] *méi*, disk-like object, piece

匕 [匕]; 匕 [匕] *bǐ*, spoon: 方寸匕 *fāng cùn bǐ*, square-inch-spoon

片 [片]; 片 [片] *piàn*, slice

个 [人]; 個 [人] *ge*, general measure word

把 [扌]; 把 [手] *bǎ*, handful

尺 [尺]; 尺 [尸] *chǐ*, chǐ, cubit

颗 [页]; 顆 [頁] *kē*, measure word for small round objects: 水上有珠子五六千颗 *shuǐ shàng yǒu zhū zǐ wǔ liù qiān kē*, there are five or six thousand water droplets on the surface of the water

遍 [辶]; 遍 [辵] *biàn*, [number of] times: 七遍 *qī biàn*, seven times

度 [广]; 度 [广] *dù*, time: 一日二三度 *yī rè èr sān dù*, 2 or 3 times a day

茎 [艹]; 莖 [艸] *jīng*, stem; a measure word: 葱白四茎 *cōng bái sì jīng*, four scallion-whites

壮 [丬]; 壯 [士] *zhuàng*: 灸少阴七壮 *jiǔ shào yīn qī zhuāng*, use seven cones [of moxa] on the lesser yīn

Other words related to numbers and quantities

第 [竹]; 第 [竹] *dì*, marker of ordinals (= nd/rd/th, but placed before number)

余 [人或入]; 餘 [食] *yú*, or more, extra, the rest: 十余日 *shí yú rì*, ten days or more

许 [讠]; 許 [言] *xǔ*, about, approximately: 一时许 *yī shí xǔ*, about an hour

多 [夕]; 多 [夕] *duō*, much, more, many more: 热多寒少 *rè duō hán shǎo*, heat [effusion] more pronounced than [aversion to cold]

少 [小]; 少 [小] *shǎo*, little, few, less, fewer: 少与调胃承气汤 *shǎo yǔ tiáo wèi chéng qì tāng*, give a little Stomach-Regulating Qì-Coordinating Decoction

数 [攵]; 數 [攴] *shù*, several: 数日 *shù rì*, several days

诸 [讠]; 諸 [言] *zhū*, all, various: 诸药 *zhū yào*, all the medicinals

各 [夂]; 各 [口] *gè*, each: 甘草、麻黄各一两 *gān cǎo, má huáng gè yī liǎng*, 1 liǎng each of licorice and ephedra

等 [竹]; 等 [竹] *děng*, equal: 等分 *děng fèn*, in equal proportions

凡 [几]; 凡 [丶] *fán*, whatever, whenever; any: 凡熨其背 *fán yùn qí bèi*, whenever a hot pack is used on the back; 凡病 *fán bìng*, in any illness

稍 [禾]; 稍 [禾] *shāo*, little; little by little, gradually: 稍加 *shāo jiā*, add little by little 稍加至二十丸 *shāo jiā zhì èr shí wán*, gradually increase to twenty pills

度 [广]; 度 [广] *dù*, time, occasion: 一日二三度 *yī rè èr sān dù*, two or three times a day

几 [几]; 幾 [幺] *jǐ*, several: 日几行 *rì jǐ xíng*, several times a day

Time

时 [日]; 時 [日] *shí*, time; a watch (equal to two-hours); sometimes: 一时许 *yī shí yǔ*, about an hour

夏 [夂]; 夏 [夂] *xià*, summer: 立夏后 *lì xià hòu*, after the beginning of summer

秋 [禾]; 秋 [禾] *qiū*, autumn: 立秋前 *lì qiū qián*, before the beginning of autumn

冬 [夂]; 冬 [冫] *dōng*, winter: 麦门冬 *mài mén dōng*, Ophiopogon

日 [日]; 日 [日] *rì*, sun, day: 数日 *shù rì*, several days

月 [月]; 月 [月] *yuè*, moon; month: 二月 *èr yuè*, second month

昼 [尺]; 晝 [日] *zhòu*, daytime: 昼日 *zhòu rì*, in the daytime

旦 [日]; 旦 [日] *dàn*, dawn: 阳旦 *yáng dàn*, yáng dawn

夜 [亠]; 夜 [夕] *yè*, night: 夜二服 *yè èr fú*, take twice at night

晡 [日]; 晡 [日] *bū*, afternoon: 日晡所 *rì bū suǒ*, late afternoon watch

朝 [𠦝]; 朝 [月] *zhāo*, morning: 朝食暮吐 *zhāo shí mù tù*, vomits in the evening food eaten in the morning

暮 [艹]; 暮 [日] *mù*, evening

早 [日]; 早 [日] *zǎo*, early: 太早 *tài zǎo*, too early

宿 [宀]; 宿 [宀] *xiǔ*, one night: 酒渍乌梅一宿 *jiǔ zì wū méi yī xiǔ*, steep the mume in wine for one night

晬 [日]; 晬 [日] *zuì*: 晬时 *zuì shí*, day (period of 24 hours)

期 [月]; 期 [月] *qī*, cycle, period: 期门 *qī mén*, Cycle Gate, LR-14

臾 [臼]; 臾 [臼] *yú* moment, while: 须臾 *xū yú*, a short time, immediately

顷 [匕]; 頃 [頁] *qǐng* moment: 一食顷 *yī shí qīng*, the time it takes to eat a meal

The twelve earthly branches

子 [子]; 子 [子] *zǐ*, B1

丑 [一]; 丑 [一] *chǒu*, B2

寅 [宀]; 寅 [宀] *yín*, B3

卯 [卩]; 卯 [卩] *mǎo*, B4

辰 [辰]; 辰 [辰] *chén*, B5

巳 [己]; 巳 [己] *sì*, B6

午 [𠂉]; 午 [十] *wǔ*, B7

未 [木]; 未 [木] *wèi*, B8

申 [申]; 申 [田] *shēn*, B9

酉 [酉]; 酉 [酉] *mǎo*, B10

戌 [戊]; 戌 [戈] *xū*, B11

亥 [亠]; 亥 [亠] *hài*, B12

Miscellaneous nouns

名 [夕]; 名 [口] *míng*, name (often followed by 曰 *yuē*, 名曰 *míng yuē* is the equivalent of the modern 叫做 *jiào zuò*): 名曰脏结 *míng yuē zàng jié*, it is called storehouse bind

声 [士]; 聲 [耳] *shēng*, voice: 声不出 *shēng bù chū*, no sound issues

意 [音]; 意 [心] *yì*, meaning: 疑非仲景意 *yí fēi zhòng jǐng yì*, [one] suspects [this is] not Zhòng-Jǐng's meaning

责 [𡗗]; 責 [貝] *zé*, duty, responsibility; to demand: 强责少阴汗 *qiáng zé shào yīn hàn*, forces shào yīn sweating

Active verbs

Physical activities

生 [丿]; 生 [生] *shēng*, live: 脉弦者生 *mài xián zhě shēng*, when the pulse is stringlike, [the patient] lives

产 [立]; 產 [生] *chǎn*, give birth, deliver: 产妇 *chǎn fù*, a woman is giving or has just given birth

死 [歹]; 死 [歹] *sǐ*, die: 欲死 *yù sǐ*, about to die

息 [自]; 息 [心] *xí*, breathe; breath: 不得息 *bù dé xī*, unable to breathe; 鼻息 *bí xī*, nose breath

食 [食]; 食 [食] *shí*, eat: 不能食 *bù néng shí*, unable to eat

饮 [饣]; 飲 [食] *yǐn*, drink: 不欲饮食 *bù yù yǐn shí*, does not desire to eat or drink

歠 [欠]; 歠 [欠] *chuò*, sip: 歠热稀粥 *chuò rè xī zhōu*, to sip hot, thin gruel

漱 [氵]; 漱 [水] *shù*, rinse the mouth: 漱水 *shù shuǐ*, rinse the mouth with water

咽 [口]; 嚥 [口] *yàn*, swallow: 不欲咽 *bú yù yàn*, not desiring to swallow [it]

含 [口]; 含 [口] *hán*, hold in the mouth: 少少含咽之 *shǎo shǎo hán yàn zhī*, hold a little in the mouth, then swallow

服 [月]; 服 [肉] *fú*, take (of medicine): 服药已 *fú yào yǐ*, after taking the medicine

顿 [页]; 頓 [頁] *dùn*, quaff: 顿服 *dùn fú*, quaff, take in a single dose

㕮 [口]; 㕮 [口] *fǔ*, chew: 㕮咀三味 *fǔ jǔ sān wèi*, chew the three ingredients

咀 [口]; 咀 [口] *jǔ*, chew (see preceding item)

寐 [宀]; 寐 [宀] *mèi*, sleep: 但欲寐 *dàn yù mèi*, desire only to sleep

眠 [目]; 眠 [目] *mián*, sleep: 眠睡 *mián shuì*, sleep; 不得眠 *bù dé mián*, unable to sleep

睡 [目]; 睡 [目] *shuì*, sleep (see preceding item)

卧 [臣]; 臥 [臣] *wò*, lie: 不能卧 *bù néng wò*, unable to lie (flat), unable to sleep

起 [走]; 起 [走] *qǐ*, get up: 卧起不安 *wò qǐ bù ān*, disquieted whether lying or sitting

立 [立]; 立 [立] *lì*, stand; establish: 立秋前 *lì qiū qián*, before the beginning of autumn

伸 [亻]; 伸 [人] *shēn*, stretch: 难以屈伸 *nán yǐ qū shēn*, difficult to bend and stretch

屈 [尸]; 屈 [尸] *qū*, bend (see preceding item)

眴 [目]; 眴 [目] *xuàn*, roll the eyes: 不能眴 *bù néng xuàn*, unable to roll the eyes

蜷 [虫]; 踡 [足] *quán*, curl up: 蜷卧 *quán wò*, lie curled up

坐 [土]; 坐 [土] *zuò*, sit: 短气但坐 *duǎn qì dàn zuò*, short of breath and only [able to] sit

持 [扌]; 持 [手] *chí*, hold: 持脉 *chí mài*, take the pulse

抱 [扌]; 抱 [手] *bào*, hold, embrace: 以手急抱 *yǐ shǒu jí bào*, hold it tightly with the hand

摇 [扌]; 搖 [手] *yáo*, shake: 振振摇 *zhèn zhèn yáo*, quivering and trembling

叉 [又]; 叉 [又] *chā*, cross: 病人手叉自冒心 *bìng rén shǒu chā zì mào xīn*, the patient has his hands crossed over his heart

取 [耳]; 取 [又] *qǔ*, take, get: 煮取三升 *zhǔ qǔ sān shēng*, boil to get three shēng

着 [羊]; 著 [艸] *zháo*, put, place: 着鸡子壳中 *zháo jī zǐ ké zhōng*, put [it] in the eggshell

引 [弓]; 引 [弓] *yǐn*, take, draw; (of pain) to stretch into: 消谷食引食 *xiāo gǔ yǐn shí*, rapid hungering and large food intake; 痛引少腹 *tòng yǐn shoǎ fù*, pain stretching into the lower abdomen

得 [彳]; 得 [彳] *dé*, get, get up: 不能得小汗出 *bù néng dé xiǎo hàn chū*, cannot get up a light sweat; 不得为少阴病 *bù dé wéi shào yīn bìng*, [it] cannot be lesser yīn disease

置 [罒]; 置 [网] *zhì*, put, place: 置大盆内 *zhì dà pén nèi*, place in a large basin

与 [一]; 與 [臼] *yǔ*, give: 可与桂枝汤 *kě yǔ guì zhī tāng*, [one] can give Cinnamon Twig Decoction

用 [冂]; 用 [用] *yòng*, use; eat: 用前法 *yòng qián fǎ*, use the previous[ly described] method; 食难用饱 *shí nán yòng bǎo*, difficulty in eating to satiation

按 [扌]; 按 [手] *àn*, press: 按之则痛 *àn zhī zé tòng*, painful when pressed

摸 [扌]; 摸 [手] *mō*, feel (as with the hands): 捻衣摸床 *niǎn yī mò chuáng*, picking at bedclothes

搅 [扌]; 攪 [手] *jiǎo*, stir: 搅之勿令焦著 *jué zhī wù lìng jiāo zhù*, stir to prevent it from burning and sticking [to the pot]

捻 [扌]; 捻 [手] *niǎn*, pinch: 并手捻作挺 *bìng shǒu niǎn zuò tǐng*, pinch with the hands so that it stands erect

绞 [纟]; 絞 [糸] *jiǎo*, wring (out the juice): 绞去滓 *jiǎo qù zǐ*, wring [out the juice] and remove the dregs

劳 [艹]; 勞 [力] *láo*, toil, exert oneself, tax onself: 劳复 *láo fù*, taxation relapse

唾 [口]; 唾 [口] *tuò*, spit: 喜唾 *xǐ tuò*, frequent spitting

Perception, thought, and speech

见 [见]; 見 [見] *jiàn*, see: 但见一证 *dàn jiàn yī zhèng*, see only one sign

视 [礻]; 視 [示] *shì*, see, look: 直视 *zhí shì*, forward-staring [eyes]

闻 [门]; 聞 [耳] *wén*, hear; smell: 两耳无闻 *liǎng ěr wú wén*, no hearing in either ear; 蚘闻食臭出 *yóu wén shí chòu chū*, roundworms come out when they smell the malodor of food

观 [又]; 觀 [見] *guān*, look: 观其脉证 *guān qí mài zhèng*, observe the pulse and signs

知 [矢]; 知 [矢] *zhī*, know: 何以知此 *hé yǐ zhī cǐ*, how [does one] know this?

了 [乛]; 瞭 [日] *liáo*, know clearly: 明了 *míng liǎo*, clear-headed

识 [讠]; 識 [言] *shì*, know, be aware: 常须识此 *cháng xū shì cǐ*, one needs always to be aware of this

裁 [𢦏]; 裁 [衣] *cái*, judge, consider: 当裁为越婢汤、桂枝汤合之 *dāng cái wéi yuè bì tāng, guì zhī tāng hé zhī*, this should be considered to be a combination of Cinnamon Twig Decoction (*guì zhī tāng*) and Spleen-Effusing Decoction (*yuè bì tāng*)

辨 [辛]; 辨 [刀] *biàn*, distinguish, identify: 辨霍乱 *biàn huò luàn*, identify sudden turmoil (cholera)

忘 [亡]; 忘 [心] *wàng*, forget: 喜忘 *xǐ wàng*, forgetfulness

疑 [匕]; 疑 [疋] *yí*, doubt, suspect: 疑非仲景意 *yí fēi zhòng jǐng yì*, [one] suspects [this is] not Zhòng-Jǐng's meaning

语 [讠]; 語 [言] *yǔ*, speak, speech: 谵语 *zhān yǔ*, delirious speech

言 [言]; 言 [言] *yán*, speak: 不能语言 *bù néng yǔ yán*, cannot speek

曰 [日]; 曰 [日] *yuē*, say, state

谓 [讠]; 謂 [言] *wèi*, to be called, to mean: 何谓藏结？ *hé wèi zàng jié*, what is storehouse bind?

云 [二]; 云 [二] *yún*, say, state

问 [门]; 問 [口] *wèn*, ask, inquire: 当问其小便 *dāng wèn qí xiǎo biàn*, [one] must inquire about urination

答 [竹]; 答 [竹] *dá*, answer

应 [广]; 應 [心] *yìng*, (cor)respond: 病皆与方相应 *bìng jiē yǔ fāng xiāng yìng*, the disease corresponds to the formula

喜 [士]; 喜 [口] *xǐ*, like to; tend to: 酒客不喜甘 *jiǔ kè bù xǐ gān*, drinkers do not like sweet [things]; 喜忘 *xǐ wàng*, forgetfulness

嗜 [口]; 嗜 [口] *shì*, like to: 嗜卧 *shì wò*, like to sleep; somnolence

恶 [亚]; 惡 [心] *xǐ*, averse to: 恶风 *wù fēng*, averse to wind

Pathological actions

咳 [口]; 咳 [口] *ké*, cough:

喘 [口]; 喘 [口] *chuǎn*, pant, panting: 喘家 *chuǎn jiā*, panting patient

呕 [口]; 嘔 [口] *ǒu*, retch, retching: 呕吐 *ǒu tù*, retching and vomiting

吐 [口]; 吐 [口] *tù*, vomiting: 水入则吐 *shuǐ rù zé tù*, vomiting of ingested fluids

噫 [口]; 噫 [口] *yī*, belching:

哕 [口]; 噦 [口] *yuē*, hiccough: 时时哕 *shí shí yuē*, frequent hiccough

痓 [疒]; 痓 [疒] *cì*, tetany:

瞤 [目]; 瞤 [目] *shùn*, twitching: 筋惕肉瞤 *jīn tì ròu shùn*, jerking sinews and twitching flesh

General movement

动 [力]; 動 [力] *dòng*, stir: 肾气动 *shèn qì dòng*, kidney qì stirs

行 [彳]; 行 [彳] *xíng*, move: 卫行脉外 *wèi xíng mài wèi*, defense moves outside the vessels

走 [走]; 走 [走] *bēn*, run: 走皮内 *zǒu pí nèi*, penetrates the skin

奔 [大]; 奔 [大] *bēn*, run, charge: 奔豚 *bēn tún*, running piglet

传 [亻]; 傳 [人] *chuán*, pass, transmit: 不传 *bù chuán*, will not pass [on to another channel]

流 [氵]; 流 [水] *liú*, flow: 谷气下流 *gǔ qì xià liú*, grain qì flows down

洪 [氵]; 洪 [水] *hóng*, swell, surge: 脉洪 *mài hóng*, the pulse is surging

漓 [氵]; 漓 [水] *lí* trickle, flow: 如水流漓 *rú shuǐ liú lí*, flow like water

漏 [氵]; 漏 [水] *lòu* leak: 漏不止 *lòu bù zhǐ*, incessantly leaking

濈 [氵]; 濈 [水] *jí*, stream: 濈然 *jí rán*,

Stopping

止 [止]; 止 [止] *zhǐ*, stop, cease: 呕不止 *ǒu bù zhǐ*, persistent retching

停 [亻]; 停 [人] *tíng*, cease: 停后服 *tíng hòu fú*, cease taking further doses

休 [亻]; 休 [人] *zuò*, to be inactive, rest: 休作有时 *xiū zuò yǒu shí*, starting and stopping periodically

罢 [罒]; 罷 [网] *bà*, cease: 柴胡证不罢 *chái hú zhèng bù bà*, the Bupleurum pattern has not ceased

尽 [尸]; 盡 [皿] *bà*, finish; do completely: 不必尽剂 *bù bì jìn jì*, need not finish the whole packet

了 [乛]; 了 [亅] *liǎo*, finish: 不了了 *bù liǎo liǎo*, no definitively, not clearly

Movement toward

来 [一]; 來 [人] *lái*, come: 经水适来 *jīng shuǐ shì lái*, the menstrual flow happens to arrive

至 [至]; 至 [至] *zhì*, arrive: 脉不至 *mài bù zhì*, the pulse does not arrive

到 [至]; 到 [刀] *dào*, 到经不解 *dào jīng bù jiě*, [the evil] reaches [the original] channel and [the disease] does not resolve

入 [入]; 入 [入] *rù*, enter: 大热入胃 *dà rè rù wèi*, great heat enters the stomach

进 [辶]; 進 [辵] *jìn*, advance; enter; ingest, take: 其病为进 *qí bìng wéi jìn*, the disease is advancing

内 [冂]; 內 [入] *nà*, put in: 内诸药 *nà zhū yào*, put in all the medicinals

Movement away

去 [去]; 去 [厶] *qù*, go, leave; remove: 寒去欲解 *hán qù yù jiě*, the cold is going and [the disease] is about to resolve; 去皮 *qù pí*, remove the skin

往 [彳]; 往 [彳] *wǎng*, go: 往来 *wáng lái*, lit. "going and coming," i.e., alternating 往来寒热 *wǎng lái hán rè*, alternating [aversion to] cold and heat [effusion]

出 [凵]; 出 [凵] *chū*, go out, issue: 蚘闻食臭出 *yóu wén shí chòu chū*, roundworms come out when they smell the malodor of food; 汗出 *hàn chū*, sweat issues, to sweat

退 [辶]; 退 [辵] *tuì*, retreat, abate: 阳气退 *yáng qì tuì*, yáng qì abates

Upward and outward movement

上 [⺊]; 上 [一] *shàng*, ascend, rise, up: 气上冲胸 *qì shàng chōng xiōng*, qì surges upward to the chest; 蚘上入其膈 *huí shàng rù qí gé*, roundworms ascend and enter the diaphragm

浮 [氵]; 浮 [水] *fú*, float: 脉浮 *mài fú*, a pulse that is floating

开 [廾]; 開 [門] *kāi*, open: 腠理开 *còu lǐ kāi*, the interstices open

发 [又]; 發 [癶] *fā*, effuse, effusion: 热自发 *rè zì fā*, heat effuses spontaneously; 发黄 *fā huáng*, yellowing; 发汗 *fā hàn*, promote sweating;

揭 [扌]; 揭 [手] *jiē*, lift, remove: 勿发揭衣被 *wù fā jiē yī bèi*, do not remove the clothes and bedclothes

散 [攵]; 散 [攴] *sàn*, spread, scatter, dissipate: 血散脉中 *xuè sàn mài zhōng*, [it will] dissipate the blood from the pulse

越 [走]; 越 [走] *yuè*, go over, stray: 津液越出 *jīn yè yuè chū*, liquid and humor stray outward

解 [角]; 解 [角] *jiǎo*, release, untie, resolve: 表未解 *biǎo wèi jiě*, the exterior has not yet resolved

举 [丶]; 舉 [臼] *jǔ*, to lift: 头重不欲举 *tóu zhòng bú yù jǔ*, head heavy [so that the patient] does not desire to lift [it]

戴 [戈]; 戴 [戈] *dài*, wear on the head: 戴阳 *dài yáng*, upcast yáng

Downward and outward movement

下 [卜]; 下 [一] *xià*, descend, precipitate: 谷气下流 *gǔ qì xià liú*, 不可下 *bù kě xià*, cannot precipitate

沉 [氵]; 沉 [水] *chén*, sink, applied to the pulse: 脉沉微 *mài chén wēi*, the pulse is sunken and faint

陷 [阝]; 陷 [阜] *xiàn*, fall, applied to evils entering the interior: 阳气内陷 *yáng qì nèi xiàn*, yáng qì falls inward

溢 [氵]; 溢 [水] *yì*, spill: 血气流溢 *xuè qì liú yì*, blood and qi flow and spill

泄 [氵]; 泄 [水] *xiè*, flow, discharge: 泄奔豚气 *xiè bēn tún qì*, discharge running piglet qi

泻 [氵]; 瀉 [水] *xiè*, flow, drain: 泻心汤 *xiè xīng tāng*, heart-draining decoction

写 [冖]; 寫 [宀] *xiě*, same as preceding item

Rotation

转 [车]; 轉 [車] *zhuǎn*, turn, shift: 转侧 *zhuǎn cèi*, turn sides; 转属阳明 *zhuǎn shǔ yáng míng*, shift to yáng brightness

旋 [方]; 旋 [方] *xuán* rotate: 旋覆花 *xuán fù huā*, inula flower

绕 [纟]; 繞 [糸] *rào*, go around; used prepositionally: 绕脐痛 *rào qí tòng*, pain around the umbilicus

Movement in normal and abnormal direction

顺 [页]; 順 [頁] *shùn*, favorably: 为顺 *wéi shùn*, means [a] favorable [outcome]; 阴阳气不相顺接 *yīn yáng qì bù xiāng shùn jiē*, yīn and yáng qì do not connect favorably

逆 [辶]; 逆 [辵] *nì*, (move) counterflow; adverse [treatment]: 客气上逆 *kè qì shàng nì*, visiting qì ascends counterflow; 下之为逆 *xià zhī wéi nì*, precipitation is an adverse treatment

厥 [厂]; 厥 [厂] *jué*, reverse, revert: 手足厥冷 *shǒu zú jué lěng*, reversal cold of the limbs; 厥阴 *jué yīn*, reverting yīn

Change

变 [亦]; 變 [言] *biàn*, transmute (change suddenly, greatly, or untowardly): 数变迟 *shuò biàn chí*, stirring and rapid [quality] changes to slow

更 [一]; 更 [日] *gēng*, change: 更衣 *gēng yī*, change one's clothes (euphemism for defecation)

化 [亻]; 化 [匕] *huà*, transform (gradually, creatively or positively): 谷不化 *gǔ bù huà*, stool remains untransformed

成 [戊]; 成 [戈] *chéng*, become: 成结胸 *chéng jié xiōng*, to become (turn into) chest bind; 捣成泥 *dǎo chéng ní*, pound into (lit. to become) a paste

Decrease

减 [氵]; 減 [水] *jiǎn*, reduce: 减二升 *jiǎn èr shēng*, reduce by two shēng

亡 [亡]; 亡 [亠] *wáng*, collapse, be ruined: 亡血 *wáng xuè*, blood collapse

绝 [纟]; 絕 [糸] *jué*, cut off, expire: 阳绝于里 *yáng jué yú lǐ*, yáng is cut off in the interior; 脉微欲绝 *mài wēi yù jué*, the pulse is faint on the verge of expiration

消 [氵]; 消 [水] *xiāo*, disperse, digest: 消渴 *xiāo kě*, dispersion-thirst; 消谷 *xiāo gǔ*, digest grain (food)

竭 [立]; 竭 [立] *jié*, be exhausted: 胃中水竭 *wèi zhōng shuǐ jié*, water in the stomach is exhausted

除 [阝]; 除 [阜] *chú*, eliminate, get rid of: 噫气不除 *yì qì bù chú*, belching is not eliminated

失 [丿]; 失 [大] *shī*, lose, fail: 失其常度 *shī qí cháng dù*, loses its normalcy; let out: 失气 *shī qì*, pass [fecal] qì (flatus)

损 [扌]; 損 [手] *sǔn*, reduce, damage: 损谷则愈, decrease food [intake and there will be] recovery.

遗 [辶]; 遺 [辵] *yí*, lose: 遗尿 *yí niào*, enuresis

阙 [门]; 闕 [門] *què*, same as 缺 *quē*, missing

Increase

增 [土]; 增 [土] *zēng*, increase: 增桂 *zēng guì*, increase the cinnamon [twig]

加 [力]; 加 [力] *jiā*, add: 加葛根 *jiā gé gēn*, add pueraria

蓄 [艹]; 蓄 [艸] *xù*, amass: 蓄水 *xù shuǐ*, water amassment

建 [廴]; 建 [廴] *jiàn*, build, in the same sense as 健 *jiàn*, fortify: 小建中汤 *xiǎo jiàn zhōng tāng*, Minor Center-Fortifying Decoction

并 [丷]; 併 [人] *bìng*, go side by side: 并病 *bìng bìng*, dragover disease

结 [纟]; 結 [糸] *jié*, bind: 结胸 *jié xiōng*, chest bind

Joining

连 [辶]; 連 [辵] *lián*, link, connect: 黄连 *huáng lián*, coptis, lit. "yellow links"

合 [人]; 合 [口] *hé*, combine, unite; entire, whole: 合病 *hé bìng*, combination disease; 面合色赤 *miàn hé sè chì*, face completely red

并 [丷]; 并 [干] *bìng*, combine: 并为六合 *bìng wéi liù gě*, combine to make six gě

接 [扌]; 接 [手] *jiē*, join, connect: 阴阳气不相顺接 *yīn yáng qì bù xiāng shùn jiē*, yīn and yáng qì do not connect favorably

续 [纟]; 續 [糸] *xù*, join, make continuous, continue; still; then, followed by: 脉续浮 *mài xù fú*, the pulse continues to be floating (is still floating); 续得下利清谷不止 *xù dé xià lì qīng gǔ bù zhǐ*, followed by persistent clear-food diarrhea

承 [→]; 承 [丿] *chéng*, inherit, carry on: 小承气汤 *xiǎo chéng qì tāng*, Minor Qì-Coordinating Decoction

附 [阝]; 附 [阜] *fù*, append: 附子 *fù zǐ*, aconite

系 [糸]; 繫 [糸] *xì*, tie, bind: 系在太阴 *xiè zài tài yì*, bound to greater yīn

缘 [纟]; 緣 [糸] *yuán*, cause, reason; continuous: 何缘得阳明病？ *hé yuán dé yáng míng bìng*, what is the reason one gets yáng brightness disease? 设面色缘缘正赤 *shè miàn sè yuán yuán zhèng chì*, the facial complexion is continuously full red

Breaking

擘 [手]; 擘 [手] *bò*, break, split: 大枣十二枚（擘） *dà zǎo èr shí méi* (*bò*), jujubes 20 pieces (broken)

捣 [扌]; 擣 [手] *dǎo*, pound: 捣筛二味 *dǎo shāi èr wèi*, pound and sift the two ingredients

筑 [竹]; 築 [木] *zhú*, pound: 若脐上筑 *ruò qí shàng zhú*, if there is pounding above the umbilicus

研 [石]; 研 [石] *yán*, grind (finely): 言如脂 *yán rú zhī*, grind until like fat

破 [石]; 破 [石] *pò*, break: 破八片 *pò bā piàn*, break into eight pieces

坼 [土]; 坼 [土] *chè*, crack: 炮令坼 *pào lìng chè*, blast-fry to make it crack

切 [刀]; 切 [刀] *qiē*, cut: 切八片 *qiē bā piàn*, cut into eight slices

断 [斤]; 斷 [斤] *duàn*, break, discontinue, stop: 经水适断 *jīng shuǐ shì duàn*, menstrual flow happens to stop

Help and nurturing

救 [攵]; 救 [支] *jiù*, eliminate; to rescue: 救邪风 *jiù xié fēng*, eliminate evil wind; 救里 *jiù lǐ*, rescue the interior

协 [十]; 協 [十] *xié*, coordinate: 协热利 *xié rè lì*, complex diarrhea

助 [力]; 助 [力] *zhù*, assist: 助药力 *zhù yào lì*, help (reinforce) the strength of the medicine

养 [丷]; 養 [食] *yǎng*, nourish: 糜粥自养 *mí zhōu zì yǎng*, [take] rice-gruel for nourishment

将 [丬]; 將 [寸] *jiāng*, nurture: 将息如前法 *jiāng xī rú qián fǎ*, care and rest as previously indicated

Control

主 [王]; 主 [丶] *zhǔ*, govern: 五苓散主之 *wǔ líng sǎn zhǔ zhī*, Poria Five governs

治 [氵]; 治 [水] *zhì*, control, direct; treat (disease): 实以虚治 *shí yǐ xū zhì*, to treat vacuity as repletion

制 [刂]; 制 [刀] *zhì*, control, restrain: 不能制水 *bù néng zhì shuǐ*, unable to control water

克 [十]; 剋 [刀] *kè*, restrain: 互相克贼 *hù xiāng kè zéi*, restraint and robbing

Pursuit

随 [阝]; 隨 [阜] *suí*, follow: 随经 *suí jīng*, follow the channel

遂 [辶]; 遂 [辵] *suì*, pursue; then, followed by: 遂发热恶寒 *suì fā rè wù hán*, then [there is] heat effusion and aversion to cold

循 [彳]; 循 [彳] *xún*, follow; grope (down, along, over): 循衣摸床 *xún yī mō chuáng*, lit. "groping [over one's] clothes and feeling the bed," i.e., picking at bedclothes

追 [辶]; 追 [辵] *zhuī*, pursue: 追虚逐实 *zhuī xū zhú shí*, seeking vacuity and pursuing repletion

逐 [辶]; 逐 [辵] *zhú*, pursue; chase out/away: 逐水气 *zhú shuǐ qì*, expel water qì

格 [木]; 格 [木] *gé*, repel: 寒格 *hán gé*, repelling cold

Violence

攻 [工]; 攻 [攴] *gōng*, attack: 不可攻痞 *bù kě gōng pǐ*, [one] cannot attack the glomus

搏 [扌]; 搏 [手] *bó*, contend: 风湿相搏 *fēng shī xiāng bó*, wind and dampness contending with each other

争 [刀]; 爭 [爪] *zhēng*, struggle: 正邪分争 *zhèng xié fēn zhēng*, right and evil struggling in turns

伤 [亻]; 傷 [人] *shāng*, damage, injure: 伤寒 *shāng hán*, cold damage

胜 [月]; 勝 [力] *shèng*, overcome: 以新虚不胜谷气故也 *yǐ xīn xū bù néng shèng gǔ qì*, because of new vacuity, [the body] cannot overcome grain qì

中 [中]; 中 [丨] *zhòng*, strike: 中风 *zhòng fēng*, wind strike

撞 [扌]; 撞 [手] *zhuàng*, surge: 气上撞心 *qì shàng zhuàng xīn*, qì surging upward to the heart

抵 [扌]; 抵 [手] *dǐ*, hit, arrive: 抵当汤 *dǐ dàng tāng*, Dead-On Decoction

犯 [犭]; 犯 [犬] *fàn*, commit (error); invade: 知犯何逆 *zhī fàn hé nì*, know what error [one] has committed; 无犯胃气及上二焦 *wú fàn wèi qì jí shàng èr jiāo*, do not assail stomach qi and the two upper burners

乘 [禾]; 乘 [丿] *chéng*, exploit: 肝乘脾 *gān chéng pí*, the liver is exploiting the spleen

掣 [手]; 掣 [手] *chè*, pull: 掣痛 *chè tòng*, pulling pain

冲 [冫]; 衝 [行] *chōng*, surge: 气上冲胸 *qì shàng chōng xiōng*, qi surges up into the chest

刺 [刂]; 刺 [刀] *cì*, prick, stab, needle: 刺风池 *cì fēng chí*, needle Wind-Pool (GB-20)

劫 [去]; 劫 [力] *jié*, pillage, force: 火劫 *huǒ jié*, fire forcing

Action of/treatment with fire

烧 [火]; 燒 [火] *shāo*, burn: 烧褌散 *shāo kūn sǎn*, Burnt Pants Powder

熨 [火]; 熨 [火] *yùn*, to iron (clothes); apply a hot pack: 熨其背 *yùn qí bèi*, apply a hot back to the back

焦 [灬]; 焦 [火] *jiāo*, parch, burn: 焦骨伤筋 *jiāo gǔ shāng jīn*, parch the bones and damage the sinews; 搅之勿令焦著 *jué zhī wù lìng jiāo zhù*, stir to prevent it from burning and sticking [to the pot]; 中焦 *zhōng jiāo*, center burner

炮 [火]; 炮 [火] *pào*, blast[-fry]: 附子一两（炮） *fù zǐ yì liǎng (pào)*, aconite 1 liǎng (blast-fried)

煎 [灬]; 煎 [火] *jiān*, cook, boil, fry: 再煎取三升 *zài jiān qǔ sān shēng*, decoct again to get three shēng

炙 [火]; 炙 [火] *zhì*, mix-fry: 甘草（炙） *gān cǎo (zhì)*, licorice (mix-fried)

熬 [灬]; 熬 [火] *áo*, slow boil: 熬黑 *áo hēi*, slow boil until black

煮 [灬]; 煮 [火] *zhǔ*, cook, boil: 微火煮 *wéi huǒ zhǔ*, boil over a mild flame

炊 [火]; 炊 [火] *chuī*, cook: 相去如炊三斗米顷 *xiāng qù rú chuī sān dǒu mǐ qīng*, after the time it takes to cook three dǒu of rice

烊 [火]; 烊 [火] *yáng*, melt, dissolve: 内阿胶烊尽 *nèi ē jiāo yáng jìn*, put in the ass-hide glue [and let it] dissolve completely

熏 [灬]; 熏 [火] *xūn*, fume: 火熏 *huǒ xūn*, to fume with fire

Action of/treatment with water

潠 [氵]; 潠 [水] *sùn*, spurt: 以冷水潠之 *yǐ lěng shuǐ sùn zhī*, spurt him with cold water

洗 [氵]; 洗 [水] *xǐ*, wash: 清酒洗 *qīng jiǔ xǐ*, wash with clear liquor

渍 [氵]; 漬 [水] *zì*, steep, soak: 渍之须臾 *zì zhī xū yú*, soak it for a while

浸 [氵]; 浸 [水] *jìn*, steep, soak: 水浸 *shuǐ jìn*, soak in water

灌 [氵]; 灌 [水] *guàn*, to pour; irrigate; to force a person to drink: 灌谷道内 *guàn gǔ dào nèi*, pour into the grain tract (here, the rectum)

淋 [氵]; 淋 [水] *lín*, drip; strangury: 淋家 *lín jiā*, strangury patient

漓 [氵]; 漓 [水] *lí*, flow: 如水流漓 *rú shuǐ liú lí*, flow like water

蒸 [艹]; 蒸 [艸] *zhēng*, steam: 蒸蒸发热 *zhēng zhēng fā rè*, steaming heat effusion

淅 [氵]; 淅 [水] *xī*, to spray, to splash: 淅淅恶风 *xī xī wù fēng*, wetted aversion to wind

Miscellaneous active verbs

作 [亻]; 作 [人] *zuò*, make, do: 作甘澜水 *zuò gān lán shuǐ*, to make worked water

为 [丶]; 爲 [火] *wéi*, make, do: 为散 *wéi sǎn*, to make a powder

教 [攵]; 教 [攴] *jiào*, teach, instruct: 教试令咳 *jiào shì lìng ké*, instructed [the students] to try to make [the patient] cough

复 [𠂉]; 復 [彳] *fù*, return, restore: 复其阳 *fù qí yáng*, restore the yáng

还 [辶]; 還 [辵] *huán*, return, be restored: 阳气还 *yáng qì huán*, yáng qì returns

及 [丿]; 及 [又] *jí*, (reach) to; as good as 不及汤 *bù jí tāng*, not as good as a decoction

受 [爫]; 受 [又] *shòu*, receive, contract, accept: 三阴当受邪 *sān yīn dāng shòu xié*, the three yīn [channels] should contract the evil; 不受食 *bù shòu shí*, will not accept food

被 [衤]; 被 [衣] *bèi*, be covered; be affected by, contract; passive particle (by): 针处被寒 *zhēn chù bèi hán*, the needling site contracts cold; 被火气劫 *bèi huǒ qì jié*, plundered by fire qì

定 [宀]; 定 [宀] *dìng*, fix, set: 屎定硬 *shǐ dìng yìng*, the stool is set hard

理 [王]; 理 [玉] *lǐ*, order, rectify: 理中汤 *lǐ zhōng tāng*, Center-Rectifying Decoction

调 [讠]; 調 [言] *tiáo*, regulate, harmonize, mix: 调胃承气汤 *tiáo wèi chéng qì tāng*, Stomach-Regulating Qì-Coordinating Decoction

试 [讠]; 試 [言] *shì*, try: 试令咳 *shì lìng ké*, try to make [the patient] cough

覆 [覀]; 覆 [襾] *fù*, cover: 覆取微似汗 *fù qǔ wēi sì hàn*, cover [with bedclothes] to obtain slight sweating

尽 [尸]; 盡 [皿] *jìn*, reach the end, to the end; all; completely: 行其经尽 *xíng qí jīng jìn*, [the evil] goes through the channels to the end

彻 [彳]; 徹 [彳] *chè*, go all the way; complete: 发汗不彻 *fā hàn bú chè*, promote sweating incompletely

负 [刀]; 負 [貝] *fù*, be defeated, lose; bear, sustain; contrary: 其脉不负 *qí mài bù fù*, the pulse is not contrary [to what is expected]

扬 [扌]; 揚 [手] *yáng*, raise, lift: 以杓扬之 *yǐ sháo yáng zhī*, lift it with a ladle

扰 [扌]; 擾 [手] *rǎo*, harass; agitate: 手足躁扰 *shǒu zú zào rǎo*, agitation of the extremities

裹 [亠]; 裹 [衣] *guǒ*, wrap: 绵裹 *mián guǒ*, wrap in cotton

鸣 [口]; 鳴 [口] *míng*, sound, rumble: 腹中雷鸣 *fú zhōng léi míng*, thunderous rumbling in the abdomen

导 [巳]; 導 [寸] *dǎo*, abduct; enema: 宜蜜煎导而通之 *yí mì jiān dǎo ér tōng zhī*, to abduct the stoool with [a] thickened honey [enema]

误 [讠]; 誤 [言] *wù*, to make a mistake: 误治 *wù zhì*, treat inappropriately

颠 [页]; 顛 [頁] *diān*, top: 颠倒 *diān dǎo*, tossing and turning

倒 [亻]; 倒 [人] *dǎo*, upside-down, reverse

迫 [辶]; 迫 [辵] *pò*, force, compel: 医以火迫劫之 *yī yǐ huǒ pò jié zhī*, the physician uses fire to force [sweating]

拒 [扌]; 拒 [手] *jù*, refuse: 拒痛 *jù tòng*, pain [that] refuses [pressure]

居 [尸]; 居 [尸] *jū*, reside: 阳明居中 *yáng míng jū zhōng*, yáng brightness resides in the center

求 [丶]; 求 [水] *qiú*, seek: 于寒湿中求之 *yú hán shī zhōng qiú zhī*, seek [to treat the disease by addressing] cold and dampness

擗 [扌]; 擗 [手] *pì*, beat the breast: 欲擗地 *yù pì dì*, about to fall (probably from the image of the chest hitting the ground)

凝 [冫]; 凝 [冫] *níng*, congeal, thicken: 凝如饴状 *níng rú yí zhuàng*, congeal to a form like malt sugar

仿 [亻]; 仿 [人] *fǎng*, follow, emulate: 诸汤皆仿此 *zhū tāng jiē fǎng cǐ*, all formulae should be used according to (lit. "following") this [method]

禁 [示]; 禁 [示] *jìn*, forbid, contraindicate: 禁生冷 *jìn shēng lěng*, cold and raw foods are contraindicated

忌 [己]; 忌 [心] *jì*, forbid, contraindicate: 禁忌 *jìn jì*, contraindication

啬 [十]; 嗇 [口] *sè*, stingy, miserly: 啬啬恶寒 *sè sè wù hán*, huddled (lit. miserly) aversion to cold

翕 [羽]; 翕 [羽] *xì*, draw the wings close to the body: 翕翕发热 *xì xì fā rè*, fearther-warm heat effusion

几 [几]; 几 [几] *shū*, stretched: 项背强几几 *xiàng bèi qiáng shū shū*, stretched rigid nape and back

翘 [羽]; 翹 [羽] *qiáo*, stick up: 连翘 *lián qiáo*, forsythia

轺 [车]; 軺 [車] *qiáo*: 连轺 *lián qiáo*, forsythia root

约 [纟]; 約 [糸] *yuē*, restrain, hold: 脾约 *pí yuē*, straitened spleen

共 [廾]; 共 [八] *gòng*, combine: 与汗共并 *yǔ hàn gòng bìng*, combines with the sweat

评 [讠]; 讝 [言] *zhān*, now written as 谵 (譫), talk deliriously, delirium: 评语 *zhān yǔ*, delirious speech

愈 [心]; 愈 [心] *yù*, to recover: 七日愈 *qī rì yù*, recover in seven days

差 [羊]; 差 [工] *chài*, to recover: 病已差 *bìng yǐ chài*, the disease is already cured

忍 [心]; 忍 [心] *rěn*, bear, endure: 忍之一日乃愈 *rěn zhī yī rì nǎi yù*, if [s/he] puts up with it for a day, s/he will recover

冒 [日]; 冒 [冂] *mào*, to obscure, veil: 眩冒 *xuàn mào*, veiling dizziness

Stative verbs

Mental states and attitudes

烦 [火]; 煩 [火] *fán*, vexed: 心烦 *xīn fán*, heart vexation

惊 [忄]; 驚 [馬] *jīng*, fright: 惊痫 *jīng xián*, fright epilepsy

狂 [犭]; 狂 [犬] *kuáng*, mania: 惊狂 *jīng kuáng*, fright mania

恐 [心]; 恐 [心] *kǒng*, fear: 恐有燥屎 *kǒng yǒu zào shǐ*, one fears [there is] dry stool

喜 [士]; 喜 [口] *xǐ*, like: 酒客不喜甘 *jiǔ kè bù xǐ gān*, drinkers do not like sweet [things]

怵 [忄]; 怵 [心] *chù*, scared: 怵惕 *chù tì*, apprehensiveness

惕 [忄]; 惕 [心] *tì*, apprehensive (see preceding item)

恍 [忄]; 恍 [心] *huǎng*, distracted, distraction; compounded with the following as 恍惚 *huǎng hū*, distracted

惚 [忄]; 惚 [心] *hū*, distracted, distraction (see preceding item)

愦 [忄]; 憒 [心] *kuì*, restiveness: 心愦愦 *xīn kuì kuì*, restiveness of the heart

嘿 [口]; 嘿 [口] *mò*, taciturn: 嘿嘿不欲饮食 *mò mò bù yǔ yǐn shí*, taciturn with no desire to eat

懊 [忄]; 懊 [心] *ào*, anguish: 心中懊侬 *xīn zhōng ào nóng*, anguish in the heart

侬 [心]; 憹 [心] *nóng*, anguish (see preceding item)

栗 [西]; 慄 [心] *lì*, shuddering: 寒栗 *hán lì*, cold shuddering

Pathological states

疼 [疒]; 疼 [疒] *téng*, painful, pain: 身疼 *shēn téng*, body pain

痛 [疒]; 痛 [疒] *tòng*, painful, pain: 腰痛 *yāo tòng*, lumbar pain

满 [氵]; 滿 [水] *mǎn*, full, fullness: 胸满 *xiōng mǎn*, fullness in the chest

胀 [月]; 脹 [肉] *zhàng*, distended, distention: 腹胀满 *fù zhàng mǎn*, abdominal distention and fullness

痞 [疒]; 痞 [疒] *pǐ*, glomus: 心下痞硬 *xīn xià pǐ yìng*, hard glomus below the heart

强 [弓]; 強 [弓] *qiáng*, stiff, rigid: 头项强痛 *tóu xiàng qiáng tòng*, stiff, painful head and nape

硬 [石]; 硬 [石] *yìng*, hard, hardness: 大便硬 *dà biàn yìng*, hard stool

固 [口]; 固 [口] *gù*, secure, firm: 固瘕 *yù zuò gù jiǎ*, a firm conglomeration

柔 [矛]; 柔 [木] *róu*, soft: 柔痓 *ròu cì*, soft tetany

拘 [扌]; 拘 [手] *jū*, hypertonicity: 两胫拘急 *liǎng jìng jū jí*, hypertonicity of the (two) lower legs

急 [心]; 急 [心] *jí*, tense, tension; urgent: 四肢微急 *sì zhī wēi jí*, the limbs are slightly tensed; 脉数急 *mài shòu jí*, the pulse is rapid and urgent

烦 [火]; 煩 [火] *fán*, vexed, vexation: 心烦 *xīn fán*, heart vexation

躁 [足]; 躁 [足] *zào*, agitated, agitation: 烦躁 *fán zào*, vexation and agitation

悸 [忄]; 悸 [心] *jì*, palpate, palpitation: 心悸 *xīn jì*, heart palpitations

窒 [穴]; 窒 [宀] *zhì*, stuffiness: 胸中窒 *xiōng zhōng zhì*, stuffiness in the chest

聋 [龙]; 聾 [耳] *lóng*, deaf, deafness: 耳聋 *ěr lóng*, deafness

噎 [口]; 噎 [口] *yē*, dysphagia

眩 [目]; 眩 [目] *xùn*, dizzy, dizziness: 头眩 *tóu xuàn*, dizzy head

重 [丿]; 重 [里] *zhòng*, heavy, heaviness: 身重 *shēn zhòng*, heavy body

痒 [疒]; 癢 [疒] *yǎng*, itch, itching: 身必养 *shēn bì yǎng*, generalized itching

肿 [月]; 腫 [肉] *zhǒng*, swell, swelling: 阴头微肿 *yīn tóu wēi zhǒng*, slight swelling of the yīn head (glans penis)

渴 [氵]; 渴 [水] *kě*, thirsty, thirst: 大渴欲饮水 *dà kě yù yǐn shuǐ*, great thirst with desire to drink water

鼾 [鼻]; 鼾 [鼻] *hān*, snoring: 鼻息必鼾 *bí xī bì hān*, the breath [from the] nose will [make a] snoring [sound]

溏 [氵]; 溏 [水] *táng*, sloppy: 大便溏 *dà biàn táng*, sloppy stool

羸 [亡]; 羸 [羊] *léi*, marked emaciation: 羸人 *léi rén*, markedly emaciated person

Size

大 [大]; 大 [大] *dà*, large; great; major: 脉大 *mài dài*, the pulse is large; 大渴 *dà kě*, great thirst; 大青龙汤 *dà qīng lóng tāng*, Major Green-Blue Dragon Decoction

小 [小]; 小 [小] *xiǎo*, small; smaller; minor: 脉小 *mài xiǎo*, the pulse is small; 小腹 *xiǎo fù*, smaller abdomen; 小柴胡汤 *xiǎo chái hú tāng*, Minor Bupleurum Decoction

细 [纟]; 細 [糸] *xì*, fine: 脉细 *mài xì*, the pulse is fine

长 [丿]; 長 [長] *cháng*, long: 长二寸许 *cháng èr cùn xǔ*, the size of a finger and about two cùn long

短 [矢]; 短 [矢] *duǎn*, short, shortness: 脉短 *mài duǎn*, short pulse

肥 [月]; 肥 [肉] *féi*, fat: 肥栀子 *féi zhī zǐ*, fat gardenia fruits

厚 [厂]; 厚 [厂] *hòu*, thick, thicken: 厚朴 *hòu pò*, magnolia bark

Weight

轻 [车]; 輕 [車] *qīng*, light, mild: 乍有轻时 *zhà yǒu qīng shí*, sudden periods of lightness

重 [丿]; 重 [里] *zhòng*, heavy, weighted; repeated: 身重 *shēn zhòng*, heavy body; 阳气重 *yáng qì zhòng*, yáng qì is weighted; 重语 *chóng yǔ*, repetitious speech

Color

黄 [艹]; 黃 [黃] *huáng*, yellow: 发黄 *fā huáng*, yellowing; 麻黄 *má huáng*, ephedra

赤 [赤]; 赤 [赤] *chì*, red: 面合色赤 *miàn hé sè chì*, face completely red; 赤小豆 *chì xiǎo dòu*, rice bean

青 [青]; 青 [青] *qīng*, green-blue: 面色青黄 *miàn sè qīng huáng*, facial complexion is green-blue or yellow; 大青龙汤 *dà qīng lóng tāng*, Major Green-Blue Dragon Decoction

白 [白]; 白 [白] *bái*, white: 白虎汤 *bái hǔ tāng*, White Tiger Decoction

黑 [灬]; 黑 [火] *hēi*, black: 去黑皮 *qù hēi pí*, remove the black skin

乌 [丿]; 烏 [火] *wū*, black: 乌梅 *wū méi*, mume

明 [日]; 明 [日] *míng*, bright, clear: 明了 *míng liǎo*, clear-headed; 阳明 *yáng míng*, yáng brightness

Temperature

温 [氵]; 溫 [水] *wēn*, warm: 温病 *wēn bìng*, warm disease

温 [氵]; 溫 [水] *yùn*, seething: 心下温温欲吐 *xīn xià yùn yùn yù tù*, seething below the heart with a desire to vomit,

暖 [日]; 煖 [火] *nuǎn*, warm: 暖水 *nuǎn shuǐ*, warm water

热 [灬]; 熱 [火] *rè*, hot, heat: 发热 *fā rè*, heat effusion

灼 [火]; 灼 [火] *zhuó*, scorch: 身灼热 *shēn zhuó rè*, scorching hot body

寒 [宀]; 寒 [宀] *hán*, cold: 恶寒 *wù hán*, aversion to cold

冷 [冫]; 冷 [冫] *lěng*, cold: 冷水 *lěng shuǐ*, cold water

凉 [冫]; 涼 [水] *liáng*, cool: 身凉 *shēn liáng*, the body is cool

凛 [冫]; 凜 [冫] *lǐn*, cold 凛冷 *lǐn lěng*, cold

沸 [氵]; 沸 [水] *fèi*, boiling: 再沸 *zài fèi*, boil again

Taste and smell

甘 [甘]; 甘 [甘] *gān*, sweet: 酒客不喜甘 *jiǔ kè bù xǐ gān*, drinkers do not like sweet [things]

甜 [舌]; 甜 [甘] *tián*, sweet: 呕家不可用建中汤，以甜故也 *ǒu jiā bù kě yòng jiàn zhōng tāng, yǐ tián gù yě*, retching patients cannot take Center-Fortifying Decoction because it is sweet

辛 [辛]; 辛 [辛] *xīn*, acrid: 细辛 *xì xīn*, asarum

苦 [艹]; 苦 [艸] *kǔ*, bitter: 口苦 *kǒu kǔ*, bitter [taste in the] mouth

腥 [月]; 腥 [肉] *xīng*, fishy smelling: 洗去腥 *xǐ qù xīng*, wash to remove the fishy smell

咸 [戊]; 鹹 [鹵] *xián*, salty: 洗去咸 *xǐ qù xián*, wash to remove the saltiness

香 [香]; 香 [香] *xiāng*, fragrant, aromatic: 熬香 *áo xiāng*, slow-boil until the aroma comes out

臭 [自]; 臭 [自] *chòu*, malodorous: 蛔闻食臭出 *huí wén shí chòu chū*, the roundworms smell the malodor of food and come out

Consistency

碎 [石]; 碎 [石] *suì*, crush

稀 [禾]; 稀 [禾] *xī*, thin (of liquids): 稀糜 *xī mí*, thin gruel

粘 [米]; 粘 [米] *nián*, sticky: 粘滑 *nián huá*, sticky and slippery

锐 [钅]; 銳 [金] *ruì*, sharp: 令头锐 *lìng tóu ruì*, make the head pointed

烂 [火]; 爛 [火] *làn*, putrefied: 口干咽烂 *kǒu gān yān làn*, mouth damage with putrefaction and redness

腐 [广]; 腐 [肉] *fǔ*, putrid: 腐秽当去 *fǔ huì dāng qù*, the putrid foulness should be eliminated

Fullness and emptiness

空 [穴]; 空 [穴] *kōng*, empty: 胃中空虚 *wèi zhōng kōng xū*, emptiness in the stomach

满 [氵]; 滿 [水] *mǎn*, full: 胸满 *xiōng mǎn*, fullness in the chest

虚 [虍]; 虛 [虍] *xū*, empty (of essential constituents), vacuous: 阴阳俱虚 *yīn yáng jù xū*, yīn and yáng are both vacuous

实 [宀]; 實 [宀] *shí*, replete: 内实 *nèi shí*, internal repletion

Speed

迟 [辶]; 遲 [辵] *chí*, slow: 脉迟 *mài chí*, the pulse is slow

数 [攵]; 數 [攴] *shuò*, rapid: 脉数 *mài shuò*, the pulse is rapid

疾 [疒]; 疾 [疒] *jí*, racing: 脉疾 *mài jí*, the pulse is racing

促 [亻]; 促 [人] *cù*, skipping: 脉促 *mài cù*, the pulse is skipping

Position, direction

直 [十]; 直 [目] *zhí*, straight, direct: 直视 *zhí shì*, looking straight [ahead], forward-staring eyes

近 [辶]; 近 [辵] *jìn*, near, get near: 近隐处 *jìn yǐn chù*, close to the private parts

高 [高]; 高 [高] *gāo*, high: 邪高痛下 *xié gāo tòng xià*, evil is high [up] and the pain is [low] down

深 [氵]; 深 [水] *shēn*, deep, severe: 热深 *rè shēn*, the heat is severe

挺 [扌]; 挺 [手] *tǐng*, stick out, stick up; erect: 并手捻作挺 *bìng shǒu niǎn zuò tǐng*, pinch with the hands so that it stands erect

纵 [纟]; 縱 [糸] *zòng*, vertical, lengthwise

横 [木]; 横 [木] *héng*, horizontal, crosswise

右 [𠂇]; 右 [口] *yòu*, right: 右五味 *yòu wǔ wèi*, the five ingredients to the right (i.e., the five ingredients above)

傍 [亻]; 傍 [人] , (at the) side (of) 脐傍 *qí páng*, the side of the umbilicus

周 [辶]; 週 [辵] *zhōu*, around; all (over): 周时观之 *zhōu shí guān zhī*, observe [the patient] the whole time

Goodness and badness

善 [羊]; 善 [口] *shàn*, good, good at; tend to: 善饥 *shàn jī*, rapid hungering

良 [艮]; 良 [艮] *liáng*, good: 甚良 *shēn liáng*, very good

佳 [亻]; 佳 [人] *jiā*, good (in quality), best: 加厚朴、杏子佳 *jiā hòu pò, xìng zǐ jiā*, it is best to add magnolia bark and apricot kernels

可 [口]; 可 [口] *kě*, satisfactory: 小便自可 *xiǎo biàn zì kě*, urination is satisfactory

纯 [纟]; 純 [糸] *chún*, 纯阴结 *chún yīn jié*, pure yīn bind

坏 [土]; 壞 [土] *huài*, bad, become bad: 坏病 *huài bìng*, aggravated disease

正 [止]; 正 [止] *zhèng*, right: 正气 *zhèng qì*, right qì

邪 [阝]; 邪 [邑] *xié*, evil: 邪风 *xié fēng*, evil wind

真 [十]; 眞 [目] *zhēn*, true: 真武汤 *zhēn wǔ tāng*, True Warrior Decoction

Ease and difficulty of action

顺 [页]; 順 [頁] *shùn*, follow, obey; favorable: 其脉不负者，为顺也 *qí mài bù fù zhě, wéi shùn yě*, when the pulse is not contrary, it means [that the disease] is [in] favorable [sequence].

逆 [辶]; 逆 [辵] *nì*, adverse; counterflow: 气逆 *qì nì*, qì counterflow

易 [日]; 易 [日] *yì*, easy: 大便乍难乍易 *dài baìn zhà nán zhà yì*, defecation is now difficult, now easy

利 [禾]; 利 [刀] *lì*, uninhibited; specifically, diarrhea: 小便不利 *xiǎo biàn bù lì*, urination is uninhibited; 下利 *xià lì*, diarrhea

通 [辶]; 通 [辵] *tōng*, free, unblocked: 气不通 *qì bù tōng*, qì is blocked

滑 [氵]; 滑 [水] *huá*, slippery: 脉滑 *mài huá*, the pulse is slippery

快 [忄]; 快 [心] *kuài*, vital, quick: 得快利 *dé kuài lì*, as soon as diarrhea occurs

难 [又]; 難 [隹] *nán*, difficult: 大便难 *dà biàn nán*, defecation is difficult

郁 [阝]; 鬱 [鬯] *yù*, be depressed: 阳气怫郁在表 *yáng qì fú yù zài biǎo*, yáng qì is depressed in the exterior

怫 [忄]; 怫 [心] *fú*, be depressed (see preceding item)

平 [一]; 平 [干] *píng*, calm: 平旦 *píng dàn*, calm dawn; 脉平 *mài píng*, the pulse is calm

濇 [氵]; 濇 [水] *sè*, rough: 脉濇 *mài sè*, the pulse is rough

涩 [氵]; 澀 [水] *sè*, rough: same as preceding character

Harmony and disharmony

谐 [讠]; 諧 [言] *xié*, concordant: 卫气不共荣气谐和 *wèi qì bù gòng róng qì xié hé*, defense qì is not in harmony with construction qì

和 [禾]; 和 [口] *hé*, harmonious, harmony, harmonize: 胃气不和 *wèi qì bù hé*, stomach qi is disharmonious; 以小柴胡汤和之 *yǐ xiǎo chái hú tāng hé zhī*, harmonize using Minor Bupleurum Decoction

静 [青]; 靜 [青] *jìng*, still: 夜而安静 *yè ér ān jìng*, by nighttime, [the patient] is tranquil

安 [宀]; 安 [宀] *ān*, quiet; peace: 心烦不得安 *xīn fán bù dé ān*, vexation that cannot be quieted; 安火上 *ān huǒ shàng*, place on the fire

乱 [舌]; 亂 [乙] *luàn*, deranged, chaotic, turmoil: 语言必乱 *yǔ yán bì luàn*, speech will be deranged; 霍乱 *huò luàn*, sudden turmoil, cholera

Wetness and dryness

枯 [木]; 枯 [木] *kū*, withered: 枯燥 *kū zào*, withered and dry

干 [二]; 乾 [乙] *gān*, dry: 干呕 *gān ǒu*, dry retching; 口干 *kǒu gān*, dry mouth

燥 [火]; 燥 [火] *zào*, dry, parched: 咽燥 *yān zào*, dry throat

濡 [氵]; 濡 [水] *rú*, soggy: 脉濡 *mài rú*, the pulse is soggy

润 [氵]; 潤 [水] *rùn*, moist: 肤润 *fū rùn*, the skin is moist

Age and duration

新 [斤]; 新 [斤] *xīn*, new: 新虚 *xīn xū*, new vacuity

旧 [日]; 舊 [艸] *jiù*, old (of things): 病人旧微溏 *bìng rén jiù wēi táng*, the patient usually has slightly sloppy stool

久 [丿]; 久 [丿] *jiǔ*, enduring; adv. for a long time: 久寒 *jiǔ hán*, enduring cold; 久按之 *jiǔ àn zhī*, press for a long time

Sameness and difference

异 [巳]; 異 [田] *yì*, different, separately: 异捣 *yì dǎo*, pound separately

他 [亻]; 他 [人] *tā*, other: 无他病 *wú tā bìng*, has no other disease

别 [刂]; 别 [刀] *bié*, different, separately: 同体别名 *tóng tǐ bié míng*, ; 别捣 *bié dǎo*, pound separately

Strength and weakness

强 [弓]; 強 [弓] *qiáng*, stiff, rigid: 头项强痛 *tóu xiàng qiáng tòng*, stiff, painful head and nape

弱 [弓]; 弱 [弓] *ruò*, weak: 脉弱 *mài ruò*, the pulse is weak

甚 [一]; 甚 [甘] *shèn*, pronounced, marked: 热甚 *rè shèn*, the heat is pronounced

微 [彳]; 微 [彳] *wēi*, faint, slightly: 脉微 *mài wēi*, the pulse is faint; 微拘急 *wēi jū jí*, slightly hypertonic

剧 [刂]; 劇 [刀] *jù*, severe, acute: 剧者必衄 *jù zhě bì nǜ*, if it is acute, there will be spontaneous external bleeding

盛 [皿]; 盛 [皿] *shèng*, exuberant: 阳盛 *yáng shèng*, yáng is exuberant

Miscellaneous stative verbs

慎 [忄]; 愼 [心] *shèn*, cautious: 慎不可灸 *shèn bù kě jiǔ*, [one must be] cautious and not use moxibustion

代 [亻]; 代 [人] *dài*, intermittent: 脉代 *mài dài*, the pulse is intermittent

结 [纟]; 結 [糸] *jié*, bound: 脉结 *mài jié*, the pulse is bound

缓 [纟]; 緩 [糸] *huǎn*, moderate: 脉缓 *mài huǎn*, the pulse is moderate

紧 [糸]; 緊 [糸] *jǐn*, tight: 脉紧 *mài jǐn*, the pulse is tight

熟 [灬]; 熟 [火] *shú*, cooked, ripe, mature: 煮米熟 *zhǔ mǐ shóu*, boil the rice until it is cooked

怪 [忄]; 怪 [心] *guài*, strange, regard as strange: 勿怪 *wù guài*, don't regard this as strange

垢 [土]; 垢 [土] *gòu*, grimy: 面垢 *miàn gòu*, grimy face

秽 [禾]; 穢 [禾] *huì*, foul: 腐秽当去 *fǔ huì dāng qù*, the putrid foulness should be eliminated

清 [氵]; 清 [水] *qīng*, clear: 清酒 *qīng jiǔ*, clear liquor

效 [攵]; 效 [攴] *xiào*, effective: 甚效 *shèn xiào*, most effective

瞑 [目]; 瞑 [目] *míng*, heavy: 其人发烦目瞑 *qí rén fā fán mù míng*, the person is vexed and the eyes are heavy

尖 [小]; 尖 [小] *jiān*, tip: 去皮尖 *qù pí jiān*, remove the skin and tips

仲 [亻]; 仲 [人] *zhòng*, 仲景 *zhòng jǐng*, Zhāng Jī's style (name)

饱 [饣]; 飽 [食] *bǎo*, satiation: 食难用饱 *shí nán yòng bǎo*, difficulty eating to satiation

饥 [饣]; 飢(饑) [食] *jī*, hunger: 饥不能食 *jī bù néng shí*, hunger with inability to eat

隐 [阝]; 隱 [阜] *yǐn*, hidden: 近隐处 *jìn yǐn chù*, close to the crotch (the hidden part)

独 [犭]; 獨 [犬] *dú*, solitary, single; alone: 阴独 *yīn dú*, yīn is solitary

Bibliography

Shāng Hán Lùn Literature

Hàn 汉 (206 B.C.E.–C.E. 220)

Zhāng Jī (张机), style Zhòng Jǐng (仲景). Circa 150–219 C.E., Eastern Hàn.
Shāng Hán Zá Bìng Lùn (伤寒杂病论 "On Cold Damage and Miscellaneous Diseases")

Three Kingdoms 三国 (220–280)

Huáng-Fǔ Mì (皇甫谧). 214–282 C.E., Three Kingdoms.
Zhēn Jiǔ Jiǎ Yǐ Jīng (针灸甲乙经 "The Systematized Canon of Acupuncture and Moxibustion")

Jìn 晋 (265–470)

Wáng Shū-Hé (王叔和). 265–316 C.E., Western Jìn
Edited the *Shāng Hán Zá Bìng Lùn* (伤寒杂病论 "On Cold Damage and Miscellaneous Diseases")
Author of *Mài Jīng* (脉经 "The Pulse Canon")

Suí-Táng 隋唐 (581–907)

Sūn Sī-Miǎo (孙思邈). 581–682 C.E., Suí-Táng.
bèi jí qiān jīn yào fāng (备急千金要方 "A Thousand Gold Pieces Prescriptions for Emergencies")
Qiān Jīn Yì Fāng (千金翼方 "Wings to the Thousand Gold Pieces Prescriptions")

Wáng Tāo (王涛). 707–772 C.E., Táng.
Wài Tái Mì Yào (外台秘要 "Essential Secrets from Outside the Metropolis")

Sòng 宋 (960–1279)

Lín Yì (林亿). Northern Sòng (960–1127). Lín et al. were entrusted by the Medical Literature Editing Bureau (校正医书局 *jiào zhèng yī shū jú*) in 1057 with the task of editing the *Shāng Hán Lùn*. The edited version subsequently printed is known as the Sòng version.

Zhū Gōng (朱肱). Northern Sòng (960–1127).
Nán Yáng Huó Rén Shū (南阳活人书 "The Nán-Yáng Life-Saving Book")

Páng Ān-Shí (庞安时), style Ān-Cháng (安常). 1042–1099, Northern Sòng.
Shāng Hán Zǒng Bìng Lùn (伤寒总病论 "A General Treatise of Cold Damage Disease")

Chéng Wú-Jǐ (成无己). 1066–1156?, Sòng.
Zhù Jiě Shāng Hán Lùn (注解伤寒论 "Annotated *Shāng Hán Lùn*")

Xǔ Shū-Wēi (许叔微). 1080–1154, Sòng.
Shāng Hán Fā Wēi Lùn (伤寒发微论 "Elaboration of the *Shāng Hán Lùn*")
Shāng Hán Jiǔ Shí Lùn (伤寒九十论 "Ninety Treatises on Cold Damage")

Míng 明 (1361–1644)

Fāng Yǒu-Zhí (方有执). 1523–? C.E., Míng.
Shāng Hán Lùn Tiáo Biàn (伤寒论条辨 "Systematized Comprehension of Cold Damage")

Lǐ Shí-Zhēn (李时珍). 1518–1593 C.E., Míng.
Běn Cǎo Gāng Mù (本草纲目 "The Comprehensive Herbal Foundation") published in 1857.

Wáng Kěn-Táng (王肯堂). 1549–1613, Míng.
Shāng Hán Zhèng Zhì Zhǔn Shéng (伤寒证治准绳 "The Level-Line of Cold Damage")

Yù Chāng (喻昌), style Jiā-Yán (嘉言). 1585–1664, Qīng.
Shàng Lùn Piān (尚论篇 "The Extolment")

Zhāng Lù (张璐), style Lù-Yǜ (路玉). 1617–1700, Míng-Qīng.
Zhāng Shì Yī Tōng (张氏医通 "Zhang's Clear View of Medicine")

Zhāng Zhì-Cōng (张志聪), style Yǐn-Ān (隐庵). 1644–1722, Qīng.
Shāng Hán Lùn Zōng Yìn (伤寒论宗印 "Verification of the *Shāng Hán Lùn* Heritage")
Shāng Hán Lùn Jí Zhù (伤寒论集注 "Collected Commentaries on the *Shāng Hán Lùn*")

Kē Qín (柯琴), style Yùn-Bó (韵伯). Circa 1662–1735, Qīng.
Shāng Hán Lái Sū Jí (伤寒来苏集 "The Cold Damage Revival Variorum")

Yè Guì (叶桂), style Tiān-Shì (天士). 1667–1746.
Yī Xiào Mì Chuán (医效秘传 "Medical Efficacy Secretly Handed Down")

Yóu Yí (尤怡), style Zài-Jīng (在泾). ?—1749, Qīng.
Shāng Hán Guàn Zhū Jí (伤寒贯珠集 "String-of-Pearls Cold Damage Variorum")

Xú Líng-Tāi (徐灵胎), style Líng-Tāi (灵胎). 1694–1771, Qīng. His numerous works include:
Shāng Hán Lèi Fāng (伤寒类方 "Categorized Formulae for Cold Damage")
Shāng Hán Yuē Biān (伤寒约编 "The Concise Book of Cold Damage")

Shěn Jīn-Aó (沈金鳌), style Qiān-Lǜ (芊绿). 1717–1776, Qīng.
Shāng Hán Gāng Mù (伤寒纲目 "The Comprehensive *Shāng Hán Lùn*")

Chén Niàn-Zǔ (陈念祖), style Xiū-Yuán (修园). 1766–1833, Qīng.
Sháng Hán Lùn Qiǎn Zhù (伤寒论浅注 "The *Shāng Hán Lùn* Simply Annotated")
Cháng Shā Gē Kuò (长沙歌括 "Cháng Shā Songs")
Shāng Hán Zhēn Fāng Gē Kuò (伤寒真方歌括 "Songs for the True Formulae of Cold Damage")
Shāng Hán Yī Fāng (伤寒医方 "Medical Remedies for Cold Damage")

Qīng 清 (1644–1911)

Gāo Xué-Shān (高学山). Early Qīng.
Shāng Hán Shàng Lùn Biàn Sì (伤寒尚论辨似 "Specious Points in the Extolment of Cold Damage")

Zhōu Yáng-Jùn (周扬俊). Early Qīng.
Shāng Hán Lùn Sān Zhù (伤寒论三注 "Three Annotations of the *Shāng Hán Lùn*")

Wáng Zǐ-Jiē (王子接), style Jìn-Sān (晋三). Early Qīng.
Jiàng Xué Yuán Gǔ Fāng Xuǎn Zhù (绛雪园古方选注 "Jiàng Xué-Yuán's Selected Notes on Ancient Formulae")

Chéng Yìng-Máo (程应旄), style Jiāo-Qiàn (郊倩). Early Qīng.

Shāng Hán Lùn Hòu Tiáo Biàn (伤寒论后条辨 "Later Systematized Comprehension of *Shāng Hán Lùn*")
Yī Jìng Gōu Cè (医径句测 "Fathoming the Paths to Medicine")

Zhāng Xī-Jū (张锡驹), style Lìng-Sháo (令韶). Early Qīng.
Shāng Hán Lùn Zhí Jiě (伤寒论直解 "Straightforward Explanation of the *Shāng Hán Lùn*")

Huáng Yuán-Yù (黄元御), style Kūn-Zài (坤载). Qīng.
Shāng Hán Xuán Jiě (伤寒悬解 "Clarification of the *Shāng Hán Lùn*")
Shāng Hán Shuō Yì (伤寒说意 "Explaining the Meaning of Cold Damage")

Wèi Lì-Tóng (魏荔彤), style Niàn-Tíng (念庭). Qīng.
Zhù Shì Shāng Hán Lùn Yì Dà Quán (注释伤寒论义大全 "The Annnotated Comprehensive Elucidation of Cold Damage")

Shěn Míng-Zōng (沈明宗). Qīng.
Shāng Hán Liù Jīng Biàn Zhèng Zhì Fǎ (伤寒六经辨证治法 "Six-Channel Pattern Identification and Treatment in Cold Damage")
Shāng Hán Liù Jīng Zuǎn Zhù (伤寒六经纂注 "Annotation of the Six Channels of Cold Damage")

Chén Bǎi-Tán (陈伯坛), style Shān-Nóng (山农). Qīng.
Shāng Hán Jìn Biān Qián Jí (伤寒近编前集 "A Modern Cold Damage Variorum I")
Shāng Hán Jìn Biān Hòu Jí (伤寒近编后集 "A Modern Cold Damage Variorum II")

Wāng Hǔ (汪琥), style Líng-Yǒu (苓友). Qīng.
Shāng Hán Biàn Zhèng Guǎng Zhù (伤寒辨证广注 "Broad Annotations on Cold Damage Pattern Identification")

Qián Huáng (钱潢), style Tiān-Lái (天来). Qīng.
Chóng Biān Zhāng Zhòng Jǐng Shāng Hán Lùn Zhèng Zhì Fā Míng Sù Yuán (重编张仲景伤寒论证治发明溯源 "Revised Exposition and Reexamination of Patterns and Treatment in Zhāng Zhòng-Jǐng's *Shāng Hán Lùn*")

Chén Píng-Bó (陈平伯).
Wēn Rè Zhǐ Nán Jí (温热指南集 "Guide to Warm-Heat Variorum")

Táng Zōng-Hǎi (唐宗海), style Róng-Chuān (容川). 1862–1918.
Shāng Hán Lùn Qiǎn Zhù Bǔ Zhèng (伤寒论浅注补正 "Plain Notes, Supplements, and Corrections to the *Shāng Hán Lùn*")

Shū Zhào (舒诏), style Chí-Yuǎn (驰远). Qīng.
Shàng Lùn Yì (尚论翼 "Wings of the Extolment")

Xú Bīn (徐彬), style Zhōng-Kě (忠可). Qīng.
Shàng Hán Yī Bǎi Shí Sān Fāng Fā Míng (伤寒一百十三方发明 "Elucidation of the 113 Cold Damage Formulae")
Shàng Hán Tú Lùn (伤寒图论 "Illustrated Treatise on Cold Damage")
Zhù Xǔ Shì Shàng Hán Bǎi Zhèng Gē (注许氏伤寒百证歌 "Xǔ's Songs on 100 Cold Damage Patterns Annotated")

Wú Yí-Luò (吴仪洛). Qīng.
Shàng Hán Fēn Jīng (伤寒分经 "Cold Damage by Channel")

Shěn Yáo-Fēng (沈尧封). Qīng.

Zhāng Nán (章楠), style Xū-Gǔ (虚谷). Late Qīng.

Sháng Hán Lùn Běn Zhǐ (伤寒论本旨 "The Basic Meaning of Cold Damage")

Republic/People's Republic 中华民国/中华人民共和国 (1911–)

Liú Dù-Zhōu (刘渡舟). 1917–. Author of many works, including:

Shàng Hán Lùn Tōng Sú Jiǎng Huà (伤寒论通俗讲话 "*Shāng Hán Lùn* Lectures")

Shàng Hán Lùn Shí Sì Jiǎng (伤寒论十四讲 "Fourteen Lectures on the *Shāng Hán Lùn*")

Shàng Hán Lùn Quán Jiě (伤寒论诠解 "Explication of the *Shāng Hán Lùn*")

Qín Zhī Zhēn (秦之桢), style Huáng-Shì (皇士). Qīng.

Shàng Hán Dà Bái (伤寒大白 "Cold Damage Made Plain")

Yú Wú-Yán (余无言). 1900–1963.

Shāng Hán Lùn Xīn Yì (伤寒论新义 "New Interpretations of the *Shāng Hán Lùn*")

Kē Xuě-Fán (柯雪帆). 1927–.

Yī Lín Duō Yīng (医林掇英 "Gathered Blooms of the Medical Grove")

Sources Used

三画

马继兴.《神农本草经辑注》. 北京: 人民卫生出版社, 1995

马继兴.《敦煌古医籍考释》. 南昌: 江西科技出版社, 1998

四画

王大观.《本草经义疏》. 北京:人民卫生出版社, 1990

丹波元坚、丹波元简.《伤寒广要、药治通义、救急选方、脉学辑要》. 北京:人民卫生出版社, 1983

丹波元坚、丹波元简.《伤寒辑义、伤寒论述义、金匮玉函要略辑义、金匮玉函要略辑义》. 北京:人民卫生出版社, 1983

五画

石国璧、陈庆平、岳湘萍.《经方要义》. 兰州:甘肃人民出版社, 1989

印会河、张伯讷.《中医基础理论》.(高等中医院校教学参考丛书). 台北:知音出版社, 1990;原版:北京:人民卫生出版社, 1989

六画

宋·成无己.《注解伤寒论》. 北京: 人民卫生出版社, 1963

刘建平等.《伤寒杂病论》. 石家庄: 河北科学技术出版社, 1993

刘渡舟.《伤寒论通俗讲话》. 上海: 上海科学技术出版社, 1980

刘渡舟.《伤寒论十四讲》. 天津:天津科学技术出版社, 1984

刘渡舟.《伤寒论校注》. 北京:人民卫生出版社, 1991

刘渡舟.《伤寒论四十讲》. 天津:天津科学技术出版社, 1984

刘渡舟、钱超尘.《伤寒论临证指要、文献通考》. 北京:学苑出出版社, 1993

刘景农.《汉语文言语法》. 北京:中华书局, 1994

关庆增、陆云平.《伤寒论古今研究》. 沈阳:辽宁科技出版社, 1994

七画

杨麦青.《伤寒论现代临床研究》. 北京:中国医药出版社, 1992.

李文瑞.《伤寒论汤证论治》. 北京: 人民军医出版社, 1989

李克光.《金匮要略译释》. 上海:上海科学技术出版社, 1993

李克光.《金匮要略》.(高等中医院校教学参考丛书). 台北:知音出版社 1990.

李培生.《伤寒论》.(高等中医院校教学参考丛书). 台北:知音出版社, 1990. 原版:北京:人民卫生出版社, 1987

李培生.《伤寒论讲义》. 长沙:湖南科技出版社, 1994

李培生.《柯氏伤寒论注疏正》. 北京:人民卫生出版社, 1996

时振声.《伤寒论串解》. 北京:中医古籍出版社, 1987

清·吴谦等编.《医宗金鉴》. 北京: 人民卫生出版社, 1963

清·何元长.《伤寒辨类》. 上海:学林出版社, 1984

张启积、王辉武.《伤寒论手册》. 重庆:重庆科技出版社, 1984

张崇、王立.《重订伤寒的临床家喻嘉言》. 北京:中国科学技术出版热, 1989

张谷才.《仲景内科学》. 上海:上海中医学院出版社, 1990

汉·张机(仲景).《仲景全书》. 台北:集文书局, 1983

张登本、武长春.《内经词典》. 北京：人民卫生出版社， 1990

张维辉.《中医的现在与未来》. 天津：天津科学技术出版社， 1994.

张树生、马长武.《神农本草经贯通》. 天津：中国医药科技出版社， 1997

陈亦人（南京中医学院）.《伤寒论译释》. 上海：上海科学技术出版社，第三版 1992 (第一版 1959)

陈伯涛.《仲景方与临床》. 北京：中国医药科技出版社， 1991

陈明、张印生.《伤寒名医验案精选》. 北京：学苑出版社， 1998

八画

罗荣汉.《医用古汉语基础》. 重庆：重庆出版社， 1991

国医编辑社编辑.《伤寒论新注》. 台北：文光图书有限公司， 1979

孟永利、沈帼男、李晓露.《伤寒论现代研究与临床应用》. 北京：学苑出版社， 1998

单玉堂.《伤寒论针灸配穴选注》. 台北：启业书局， 1986

九画

清 · 柯琴.《伤寒来苏集》. 台北县：旋风出版社， 1973

赵存义.《中医古方名考》. 北京：中国中医药出版社， 1994

段德森.《实用古汉语虚词》. 太原：山西教育出版社， 1990

姜春华.《伤寒论识义》. 上海：上海科学技术出版社， 1985

姜建国.《伤寒思辨》. 济南：山东大学出版社， 1995

十画

清 · 秦之桢.《伤寒大白》. 北京：人民卫生出版社， 1982

钱超尘.《唐本伤寒论》. 北京：中国医药科技出版社， 1994

徐凌云、高荣林.《典要仲景学说的尤怡》. 北京：中国科学技术出版社， 1989

郭秀梅.《日本医家伤寒论注解辑要》. 北京：人民卫生出版社， 1996

郭霭春、张海玲.《伤寒论校注语译》. 天津：天津科学技术出版社出版， 1996

唐关锐.《新编中医温病学心法要诀注解》. 北京：人民卫生出版社， 1985

唐宗海.《伤寒论浅注补正》. 台北：力行书局， 1993

十一画

曹炳章.《中国医学大成》. 上海：上海科学技术出版社， 1990

十二画

傅延龄.《伤寒论研究大词典》. 济南：山东科技出版社， 1994

程昭寰.《伤寒心悟》. 北京：学苑出版社， 1989

十四画

蔡德元.《古本伤寒论杂病论校评》. 郑州：江西科技出版社， 1992

十七画

戴玉等.《仲景辨证治疗学》. 北京：中国中医药出版社， 1995

十八画

清 · 魏荔彤.《金匮要略方论本义》. 北京：人民卫生出版社， 1997

Sòng Version Line Number Index

Since in chapters 1–8 the lines are presented in a modern order (see Introduction, p. 9), but are numbered according to their sequence in the Sòng version, the present index has been added to allow readers to locate a known Sòng line (l.) number in the present volume.

English Index of Terms

Pīnyīn Index of Terms

English Index of Medicinals & Formulae

Pīnyīn Index of Medicinals & Formulae